Statistical Methodology in the Pharmaceutical Sciences

STATISTICS: Textbooks and Monographs

A Series Edited by

Vol. 1: The Generalized Jackknife Statistic, *H. L. Gray and W. R. Schucany*
Vol. 2: Multivariate Analysis, *Anant M. Kshirsagar*
Vol. 3: Statistics and Society, *Walter T. Federer*
Vol. 4: Multivariate Analysis: A Selected and Abstracted Bibliography, 1957-1972, *Kocherlakota Subrahmaniam and Kathleen Subrahmaniam* (out of print)
Vol. 5: Design of Experiments: A Realistic Approach, *Virgil L. Anderson and Robert A. McLean*
Vol. 6: Statistical and Mathematical Aspects of Pollution Problems, *John W. Pratt*
Vol. 7: Introduction to Probability and Statistics (in two parts), Part I: Probability; Part II: Statistics, *Narayan C. Giri*
Vol. 8: Statistical Theory of the Analysis of Experimental Designs, *J. Ogawa*
Vol. 9: Statistical Techniques in Simulation (in two parts), *Jack P. C. Kleijnen*
Vol. 10: Data Quality Control and Editing, *Joseph I. Naus* (out of print)
Vol. 11: Cost of Living Index Numbers: Practice, Precision, and Theory, *Kali S. Banerjee*
Vol. 12: Weighing Designs: For Chemistry, Medicine, Economics, Operations Research, Statistics, *Kali S. Banerjee*
Vol. 13: The Search for Oil: Some Statistical Methods and Techniques, *edited by D. B. Owen*
Vol. 14: Sample Size Choice: Charts for Experiments with Linear Models, *Robert E. Odeh and Martin Fox*
Vol. 15: Statistical Methods for Engineers and Scientists, *Robert M. Bethea, Benjamin S. Duran, and Thomas L. Boullion*
Vol. 16: Statistical Quality Control Methods, *Irving W. Burr*
Vol. 17: On the History of Statistics and Probability, *edited by D. B. Owen*
Vol. 18: Econometrics, *Peter Schmidt*
Vol. 19: Sufficient Statistics: Selected Contributions, *Vasant S. Huzurbazar (edited by Anant M. Kshirsagar)*
Vol. 20: Handbook of Statistical Distributions, *Jagdish K. Patel, C. H. Kapadia, and D. B. Owen*
Vol. 21: Case Studies in Sample Design, *A. C. Rosander*
Vol. 22: Pocket Book of Statistical Tables, *compiled by R. E. Odeh, D. B. Owen, Z. W. Birnbaum, and L. Fisher*
Vol. 23: The Information in Contingency Tables, *D. V. Gokhale and Solomon Kullback*

Vol. 24: Statistical Analysis of Reliability and Life-Testing Models: Theory and Methods, *Lee J. Bain*
Vol. 25: Elementary Statistical Quality Control, *Irving W. Burr*
Vol. 26: An Introduction to Probability and Statistics Using BASIC, *Richard A. Groeneveld*
Vol. 27: Basic Applied Statistics, *B. L. Raktoe and J. J. Hubert*
Vol. 28: A Primer in Probability, *Kathleen Subrahmaniam*
Vol. 29: Random Processes: A First Look, *R. Syski*
Vol. 30: Regression Methods: A Tool for Data Analysis, *Rudolf J. Freund and Paul D. Minton*
Vol. 31: Randomization Tests, *Eugene S. Edgington*
Vol. 32: Tables for Normal Tolerance Limits, Sampling Plans, and Screening, *Robert E. Odeh and D. B. Owen*
Vol. 33: Statistical Computing, *William J. Kennedy, Jr. and James E. Gentle*
Vol. 34: Regression Analysis and Its Application: A Data-Oriented Approach, *Richard F. Gunst and Robert L. Mason*
Vol. 35: Scientific Strategies to Save Your Life, *I. D. J. Bross*
Vol. 36: Statistics in the Pharmaceutical Industry, *edited by C. Ralph Buncher and Jia-Yeong Tsay*
Vol. 37: Sampling from a Finite Population, *J. Hajek*
Vol. 38: Statistical Modeling Techniques, *S. S. Shapiro*
Vol. 39: Statistical Theory and Inference in Research, *T. A. Bancroft and C.-P. Han*
Vol. 40: Handbook of the Normal Distribution, *Jagdish K. Patel and Campbell B. Read*
Vol. 41: Recent Advances in Regression Methods, *Hrishikesh D. Vinod and Aman Ullah*
Vol. 42: Acceptance Sampling in Quality Control, *Edward G. Schilling*
Vol. 43: The Randomized Clinical Trial and Therapeutic Decisions, *edited by Niels Tygstrup, John M. Lachin, and Erik Juhl*
Vol. 44: Regression Analysis of Survival Data in Cancer Chemotherapy, *Walter H. Carter, Jr., Galen L. Wampler, and Donald M. Stablein*
Vol. 45: A Course in Linear Models, *Anant M. Kshirsagar*
Vol. 46: Clinical Trials: Issues and Approaches, *edited by Stanley H. Shapiro and Thomas H. Louis*
Vol. 47: Statistical Analysis of DNA Sequence Data, *edited by B. S. Weir*
Vol. 48: Nonlinear Regression Modeling: A Unified Practical Approach, *David A. Ratkowsky*
Vol. 49: Attribute Sampling Plans, Tables of Tests and Confidence Limits for Proportions, *Robert E. Odeh and D. B. Owen*
Vol. 50: Experimental Design, Statistical Models, and Genetic Statistics, *edited by Klaus Hinkelmann*
Vol. 51: Statistical Methods for Cancer Studies, *edited by Richard G. Cornell*
Vol. 52: Practical Statistical Sampling for Auditors, *Arthur J. Wilburn*
Vol. 53: Statistical Signal Processing, *edited by Edward J. Wegman and James G. Smith*
Vol. 54: Self-Organizing Methods in Modeling: GMDH Type Algorithms, *edited by Stanley J. Farlow*
Vol. 55: Applied Factorial and Fractional Designs, *Robert A. McLean and Virgil L. Anderson*
Vol. 56: Design of Experiments: Ranking and Selection, *edited by Thomas J. Santner and Ajit C. Tamhane*
Vol. 57: Statistical Methods for Engineers and Scientists. Second Edition, Revised and Expanded, *Robert M. Bethea, Benjamin S. Duran, and Thomas L. Boullion*
Vol. 58: Ensemble Modeling: Inference from Small-Scale Properties to Large-Scale Systems, *Alan E. Gelfand and Crayton C. Walker*
Vol. 59: Computer Modeling for Business and Industry, *Bruce L. Bowerman and Richard T. O'Connell*
Vol. 60: Bayesian Analysis of Linear Models, *Lyle D. Broemeling*

Vol. 61: Methodological Issues for Health Care Surveys, *Brenda Cox and Steven Cohen*

Vol. 62: Applied Regression Analysis and Experimental Design, *Richard J. Brook and Gregory C. Arnold*

Vol. 63: Statpal: A Statistical Package for Microcomputers – PC-DOS Version for the IBM PC and Compatibles, *Bruce J. Chalmer and David G. Whitmore*

Vol. 64: Statpal: A Statistical Package for Microcomputers – Apple Version for the II, II+, and IIe, *David G. Whitmore and Bruce J. Chalmer*

Vol. 65: Nonparametric Statistical Inference, Second Edition, Revised and Expanded, *Jean Dickinson Gibbons*

Vol. 66: Design and Analysis of Experiments, *Roger G. Petersen*

Vol. 67: Statistical Methods for Pharmaceutical Research Planning, *Sten W. Bergman and John C. Gittins*

Vol. 68: Goodness-of-Fit Techniques, *edited by Ralph B. D'Agostino and Michael A. Stephens*

Vol. 69: Statistical Methods in Discrimination Litigation, *edited by D. H. Kaye and Mikel Aickin*

Vol. 70: Truncated and Censored Samples from Normal Populations, *Helmut Schneider*

Vol. 71: Robust Inference, *M. L. Tiku, W. Y. Tan, and N. Balakrishnan*

Vol. 72: Statistical Image Processing and Graphics, *edited by Edward J. Wegman and Douglas J. DePriest*

Vol. 73: Assignment Methods in Combinatorial Data Analysis, *Lawrence J. Hubert*

Vol. 74: Econometrics and Structural Change, *Lyle D. Broemeling and Hiroki Tsurumi*

Vol. 75: Multivariate Interpretation of Clinical Laboratory Data, *Adelin Albert and Eugene K. Harris*

Vol. 76: Statistical Tools for Simulation Practitioners, *Jack P. C. Kleijnen*

Vol. 77: Randomization Tests, Second Edition, *Eugene S. Edgington*

Vol. 78: A Folio of Distributions: A Collection of Theoretical Quantile-Quantile Plots, *Edward B. Fowlkes*

Vol. 79: Applied Categorical Data Analysis, *Daniel H. Freeman, Jr.*

Vol. 80: Seemingly Unrelated Regression Equations Models : Estimation and Inference, *Virendra K. Srivastava and David E. A. Giles*

Vol. 81: Response Surfaces: Designs and Analyses, *Andre I. Khuri and John A. Cornell*

Vol. 82: Nonlinear Parameter Estimation: An Integrated System in BASIC, *John C. Nash and Mary Walker-Smith*

Vol. 83: Cancer Modeling, *edited by James R. Thompson and Barry W. Brown*

Vol. 84: Mixture Models: Inference and Applications to Clustering, *Geoffrey J. McLachlan and Kaye E. Basford*

Vol. 85: Randomized Response: Theory and Techniques, *Arijit Chaudhuri and Rahul Mukerjee*

Vol. 86: Biopharmaceutical Statistics for Drug Development, *edited by Karl E. Peace*

Vol. 87: Parts per Million Values for Estimating Quality Levels, *Robert E. Odeh and D. B. Owen*

Vol. 88: Lognormal Distributions: Theory and Applications, *edited by Edwin L. Crow and Kunio Shimizu*

Vol. 89: Properties of Estimators for the Gamma Distribution, *K. O. Bowman and L. R. Shenton*

Vol. 90: Spline Smoothing and Nonparametric Regression, *Randall L. Eubank*

Vol. 91: Linear Least Squares Computations, *R. W. Farebrother*

Vol. 92: Exploring Statistics, *Damaraju Raghavarao*

Vol. 93: Applied Time Series Analysis for Business and Economic Forecasting, *Sufi M. Nazem*

Vol. 94: Bayesian Analysis of Time Series and Dynamic Models, *edited by James C. Spall*

Vol. 95: The Inverse Gaussian Distribution: Theory, Methodology, and Applications, *Raj S. Chhikara and J. Leroy Folks*

Vol. 96: Parameter Estimation in Reliability and Life Span Models, *A. Clifford Cohen and Betty Jones Whitten*

Vol. 97: Pooled Cross-Sectional and Time Series Data Analysis, *Terry E. Dielman*

Vol. 98: Random Processes: A First Look, Second Edition, Revised and Expanded, *R. Syski*

Vol. 99: Generalized Poisson Distributions: Properties and Applications, *P.C. Consul*

Vol. 100: Nonlinear L_p-Norm Estimation, *René Gonin and Arthur H. Money*

Vol. 101: Model Discrimination for Nonlinear Regression Models, *Dale S. Borowiak*

Vol. 102: Applied Regression Analysis in Econometrics, *Howard E. Doran*

Vol. 103: Continued Fractions in Statistical Applications, *K.O. Bowman and L.R. Shenton*

Vol. 104: Statistical Methodology in the Pharmaceutical Sciences, *Donald A. Berry*

Vol. 105: Experimental Design in Biotechnology, *Perry D. Haaland*

ADDITIONAL VOLUMES IN PREPARATION

Statistical Methodology in the Pharmaceutical Sciences

Edited by

DONALD A. BERRY

School of Statistics
University of Minnesota
Minneapolis, Minnesota

MARCEL DEKKER, INC. New York and Basel

Library of Congress Cataloging-in-Publication Data

Statistical methodology in the pharmaceutical sciences / edited by Donald A. Berry.
p. cm. — (Statistics, textbooks and monographs ; vol. 104)
Includes index. ISBN 0-8247-8117-1 (alk. paper)
1. Drugs—Testing—Statistical methods. 2. Clinical trials–
–Statistical methods. 3. Pharmacy—Research—Statistical methods.
I. Berry, Donald A. II. Series: Statistics, textbooks, and monographs ; v. 104.
[DNLM: 1. Clinical Trials—methods. 2. Drug Industry.
3. Pharmacy—methods. 4. Statistics. QV 25 S797]
RM301.27.S73 1989
615′.1901—dc20
DNLM/DLC
for Library of Congress 89-16852
CIP

This book is printed on acid-free paper.

MARCEL DEKKER, INC.
270 Madison Avenue, New York, New York 10016

Current printing (last digit):
10 9 8 7 6 5 4 3 2 1

PRINTED IN THE UNITED STATES OF AMERICA

Preface

This work presents a variety of statistical methods that are useful in pharmaceutical research. We write for applied statisticians and others who use statistical methods in their professional life. Although primarily a reference, this volume is an ideal textbook. By selecting various chapter combinations an instructor can use it for a variety of types of undergraduate and graduate courses. An undergraduate course in statistical theory and methods will provide the necessary background for most of the chapters.

Our objective is to teach, and we teach mostly by example. A typical chapter begins with actual settings or real data sets. The author then guides the reader through the development of the methods in question while relating to these examples. When appropriate, the author refers the reader to the relevant parts of the most common statistical packages, especially SAS.

Each chapter starts from first principles and proceeds to state-of-the-art techniques. Our goal has been to create a standard handbook of statistical analysis for use in the pharmaceutical industry. We address controversies when they exist, and make recommendations after presenting all sides. These recommendations are consistent with good statistical practice and with the notion that statisticians must be able to persuade nonstatisticians as to the correctness of their conclusions. To this end we accent pictorial presentations that are backed up by the appropriate mathematical analyses.

Donald A. Berry

Contents

Contributors

INGRID A. AMARA Quintiles, Inc., Chapel Hill, North Carolina

DONALD A. BERRY School of Statistics, University of Minnesota, Minneapolis, Minnesota

JAMES A. BOLOGNESE Merck Sharp & Dohme Research Laboratories, Rahway, New Jersey

GREGORY J. CARR School of Public Health, University of North Carolina, Chapel Hill, North Carolina

R. DENNIS COOK School of Statistics, University of Minnesota, St. Paul, Minnesota

RICHARD G. CORNELL University of Michigan, Ann Arbor, Michigan

WILLIAM DuMOUCHEL BBN Software Products Corporation, Cambridge, Massachusetts

BRUCE P. EKHOLM 3M/Riker, 3M Health Care, St. Paul, Minnesota

TERRANCE L. FOX 3M/Riker, 3M Health Care, St. Paul, Minnesota

JUDITH D. GOLDBERG Lederle Laboratories, American Cyanamid Company, Pearl River, New York

A. P. GRIEVE* CIBA-GEIGY Pharmaceuticals, Horsham, West Sussex, England

ROBERT V. HOGG The University of Iowa, Iowa City, Iowa

JOHN D. KALBFLEISCH University of Waterloo, Waterloo, Ontario, Canada

GARY G. KOCH School of Public Health, University of North Carolina, Chapel Hill, North Carolina

KENNETH J. KOURY Lederle Laboratories, American Cyanamid Company, Pearl River, New York

DAVID A. LANE School of Statistics, University of Minnesota, Minneapolis, Minnesota

GEORGE A. MILLIKEN Kansas State University, Manhattan, Kansas

PETER C. O'BRIEN Mayo Clinic, Rochester, Minnesota

AMY RACINE-POON CIBA-GEIGY AG, Basel, Switzerland

NIGEL S. B. RAWSON* Drug Safety Research Unit, Southampton, England

BRUCE E. RODDA† Wyeth-Ayerst Research, Inc., New York, New York

STEPHEN J. RUBERG Merrell Dow Research Institute, Cincinnati, Ohio

ADRIAN F. M. SMITH University of Nottingham, University Park, Nottingham, England

MAURA E. STOKES SAS Institute, Inc., Cary, North Carolina

JAMES O. STREET Boehringer Ingelheim Pharmaceuticals, Inc., Ridgefield, Connecticut

THOMAS J. URYNIAK Fisons Corporation, Bedford, Massachusetts

SANFORD WEISBERG School of Statistics, University of Minnesota, St. Paul, Minnesota

LIANNG YUH Merrell Dow Research Institute, Cincinnati, Ohio

*Current affiliation: Institute of Cancer Research, Royal Cancer Hospital, Belmont, Surrey, England

†Current affiliation: The Squibb Institute for Medical Research, Princeton, New Jersey

1

Basic Principles in Designing and Analyzing Clinical Studies

DONALD A. BERRY University of Minnesota, Minneapolis, Minnesota

The goal of this chapter is to present the design and analysis of clinical trials in rather general terms, with emphasis on trials sponsored by pharmaceutical companies. Many topics discussed here are subjects of entire chapters elsewhere in this volume; my coverage of these topics will be especially brief and will serve mainly to set the context for these other chapters. My goal is not to give a compendium of designs and analyses. Rather, I focus on design and analysis issues that are most important to pharmaceutical statisticians. My approach is rather basic, assuming only a rudimentary knowledge of statistics. But I hope that even accomplished statisticians will find the discussion enlightening. I discuss philosophical issues, inevitably coming down on the side of practicality.

Most designs used in pharmaceutical studies are simple to describe. This is quite appropriate. Complex designs can muddle issues. Suitably complicated statistical analyses can sometimes retrieve valuable information from complex studies, but they frequently involve assumptions that may be questionable. In any case, a complicated analysis can seem like voodoo to physicians and other nonstatisticians.

Along the lines of keeping things simple, I want to make a point of practical importance, one that the reader should keep in mind while perusing the remainder of this book and in the practice of statistics generally: Statisticians are too statistical! The essence of statistical practice is communication. Statistical lingo handicaps interacting with nonstatisticians. P-values, chi-square tests, regression analyses, and so on, may be the icing but they are not the cake. Pictures and simple charts are the stuff of enlightened discourse.

To give an especially easy example, suppose that patients have been administered various doses of a drug. A hypothesis test suggests that any dose-response relationship is nonlinear. Don't give a p-value (except parenthetically). Show a plot of responses versus dose, perhaps using box plots or histograms for each dose level if the data set is unwieldy. [The excellent monograph by Cleveland (1985) gives other graphing methods.] Rebel against fitting into tired formats for reports and presentations: keep it simple but be creative. If you must emulate someone else's style, try your favorite weekly news magazine. Unfortunately, to have a major impact on policymaking, one has to shed part of the label "statistician."

Although simplicity is an appropriate goal, many designs that are used in pharmaceutical studies are *too* simple. There can be many important factors in predicting drug effect: dose, diagnostic and demographic variables, concomitant treatment, and so on. A study that considers only one level of each factor can be an extremely inefficient use of resources. Factorial designs [see Snedecor and Cochran (1980, Chap. 16)] should perhaps be used more than they are currently.

This chapter is organized as follows. I first discuss the various phases of drug development. Then I consider the types of controls used in clinical trials. I then discuss the designs commonly used in pharmaceutical trials, relating these to the phases of drug development and to types of control. Finally, I discuss the analysis of the results from clinical trials.

1 THREE PHASES OF DRUG DEVELOPMENT

Early in its development, a drug is used in animals to try to understand its action in animal systems. Many drugs are abandoned at this stage for lack of effect or because of serious toxic effects. Those that show promise are introduced into the clinic. (See Section 3.9 for a method for deciding under what circumstances to continue with drug development.) Animal studies give some notion of dose-response/dose-toxicity in animals (Chapter 4). They also give information for starting doses in humans. Normalized by weight or body surface area, these are usually small fractions of doses that are toxic for animals; extrapolating from animals to humans is chancy and conservatism is in order.

It is standard to categorize pharmaceutical trials into early, middle, and late: phases 1, 2, and 3. [Postmarketing surveillance (Chapter 16) is sometimes called phase 4.] The first two phases are concerned mainly with clinical pharmacology and the third is to demonstrate safety and effectiveness:

> Phase 1 starts when the new drug is first introduced into man—only animal and in vitro data are available—with the purpose of determining human toxicity, metabolism, absorption, elimination, and other pharmacological action, preferred route of administration, and safe dosage range; phase 2 covers the initial trial on a limited number of patients for specific disease control or prophylaxis purposes.... phase 3 provides the assessment of the drug's safety and effectiveness and optimum dosage schedules in the diagnosis, treatment, or prophylaxis of groups of subjects involving a given disease or condition. (Code of Federal Regulations, April 1, 1986, p. 63.)

There is always overlap between phases. This is true in part because trials are planned long before they are initiated. In addition, to fill gaps in knowledge or to experiment with new formulations of a drug, some phase 1 trials may actually be initiated after some phase 3 studies have ended. For these and other reasons that will become clear, there may be no conscious labeling of the phase of a clinical trial by a pharmaceutical company. Still, this trichotomy provides a good starting point for this chapter. I give a brief description of the three phases here; the design and analysis of clinical trials during these phases are discussed later in this chapter and in other chapters.

1.1 Phase 1 Trials

There are many important questions to be addressed in the early stages of clinical development. These include the following: Which doses and drug plasma levels are associated with therapeutic effect? toxicity? serious side effects? What is the drug's plasma half-line in humans? How does this half-life vary among subjects? among different types of patients? Is the half-life different after a single dose than after chronic dosing? How is the drug eliminated from the body? Does it have active metabolites? Is the drug's metabolism, effectiveness, or toxicity affected by other drugs that might be taken concomitantly? by food?

Such questions are of paramount importance and will be addressed at numerous times during a drug's clinical development; phase 1 answers (as all answers) are only tentative. Generally, the purpose of phase 1 is to provide a rather complete picture of a drug, but one that will require substantial focusing during phases 2 and 3. For example, phase 1 studies do not generally involve long-term treatment or long-term follow-up.

A drug may be used in various formulations (capsules, tablets, liquid, intravenous, etc.) over the course of its development and marketing phases. Since the drug may be marketed in a form different from that used in clinical trials, it is incumbent on the company to show that the various forms are bioequivalent. Bioequivalence studies occur in phase 1. Chapter 2 gives a thorough discussion of the issues. An interesting aspect of bioequivalence studies is that the statistical problem differs from the standard test of a hypothesis: the objective is to show equality rather than inequality.

1.2 Phase 2 Trials

These are intermediate between the exploratory trials of phase 1 and the definitive trials of phase 3. The goals of phase 2 are (1) to identify accurately the patient population that can benefit from the drug, and (2) to verify and estimate the effectiveness of the dosing regimen determined in phase 1. These goals are by no means unique to phase 2; they really carry over from phase 1 and into phase 3. Although there are no clear distinctions, phase 2 is somewhat more focused and less exploratory than is phase 1. In addition, phase 2 trials are smaller than phase 3 trials and may not compare drug with placebo or standard therapy.

Actually, phase 2 could be skipped entirely! But there would be danger in so doing. First, there are economic concerns for the company. Large-scale comparative trials of phase 3 are more expensive to sponsor and manage than are the smaller trials of phase 2. Second, since more patients are administered experimental treatment in a larger trial, more patients are at risk should the drug turn out to be ineffective or harmful. Having a phase 2 before phase 3 is a "walk before you run" philosophy (phase 1 is the crawl). Phase 2 should be skipped only if there is a compelling humanitarian reason for doing so; an example is the Burroughs-Wellcome drug zidovudine (AZT) for the treatment of AIDS.

Goals 1 and 2 of phase 2 trials are related since the optimal dosing regimen may well depend on the patient subgroup. For example, sicker patients may require more drug or may be able to tolerate smaller doses.

Patient Population

In setting up phase 2 trials, there are two extreme attitudes that a company might reasonably have regarding goal 1. One attitude is *narrow* and the other is *broad*. In practice, an intermediate course may be best.

The broad approach in phase 2 is to admit all comers, possibly stratifying on the basis of disease state and other important prognostic variables. Even without stratifying, the patient's responses should be analyzed as a function of the various predictor variables (see Example 3). This approach has obvious implications on sample size (see Section 3, especially Section 3.1). The idea is to learn as much as possible early on about the population of patients who might benefit from the drug. Those for whom the drug seems beneficial can be continued into phase 3 [assuming that the results are sufficiently beneficial to warrant continuing into phase 3 (see Section 3.9)]. Those categories of patients who do not respond well, or for whom there may be problems with side effects, could be kept in phase 2 for further study or simply dropped from consideration (see Chapter 9).

The narrow approach is to study a single subgroup of patients, at least initially. For example, the study subgroup might consist of those patients whose prognosis is fair: neither the sickest nor the least sick. Such a middle ground avoids the risks of possibly greater drug toxicity among the sickest patients. It also avoids the possibility of being unable to demonstrate effectiveness on the least sick patients. But a balance must be sought between clearly showing the drug's effect and maximizing its economic potential.

Once the effect of the drug has been verified in the study subgroup and phase 3 studies are planned or under way in that subgroup (assuming that the early results warrant this), phase 2 studies may be initiated on other subgroups. This strategy is conservative since fewer patients are exposed to an experimental drug during the earliest, most risky stages.

In addition, the narrow approach allocates a smaller portion of the company's resources to the drug early in its clinical development. So if something untoward happens (a serious side effect may show up after long-term use) and the drug's development is abandoned, less will be lost.

The broad approach will be necessary if the disease or condition being treated is quite rare. For then patient admission rates using the narrow approach may be too low to make the drug development program economically feasible.

Choosing between the narrow and broad approaches is an important decision for a pharmaceutical company. The narrow approach will usually be better: it involves less risk and it will probably lead to earlier approval of the drug by regulatory agencies. Of course, such approval may be limited initially to patients in the study subgroup. But such a restriction may be lifted when phase 3 trials are conducted in the other subgroups. If phase 2 results for the other subgroups are similar to those of phases 2 and 3 for the study subgroup, the drug may actually be approved for these subgroups without relevant phase 3 trials.

Dosing Regimen

Goal 2 of phase 2 trials is to establish firm dosing regimens for use in phase 3. It is a mistake to suppose that the effects of the various dosing regimens are understood completely after the preliminary studies of phase 1. Rather, the body of knowledge available at the time gives estimates of effects, estimates that are subject to error. There is the usual between-patient sampling variability. But there is also between-study variability, which is much more difficult to deal with (see Chapters 7 and 15).

These errors are obviously not limited to phase 1 but apply to all phases. However, while learning goes on throughout the clinical development of a drug (and even into the postmarketing phase—Chapter 16), these errors become smaller as development continues. By the time a company seeks approval to market a drug, its optimal dosing regimen should be reasonably firmly established; in practical terms, this is the meaning of goal 2.

1.3 Phase 3 Trials

To be approved for marketing, a drug must be shown to make a worthwhile contribution to medical treatment. Phase 3 studies are designed to identify a set of patients who are better treated with the drug (possibly in combination with other drugs) than in any other available way—if, in fact, there are such patients! They should also identify patients who are badly treated with the drug. This includes the possibility of identifying such patients during the course of treatment, perhaps with low doses but in any case before a high level of toxicity develops. The eventual goal is to recommend treatment strategies for the various patient types to the practicing physician.

In August 1988, the FDA began examining a proposal to eliminate phase 3 for certain drugs designed to treat life-threatening diseases. The point is to get important advances into the hands of physicians sooner.

Patient Population

Phase 1 identifies the patient population to be considered in phase 2, and phase 2 identifies the patient population to be considered in phase 3. The ideal circumstance is to consider the same population in phase 3 that was considered in phase 2, but this is not possible when doubts arise concerning the appropriateness of the drug for a subset of the phase 2 patient population. For example, hypertensive patients might have to be eliminated going into phase 3 if existing data suggest that the drug, an antibacterial agent, tends to elevate blood pressure in hypertensive patients. In any case, types of patients not considered in phase 2 should not be added in phase 3. As indicated in Section 1.2, once the drug is shown to be beneficial for the patients considered in phase 3, phase 2 studies on other subsets of patients may be sufficient to obtain marketing approval for these sets of patients as well.

Comparative Trials

To demonstrate that a drug has a place in medical practice, it must be compared with standard therapy. Just what constitutes "standard therapy" may not be clear. And even if it is clear, the standard therapy may not be widely recognized as effective.

The safest way to address the effectiveness of an experimental drug is to compare it with placebo or with no therapy. The comparison with placebo in a clinical trial directly addresses the question of the effect of the drug. This effect can then be compared with that of standard therapy indirectly through previous studies involving the standard. Better yet is to compare the experimental drug directly with *both* standard and placebo. This can be done in two separate clinical trials (experimental versus placebo and experimental versus standard) or in one trial involving all three treatments (experimental, standard, and placebo).

There is no unanimity of opinion as to which of these strategies is preferable. In my view, the first is usually better. Although two trials are more expensive, they give substantially more information about the experimental treatment per unit cost. Two trials also address the issue of trial effect and the reproducibility of experimental results. They should involve the same population of patients. If the results for those patients on the experimental treatment are consistent in the two studies (perhaps adjusting for any observed differences in patient populations), this speaks for the predictability of results if and when the drug is used in clinical practice. On the other hand, if the results are very different in the two studies (and adjusting for the various covariates does not adequately explain this difference), more trials may be necessary. But the strategy of conducting two separate comparative trials usually gives added weight to a claim of safety and efficacy.

In any comparison of experimental with standard therapy, both should be given optimally. This is one reason that phases 1 and 2 are so important: it would be folly for a pharmaceutical company to sponsor a large-scale comparison study involving an experimental drug for which the dose-response relationship is not well understood.

2 CONTROLS

The term "controlled study" has two meanings consistent with the English word "control": (1) one that is closely managed, regulated, or monitored, and (2) one that includes some subjects who are treated the same as the experimental subjects for the omission of or substitution for the experimental therapy. This section addresses meaning (2).

The reason for using controls in a study is to have a standard or comparison with the experimental therapy. A controlled study

> provides a comparison of the results of treatment or diagnosis with a control in such a fashion as to permit quantitative evaluation. Generally, four types of comparison are recognized:
>
> (i) No treatment: Where objective measurements of effectiveness are available and placebo effect is negligible, comparison of the objective results in comparable groups of treated and untreated patients.
>
> (ii) Placebo control: Comparison of the results of use of the new drug entity with an inactive preparation designed to resemble the test drug as far as possible.
>
> (iii) Active treatment control: An effective regimen of therapy may be used for comparison, e.g., where the condition treated is such that no treatment or administration of a placebo would be contrary to the interest of the patient.
>
> (iv) Historical control: In certain circumstances, such as those involving diseases with high and predictable mortality (acute leukemia of childhood), with signs and symptoms of predictable duration or severity (fever in certain infections), or in case of prophylaxis, where morbidity is predictable, the results of use of a new drug entity may be compared quantitatively with prior experience historically derived from the adequately documented natural history of the disease or condition in comparable patients or populations with no treatment or with a regimen (therapeutic, diagnostic, prophylactic) the effectiveness of which is established. (Code of Federal Regulations, April 1, 1982, p. 106.)

I prefer a different categorization, listed in order or preference of most biostatisticians:

a. Concurrent controls assigned and followed in a double-blind manner
b. Concurrent controls without blinding
c. Historical controls, based on the investigator's own experience
d. Literature controls, based on the experience of others

Depending on the circumstances, type c can be better than type b. Well-designed studies combine several types of controls: for example, types a, c, and d. The task of analysis is made difficult by multiple levels of controls, especially as regards the weights given to the different levels. But no study exists in a vacuum. Comparisons with historical and literature controls can only enhance conclusions from a study. Consumers of the results of a study will make comparisons with the results of previous studies, *as they perceive these results.* An explicit comparison will help consumers and will improve this process. (see Chapter 15 for a formal method of combining results from many studies.)

Uncontrolled studies have dubious value, but they are not worthless:

> Uncontrolled studies or partially controlled studies are not acceptable as the sole basis for the approval of claims of effectiveness. Such studies, carefully conducted and documented, may provide corroborative support of well-controlled studies regarding efficacy and may yield valuable data regarding safety of the test drug. Such studies will be considered on their merits in the light of the principles listed here, with the exception of the requirement for the comparison of the treated subjects with controls. Isolatea case reports, random experience, and reports lacking the details which permit scientific evaluation will not be considered. (Code of Federal Regulations, April 1, 1982, p. 107.)

2.1 Baseline Controls

A type of control not mentioned above is perhaps the most basic: the patient's baseline condition. It was not mentioned because it is not a sufficient form of control in a "controlled" clinical trial. Any improvement that a patient experiences may indeed be due to therapy, but it may also be spontaneous and unrelated to therapy: it is an irrefutable empirical fact that patients with extreme baseline measurements *tend* to improve even without therapy (cf. Section 4.7). Therefore, any improvement may be mistakenly attributed to treatment.

When possible, studies should call for predrug (baseline) measurements to be compared with the corresponding postdrug measurements. The analysis of the results then involves either change from baseline or percent change from baseline, or uses baseline as a covariate (see Section 4.4). In some studies (e.g., phase 1 studies) this will be the only control. In others, especially phase 3, changes from baseline will be the principal measurement being analyzed, but in the context of drug versus other forms of control.

2.2 Concurrent Controls

Most pharmaceutical studies use concurrent controls. For parallel studies (Section 3.6 and Chapter 8) the same protocol should be followed for the control and experimental groups. For crossover studies (Section 3.7 and Chapter 8) the same protocol should be followed in the two (or more) stages of the study. This allows for direct comparisons between the experimental and control data.

Randomization

In a study with concurrent controls, therapy can and should be assigned randomly. When there are two therapy groups, this can be accomplished by generating a single random sequence of 1's and 2's and assigning patients accordingly. To minimize problems with drop-outs, randomization should occur as close to the time of administering drug as possible.

Randomization does not guarantee that the 1's and 2's will be adequately balanced with regard to important prognostic factors. For example, consider a trial in which the endpoint (variable of interest) is death. Some patients in the trial have congestive heart failure (CHF) and some do not. Since CHF patients are at greater risk of death, a therapy that happened to be assigned to more CHF patients would be unfairly disadvantaged in comparison with the other therapy. This possibility can be avoided by stratifying: generate two random sequences of 1's and 2's and use one for CHF patients and the other for non-CHF patients.

Stratifying can be carried out on a finer partition of patients. For example, a patient with a mild case of CHF usually has a longer life expectancy than that of one with a severe case. CHF patients are classified from least to most severe into grades I, II, III, and IV. So all patients can be partitioned into five categories (including those with no CHF); each can have its own therapy assignment sequence of 1's and 2's.

Many statisticians caution against having too many categories; indeed, many [e.g., Peto et al. (1976)] recommend against all stratification schemes. One reason they give is that statistical power for individual categories is less than for the study as a whole; sometimes it is much less. Another reason is that a greater number of hypothesis tests (one for each category) can require a greater adjustment in reported statistical significance levels. Further, it is not legitimate to stratify to achieve balance across treatments and then ignore the stratification in the analysis—the resulting significance levels are incorrect. In my view, this awkwardness does not reflect an inherent weakness in stratification but results from the inverted nature of the classical statistical approach to hypothesis testing. Approaches consistent with the "likelihood principle" (Berger, 1986; Berry, 1987a) are not subject to such difficulties, and therefore allow and even encourage stratification.

In the presence of an important prognostic variable, analysis of covariance is appropriate, especially if stratification is not used. Of course, the conclusion that an experimental drug saves lives even though a greater proportion of patients died on the drug than on placebo will raise some eyebrows! This might happen if the experimental drug happened to be assigned to a disproportionate number of very sick patients. But presenting the data in tables and figures will convince most skeptics.

In a randomized trial, treatment assignment should be *nonpredictable* in the sense that admitting clinicians cannot reasonably guess which therapy the next patient will be assigned. If patients are randomly assigned to treatment in pairs (resulting in 12, 12, 21, 12, ..., say), and if the therapies previously assigned may become known after being assigned (through characteristic side effects, say), then the therapy assigned to even-numbered patients is predictable. If an assignment scheme is predictable, a clinician may be able to bias the results (perhaps subconsciously) by juggling the order of admission and thereby assigning sicker patients, say, to the experimental therapy.

In a completely randomized assignment scheme, a patient is assigned therapy independent of previous assignments. Such a scheme is nonpredictable. But it can result, by chance, in an imbalance in the sizes of the experimental and control groups. For example, 20 of the first 50 patients may be assigned to experimental and the other 30 to control, even though a 50-50 randomization scheme was used. This can be particularly troublesome in multicenter trials (Section 3.8 and Chapter 7) because therapy can become partially confounded with center.

There are several possible resolutions. One is to assign treatment by sampling without replacement from k 1's and k 2's. If $2k$ is the study size (within a center, say), the treatments will be perfectly balanced, although, depending on the particular scheme that results, there may be some predictability present toward the latter part of the assignment. If $2k$ is greater than the study size, the assignment will be less predictable; the study may not be perfectly balanced, but it will tend to be more balanced than a completely randomized scheme (which corresponds to $k \to \infty$). If $2k$ is less than the study size, it can be repeated until the study is complete—this corresponds to randomizing in blocks of size $2k$. Randomized block designs are more predictable for smaller k, randomized pairs corresponding to $k = 1$.

A neat modification of randomized blocks that avoids predictability is what I call "moving blocks." Assume $k = 10$ to be specific—generalizations will be clear. Start with ten 1's and ten 2's. After assigning the first 10 patients, say, by sampling without replacement, add 10 more 1's and 10 more 2's. Then assign the next 20 patients by sampling without replacement. Repeat the preceding step as necessary. Unbalanced randomization can be effected by changing the proportion of 1's. (Complete randomization is the case in which assignments are made by sampling with replacement.)

Randomizing minimizes the possibility of assignment bias. If clinicians assign treatment on the basis of an examination of the patient, the patients' prognoses may be confounded with treatment. Even a clinician who has no conscious bias may unknowingly feel that one drug is better than the other for certain patients, those who are most seriously ill, say. If a preponderance of such patients are assigned to one drug, the results on the two drugs cannot be fairly compared. An attempt should be made to adjust for the patients' prognoses and other covariates in analyzing the results, but the important covariates may not be measurable. Such assignment makes legitimate inferences difficult or impossible and should be avoided. If clinicians feel that certain types of patients should not receive one of the treatments, these patients should be excluded from the trial. Properly selected historical controls (Section 2.3) allow safer inferences than do controls assigned by the examining clinician.

In the United States, as in many other countries, patients in a randomized clinical trial must be informed that they will be randomized to therapy. Many potential patients will refuse to participate. This may create a bias because, for example, there may be correlations between treatment responses, prognoses, and willingness to participate. Also, many physicians refuse to take part in a randomized clinical trial. There is no doubt that such trials present ethical dilemmas for physicians and for statisticians as well (see Section 3.9).

An alternative to randomized controls that is seldom used is to have patients choose their own therapy. (Prior approval and close coordination with regulatory officials is essential here.) Selection bias may still be present, but it varies from one patient to the next. The patient can be informed about the various treatments (including estimates of efficacy and safety, costs, inconveniences, cosmetic effects, etc.) and choose accordingly. A distinct advantage over randomization is that the clinicians avoid ethical dilemmas. Data analysis requires taking account of all possible covariates. This type of study will be controversial. To make it more acceptable to some people, the design might include one group (selected randomly!) who are randomized to treatment and a second group who are offered their choice of treatment. (Letting patients choose whether or not to be randomized would probably yield a very small randomized group.) The groups might be pooled if their responses are similar (within treatment subgroups), but should the two groups turn out to have very different results, the group of patients who were offered their choice might be wasted insofar as inference is concerned.

Blinding

A critical aspect of modern clinical trial dogma is that studies should be double-blind: neither patient nor clinician is aware of the treatment assigned. A patient may respond differently knowing his or her treatment than not knowing it. The idea of blinding is to make the treatment and control groups as alike as possible except for treatment; both know that they could be receiving treatment and that they could be receiving control. Similarly, a clinician who is not blinded may give different collateral treatment to a patient known to be a control than to one known to be receiving the experimental drug.

It may not be possible to blind clinicians. For example, part of treatment may involve a surgical procedure. Or one treatment may have a universal side effect that effectively reveals which treatment was assigned. When a trial is not double-blind, patients must be admitted before treatment is assigned. For otherwise a clinician could subconsciously let knowledge of the treatment to be assigned affect whether the patient is admitted. This could easily bias the results. (However, provisions must be made to allow clinicians to break the treatment assignment code in case of an emergency.) Once patients are admitted they become part of the study and are analyzed as such even if they subsequently drop out (Chapter 9).

Matched Pairs

A special kind of parallel design (Section 3.6) is to pair patients on the basis of important demographic variables and other covariates: age, sex, disease state, time of enrollment, and so on. One member of each pair is assigned the experimental therapy and the other serves as a control. A single-sample analysis based on paired differences is appropriate (see Section 4.4).

Active Therapy or Placebo?

Most clinical trial specialists and regulatory agencies recommend placebo-controlled trials. The point of such a trial is to show that the experimental therapy does something, and to assess just what it does. As I indicated previously, multiple levels of controls enhance any study. Inevitably, an experimental therapy must be compared with the various standard therapies. The results from a placebo-controlled study should be compared formally with results from previous studies (Chapter 15). (Such a comparison is far from easy and a reasonable comparison may be impossible.) If there is a previous study that compared standard with placebo, an experimental-placebo comparison can be used to compare the experimental with the standard; the value of this comparison will be enhanced if the placebo results were similar in the two studies. Obviously, any comparison will be made easier if the same variables were measured in both studies; this should be kept in mind when designing a study.

There are obviously circumstances that mitigate against a placebo control. For example, it may be unethical not to treat the disease or condition in question. But even in the case of relatively benign conditions, studies with active controls enjoy a very pragmatic advantage over those with placebo as control: the experimental therapy is compared head to head with the competition! As suggested earlier, the best strategy may be to have two studies, one with placebo and one with active control.

2.3 Historical Controls

As indicated in the introduction of this section, it is important to distinguish between two types of historical control studies: (1) those in which the controls were treated at the same institution and by the same clinicians as the experimental patients, and (2) those in which the controls were treated at different institutions. Literature controls are included in the latter group.

The controls in (2) should serve only to supplement other types of controls. The differences among protocols/institutions/clinicians are usually too great to place much faith in the controls in (2) as a comparison group. So I will focus on type (1).

Historical controls should be similar to experimental patients—except for therapy. And they should be as close in time as possible. The same inclusion-exclusion criteria should be used in both groups.

An important consideration is that the same variables be measured on controls as on experimental patients. Also, these measurements should be at similar times after treatment in both groups. The availability and quality of control data are prime considerations in choosing centers to participate in a multicenter study with historical controls.

Gehan (1984) discusses the advantages and disadvantages of historical controls in cancer trials. I modify his lists below.

Advantages over Randomized Controls

Cost. Historical control studies can cost less than half as much as randomized studies with comparable sample sizes.
Power. There may be many more control patients available historically than concurrently.
Ethics. A clinician who believes (however weakly) that the experimental therapy is better than the control faces no ethical dilemma in admitting patients for treatment.
Recruitment. Patients are more apt to enlist for a study in which treatment assignment is not randomized. And since all patients will receive experimental therapy, patient recruitment can proceed at least twice as fast.

Disadvantages of Historical Controls

Comparability. Historical controls are less likely to be similar to experimental patients than are randomized controls. There are various reasons for this, the most important being differences in time and in entry criteria.
Believability. Randomized studies are generally accepted as being scientific; historical control studies are regarded by some as less than scientific. So regulatory agencies and practicing physicians will usually be more convinced by randomized studies.
Inflexibility. The form of control (active or placebo, say) can be chosen as part of the study design in randomized studies. In historical control studies, the treatment of control patients is fixed.

3 DESIGNS

In this section I describe some of the designs most commonly used in pharmaceutical clinical trials. Designs and types of control are related, the control being an integral part of the design. Sample size is addressed in many of the individual subsections; general considerations of sample size are discussed in Section 3.1. Some examples of the various designs are given in the data analysis section (Section 4). The final topic treated in this section is the ethics of clinical trials.

3.1 Sample Size

To calculate classical statistical measures of inference such as P-values, the trial design must be laid out completely in advance (see Section 4.1). This includes specifying sample size, since it is a design consideration. In practice it can be difficult to adhere to a previously specified size—there may be dropouts, slower patient acquisition than expected, and other problems. Moreover, interim data may seem to give sufficient information and suggest that stopping can occur sooner than expected. Such a cavalier attitude toward stopping can invalidate classical inferences (Section 3.9 and Chapter 10). Many biostatisticians object to a fixed-sample-size analysis when stopping occurs because of extreme interim results. (But few complain of such an analysis when the eventual sample size is affected by dropouts, deleting protocol violations, etc.) Even if the design/analysis does not meet the rigorous formalism of classical statistics, some analysis must be done!

There are various approaches to choosing sample size. The basic idea is to balance information gained with the costs of obtaining the information. These costs include time and resources as well as the cost of treating patients less than effectively. It the study size required to obtain necessary information is inordinately expensive, and alternative sources of information are unavailable, the company should consider abandoning development of the drug (in Section 3.9 I describe how to make the appropriate calculations).

Size of Phase 1 Trials

Phase 1 studies tend to be small. A phase 1 study seldom includes more than 20 subjects or patients, but it can include fewer. The size of a phase 1 study is frequently determined more by tradition than by science (but see Chapter 2 regarding bioequivalence studies), with current studies copying previous studies of the same general type. This is not bad. These studies are supposed to shed light on the issues; they are not meant to be definitive. If more evidence is required than that provided by the current study or from studies in phases 2 or 3, another phase 1 study of the same type can be carried out.

Size of Phase 2 Trials

Some statisticians recommend choosing sample sizes in phase 2 based on considerations of power (see below). Keep in mind that phase 2 trials are not supposed to be definitive. Although power calculations can help, other considerations are more important. One such consideration is economics. A large study can be financial drain. It may be financially wise to string several small studies together (perhaps analyzing them using the methods of Chapter 15).

As a rule of thumb, there should be at least 10 patients per treatment group per center; a smaller number leaves virtually no ability to discern center differences. This means at least 10 patients per center for crossover studies, for example, and twice this number for two-treatment parallel studies (although the expense of a parallel study with 20 patients may not be much greater than that of a crossover with ten). If trials involving the drug in question are inexpensive, substantially more than 10 per treatment per center may be quite appropriate.

Size of Phase 3 Studies

Phase 3 studies are confirmatory. As such they are usually quite large. Regulatory and granting agencies usually require "power calculations." Suppose first that the patients serve as their own controls (as in crossover designs or comparison with baseline) or are matched in pairs. Then the problem is to choose a single sample size n. We are interested in testing the mean improvement μ of drug over control; the null hypothesis is no improvement, H_0: $\mu = 0$. Let σ be the standard deviation of an individual difference and assume that σ is known. Also assume that n will be large enough that the sample mean will be close to normally distributed.

Let δ stand for the value of μ that is regarded to be a "clinically important" improvement over control. (Suppose that a positive difference is favorable for the drug so that $\delta > 0$.) Choosing δ is a difficult task: small μ may not mean much and large μ means a lot, but how to decide where in between it becomes important? In practice the choice of δ is at least somewhat arbitrary. (Statisticians have been known to calculate backwards—they know what n they want and they choose δ to give that value of n! This of course makes a mockery of the process, but the process invites such abuse: no one will ever know! I am not condoning this activity; rather, I am criticizing an approach that allows and even encourages it.)

Consider two simple hypotheses: H_0: $\mu = 0$ versus H_1: $\mu = \delta$. Let α and β denote the sizes of types I and II error for these hypotheses. Let Z_α denote the standard normal deviate with significance level α: $P(Z > Z_\alpha) = \alpha$. Snedecor and Cochran (1980, pp. 102–105) show that

$$n = \frac{(Z_\alpha + Z_\beta)^2 \sigma^2}{\delta^2}.$$

For two-tailed tests,

$$n = \frac{(Z_{\alpha/2} + Z_{\beta/2})^2 \sigma^2}{\delta^2}.$$

For two independent samples (as in parallel designs), each of size n from populations with variances σ_2^1 and σ_2^2, the formulas above apply with $\sigma^2 = \sigma_1^2 + \sigma_2^2$.

There are similar expressions for sample size in other settings. For example, consider a proportion p and tests for H_0: $p = p_0$ versus H_1: $p = p_1$. In the one-sided case, assuming that the resulting n is large enough that the normal approximation to the binomial is adequate,

$$n = \frac{[Z_\alpha \sqrt{p_0(1-p_0)} + Z_\beta \sqrt{p_1(1-p_1)}]^2}{(p_0 - p_1)^2}.$$

The foregoing determinations of sample size assume a single measure of interest. In many trials there are several important measures of efficacy; and there are always safety considerations, which in a sense are of infinite dimension. One approach in this more complicated setting is to calculate the required sample size for each efficacy measurement and use the largest. But this may be too conservative in that the resulting sample size may be enormous; some good economic sense is in order. And if the required sample size turns out to be very small (a high degree of improvement is expected, and this is coupled with small variance), the sample size should probably be increased to have the possibility of detecting side effects that occur infrequently but are very serious.

Finally, however the sample size is determined, once the study is run and the results are in, power considerations are irrelevant. I return to this controversial issue in Section 4.2.

3.2 Drug Versus Baseline

The simplest design for a clinical trial is to admit subjects, establish baseline measurements (perhaps after administering a placebo), and then measure the same variables after administering the drug. These two measurements are then compared in pairs. The null hypothesis is usually that there is no change on average from baseline.

The assumption implicit in such a design is that any drug effect is not confounded with time. Since it is difficult to have much confidence in this assumption, such a design is usually restricted to phase 1 trials. The simple device of exchanging the order of drug and placebo in some of the patients allows for a test of any confounding of time (see crossover trials in Section 3.7 and Chapter 8).

A variant of the drug versus baseline design is to have several baseline measurements of the same quantity in the same subject and several measurements on drug. This gives a more accurate picture of the drug response in each subject. It is particularly appropriate when the measurement is quite variable within subjects, due either to inherent variability of the quantity being measured or to variability in the measuring process.

Another variant is to make repeated measurements on drug, say at 0, 1/2, 1, 2, 3, 4, and 8 hours after administering the drug. This gives information about the effect of the drug over time. Again, such a design is most useful in phase 1. Repeated measures designs are the subject of Chapter 3.

Drug versus baseline studies tend to be small. A small drug versus baseline trial can provide substantial information because within-subject variances are frequently very small. Suppose that a drug is administered to ten patients who have been at rest for 2 hours. All their blood pressures drop by 8 to 10 mmHg in the first 30 minutes. It is not unreasonable to attribute this decrease to the drug, but this must be verified in a controlled setting.

3.3 Titration Studies

Titration designs are used in phases 1 and 2, and sometimes in phase 3. In such a design each patient's dose is increased until achieving a satisfactory balance between beneficial and maleficent effects. The purpose is usually to determine the optimal dose or dose range of the drug. Not all types of drugs are candidates for such a design. Generally speaking, agents that require chronic dosing to control a disease or condition (e.g., hypertension) are candidates for a titration study. In fact, a drug whose response is highly variable may *require* titration dosing throughout its clinical development and after it is approved for marketing. On the other hand, it is difficult to set up a titration study for an agent that is designed to cure a disease or condition (e.g., infection) rather than to control it.

Although a good titration study is difficult to conduct, it gives important information in a very efficient manner. Upon admission to a titration study, the patient's condition is assessed by establishing baseline measurements; these will be compared with later measurements on the drug. Baseline measurements should not be used to decide which patients are admitted to the study; for this purpose there should be an earlier screening period. Using the same measurements for analysis and to determine admission can invalidate the conclusions of the study (see Section 4.7).

The rest of the course of the patient's treatment is partitioned in advance into a number of roughly equal periods, a period being chosen large enough to show a response to that dose of the drug. During the first period the patient is administered the drug at the lowest dosage associated with some efficacy in earlier studies. The measurements taken at baseline are repeated at the end of the first period. Perhaps using predetermined criteria, the clinician decides whether a patient's response is satisfactory. If it is, the patient stays at the same dose during the next period. If it is not, the patient's dose is increased during the next period, to a level prescribed in advance.

This process is repeated in each period, up to the maximum specified dose (perhaps one clearly associated with toxicity in earlier studies). A patient whose dose stayed the same in an early period may be increased in a later period. The dose of a patient who experiences limiting side effects can be decreased, or if necessary, the patient can be dropped from the study and considered a failure in any subsequent analyses (see Chapter 9). For reasons discussed in Section 4.7, a patient who responds satisfactorily should *never* be dropped prematurely from the study.

Results from a titration study give information about the doses that will be required in clinical practice, and also about the success rates at the various doses. But the results do not give direct information about the levels of response and frequencies of side effects at dosing regimens other than the lowest. For, only those patients who did not respond satisfactorily at the low dose reach the next dose. So the average response of those patients who received the second-lowest dose is biased, and this bias can be substantial. If direct information concerning response at the various doses is desired, the design should be modified to have *every* patient's dose increased from one period to the next.

Titration studies are not limited to settings in which comparisons are made with baseline measurements. In particular, titration comparisons with standard therapy are possible in parallel or crossover double-blind studies (Sections 3.6 and 3.7), even if the dosing intervals on the two drugs are different. For example, suppose that the effective dose for experimental drug ranges from 100 to 300 mg, while that for the standard ranges from 300 to 500 mg. Identical capsules containing 100, 200, and 300 mg of the first drug and 300, 400, and 500 mg of the second can be used in the study. Patients randomized to the first drug start at 100 mg and those on the second start at 300 mg. A patient who responds sufficiently well during the first week is kept at that dose. One who does not respond is increased to the next dose (of the same drug). Similarly, nonresponders during the second week (at the middle dose) can be increased to the high dose for the third and final week. [Responders continue in the study at the same dose (see Section 4.7 and Chapter 9 for dangers in dropping responders).]

There are no special concerns for sample size of titration studies. Exploratory studies (phase 1) tend to be small, and sample size may be only roughly specified in advance. Confirmatory studies tend to be large.

3.4 Using Historical Controls

A study in which experimental drug is compared with historical controls is relatively easy to design and carry out: every patient who is admitted to the study is given the experimental drug. The patients' responses are measured and compared with the responses of controls. The protocol for obtaining measurements and their timing should be the same for the experimental patients as for controls.

Sample sizes can be calculated as described in Section 3.1. If the historical control group is very large, the effect of control may be assumed known. Otherwise, the sample size for the control group is assumed to be given. In any case, the required treatment sample size can be calculated using methods similar to those in Section 3.1. Advantages and disadvantages of historical controls are discussed in Section 2.3.

3.5 Matched Pairs

A problem that faces every study designer is variability in the population. Sometimes it is possible to minimize variability. One way is to use the various treatments on the same patient (see Section 3.7). (In Chapter 2 the intriguing possibility of using two or more treatments on the same patient at the same time is discussed.) Another way to decrease variability for between-treatment comparison is to match individuals in pairs (for two-treatment studies) to ensure that they have similar values of prognostic and demographic variables, and administer one treatment to one member of each pair (selected randomly) and the other treatment to the other member.

The success of a matched-pair study depends on the availability of a sufficient number of patients who can be matched with other patients. Inferences will be better if the matching does in fact decrease the biological variability within pairs. Sample size is determined as in the one-sample case, where pairs are the observational units.

3.6 Parallel Studies

Phase 3 studies generally have parallel designs. Usually, there are two treatment groups: experimental and control. The controls must be concurrent in a parallel design. Control may be placebo, standard therapy, no therapy, or another experimental therapy. Patients are assigned to one of the two treatment groups upon entering the study—usually the assignment is random.

If the dosing intervals of the two drugs differ, this can be accommodated without compromising the blind by using placebo capsules that are identical in appearance with those containing drug. For example, suppose that the first drug is to be taken every 8 hours and the second every 12 hours. The capsules taken at 0800, 1600, and 2400 hours by those patients on the first drug can contain drug, while those taken at 2000 hours contain placebo. For the other drug, capsules taken at 0800 and 2000 hours contain drug, while those taken at 1600 and 2400 hours contain placebo.

Traditionally, equal numbers of patients are assigned to the two treatment groups. For fixed total number of patients, this allows for maximum information concerning the difference between the treatment means in the following sense. Suppose that σ_1 and σ_2 are the two population standard deviations and n_1 and n_2 are the respective sample sizes. The variance of the difference in sample means is

$$\frac{\sigma_1^2}{n_1} + \frac{\sigma_2^2}{n_2}.$$

An easy calculation shows that for fixed $n_1 + n_2$, this variance is minimized by taking

$$\frac{n_1}{n_2} = \frac{\sigma_1}{\sigma_2}.$$

In particular, if $\sigma_1 = \sigma_2$, then $n_1 = n_2$ minimizes the variance of the difference in sample means.

However, the utility of equal allocation is greatly exaggerated by tradition. Pharmaceutical companies should entertain using unbalanced designs, perhaps weighted 2:1 or 3:1 in favor of the experimental treatment [for a similar view, see Peto et al. (1976)]. Such an imbalance gives more information concerning the experimental drug per unit cost. This is especially appropriate when information concerning the standard therapy can be supplemented using historical or literature controls (see Section 2.3 and Chapter 15).

3.7 Crossover Studies

The treatment groups in parallel studies are independent. In crossover studies they are paired. Just as in baseline versus drug studies, the pairing in crossover studies is provided by the individual patient. Most crossover studies involve two treatments and two treatment periods. Half the patients receive drug 1 followed by drug 2; the other half receive drug 2 followed by drug 1. The order (12 versus 21) can be assigned randomly and the assignment can be double-blind. There must be ample time between the two periods to allow the effects of the first drug to wear off—obviously, if a cure is possible, this design is inappropriate. If dosing intervals are different for the two drugs, the blind can be preserved just as described in Section 3.6. There are variants of the two-period crossover design in which three or four treatment periods are employed (see Chapters 2 and 8), but multiple periods are usually avoided because they have higher patient dropout rates.

Crossover designs can be considered when there is less within-subject variability than there is between subjects. But when there is just as much variability within the same subject at different times as between two different subjects, a crossover has no advantage (see Example 5). A thorough discussion of the role of crossover designs is provided in Chapter 8.

The use of baseline measurements in crossover studies is problematic [cf. Fleiss et al. (1985)]. Suppose that both treatment periods have baseline measurements. Should the second-period measurements be compared with the second baseline or with the original baseline? A simpleminded but generally satisfactory procedure is to compare all treatment measurements with the average of all baseline measurements. Also, the baseline measurements may themselves be analyzed for time and carryover effects or integrated with the drug measurements in a single comprehensive analysis (Section 4.2 of Chapter 8). The number and timing of baseline measurements should be addressed carefully: there should be good reasons to have more than one set of baseline measurements, and having none at all is not out of the question in a crossover trial. Sample size is determined as in the one-sample case, where an observational unit is the individual patient.

3.8 Many Centers

Many phase 2 and essentially all phase 3 studies involve more than one clinic. The purpose of having more than one center is to demonstrate that the effective use of the drug is not limited to a single, restricted setting. Center effect is an important unknown that can complicate a drug development program. Phase 2 studies can help shed light on center effect. But too many centers can obscure other issues. So, while phase 2 trials should involve more than one center, the number should be small—perhaps two to four.

Phase 3 trials may include 20 or more centers. A large number of centers can make analysis difficult. Some statisticians insist that if the results vary substantially among the centers, they cannot be pooled into a single analysis. Others would simply incorporate the possibility of center effect and do a single analysis on the combined data (compare Chapters 7, 13, and 15). If the data cannot be pooled, then, it is said, each center has to "stand on its own." I have never understood this attitude: after analyzing individual centers, the results of the various analysis *have to be* pooled in order to come to a conclusion concerning the safety and efficacy of the drug. I mention this attitude here because it is held by some influential statisticians, including some at regulatory agencies. If statistics cannot make a single inference from multifarious sources, there is something wrong with statistics.

I would prefer to see eight centers with 50 patients each to 20 centers with 20 patients each. Some statisticians go further and recommend as few as three centers; this allows a single center to "stand alone" more easily. While I prefer three to 20, three centers may too easily fail to represent the population of centers. In practice, statisticians have to live with circumstances that are less than ideal. For example, the rate of patient acquisition may be completely inadequate when dealing with a small number of centers.

In a multicenter trial, each center should have its own randomization schedule so as to avoid treatment-center confounding. Ideally, each center should contribute the same number of patients. This may not be possible. But suppose that the trial is to stop when a total of 400 patients have been treated in 20 centers (200 per drug, say). The majority of the patients will probably be contained in only three to five of the 20 centers. At the other end of the spectrum, five centers will probably contribute fewer than five patients each. Such small centers may be more trouble than they are worth.

The study protocol could specify upper and lower limits on the number of patients per center, but a lower limit may drag out the study longer than is reasonable. The key is to use only centers that are reasonably able to provide a moderate number of patients; questionable centers should not be included. See Chapter 8 for a detailed discussion of the design and analysis of multicenter studies.

3.9 Sequential Designs

All designs discussed above are characterized as follows: (i) the treatment assignment sequence is set in advance (perhaps randomly), and (ii) the study is to include a fixed number of patients. In particular, the treatment assignment scheme cannot depend on the interim results and the trial cannot be stopped prematurely based on interim results. A *sequential* design allows interim results to affect treatments assigned to later patients or to allow for early stopping.

Adaptive Treatment Assignment

The usual goal of sequential (or adaptive) treatment assignment schemes is to use early results to better treat those patients who arrive later in the study. So if early results suggest that standard therapy is better than experimental therapy, say, standard will be used more than will experimental for patients later in the study. This state of affairs would not be in the best interests of a sponsoring pharmaceutical company. Rather, if the results are sufficiently convincing that experimental therapy is inferior, the company would be better advised to stop the study altogether (see below). So, while adaptive assignment schemes may have a place in studies conducted by the National Institutes of Health, say, they do not have a place in studies sponsored by pharmaceutical companies. The reader interested in adaptive assignment schemes is referred to Berry and Fristedt (1985), especially its annotated bibliography.

Sequential Stopping

Suppose that a trial is stopped prematurely because accumulating data suggest that one of the treatments is better than or safer than the other. Then p-values and confidence intervals are affected (see Chapter 10). In general, it is not enough to know the data when making classical statistical inferences. One also needs to know all the details of the design, including a complete specification of the interim data that would have called for stopping.

The luxury of *being able* to stop early has a price: whether or not the trial is stopped prematurely, p-values and confidence intervals are affected (Chapter 10). As a result, few clinical trials sponsored by pharmaceutical companies allow explicitly for early stopping. (However, many investigators in phase 1 and phase 2 trials examine accumulating data periodically with the possibility of stopping or otherwise modifying the trial. Such behavior renders p-values calculated at the end of the trial meaningless.) In the Bayesian and likelihood approaches to statistics there is no price paid for examining accumulating data (Berry, 1985, 1987a, 1988). But these approaches have thus far had little impact on biostatistical practice.

A thorough treatment of the statistical issues involved with sequential stopping rules is presented in Chapter 10. In Section 3.11 I address ethical issues related to the use of such rules.

Stopping Drug Development

The heading of this section seems out of place under "sequential designs" and even out of place under "designs." It is included here because it deals with the analysis of accumulating data, either within a single trial or over the course of the various trials in a drug development program.

A question of paramount concern to a pharmaceutical company is whether and when to stop a drug development program because the available data suggest that the drug has insufficient efficacy. This decision involves monetary considerations. If the drug is eventually approved for marketing, the company will probably make money. But if development continues now, only to be stopped one year from now, say, or if it is not stopped but the drug is not approved for marketing, the company will lose its interim investment. If development is stopped, the associated costs will be saved, but of course there is no chance for future profits. The question of stopping or not is a typical problem in statistical decision theory.

The design of a trial can specify periodic analyses to determine whether or not to stop the trial and in so doing to stop future development. The trial will not be stopped for positive efficacy results. This is consistent with the need for safety information regarding any experimental drug; the trial will continue as planned to obtain this information even if interim efficacy results are very favorable. There is no issue related to adjusting p-values for early stopping, for example, because the trial results would not then be used to convince anyone of the drug's efficacy: by stopping the trial the company effectively gives up the possibility of obtaining marketing approval for the drug. The stopping problem is not one that involves testing statistical hypotheses. The pharmaceutical company must have a collateral process of data analysis for preparing a submission to a regulatory agency should the internal decision continue to be that the drug's development is worth pursuing.

Berry and Ho (1988) [see also Berry (1987c)] show how to resolve this problem and carry out an example; I will not go into specifics here. Qualitatively, one proceeds as follows. Assess the various expected costs, gains, and losses of continuing as a function of the drug's safety and efficacy, which are as yet not completely known. Assess the information present about safety and efficacy; this information will be updated using Bayes's theorem as the data accumulate. The expected total gain of continuing depends on the minimum expected total future gain at the next interim analysis and on the intervening costs. The first of these is random since it depends on data not yet observed. This can be resolved by averaging over these data, averaging with respect to their (predictive) probability distribution.

The biggest calculational difficulty to overcome is that future expected gains at the next analysis are not known, even conditioning on the intervening data, any more than the current future expected gains are known. This can be resolved using backward induction (dynamic programming) as follows. Start at the last analysis period when all the data are available. Find the best decision for all possible data. Evaluate the expected future total gain of that decision. Now consider all possible data available at the next-to-last period. Evaluate the expected gain of continuing by averaging over the as yet unobserved data, deciding whether to stop or continue. Proceed backwards in this way through time to the present, always evaluating the expected future gain of continuing and comparing it with the expected future gain of stopping (usually zero). This gives the optimal current decision.

Explicit monetary considerations in health-related settings bother some people. But pharmaceutical companies that strive to maximize expected profit are not behaving inconsistently with delivering good medicine (cf. Section 3.11). Only a very shortsighted company would market a drug it knows to be ineffective or unsafe. A company that markets an ineffective drug risks losing marketing and other developmental costs; in this age of litigation, marketing an unsafe drug risks being forced into bankruptcy.

An important message in this section is that major decisions, such as whether to continue with drug development, are *statistical*. For each possible decision, future gains and losses can be weighed by their probabilities. This provides for a numerical comparison (expected monetary gain) of the available decisions.

Statistics is much more than a set of tools for data analysis. In a larger sense, statistics is making decisions under uncertainty. This seems to be a well-kept secret. Biostatisticians should be involved in a leadership capacity in major pharmaceutical company decisions [cf. Berry (1987c)]. But no one is going to offer them this role—biostatisticians must seize the available opportunities.

3.10 Drug Interaction Studies

Patients on experimental therapy may be taking other drugs. It is not possible to assess how an experimental drug is affected by all other marketed drugs. But such an assessment is necessary for those drugs that are likely to be used in association with the experimental drug.

There are basically two ways for making this assessment. One is to conduct a trial designed expressly for the purpose. The other is to keep track of each patient's concomitant therapy in all clinical trials involving the experimental drug (this procedure should be standard in clinical trials) and compare patients on the concomitant drug in question with those not on it.

The latter is the usual path because it is relatively easy to follow. And it has the following advantage. The incidence of use of concomitant drugs in clinical trials should be roughly similar to that of clinical practice. So there is a natural self-selection of drugs when using the latter method; in particular, a drug not encountered as concomitant therapy in clinical trials will probably not be encountered after marketing.

The other way to assess interaction is more interesting. There is a relatively small but rapidly growing literature dealing with prospectively designed interaction studies [e.g., Holtzman et al. (1987)]. (Although nominally a phase 1 study, such an investigation might reasonably be delayed until such time that the drug seems likely to be approved for marketing.) I will confine my discussion here to some very basic ideas.

Suppose that a trial is designed to assess the interaction of an experimental drug (A) with digitalis therapy (B) in patients with congestive heart failure. A 4-week study might be used: in the first week patients receive no drug, in the second they receive B, in the third $A + B$, and in the fourth only A. (These might be given in crossover fashion. Suppose that there are 24 patients in the study; one can be assigned to each of the 24 possible sequences of $\emptyset$, A, B, $A+B$. Various incomplete versions are possible for a smaller number of patients.) Clinical measurements and blood samples are taken on the seventh day of each week. One can then test whether the clinical effects of the drugs are *additive* [$(A)-(\emptyset)+(B)-(\emptyset) = (A+B)-(\emptyset)$, or $(A+B)-(A)-(B)+(\emptyset) = 0$], *subadditive*, or *superadditive* (i.e., *synergistic*). Also, one can test whether the plasma levels and plasma clearances of the drugs are affected by the presence of the other drug (Holtzman et al., 1987).

As pointed out by Chi (1984), there are dangers in using combination therapy on subsets of patients that are determined by their response to the drugs given individually. Ideally, all patients should receive $\emptyset$, A, B, and $A + B$. If this is not possible, the patient group should be divided in two in advance; half of the patients receive A and $A + B$ and the other half, B and $A + B$. If even this is not possible, the patients can be divided in thirds in advance; one-third receive A, one-third B, and one-third $A + B$. Inferences concerning the effect of combination therapy will be difficult with such a parallel design unless the trial is very large.

One can use designs with multiple periods for comparing various combinations of single and chronic dosing of two drugs [e.g., Holtzman et al. (1984)]. These designs are somewhat complicated for standard use. A better way to use resources is to design a trial involving only single doses. Then, based on the results of the first study, a second study involving chronic dosing can be more efficiently designed. But a second study may be unnecessary if data concerning the interaction of these two drugs used chronically derive from studies in phases 2 and 3.

3.11 Ethics of Randomized Clinical Trials

In discussing concurrent controls and randomization (Section 2.2) I referred to a fundamental ethical dilemma. Randomized clinical trials are wonderful inferential tools. As such, they allow clinicians to make reasonably informed choices in treating patients who present themselves after the trial. But they may expose patients *in* the trial to inoptimal therapy.

Suppose that results from studies in phases 1 and 2 are quite positive. Drug development enters phase 3. Regulatory agencies require a randomized controlled study. The endpoint is death. Placebo controls are ruled out and standard therapy is used as a control. Early results from the trial *suggest* that the new drug is superior to the standard (*inferior* also presents a dilemma). Is it ethical to continue the trial, giving half the patients apparently inferior treatment?

First I address this question from the point of view of society. Of course, societies operate under a set of rules that answer the question; for example, in the United States, laws passed by Congress guide the Food and Drug Administration (FDA) in regulating pharmaceutical clinical trials.

Next I address the question within the context of current FDA regulations. Statistical issues have a substantial impact on public policies regarding clinical trials. So while pharmaceutical statisticians are concerned with abiding by FDA regulations, they should also be interested in whether these regulations serve society well.

Setting Public Policy

Consider the next patient in the above-described trial. This patient would obviously prefer the treatment that has performed better so far. But if every patient were given the currently better-performing therapy, one of the two therapies would be given to the overwhelming majority of patients. A great imbalance in a trial limits the ability to decide which drug is better. So the treatment of patients presenting themselves after the trial will not be as well informed.

This is the great dilemma of clinical trials: if each patient is treated as well as possible, patients as a whole are not. There is an inherent conflict between the *éthique individuelle* and the *éthique collectif.* Society must decide between them, or how much each is to be weighed. The challenge for statisticians is to provide methodology that allows for legitimate inferences outside the rigid structure of randomized controlled trials. This would move into the direction of the *éthique individuelle* without sacrificing the *éthique collectif.* There have been attempts in this direction [e.g., Kadane (1986)], but none has been widely accepted by biostatisticians.

Many clinicians and statisticians feel that randomized clinical trials are perfectly ethical. One argument to this effect is that we really do not know which drug is better else we would not be conducting a clinical trial. But we never really *know* anything—we have varying degrees of information. And we could easily feel more strongly about a drug comparison based on interim data on 20 patients than we could about another drug comparison based on the complete results from a trial involving 200 patients.

Another argument advanced is that if we do not look at interim results we will not know any more than when we started, and we cannot act on what we do not know. Although true, I think it is preposterous to claim that ignoring information somehow avoids the ethical dilemma: Is a clinician who refuses to examine a patient innocent when the patient dies?

A related issue of particular interest to statisticians is group sequential design. As indicated in Section 3.9 (see Chapter 10), the more times accumulating data are analyzed, the more adjustment is required in the final significance level. Consequently, some statisticians recommend few or no interim analyses. Or they suggest designs in which it is difficult to stop early (see Chapter 10); for then, if there is no early stopping, the actual significance level is only slightly larger than the apparent level. So while these designs are more ethical (and also more economical) than non-sequential designs, they are limited by the confines of classical statistical inference. Any substantial progress made toward satisfying the *éthique individuelle* without compromising the *éthique collectif* will have to break out of these confines. Both Bayesian and likelihood approaches to statistics

(Berry, 1985, 1987a, 1988) are possible candidates because they have much greater flexibility; in particular, they do not require adjusting inferences for interim analyses.

Ethics Under FDA Regulations

Individual pharmaceutical statisticians do not set policy, they abide by it. In the United States, they must live within FDA guidelines. So many of the ethical issues discussed above are moot. But there is substantial leeway within these guidelines. In particular, while the FDA must approve the size of a planned trial, along with other design aspects, a wide range of sizes is usually acceptable. And if the eventual size is not radically different, a fixed-size analysis will be acceptable.

There is much flexibility in the design and analysis of studies during phases 1 and 2. A pharmaceutical company wants to pursue its drug's development, but only if it will be a financial success. It will not be a success if it is not efficacious and safe; in particular, it will probably not be approved for marketing. It is not difficult for the company to meet its ethical obligation during these phases by proceeding cautiously while getting information about efficacy and safety. The pharmaceutical statistician can help the company meet its ethical obligations while maximizing its expected future profit using analyses similar to that outlined in Section 3.9.

To get FDA approval for marketing a drug usually requires randomized clinical trials; these occur during phase 3. So [provided that the need for phase 3 has not been eliminated (see Section 1.3)] a pharmaceutical company is forced to adopt an *éthique collectif*—but only in one direction. Namely, even if the experimental drug is performing much better than the control, the company on its own cannot stop the trial and give everyone the experimental. But it can stop the trial if the drug is performing sufficiently worse than control—Section 3.9 shows how to decide what is "sufficiently worse." (As indicated in that section, there is no need to adjust significance levels when using such one-sided stopping boundaries.)

Although a pharmaceutical company cannot stop a trial and proclaim its drug superior, if phase 3 studies are incredibly promising, there is something it can do. First, for legitimate classical inferences such a possibility must be specified in advance (along the lines of Chapter 10). More important, it must be agreed to by the FDA—this is quite appropriate, for the company is hardly an unbiased observer. Somewhat ironically, early stopping for very promising results might mean *less* effective therapy for patients who have been in the trial continuation. Had the trial continued, they had a 50% chance of getting the experimental therapy. It will take a substantial period of time for marketing approval and subsequent marketing—more than a year even in the best of circumstances. So they may be deprived of this therapy during the approval/marketing process. What early stopping does is start this process sooner, thereby making the drug available to a larger number of patients sooner.

The FDA may reasonably disallow early stopping for promising results. The effect of a drug is multidimensional. It may be obvious that it is the best drug of its type after very few patients, but safety is another matter. Rare but serious adverse experiences may require observing many more patients. There is an obvious trade-off: A very efficacious drug for a serious disease or condition might be approved on the basis of very limited safety information, while a similarly efficacious drug for a less serious ailment would not.

Monitoring efficacy results with the possibility of early stopping requires adjusting significance levels, and so is discouraged by some statisticians. But monitoring for safety is essential. Berry (1989) describes a method for continual monitoring with the possibility of stopping a trial on the basis of the incidence of serious adverse experiences. If adverse experiences are correlated with efficacy, significance levels may be affected, but in ways that are nearly impossible to evaluate. However, in no case is this sufficient reason to discourage monitoring for safety.

4 ANALYSIS

Most of the chapters in this book deal with the analysis of pharmaceutical data. I confine my discussion here to the most basic ideas of data analysis. This will serve to introduce some of the later chapters, but some of the points I make are not discussed later in the book.

4.1 Design and Analysis: A Tandem?

"The design determines the analysis," statisticians say. This is certainly true when using classical statistical inferences such as p-values.

To use a simple example, consider a study involving matched pairs with drug (D) and control (C). Responses are dichotomous: either D or C is better in each pair. The null hypothesis is that these are equally likely. The data are

$$DCDDDDCCDDDDC.$$

If the sample size had been fixed in advance at $n = 13$, the two-sided p-value is the null probability of observing 0, 1, 2, 3, 4, or 9, 10, 11, 12, 13 preferences for D: $p = 0.049$. So the results are statistically significant.

Had the design been different and the same data observed, the p-value would (usually) also be different. For example, suppose that the plan had been to stop upon observing at least 4 Ds and 4 Cs. Then the (two-sided) p-value is the null probability of observing 13, 14, 15, ... pairs: $p = 0.021$. If there were no plan at all—or if there were dropouts—no p-value could be calculated! Similarly, confidence intervals could not be calculated. Obviously, "the design determines the analysis."

A real example is provided in Freireich et al. (1963) [see also Berry (1987a)]. Of 21 pairs, 18 were preferences for drug over placebo. The two-sided fixed sample ($n = 21$) p-value is 0.0015. But the design was sequential (Section 3.9 and Chapter 10), so the significance level reported was much larger: 0.05.

This state of affairs may make sense to many statisticians, but it can baffle nonstatisticians: Why isn't it enough to know that D won 9 of the 13 (or 18 of the 21) head-to-head comparisons? The safest approach is not to tell nonstatisticians that it isn't enough.

Some compromise regarding this issue is almost always necessary. There *are* dropouts, protocol violations, and similar problems. It is not possible to take all possibilities into account in the study protocol. Statisticians usually proceed as though the actual sample size (and other aspects of the resulting design) were planned in the protocol. Although not strictly correct, such pragmaticism is required: the alternative is to refuse to make any calculations.

In summary, my answer to the section heading is a highly qualified "yes." The design-analysis tandem is frequently broken and the resulting tandem is not always the one planned.

4.2 Pre- Versus Postdata Precision

This section is devoted to a very important but rather simple question: How relevant are power considerations in analyzing data? I would not have included such a section at all except that many statisticians believe they are of utmost importance. I want to argue against that perception.

Consider a matched-pair design as in Section 3.5 and the example in Section 4.1. Let p be the probability that D is better than C for a randomly selected pair. The null hypothesis is H_0: $p = 1/2$. We would regard D as an important treatment if it is an effective improvement over control in 40 percent of patients; this corresponds to $p = 0.7$ (this allows for half of the remaining 60% of the patients to respond better on D by happenstance alone). For a one-sided test, $\alpha = \beta = 0.05$, and the normal approximation to the binomial, we find from Section 3.1 that we require

$$n = \frac{[1.645\sqrt{(0.5)(0.5)} + 1.645\sqrt{(0.7)(0.3)}]^2}{(0.2)^2} \doteq 63$$

pairs.

The study was actually run with only 25 pairs (we came upon this study after the fact, or perhaps our advice concerning sample size was ignored). There were 23 preferences for D. Assuming that $n = 25$ was fixed in advance, the exact (one-sided) p-value is

$$p\text{-value} = \left[\binom{25}{23} + \binom{25}{24} + \binom{25}{25}\right]\left(\frac{1}{2}\right)^{25} \doteq 10^{-5}.$$

So the results are very suggestive that H_0 is false.

Some statisticians would say that the study was "inadequate" because it "lacked power." But the data not only contradict H_0, they also suggest that $p \neq 0.7$ [a 95% confidence interval for p is $(0.750, 0.978)$—Lindgren et al. (1978, p. 165)]. So the results were somewhat unexpected, but they are the results! The alternative hypothesis $p = 0.7$ is now irrelevant. More relevant is $\hat{p} = 0.92$. Had this been the alternative considered at the design stage, the required sample size would be

$$n = \frac{[1.645\sqrt{(0.5)(0.5)} + 1.645\sqrt{(0.92)(0.08)}]^2}{(0.42)^2} \doteq 10.$$

The normal distribution is not a very good approximation to the binomial when n is as small as 10 and $p = 0.92$. While $n = 10$ is not sufficient, $n = 13$ is: with rejection region $\{10, 11, 12, 13\}$, $\alpha = 0.046$ and $\beta = 0.016$. So the *observed* power is quite sufficient, and the study was quite "adequate."

The data in the example above were (I hope) dramatic enough to make my point. But the conclusion is valid when the data are not as extreme. Namely, once the data are in hand, any preconceptions about them become irrelevant. And if you plan to argue the contrary with nonstatisticians, you are likely to convince them only that there is something wrong with statistics.

4.3 P-Values: One-Sided or Two-Sided?

This is another rather small question. I include it because it is controversial. Some biostatisticians claim that all p-values should be two-sided since one can never be sure just what effect an experimental drug has. Whether p is one- or two-sided is not important. But it is important to state how the

p-value was calculated. If it is one-sided and the reader prefers two-sided, the reader can simply multiply it by 2.

The exact p-value should never be taken too seriously; for example, $p = 0.01$ does not mean that H_0 is false—it does not even mean that H_0 is probably false. It does provide more evidence against H_0 than does $p > 0.01$ in the same setting. But when the setting changes, the same p-value can give very different evidence against H_0.

4.4 One-Sample Analyses

One-sample analyses are appropriate when data are paired. Examples include drug versus baseline and matched pairs. Another example wherein one-sample analyses apply is the comparison of drug with an historical control with sufficient data that its effects are assumed to be completely known. I will discuss the analysis of one-sample data using two examples taken from Berry (1987b).

EXAMPLE 1 Twelve patients who experienced frequent premature ventricular contractions (PVCs) were administered a drug with antiarrhythmic properties. One-minute EKG recordings were taken before and after drug administration. The PVCs were counted on both recordings. The results are shown in Table 1.

By far the most common method of analysis for drug versus baseline data is the paired t-test, which is the one-sample t-test for the hypothesis that the mean change is zero. Such reliance on the t-test is inappropriate. The t-test is designed for normal populations; in this case the differences in response are assumed to be normal. But the t-test is not very robust when there are unusually large or small observations. Chapter 12 presents better procedures.

Other procedures that are more robust than the t-test are nonparametric methods (such as the signed-ranks test) and the t-test on transformed data. A transformation that lessens the influence of large observations is the logarithm. But it can unduly increase the influence of small observations. See Berry (1987b) for a method of adding a constant before taking logarithms that attempts to balance these two extremes by making the residuals close to normal. Other transformations that turn the t-test into a robust procedure are the rank transformations of Conover and Iman (1981). For example, using rank transformation-1 (RT-1), all the data are ranked from 1 to the number of data points, and then a t-test or other parametric procedure is carried out.

Table 1 Data for Example 1

Patient number	PVCs per minute Baseline	Postdrug	Change
1	6	5	−1
2	9	2	−7
3	17	0	−17
4	22	0	−22
5	7	2	−5
6	5	1	−4
7	5	0	−5
8	14	0	−14
9	9	0	−9
10	7	0	−7
11	9	13	+4
12	51	0	−51
Mean	13.4	1.9	−11.5
SD	—	—	14.3

The average decrease for the 12 patients in Example 1 is 11.5 PVCs per minute with standard deviation 14.3. So $t = -2.79$ and two-sided $p = 0.018$. (The SDs of predrug and postdrug responses are irrelevant for this and for all other inferences; it is better not to give them at all.) This investigator actually calculated t after every patient [see Berry (1985) for a discussion of this practice from various points of view] and found that t increased (from $t = -3.56; p = 0.005$) when patient 12 was included, even though this patient's response was the most favorable in the experiment! The reason should be evident to a statistician: although the mean is somewhat closer to zero (−7.91 instead of −11.5) without patient 12, the standard deviation is almost halved (7.37 instead of 14.3).

It is obvious that the assumption of normality required for the t-test is not appropriate for this experiment. Table 2 gives p-values for various nonparametric tests and for t-tests using transformed data. Table 3 lays out the calculations for RT-1. The constant 2.8 added to the data before taking logarithms makes the residuals as normal as possible in a sense described by Berry (1987b).

Table 2 p-Values for Example 1

Test	t	df	p
t-test	−2.78	11	0.018
t-test on $\log(x + 2.8)$	−4.23	11	0.001
t-test on RT-1	−5.03	11	0.0004
Sign test	—	—	0.006
Signed-rank test	—	—	0.002

In analyzing pre-post data, percent change from baseline is sometimes used instead of absolute change:

$$PC = \frac{\text{postdrug} - \text{baseline}}{\text{baseline}} \times 100.$$

This transformation treats decreases from 30 to 10 PVCs per minute and from 6 to 2 PVCs per minute as identical evidence of drug effect, whereas taking differences treats the former as greater evidence of effect (20 versus 4). Percent change is appropriate if the effect of the drug is multiplicative

Table 3 Ranks of Data in Table 1

Patient number	Baseline rank	Postdrug rank	Change in rank
1	14	12	−2
2	18	9.5	−8.5
3	22	4	−18
4	23	4	−19
5	15.5	9.5	−6
6	12	8	−4
7	12	4	−8
8	21	4	−17
9	18	4	−14
10	15.5	4	−11.5
11	18	20	+2
12	24	4	−20
Mean	17.8	7.3	−10.5
SD	—	—	7.2

rather than additive; whether it is multiplicative or additive or neither is, of course, unknown.

Percent change is not symmetric in baseline and postdrug measurements. In particular, it is bounded below by −100 (assuming that the measurements are positive), but it is unbounded above. Subjects with small baseline values can have a greatly inflated influence on the analysis. For example, if the baseline measurement is 20 and the postdrug measurement is 80, the percent increase is 300. But if the baseline is 120 and the postdrug is 180, giving the same absolute increase, the percent increase is only 50.

For the purpose of data analysis, I prefer replacing percent change with "symmetrized percent change":

$$\begin{aligned}\mathrm{SPC} &= \frac{\text{postdrug} - \text{baseline}}{\text{postdrug} + \text{baseline}} \times 100 \\ &= \frac{100 \times PC}{200 + PC}.\end{aligned}$$

This number is no further from 0 than is percent change, and it is typically closer. SPC is bounded between −100 and +100. So the effect of subjects with small baseline measurements is lessened. In the example in the preceding paragraph, 80 is a 60 symmetrized percent increase from 20, while 180 is a 20 symmetrized percent increase from 120.

A disadvantage of symmetrized percent change is that researchers and consumers are conditioned to thinking about percent change. To overcome this, one can analyze the data in the transformed scale SPC and then report averages in the original PC scale. This gives a "robust percent suppression":

$$\mathrm{RPC} = \frac{200 \times \mathrm{SPC}}{100 - \mathrm{SPC}}.$$

I want to stress that while analysis in the SPC scale is better than in the PC scale, absolute change from baseline or other transformations may be preferred to both. One way to decide is to plot the data (or the residuals in ANOVA) and choose the transformation for which the data are most nearly normal [see Berry (1987b)].

EXAMPLE 2 This example shows how misleading percent change can be; it also shows how analysis using symmetrized percent change can be better (although perhaps not best). An antiarrhythmic drug [Drug B in Example 3 of Berry (1987b), a different drug from the one in Example 1] was administered to 12 patients. PVCs were counted in 24 hours predrug and in a second 24-hour period while on drug. Table 4 shows the data along with the PC and SPC transformations.

Table 4 Data and Transformations for Example 2

Patient number	Average PVCs per hour: Baseline	Postdrug	Change	Percent change	Symmetrized PC	Change in rank
1	227	7	−220	−97	−94	−11.5
2	328	1.4	−326.6	−100	−99	−16
3	245	205	−40	−20	−9	−2
4	18	0.3	−17.7	−98	−97	−6
5	299	0.2	−298.8	−100	−100	−18
6	68	33	−35	−51	−35	−4
7	67	37	−30	−45	−29	−2
8	496	9	−487	−98	−96	−15
9	0.1	0.6	+0.5	+500	+71	+3
10	7	63	+56	+800	+80	+6.5
11	360	145	−215	−60	−43	−6
12	21	0	−21	−100	−100	−10
Mean	178	42	−136	+44	−46	−6.8
SD	—	—	169	291	66	7.6
t	—	—	−2.80	+0.53	−2.42	−3.07
p	—	—	0.017	0.61	0.034	0.011

The mean percent change is +44 even though 10 of the 12 changes were negative. The mean symmetrized percent change is −46, which is statistically significant. Converting this back to percent change gives robust percent change:

$$\text{RPC} = \frac{200 \times (-46)}{100 + 46} = -63.$$

This compares with a percent mean change of −76 and a median percent change of −78.

Rankit plots and Wilk–Shapiro statistics for absolute change, percent change, symmetrized percent change, and changes in ranks are shown in Figure 1. PC is dramatically nonnormal. The other transforms are clearly better. If the choice is restricted to analyzing either absolute change or percent change, there is no question that the former is to be preferred for these data. Of the four, change in rank is most nearly normal; the disadvantage of using ranks is that it is difficult to intuit an average drop in rank of 6.8, say.

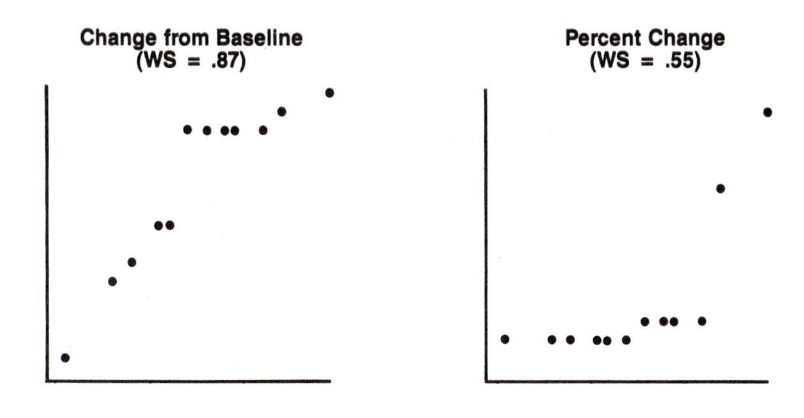

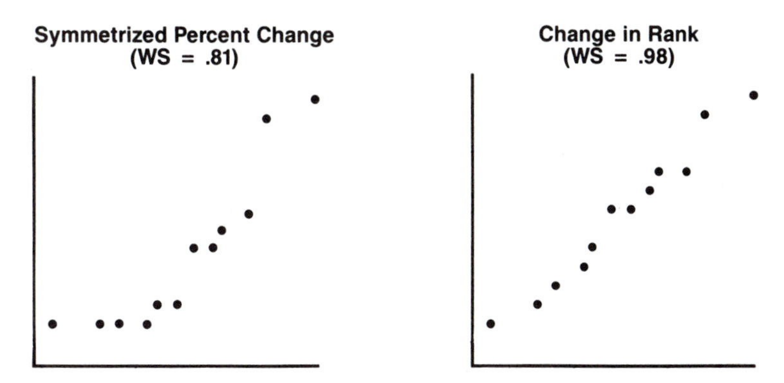

Figure 1 Rankit plots and Wilk–Shapiro statistics for Table 4.

4.5 Two-Sample Analyses

Testing the effectiveness of an experimental drug versus control in a parallel study is a typical two-sample problem. The usual method of analysis is the two-sample t-test. When there are multiple centers or covariates present, the usual method is analysis of variance (ANOVA). Just as I suggested in Section 4.4, so too here, robust methods may be more appropriate (cf. Chapter 12). The next example concerns a small study, but one with two interesting aspects: it involves two investigators and a covariate that measures state of disease.

EXAMPLE 3 Salsburg (1987) gives data concerning an "experimental measure of efficacy" from a small congestive heart failure (CHF) study. (CHF is the failure of the heart to pump an adequate supply of blood to the body.) Namely, he gives the rates of change per week in distance walked after being administered therapy, experimental drug (D) or placebo (P). These are shown (in hundredths of miles) in Table 5. Distance was measured using a pedometer. There were two investigators. Baseline left ventricular ejection fraction (LVEF) was regarded as a possibly important covariate. (LVEF is the percent of blood in the left ventricle that is ejected with a single heartbeat. So lower LVEF indicates more serious CHF.) The categorization by baseline LVEF shown in Table 5 was made after the study; it was not a stratification variable.

Temporarily ignore the possibility of investigator and baseline LVEF effects. The means, standard deviations, and sample sizes are

$$\bar{X}_D = 240.6, \qquad S_D = 451.2, \qquad n_D = 32,$$
$$\bar{X}_P = -98.5, \qquad S_P = 322.4, \qquad n_P = 31.$$

The two-sample t with d.f. $= 61$ is

$$T = \frac{\bar{X}_D - \bar{X}_P}{\sqrt{S_D^2/n_D + S_P^2/n_P}} = 3.43$$

(pooling the variances gives $T = 3.37$). So the (two-sided) p-value is 0.001, suggesting that the drug has an effect on this measurement.

Table 5 Rate of Change in Distance Walked per Week (Hundredths of Miles) by Drug, Investigator, and Baseline LVEF

	LVEF ≤ 15		15 < LVEF ≤ 25		25 < LVEF ≤ 30		30 < LVEF	
Investigator	D	P	D	P	D	P	D	P
1	0	69	842	−451	319	−178	165	−141
	56	1276	107	−132	−59	8	−342	−533
	327	−20	−131		1075	191	173	−244
	−255	−109			1173	−181		
		−107			−5	−220		
2	−144	−248	228	−84	168	−286	−59	−383
	604	−71	−657	−316	885	155	291	−631
	1221	144	−211	−90	745	30	0	−397
	497		75	37		−123	540	10
	168		−96					−27

Is it appropriate, as in the calculation above, to compare with placebo? That is the purpose of having a control. But the effect of the drug may be artificially inflated by the presence of placebo: $\bar{X}_D - \bar{X}_P = 3.4$ miles per week (mi/wk), while $\bar{X}_D$ itself is only 2.4 mi/wk. The difference, $\bar{X}_P = -1.0$ mi/wk, could well be random error. Is it conceivable that placebo could have a deleterious effect on the distance patients walk? Yes, but the scenarios required seem farfetched. It happens that $\bar{X}_D$ is significantly different from 0:

$$T = \frac{240.6}{451.2/\sqrt{32}} = 3.02, \qquad p = 0.005.$$

Although many statisticians think my attitude is wrong, I would be reluctant to say that the results are statistically significant otherwise. I return to this issue later in this example.

Now consider the possibility of investigator and baseline LVEF effects. Investigator is a categorical variable and LVEF is continuous, although it is categorized in Table 5. Assume that LVEF = 12.5 for the first category, and 20, 27.5, and 35 for the second through fourth categories; I will include it as such in a linear model. Table 6 is the ANOVA table for main effects and interactions. The value of T for drug effect is essentially unchanged from ignoring all other factors ($T = \sqrt{11.66} = 3.41$). Indeed, none of the other factors is significant.

For comparison, the data were ranked from 1 to 63 [RT-1 of Iman and Conover (1981)] and an ANOVA was carried out on the ranks in the same way as above. The results are also shown in Table 6. Drug is even more significant, but the ANOVA table for the ranks is really quite similar to that for the original data. The residuals in the case of the ranked data are more nearly normally distributed: Wilk–Shapiro = 0.99 as opposed to 0.92.

Table 6 ANOVA for Example 3

		Original data		Rank transform	
Source	d.f.	F	p	F	p
Drug	1	11.66	0.001	15.96	0.0002
Investigator	1	0.09	0.77	0.02	0.90
LVEF	1	1.48	0.23	1.18	0.28
Inv. × drug	1	0.21	0.65	0.06	0.81
LVEF × drug	1	1.76	0.19	2.63	0.11

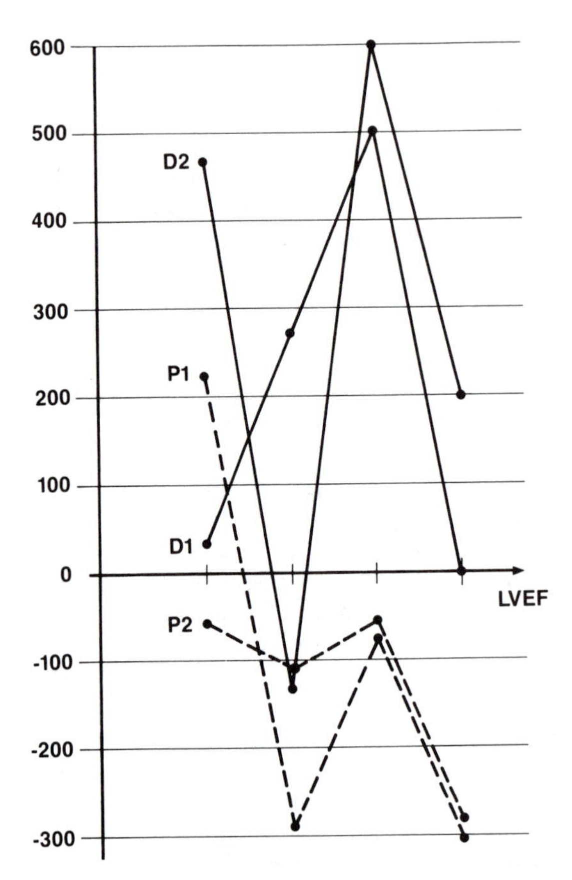

Figure 2

Suppose that instead of incorporating LVEF as a numerical variable, it is included as a categorical variable. Then for LVEF, the F-statistic is $F = 3.34$ ($p = 0.03$) for the original data and $F = 2.98$ ($p = 0.04$) for the ranked data. The reason that LVEF is now significant but was not significant before is that there appears to be an effect of LVEF (see Figure 2 to 4 discussed below), but that effect is not linear—or even monotone. The question of whether to treat a covariate as categorical or as numerical (in a linear mode) is problematic. Since LVEF seems so unlikely to have an effect that is not monotone, I think treating it as numerical is better. My view of the statistical significance of categorical LVEF in this example is that it is simply happenstance.

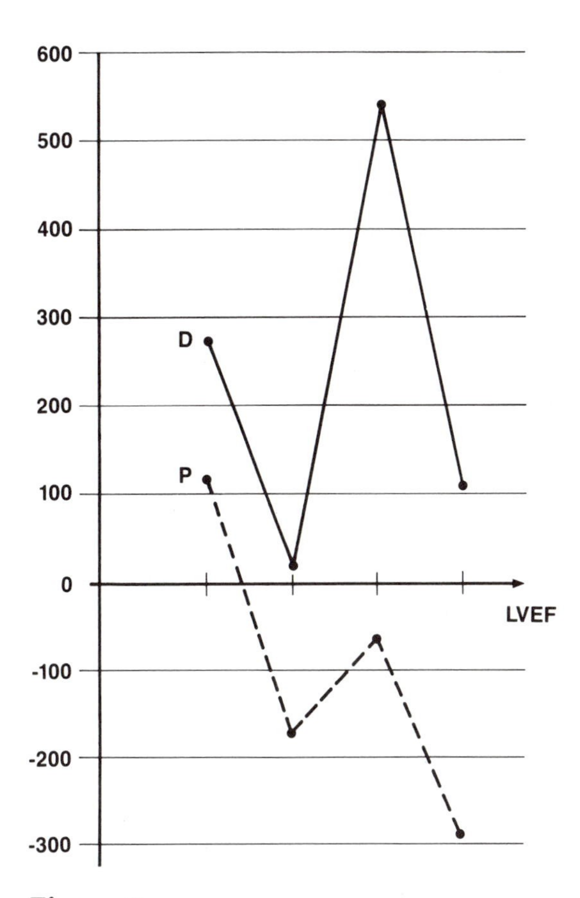

Figure 3

Pictures are more important than ANOVA tables for communicating with nonstatisticians. Figure 2 shows the mean rate of increase in distance walked as a function of LVEF and by investigator/drug groups. The investigator effect is minimal (cf. Table 6), so the investigators are combined in Figure 3. There seems to be little effect of LVEF in the drug group, and the possibility of a negative effect in the placebo group. Taking the difference in the two groups (Figure 4) shows a substantial positive effect for both of the high-LVEF groups, and only a modest positive effect for the two low-LVEF groups.

Is the effect shown in Figure 4 real? Or does the drug group in Figure 3 tell a more accurate story? There are two reasons to doubt Figure 4's message. One is that we got to Figure 4 by a process of data dredging

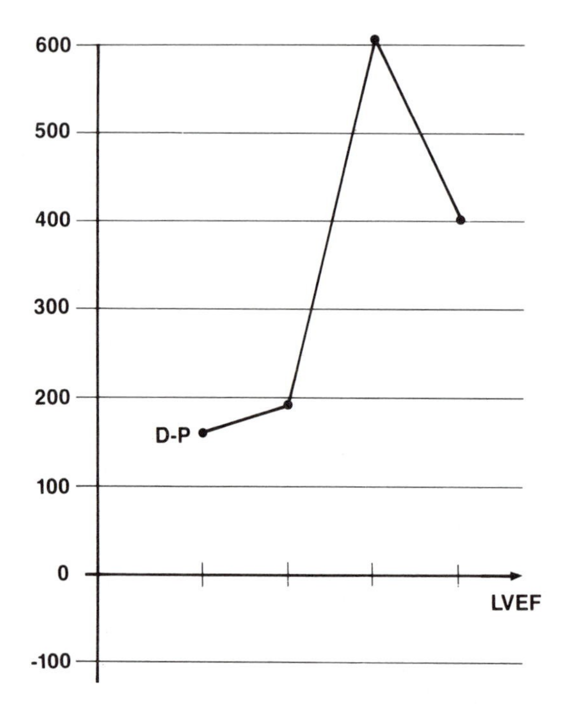

Figure 4

(Salsburg, 1987; Berry, 1988). The other is that the impact of Figure 4 is very much affected by the placebo group. As I suggested earlier, it is difficult to imagine a negative placebo effect in this study. It is even more difficult to believe a placebo effect that differentiates among the various degrees of LVEF. These two reasons are related: if a differential placebo effect were believable a priori and data dredging turned it up, the story suggested by Figure 4 would be more credible.

EXAMPLE 4 Two antiarrhythmic drugs (A = flecainide acetate, B = quinidine sulfate) were compared in a 16-center, double-blind, parallel study (Flecainide-Quinidine Research Group, 1983). The principal efficacy measurement was percent suppression of PVCs (see Example 1) from baseline after 2 weeks of drug therapy. The ANOVA table (Table 7) shows that the difference in percent suppression for the two drugs was not significant. Neither were center and drug $\times$ center interaction.

The story does not stop here. Figure 5 compares the empirical CDFs of percent suppression for the two drugs. (The values for drug B to the left

Table 7 ANOVA for Percent Suppression in Example 4

Source	d.f.	F	p
Drug	1	2.75	0.10
Center	15	0.84	0.63
Drug × center	15	0.82	0.66

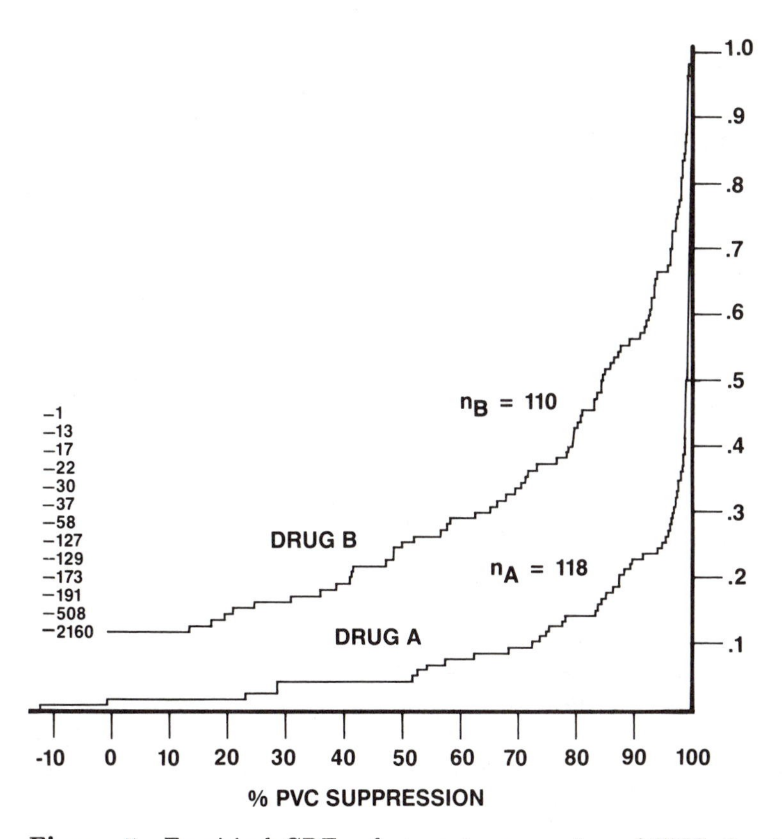

Figure 5 Empirical CDFs of percent suppression of PVCs by drugs A and B.

Table 8 ANOVA for Symmetrized Percent Suppression in Example 4

Source	d.f.	F	p
Drug	1	20.18	7×10^{-6}
Center	15	0.43	0.97
Drug × center	15	0.54	0.92

Table 9 Estimate of Percent Suppression

	Mean	Median	Robust[a]
Drug A	91.0	99.6	93.4
Drug B	39.2	84.7	74.9

[a]Inverted mean symmetrized percent suppression.

of 0 are listed on the figure.) There is a dramatic difference between the two: the Kolmogorov–Smirnov p-value is about 10^{-9}.

The difficulty with doing a parametric analysis such as that shown in Table 7 is that it is so greatly affected by the extreme negative percent suppressions on drug B. Rejecting these as outliers would bias the results toward drug A. There are many reasonable alternatives. Some are given in Chapter 12. Another is a parametric analysis using symmetrized percent suppression as defined in Section 4.4. The ANOVA table using SPC (Table 8) verifies the difference that is evident in Figure 5.

Table 9 compares various measures of central tendency. The mean is greatly affected by the several very small percent suppressions (see Figure 5). On the other hand, the median is not much affected by these extreme values. Mean symmetrized percent suppression (inverted to form a robust percent suppression as in Section 4.4) takes a middle course.

4.6 Crossover Studies

Chapter 8 gives a thorough discussion of the analysis of crossover studies. My objective here is to make a few elementary points using an example.

EXAMPLE 5 Brown (1980) analyzes data from Zinner et al. (1971) concerning "decrease" in an oral hygiene index among patients with gingivitus for a test compound (oxygen gel) as compared with a placebo gel. These are shown in Table 10. I stress that these are changes from individual period baselines; Fleiss et al. (1985) show that the usual analysis of such differences may produce bias between residual and treatment effects.

I have modified the table reported by Brown in two ways. First, he gives the data shown in Table 10 divided by 6 and rounded to the nearest hundredth. As an example, his entry for group 1, subject 1, period 1 is 0.83 instead of 5. (The index in question probably had six components and the investigators added them and divided by 6. This division creates round-off problems and complicates data display, but it does not change any inferences. Curiously, Brown gives various statistics with five-digit accuracy, while the earlier rounding gives him the right to only two-digit accuracy.) I have also modified his table by giving the changes (test minus placebo) for each subject and the means and standard deviations for each column.

In Section 3.7, I indicated that a crossover design should not be used when there is as much within- as between-subject variability. In particular, to make a crossover design worthwhile, the correlation between test and placebo should be large, surely positive. It is easy to calculate the correlation coefficient using the statistics given on Table 10. Since

$$\operatorname{var}(X-Y) = \operatorname{var}(X) + \operatorname{var}(Y) - 2\operatorname{cov}(X,Y),$$

the covariance between test and placebo for group I is

$$(1/2)[(4.6)^2 + (3.6)^2 - (6.9)^2] \doteq -6.7.$$

Therefore,

$$r_I \doteq \frac{-6.7}{(4.6)(3.6)} \doteq -0.4.$$

Similarly, for group II,

$$r_{II} \doteq \frac{0.2}{(3.7)(2.3)} \doteq 0.0.$$

So r_{II} is very nearly 0 and r_I is actually negative. The magnitude of r_I is somewhat misleading; it is greatly influenced by subject 28, without whom r_I would be -0.2. [Grieve (1985) shows that using change from baseline within each period induces zero correlation between the derived values.]

Brown concludes that a crossover analysis is not appropriate because the residual effect is statistically significant ($p = 0.09$), and therefore

Table 10 Improvement in Oral Hygiene Index

Group I				Group II			
Subject	Period 1 placebo	Period 2 test	$T-P$	Subject	Period 1 test	Period 2 placebo	$T-P$
1	5	11	6	1	10	2	8
2	6	13	7	2	15	3	12
3	4	10	6	3	6	−1	7
4	3	9	6	4	10	3	7
5	3	14	11	5	11	3	8
6	5	11	6	6	3	2	1
7	6	3	−3	7	8	4	4
8	4	2	−2	8	8	0	8
9	4	3	−1	9	3	1	2
10	2	4	2	10	13	5	8
11	0	5	5	11	10	2	8
12	7	8	1	12	9	0	9
13	0	4	4	13	8	3	5
14	3	11	8	14	9	3	6
15	2	9	7	15	8	0	8
16	2	9	7	16	4	−1	5
17	3	7	4	17	10	3	7
18	6	10	4	18	15	4	11
19	0	8	8	19	11	0	11
20	3	9	6	20	5	4	1
21	−3	17	20	21	14	1	13
22	1	14	13	22	7	3	4
23	6	8	2	23	8	0	8
24	6	10	4	24	8	5	3
25	8	4	−4	25	2	8	−6
26	2	5	3	26	13	7	6
27	12	6	−6	27	6	2	4
28	24	1	−23	28	2	6	−4
29	5	10	5	29	7	1	6
30	3	8	5	30	3	3	0
31	3	9	6				
32	3	10	7				
33	13	8	−5				
34	4	7	3				
Mean	4.6	8.1	3.6	Mean	8.2	2.5	5.7
SD	4.6	3.6	6.9	SD	3.7	2.3	4.3

that conclusions must be based on first-period data alone. (A manifestation of the residual effect is that the mean of the placebo data in group II is different from that in group I.) One can easily make a case for not collecting data (e.g., not crossing subjects over to another therapy), but ignoring data is another matter. Data that were collected honestly should be analyzed; to discard evidence is to admit that one's ability to analyze it is limited. Moreover, regulatory agencies will look askance at an analysis of only a portion of the data. In the case at hand, if the usual crossover analysis is ruled out by the possibility of a residual effect, one should build a model or use an analysis that is appropriate. For example, a judiciously chosen transformation may lessen the apparent residual effect and also more nearly satisfy the ANOVA assumptions.

To see that a transformation is in order from the point of view of satisfying the ANOVA assumptions, let us examine Brown's claim (1980, p. 77) that "fortunately, the study was large enough to provide a precise estimate of the treatment effect from the first-period data alone. If the study had been smaller no definitive conclusion would have been possible." He finds that $T = 3.43$ for the first-period data (two-sided $p = 0.001$). Suppose that we consider the first-period data for only the first 20 subjects in each group (5/8 of the complete first-period data). Then $T = 6.02$ ($p = 5 \times 10^{-7}$). So the conclusion is much *more* definitive. Further, suppose that we consider the first-period data for only the first 10 subjects in each group. Then $T = 3.42$ ($p = 0.003$)—about the same definiteness with less than one-third the study size, thus refuting Brown's claim.

In carrying out a t-test Brown has not only discarded all of the second-period data, but has effectively discarded two-thirds of the first period as well. Group I subjects 27, 33, and especially 28 are outliers and are extremely influential (it happens that all are near the end of the study). A simple rank transformation [RT-1 of Conover and Iman (1981)] lessens their effect; ranking the first-period data gives $T = 4.50$ ($p = 3 \times 10^{-5}$).

4.7 The Regression Effect

The regression effect rears its head in essentially every inferential setting. In sports, players who do very well in one year usually do worse in the following year, and those who did badly tend to improve. In medicine, patients who are very sick tend to get better (excepting those with degenerative diseases, for example). In business, companies that do very badly in one period tend to do better in the next. In education, students who do the best on one exam tend to do relatively worse on the next—not as bad as the average student but worse than their previous standard.

What causes these changes? Companies that do badly may try harder or they may make tactical or personnel changes. The sports player who had excelled may become overconfident or may change the way she does something. The very sick patient may have been treated. Such active steps may or may not be responsible for the changes. But they are almost always given credit. Suppose that a golfer is playing badly and so takes a lesson; any improvement is attributed to the lesson. Suppose that a person has an attack of severe lower backpain, has surgery, and the pain lessens in severity or goes away completely; the surgery is given credit.

There are other possible explanations. The most likely is the regression effect, sometimes called regression to the mean. Consider two measurements, say X and Y, of the same quantity on the same subject but at different times. There is variation over time but there is a correlation $r > 0$ between X and Y since the subject is the same in both cases. Suppose that X and Y are jointly normally distributed—the regression effect is present more generally but it is not as easy to quantify outside the normal case. Also suppose that the means of X and Y and the standard deviations of X and Y are the same, say μ and σ; similar results hold when the means and standard deviations are different. When X is observed to be x_0, say, the expected value of Y is

$$\mu + r(x_0 - \mu) = (1 - r)\mu + rx_0,$$

the "regression function" of Y on X. This is between x_0 and μ, the latter being what we would expect without knowing $X = x_0$, the weights being r and $1 - r$, respectively. So if x_0 is larger than μ—the athlete does better than average, the patient's blood pressure is higher than average, and so on—then Y tends also to be larger than μ—the athlete is probably good, the patient is probably hypertensive, and so on. But—and this is the "regression effect"—we do not expect Y to be as large as x_0. Similarly, if $x_0 < \mu$, we expect Y also to be smaller than μ, but not as small as x_0. Clearly, the closer r is to 0, the more pronounced is the regression effect. (Incidentally, the standard deviation of Y given that $X = x_0$ is $\sigma\sqrt{1 - r^2}$, constant in x_0 and less than the unconditional standard deviation of Y.)

Although there is no way to tell for sure, my suspicion is that essentially all instances of "placebo effect" (improvement in the condition of a sick person that occurs in response to a specific nontreatment) are really instances of regression effect.

Baseline Restrictions

When there are baseline restrictions, it can be extremely difficult to draw conclusions from a study. The following excerpt is a dramatic demonstration of this; it was reported in *Science News* (June 27, 1987, p. 405) under the heading, "getting the drop on blood pressure."

> Several recent studies have suggested that muscle-relaxation training and bio-feedback techniques that promote relaxation reduce the blood pressures of some hypertensives. But scientists at SRI International, a nonprofit research organization in Menlo Park, Calif., now report that there is a simpler alternative for newly diagnosed mild hypertensives: no relaxation training, no medication, just regular blood pressure monitoring for at least one year.
>
> "We were surprised by the results," says project director Margaret A. Chesney. "It appears that before physicians make decisions about medications or other treatments for mild hypertensives, the first step might be systematic blood pressure monitoring."
>
> The researchers recruited unmedicated persons with mild hypertension, whose diastolic blood pressure (when the heart expands) ranged from 90 to 104 mmHg, from two large companies near San Francisco. They randomly assigned 40 mild hypertensives to blood pressure monitoring every nine weeks at both a company medical clinic and each participant's worksite. Another 118 hypertensives received 13 weekly instruction sessions in a behavioral treatment, either muscle-relaxation procedures alone or in combination with biofeedback measures of muscle relaxation, "cognitive restructuring" aimed at identifying stressful situations and thoughts, and advice on exercise and dietary changes.
>
> In company clinics, significant blood pressure reductions for both behavioral treatment and monitoring groups appeared after 18 weeks, report Chesney and her co-workers in the May/June *Psychosomatic Medicine.* Systolic blood pressure (when the heart contracts) fell an average of 7.4 mmHg for those receiving behavioral treatment and 9.0 mmHg for subjects being monitored. Diastolic blood pressure declined an average of 4.5 mmHg for the former group and 5.9 mmHg for the latter group. *These reductions remained 36 weeks later.* [Italics added.]
>
> Both groups also displayed significant blood pressure reductions at the worksite by the end of the year-long study.
>
> Reasons for the equal effectiveness of behavioral treatments and blood pressure monitoring are unclear, says Chesney. The percentage of individuals whose personal physicians prescribed antihypertensive medication during treatment did not differ between the two conditions, and neither group showed significant changes in weight. These factors, notes Chesney, are unlikely to have accounted for the results.

> But there are several possible explanations. "When blood pressure is repeatedly measured," she says, "there may be a desensitization to anxiety that often elevates the blood pressures of mild hypertensives in clinic settings." Expectations that blood pressures will drop as a result of monitoring may also be critical. Furthermore, monitoring may serve as a form of biofeedback, since participants see their blood pressure readings at each measurement session.
>
> "We need to study more closely what repeated blood pressure measurements do to the sense of control over one's body," says Chesney.

A person's blood pressure varies considerably over time. Some people have high diastolic blood pressure (90 to 104 mmHg, say) at any given time by happenstance; the next time it will tend to be less—even with no intervening therapy. So the baseline restriction created an artificial "nontreatment effect." The conclusions made in this study are unwarranted, and it is likely that monitoring has no effect whatever.

Here is a case in which it is impossible to have a control: the measuring process is itself the treatment. But it is easy to design a study not subject to the regression effect. Namely, have no restrictions on the baseline measurement for admission to the study; that is, take all comers. The highs will tend to get lower, but this will be balanced by the lows getting higher.

This is usually an impractical design since the purpose of a clinical trial is to treat people who are sick. A more practical solution is to use a screening process for admissions and then, at a later time, obtain baseline readings that will be used for purposes of analysis. Never analyze screening measurements. Notice that in the monitoring study described above, "these reductions remained 36 weeks later." So if the initial measurement had been used only to select candidates for admission to the study, no improvement due to monitoring would have been observed.

Dropping Responders

A problem related to that discussed above is caused by calling a patient a "success" at some point during a trial and dropping that patient from the trial. Consider a trial comparing an experimental antihypertensive drug with placebo. The dose of drug or placebo is to be increased until the patient's diastolic blood pressure drops below 90 mmHg, at which time the patient is labeled a success and is discontinued from the study. Most patients will eventually meet this criterion simply because of the randomness in blood pressure and the measuring process. It is almost impossible to make sense out of a comparison between two "success" curves as a function of increasing dose. And even if it is possible to adjust for random variability, few people will be convinced. The obvious way to fix up the study design is to keep everyone in the study, responders included. Then the two dose-response curves can be compared as usual (see Chapter 6, for example).

Differential Drug Effect

Suppose that a large clinical trial has been conducted comparing an experimental antibacterial agent with placebo. Routine safety tests after 1 week on drug show an average increase in diastolic blood pressure of 6 mmHg, while the average change on placebo was zero. The data are sufficiently convincing that there seems little doubt that the drug was responsible for the increase. This is somewhat alarming; at the very least, hypertension should be a contraindication for the drug. But there seems to be redeeming aspect of this effect: patients with the highest blood pressures experienced no change on average, while those with the lowest blood pressures experienced an average increase of 12 mmHg. So the drug may be safe after all. Is this observed differential effect real? Or will the drug increase everyone's blood pressure by about 6 mmHg?

The answer is that at least part of the observed differential effect is due to the regression effect. Patients with the highest blood pressures would be expected to have lower readings the next time, perhaps about 6 mmHg lower. The fact that they did not decrease is a result of the drug. Patients with low blood pressure would be expected to increase, perhaps about 6 mmHg. The fact that their increase was 12 mmHg represents an added effect of the drug. So it is possible that any increase caused by the drug is the same for all patients. Berry et al. (1984) show how to decide what portion of the change is due to the regression effect; they give data from a clinical trial in which there is an apparent differential effect and show that the data are due entirely to the regression effect.

5 CONCLUSION

Our purpose in this chapter was merely to scratch the surface of the design and analysis of clinical studies. Some of the later chapters deal in much greater detail with designs and analyses presented here. Others discuss special types of analyses and related issues of statistical inference not touched upon here.

Acknowledgments. I am indebted to Andrew P. Grieve for straightening out some issues dealing with crossover studies. I thank Joseph L. Fleiss for his very detailed and intelligent comments on an earlier version of this chapter; in the few cases in which I did not take his advice, my view represents a minority of biostatisticians.

REFERENCES

Berger, J. O. (1986). *Statistical Decision Theory and Bayesian Analysis*, 2nd ed. Springer-Verlag, New York.

Berry, D. A. (1985). Interim analysis in clinical trials: classical vs. Bayesian approaches. *Statist. Med. 4*, 521–526.

Berry, D. A. (1987a). Interim analysis in clinical trials: the role of the likelihood principle. *Amer. Statist. 41*, 117–122.

Berry, D. A. (1987b). Logarithmic transformations in ANOVA. *Biometrics 43*, 439–456.

Berry, D. A. (1987c). Statistical inference, clinical trials, and pharmaceutical company decisions. *Statistician 36*, 181–189.

Berry, D. A. (1988). Interim analysis in clinical research. *Cancer Invest. 5*, 469–477.

Berry, D. A. (1989). Monitoring accumulating data in a clinical trial, unpublished manuscript.

Berry, D. A., and B. Fristedt (1985). *Bandit Problems: Sequential Allocation of Experiments*. Chapman & Hall, London.

Berry, D. A., and C.-H. Ho (1988). One-sided sequential stopping boundaries for clinical trials: a decision-theoretic approach. *Biometrics 44*, 219–227.

Berry, D. A., M. L. Eaton, B. P. Ekholm, and T. L. Fox (1984). Assessing differential drug effect. *Biometrics 40*, 1109–1115.

Brown, B. W. (1980). The crossover experiment for clinical trials. *Biometrics 36*, 69–79.

Chi, G. Y. H. (1984). Design considerations for some combination drug trials in the treatment of hypertension. *Proceedings of the Biopharmaceutical Section*. American Statistical Association, Washington, D. C., pp. 81–86.

Cleveland, W. S. (1985). *The Elements of Graphing Data*. Wadsworth, Belmont, Calif.

Conover, W. J., and R. L. Iman (1981). Rank transformations as a bridge between parametric and nonparametric statistics (with discussion). *Amer. Statist. 35*, 124–133.

Flecainide-Quinidine Research Group (1983). Flecainide versus quinidine for treatment of chronic ventricular arrhythmias: a multicenter trial. *Circulation 67*, 1117–1123.

Fleiss, J. L., S. Wallenstein, and R. Rosenfeld (1985). Adjusting for baseline measurements in the two-period crossover study: a cautionary note. *Controlled Clin. Trials 6*, 192–197.

Freireich, E. J., E. Gehan, E. Frei, L. R. Schroeder, I. J. Wolman, R. Anbari, E. O. Burgert, S. D. Mills, D. Pinkel, O. S. Selawry, J. H. Moon, B. R. Gendel, C. L. Spurr, R. Storrs, F. Haurani, B. Hoogstraten, and S. Lee (1963). The effect of 6-mercaptopurine on the duration of steroid-induced remissions in acute leukemia: a model for evaluation of other potentially useful therapy. *Blood 21*, 699–716.

Gehan, E. A. (1984). The evaluation of therapies: historical control studies. *Statist. Med. 3*, 315–324.

Grieve, A. P. (1985). A Bayesian analysis of the two-period crossover design for clinical trials. *Biometrics 42*, 979–990.

Holtzman, J. L., D. A. Berry, D. C. Kvam, L. Mottonen, and G. Borrell (1984). The application of second-order polynomial equations to the study of pharmacodynamic interactions: the effect of flecainide acetate and propranolol on cardiac output and vascular resistance. *J. Pharmacol. Exp. Ther. 231*, 286–290.

Holtzman, J. L., D. C. Kvam, D. A. Berry, L. Mottonen, G. Borrell, L. I. Harrison, and G. J. Conrad (1987). The pharmacodynamic and pharmacokinetic interaction of flecainide acetate and propranolol: effects on cardiac function and drug clearance. *European J. Clin. Pharmacol. 33*, 97–99.

Kadane, J. B. (1986). Progress toward a more ethical method for clinical trials. *J. Med. Philos. 11*, 385–404.

Lindgren, B. W., G. W. McElrath, and D. A. Berry (1978). *Introduction to Probability and Statistics*, 4th ed., Macmillan, New York.

Peto, R., M. C. Pike, P. Armitage, N. E. Breslow, D. R. Cox, S. V. Howard, N. Mantel, K. McPherson, J. Peto, and P. G. Smith (1976). Design and analysis of randomized clinical trials requiring prolonged observation of each patient: I. Introduction and design. *British J. Cancer 34*, 585–612.

Salsburg, D. (1987). Situations where formal confirmatory analysis (based on the Neyman–Pearson formulation of hypothesis testing) is inappropriate, unpublished manuscript. Pfizer Central Research, Groton, Conn.

Snedecor, G. W., and W. G. Cochran (1980). *Statistical Methods*, 7th ed. Iowa State University Press, Ames.

Zinner, D. D., L. F. Duany, and N. W. Chilton (1970). Controlled study of the clinical effectiveness of a new oxygen gel on plaque, oral debris and gingival inflammation. *Pharmacol. Ther. Dent. 1*, 7–15.

2

Bioavailability: Designs and Analysis

BRUCE E. RODDA*† Wyeth-Ayerst Research, Inc, New York, New York

1 INTRODUCTION

1.1 History

Throughout the development process, many changes are made in the formulation of new pharmacological agents. The final formulation which is marketed rarely is the same as that used in the controlled clinical trials. Clearly, there needs to be assurance that the dosage form that we buy at our neighborhood pharmacy is therapeutically identical to that which underwent study for safety and efficacy.

The most relevant way of providing this assurance is to conduct controlled clinical trials in the target population with various formulations throughout the development process. However, testing every necessary step in this evolution with controlled trials is prohibitively expensive in

*Current affiliation: The Squibb Institute for Medical Research, Princeton, New Jersey

†With the technical assistance of Carol Shirley, Merck Sharp & Dohme Research Laboratories, Rahway, New Jersey.

terms of the time required, exposure of patients to experimental drugs, and the economic resources that would be necessary to implement these trials. Since this is a practical impossibility, methods had to be developed that would provide assurance of the similarity of succeeding formulations throughout development. The consensus among both medical and pharmaceutical scientists was that if the rate and extent to which the active pharmaceutical moiety reached the site of action was similar from one formulation to another, this would be convincing evidence that the clinical response would be the same.

1.2 Rationale

Developmental changes are often substantial, and the need for a true measure of therapeutic similarity is very important. In each step of development, many different variables are introduced. Examples of these include various excipients and their concentrations, the various milling procedures that might be used, tablet coatings, and different compressions used during manufacture. Any of these factors, either alone or in combination, can affect the rate and extent to which the active drug product reaches the site of action. To ensure that the clinical effect is not changed by a modification in the formulation, certain assurances must be developed to guarantee that each modification has no clinical importance.

In addition, most clinical trials employ capsule formulations, because capsule formulations are usually more predictable and have fewer variables than tablet formulations. Capsules are easier to manufacture on a small scale and provide much more flexibility in double-blind clinical trials. On the other hand, tablets are most often the final dosage form that is marketed.

In the 1970s the U.S. Food and Drug Administration (FDA) provided a list of four acceptable ways in which bioavailability could be estimated (*Federal Register*, 1977; Food and Drug Administration, 1977). These were:

1. Measuring the plasma or serum concentration of a drug and/or its metabolite over a period of time
2. Measuring a therapeutic or acute pharmacologic effect
3. Conducting clinical trials that establish the safety and effectiveness of the drug
4. Other techniques or methodologies as agreed upon by the regulatory agency and the applicant

These definitions provide a sense of the problems associated with estimating and comparing bioavailability. The last point identifies bioavailability as having a significant regulatory component. In fact, regulatory concern was the initial motivation for the interest in the topic of bioavailability.

It is important to note that the three specific techniques suggested (and these were suggested by the FDA in this order) are in the inverse order of clinical relevance. Although measuring blood levels is the first technique suggested, the last technique, conducting clinical trials, is clearly much more relevant. If we can demonstrate the safety and effectiveness of a drug using a clinical trial, other issues are less relevant. Whether there is a relationship between blood levels and pharmacologic effect is an assumption, rather than a point that can be demonstrated for most drugs.

Although estimating bioavailability by determining concentrations in blood or urine over one or more dosing intervals may not be the most relevant means to accomplish this task, this is the norm, and in the remainder of the chapter we presume that bioavailability is measured only by these techniques.

2 DEFINITIONS AND CONCEPTS

2.1 Definitions

Bioavailability is the rate and extent to which the active drug ingredient or therapeutic moiety is absorbed from a drug product and becomes available at the site of action. This sounds deceptively simple, and it is, because we can never identify the rate and extent to which the drug is available at the site of action. We can never observe the site of action, but can only estimate the rate and extent to which the drug appears in the blood or urine or other body fluids.

Thus we must *assume* that there is a relationship between the concentration in the blood and the concentration at the site of action. This may be more tenable than the more necessary and fundamental assumption that a relationship also exists between the concentration in the blood and the therapeutic response. There is but a handful of drugs for which this assumption has been demonstrated with any scientific validity.

For all new drugs, there needs to be a characterization of their bioavailability. There is usually a requirement that this be done in an absolute sense, since the definition of bioavailability is the rate and extent to which the drug reaches the systemic circulation. Placing the active drug in the plasma by intravenous injection provides a determination of the absolute availability of the product, since the entire dose is placed in the systemic circulation and is not subject to any of the confounding influences, such as first-pass effects (where the drug is metabolized in the liver before reaching the general circulation), metabolism at the injection site, or differences in formulations. However, with the exception of this initial characterization, literally all subsequent bioavailability investigations are comparative. Formulations are compared with the absolute bioavailability determined early in the development process, or formulations are compared with each other to assure the manufacturer that no important differences are developing with the periodic changes in formulations that occur in the development process.

Detailed discussions of the concept of bioavailability and the biopharmaceutical and pharmacologic considerations which are important to this topic can be found in a variety of books [e.g., Wagner (1970)]. We do not attempt to discuss these in detail in this chapter, but relate more to the statistical aspects of these bioavailability studies.

2.2 Factors That Affect Bioavailability

There are many factors that will change the rate and extent to which a drug appears in the systemic circulation; some of these were discussed earlier in this chapter. Figure 1 provides an intuitive overview of some of the more mechanical factors that are important in determining the rate and extent of absorption following ingestion of an orally administered dosage form.

Tablets, in particular, have a number of opportunities for reduction in bioavailability. Upon ingestion, a tablet must first disintegrate, and the rate of disintegration can be a function of the compaction, the coating, and other controllable elements. Following disintegration, dissolution must take place. The excipients mixed with the active drug can affect the environment of the gastrointestinal tract, and result in either increased or decreased rate of appearance in the systemic circulation. In some cases, delay of this dissolution step can totally restrict the absorption of the product. Once dissolution has occurred, the drug must be absorbed and then passed through the portal circulation before reaching the systemic circulation. The rate at which the active agent enters the liver can affect the metabolism (the first-pass effect), and thus result in a greater or lesser bioavailability of the product. Clearly, having the same amount of active drug in a particular formulation does not guarantee identical bioavailability.

2.3 Curve Definition and Characterization

The principal source of data in a bioavailability study is the plasma (or serum or blood) concentration-time curve. In a typical study, a subject is given the dosage form under consideration and has blood samples taken at several points over a defined period thereafter. This period is often long enough to cover several plasma half-lives of the drug, so that a charac-

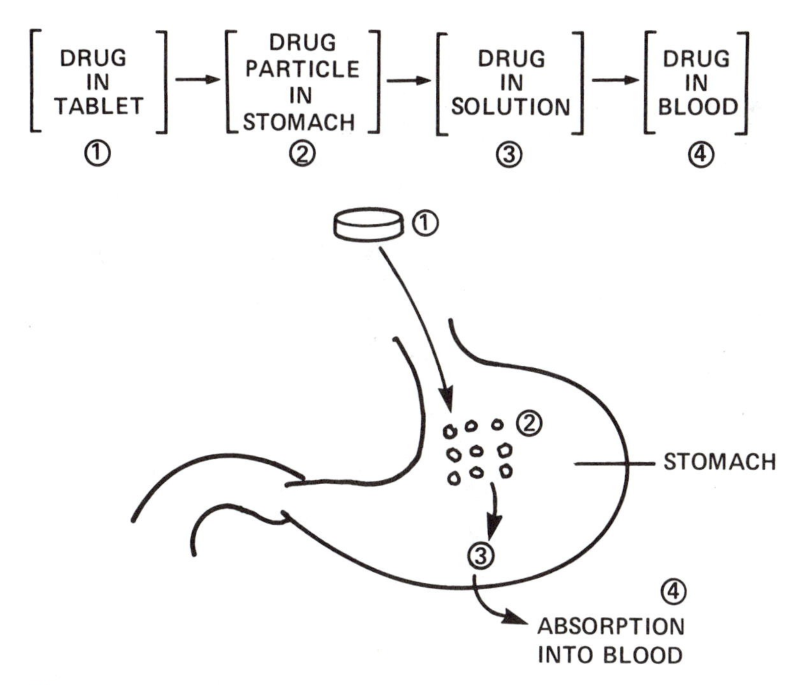

Figure 1

terization of the entire curve can be made with confidence. More points are sampled during the absorption phases, and fewer are taken at the latter points, where the elimination process is dominant. The absorption phase refers to those concentrations observed while the concentrations are increasing. Distribution, while also a continuous process, is conceptually associated with the points that are in the neighborhood of the maximum concentration. Two typical plasma concentration-time curves are presented in Figure 2, and these curves simply connect the observed serum concentrations for each formulation.

There are at least three characteristics of concentration curves that are independent of any mathematical model that might be considered to describe the data. They are the observed peak plasma concentration, the time at which this peak concentration was observed, and the area under the curve over the observation period. The importance of these measures should be evident. For example, if the rate and/or extent of absorption is reduced to the point where the peak concentration never reaches the minimum effective concentration (MEC), the therapeutic effect of the product will not be observed. In contrast, if the rate and extent of the appearance

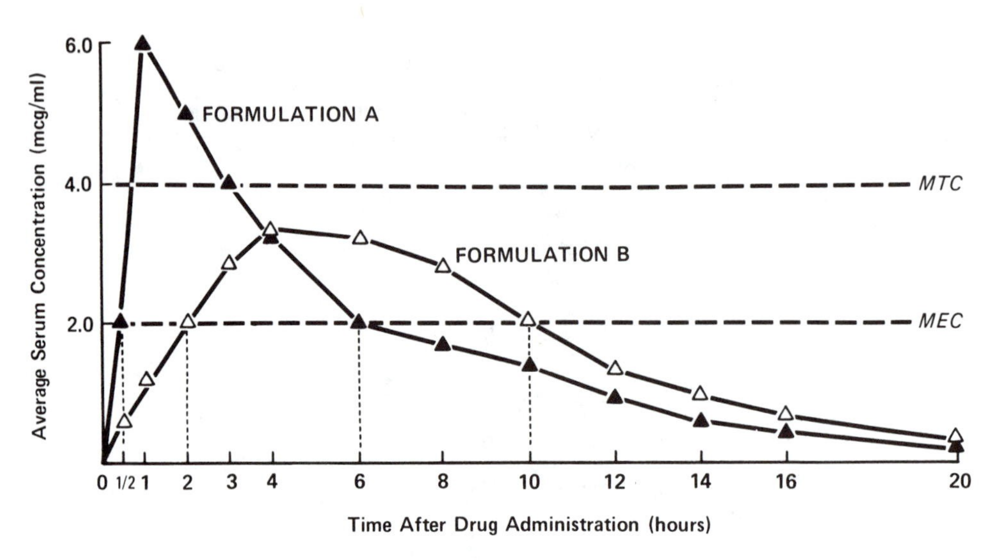

Figure 2

in the plasma are increased to the point where the maximum tolerated concentration (MTC) is exceeded, adverse experiences will become manifest and may overshadow the beneficial effect of the drug. It is important to understand that both MEC and MTC are random variables and will be different for different patients. The relationship between plasma concentration and clinical effect is usually imprecise, but estimation of the minimally effective dose is required in many cases (see Chapter 4).

The rate of absorption can be measured by the time it takes to reach the peak plasma concentration, or if pharmacokinetic models are assumed, by the absorption rate constant. This constant (k_a) is the proportionality factor relating the amount of drug available for absorption in the gut (k_g) with the rate of appearance in the plasma (dX_p) assuming a first-order process, that is,

$$\frac{dX_p}{dt} = k_a X_g.$$

The extent of drug absorption can be estimated in a number of ways. The peak plasma concentrations are related to absorption since they will tend to be higher if the extent of absorption is greater, and peaks will be lower if the converse is true. Also, the integral of the plasma concentration-time curve (the area under that curve) is proportional to the total amount of drug that has appeared in the plasma. Urinary recovery will also provide an index of the amount of drug that has been absorbed into the systemic circulation, since the only route to the kidneys is through that circulation. However, the bioavailability of drugs that are highly metabolized will be poorly estimated by urinary recoveries. In addition, certain composite indices have been suggested, which may combine the information from both the blood and the urine.

2.4 Role of Pharmacokinetics

Bioavailability can be described both from a model-free standpoint in which indices such as area, peak plasma concentration, and time of peak plasma concentration are measured, or it can be defined in terms of pharmacokinetic models. Pharmacokinetics is the effect of the human body on the disposition of a drug product. Mathematical modeling is used to characterize and estimate various clinically relevant parameters associated with the absorption, distribution, metabolism, and elimination of the product. Pharmacokinetic models and their associated parameters have a number of attractive attributes [see Gibaldi and Perrier (1975)]. First, they give actual rates of absorption, accumulation, and elimination; and second, they allow for modeling of potentially important factors. For example, the simplest pharmacokinetic model for describing the plasma concentrations over time following oral administration is as follows:

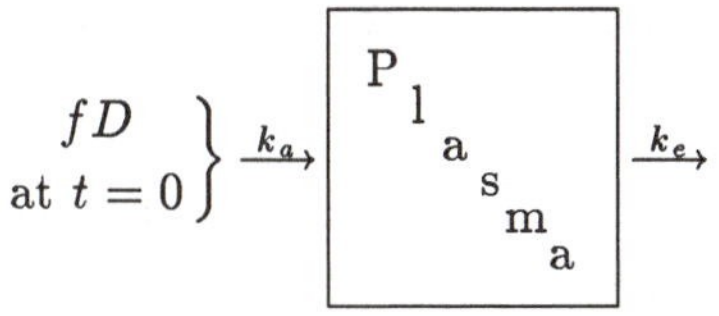

$$\left.\begin{matrix} fD \\ \text{at } t=0 \end{matrix}\right\} \xrightarrow{k_a} \boxed{\text{Plasma}} \xrightarrow{k_e}$$

In this model, a fraction (f) of the administered dose (D) appears in the plasma according to a first-order process with absorption rate constant k_a. Disappearance from the plasma also occurs by first-order kinetics, with the rate of disappearance being proportional to the plasma concentration. The mathematics of most pharmacokinetic models are relatively simple. The reader is referred to Chapter 5 for related discussions.

If renal clearance is an important factor for a particular drug product and there is concern that by modifying the formulation this renal clearance will be changed, pharmacokinetic models can permit evaluation of this, whereas simple model-free methods cannot. In the same vein, there is an opportunity for the identification of mechanisms of action and the degree to which the data fit or deviate from various pharmacodynamic assumptions. These models can provide useful information about mechanisms of actions.

FDA guidelines specifically suggest the use of pharmacokinetic models for evaluation of some bioavailability studies. They recommend that the absorption rate constant (k_a), the maximum concentration (C_{max}), the time of this concentration (t_{max}), the elimination rate constant (k_e), the area under the curve (AUC), and the fraction of dose appearing in the plasma (f) be computed. They also suggest estimating other pharmacokinetic parameters.

3 BIOEQUIVALENCE

3.1 Rationale

Some of the reasons for conducting bioequivalence studies were discussed earlier. An additional issue that has gained great prominence in the pharmaceutical industry and in the public eye is the concept of generic drugs.

Following expiration of patent protection for a new drug, any company can manufacture and market the agent if it can demonstrate that its product is safe and effective. The regulations permit the assumption of safety and effectiveness if later manufacturers can demonstrate that their formulation is bioequivalent to the original product. This requires satisfying certain regulations concerning control and manufacturing, and a demonstration that the safety and efficacy of the generic formulation are the same as those of the original product.

This comparison is, of course, a variation on the theme discussed previously. But it is politically much more sensitive because of intercompany competition and the price differential that usually exists between a generic drug and the original. In many cases, the generic agent will be less expensive than that of the original, because the risks and development costs incurred in the initial demonstration of safety and efficacy for a pharmaceutical product are borne by the innovator. These expenses do not need to be recouped by a generic manufacturer, resulting in an opportunity for lower pricing for products introduced later.

3.2 Definition of Bioequivalence

Clearly, there are many reasons for conducting bioequivalence studies, but the essential definition must be understood. The textbook definition of bioequivalence is: "Two drug products are bioequivalent if their bioavailabilities are the same." This is a straightforward definition, but begs the issue. The important question is: What does it mean to be the same?

The accepted standards at the FDA and at pharmaceutical regulatory agencies in most other countries permit a product to be considered bioequivalent to the standard if its bioavailability is within 80 to 120% of the standard's bioavailability. This permits three mathematically equivalent formulations of the concept of bioequivalence. One is that the true mean bioavailability of the test formulation must be between 80 and 120% of the true bioavailability of the standard. The second is that the absolute difference between the true bioavailabilities of the standard and the test is less than 20% of the standard. The third is that the ratio of the bioavailabilities of the test to the standard is between 80 and 120%. These are presented schematically below.

$$0.8\mu_s < \mu_t < 1.2\mu_s$$
$$|\mu_s - \mu_t| < 0.2\mu_s$$
$$0.8 < \frac{\mu_t}{\mu_s} < 1.2$$

Although these are mathematically equivalent, they are not equivalent from a statistical standpoint. This is because the various distributional properties of the data and the different models necessary for analysis can provide different results.

4 EXPERIMENTAL DESIGN

4.1 Design Considerations

The great majority of bioavailability studies are comparative and use blood-level curves as the principal data source. The initial involvement of statisticians with these studies is in their design, and these considerations are similar to those of any other type of clinical program. General design issues are discussed in Chapter 1.

The unique aspects of blood-level curves require the planner to determine the number of sampling points over time; where these sampling points are to be located; the number of subjects or patients; whether or not a pharmacokinetic model is to be used and if it is, what its effects will be on the number and location of sampling points; and the experimental layout.

There has been much recent activity in developing optimal sampling strategies for pharmacokinetic models; however, the inherent uncertainty in bioavailability studies will probably continue to make us "sample where the action is," which is basically what optimal strategies suggest.

In designing a bioequivalence study, as in designing any clinical trial, the optimal design depends on the objective of the study. In most bioequivalence studies, the objective is to determine whether a clinically important difference exists between the mean bioavailability of a test formulation compared with a standard formulation. This can be done using either differences or ratios, and for the purposes of design, these are equivalent.

A second objective, which has not received the same degree of attention but which is becoming relatively more important, is a comparison of variabilities between the test formulation and the standard. If a formulation has less subject-to-subject variability than another, or has less intrasubject variability than another, it would be more predictable and therefore more advantageous therapeutically.

A third objective, and one that has recently become much more important, relates to the concept of interchangeability. With the advent of multi-source drugs, patients often receive the same prescription but have it filled with different formulations from different manufacturers. Thus it is important that all sources of a particular drug be interchangeable. To provide assurance that this is so, studies must be defined to characterize patient $\times$ treatment interaction.

Each of these very different but related objectives requires different considerations in terms of experimental design.

4.2 Specific Designs

Most experimental designs for estimating central tendency or mean bioavailability and for the comparison of mean bioavailability between two or more formulations utilize a crossover design [e.g., see Chapter 8; Brown (1980); Grizzle (1965)]. In a standard two-way crossover design the model elements include order, subjects nested within order, period effect, and the formulation effect. Obviously, the period $\times$ formulation interaction and the order effect are completely confounded and thus, in this simple design, there is no clear estimate of carryover effect. For investigations of more than two agents, variations of Latin square designs are usually employed.

When it is necessary to characterize and compare the bioavailabilities of several formulations, such as in a dose-response study, it may be infeasible to conduct a study where every patient receives all the doses. In this case, balanced incomplete block designs are appearing more and more commonly in early dose-response studies (Westlake, 1974). These studies are also very useful when the patient cannot tolerate multiple experiences in the study, such as when using children in bioequivalence studies.

There are clear limitations to these types of designs. Their greatest value has been in dose-response studies where the objective is to compare a range of doses but where a complete repeated-measures design (see Chapter 3) is impractical because of patient withdrawal. A balanced incomplete block design in this case provides a relatively efficient means of obtaining information that may not be obtainable otherwise.

Studies designed to compare variabilities of formulations require different considerations. Variability can be both intrasubject and intersubject. Most designs, including those mentioned earlier, will allow a clear estimate of intersubject variability. However, the standard crossover designs that are used for most studies do not permit a true estimate of intrasubject variability. For this reason, the design presented schematically below is one that has been used to estimate not only intrasubject variability but also subject by formulation interaction.

	Period			
Order	1	2	3	4
1	A	A	B	B
2	A	B	A	B
3	B	B	A	A
4	B	A	B	A
5	A	B	B	A
6	B	A	A	B

The order can be replicated so that the study can include 6, 12, 18, ... subjects. This design, although twice as long as a standard crossover, has each subject receiving each formulation twice. Thus there is a clean estimate of the intrasubject variability for each of the formulations. In addition, the subject $\times$ formulation interaction can be estimated using this design. Both these components are given inadequate consideration in many bioavailability studies, even though regulatory guidelines recommend that they be examined.

The consistency of bioavailability within a subject from one tablet to another tablet of the same formulation is a true index of both content uniformity and the consistency of clinical response that can be expected from that formulation. Formulation $\times$ subject interaction, on the other hand, is the measure of intersubject consistency of the difference between the bioavailability of one product and another. Although it may be relatively simple to simulate the mean bioavailability of an innovator's product, matching the intrasubject variability and the intersubject variability may be a more difficult technological challenge. Thus in cases where the objective is to determine whether a new formulation is, in fact, similar with respect to both mean and consistency of bioavailability, this type of design may be more appropriate.

Most statisticians are very comfortable in estimating the number of subjects required for participation in a clinical program. The considerations necessary for determining the number of subjects required in a bioequivalence study are very straightforward if the objective is to compare means. The FDA usually requests that the number of patients enrolled be adequate to provide 80% power of detecting a 20% difference in mean bioavailability at the 0.05 significance level using a two-tailed test. However, there are no suggestions for what equivalence means in terms of inter- or intrasubject variability. In addition, the number of subjects that must be examined to provide any assurance of comparable variabilities is much larger than that needed to provide such an assurance concerning means. Although these sample sizes may be very large, the consequences of designing a study that will not provide assurances of interchangeability must be considered, and if necessary, the appropriate price paid in terms of the magnitude of the clinical studies.

4.3 Sources of Variability

All experimental designs are subject to many sources of variation. Some of these are inescapable and others are controllable. A brief summary of some of these considerations is presented in Table 1.

Sources of variability that are inescapable include the variability associated with the individuals who participate in the study (both inter- and intrasubject), differences among formulations, subject × formulation interaction, and random variability. Although these are inescapable, their effects can be estimated by appropriate modeling, and thus can be used in interpreting the analysis.

There are also sources of variation that are controllable. These include the carryover effects that most drugs have. Reasons for these carryover effects include drug or metabolite residue, metabolic induction or inhibition, and gastric irritation that might enhance absorption or might increase intestinal motility, and thus decrease bioavailability. Many carryover effects can be controlled by extending the period between treatments sufficiently.

Time factors are also controllable, because we can select the sampling times. In addition, handling of the samples after they have been taken is very important. Although statisticians tend not to worry about this, it is sometimes critical to consider the timing of assays in the experimental design. The blood samples of patients who enter the study early man deteriorate compared with those of patients who enter the study later. It can be very important to assay samples according to a particular design so that these effects and those due to individual laboratory technician, time

Table 1 Sources of Variation in Bioavailability Studies

- Inescapable Variation
  - Subject differences
    - Among
    - Within
  - Medication differences
  - Subject × formulation interaction
  - Random error
- Controllable variation
  - Carryover effects
    - Drug/metabolite residue
    - Induction
    - Inhibition
    - Irritation
  - Time factors
    - Sampling time
    - Storage factors
  - Physiological factors
    - Gastric emptying
    - Food, fluid, other drugs

of day, time of sample receipt, and so on, can be balanced and therefore minimized.

A third type of controllable factor includes those associated with physiology, gastric emptying, concomitant administration of fluids or other drugs, and other such factors. For example, using indices of renal function, such as creatinine clearance, as covariates may be important in evaluating drugs that are cleared by the kidney. Physiological factors can be included in the experimental design and their effects on the formulations of interest can be evaluated.

A relatively new procedure that substantially reduces all elements of variability is the simultaneous administration of two therapeutic entities using cold radiolabeled techniques. The concept underlying this is as follows. Formulation A is labeled with a particular stable isotope and formulation B is labeled in the same place, but with a different isotope. Both formulations are then administered simultaneously. When the samples are taken, it is straightforward to identify what the concentration of the drug in the blood due to the administration of formulation A is, and also to determine the concentration due to formulation B. Thus the sources of variability due to intersubject variation, time-to-time variation within the same subject, and any type of external factors are all eliminated; we observe the relative bioavailability of two products simultaneously within the same experimental unit. Although there are problems associated with this procedure, it provides an extremely efficient way of comparing the bioavailabilities of two formulations.

5 OBJECTIVES OF BIOEQUIVALENCE STUDIES

Recall that two formulations are bioequivalent if their bioavailabilities are the same. This means that both the rate of absorption and the total amount of drug appearing in the systemic circulation are the same for two formulations. Thus the objective of the great majority of bioequivalence studies is to prove, beyond reasonable doubt, that two formulations are the same, not to prove that they are different.

In contrast, the objective of most clinical trials is to demonstrate that a new formulation is superior in some respect to a standard regimen of therapy. In these studies, a philosophical conception of the objective would be to find significant differences. The smaller the p-value, the more confident we are that the new formulation is superior to the standard. However, in bioequivalence studies we are not trying to find treatment differences. We are trying to show that the treatments are the same. Thinking of our basic data source as a plasma concentration-time curve, we want to determine whether two formulations have equivalent curves.

Early in the history of the analysis of bioequivalence studies, the standard approach was to use a simple analysis of variance on variables derived from the plasma concentration-time curve. In fact, this approach was recommended in the FDA bioavailability guidelines. This was usually an analysis of the plasma concentrations at each time point, an analysis of the area under the plasma concentration-time curve, the peak plasma concentration, and the time that the peak concentration was observed. The result of the analysis was that the difference between the two formulations was either significant or not significant for each of the variables analyzed.

The problem associated with this type of analysis is in reaching a conclusion. It was often the case that small differences were statistically significant but did not reach the 20% deviation to be declared biologically inequivalent, or that large differences were observed but the power of the particular design was so low that little confidence could be had that the difference observed represented a true difference between the formulations. Given this apparent inconsistency, it is clear that if the objective is to determine similarity, conventional hypothesis testing is not very relevant and other methods must be explored.

Because most conventional statistical methodologies are designed to demonstrate differences rather than similarities, they are inappropriate for the evaluation of bioequivalence studies. For this reason, a variety of alternative methods have been suggested by a variety of investigators to address the issue of similarity. Thus, as Metzler (1974) stated, the problem of bioavailability is a problem in equivalence.

6 ANALYTIC ALTERNATIVES

The need to demonstrate bioequivalence in a scientifically accepted manner is extremely important—it is important for many drugs produced by many companies and for a variety of reasons. The methodologies that accomplish this cannot be dictated by regulatory agencies; they must be based on good statistical and scientific principles. It is impossible in a chapter of this length to explain each of these methodologies in detail. In this section we outline several of the approaches that have been suggested and provide references that will allow the reader to investigate them in greater detail. Excellent, more extensive summaries are provided in Westlake (1979a, 1979b) and Metzler and Huang (1983).

6.1 Power Evaluation

As outlined in Section 5, one of the approaches that is recommended, and certainly one that has been viewed as necessary by the FDA is an analysis of variance derived from the plasma concentration-time curve. Analysis of variance can also be performed on the raw data or on a transformation of the raw data. The analysis itself is usually straightforward but poses the problems of interpretation as described earlier. In particular, a clinically important difference may not be statistically significant, while a statistically significant difference may be clinically unimportant.

To address this issue, the FDA has requested a retrospective evaluation of the power of bioequivalence studies. If a study, in retrospect, has an 80% assurance of declaring a 20% difference significant, but the observed difference was not significant, the study usually is accepted by the FDA as confirming bioequivalence. On the other hand, studies that have less than 80% power to detect such a difference may be held in question. Although the rationale for such a post hoc evaluation makes some sense, the statistical theory underlying it may be questioned, since when the study is completed, the concept of power is no longer relevant (see Chapter 1). To avoid this potential problematic situation, several authors have suggested approaches that address the problem more directly. These are discussed in subsequent sections.

6.2 Confidence Intervals

Early in the 1970s, Westlake and others (Westlake, 1972, 1973, 1976; Kirkwood and Westlake, 1981; Levy, 1972; Mantel, 1977; Steinijans and Diletti, 1983) suggested using confidence intervals, rather than hypothesis tests, to evaluate the results of bioavailability studies. Although several variations have been proposed and are noted in the bibliography, the general approach was to calculate confidence intervals about the observed relative bioavailability.

There have been various approaches to constructing confidence intervals. Intervals have been symmetric and asymmetric; they have been computed for differences and for ratios; and they have been for transformed and untransformed variables. Usually, a 95% confidence interval has been recommended; and if this interval falls completely within the interval from 0.8 to 1.2 (or sometimes 1.25), the two products are accepted as being bioequivalent.

The difficulty associated with this is that the frequency with which such intervals cover either 0.8 or 1.2 is very large, even when the two formulations are identical. Studies have suggested that the frequency with which at least one of the confidence limits falls outside the range 0.8 to 1.2 can be upwards of three times as great as the putative 5% alpha level. Thus, using these procedures provides a very conservative decision-making approach, but one that may not be optimal for comparing the similarity of two products.

6.3 Interval Approach Suggested by Mandallaz and Mau

A number of new approaches have been suggested recently for the evaluation of bioequivalence studies. Mandallaz and Mau (1981) [see also Fluehler et al. (1981, 1983)] suggested an analytic approach based on an interval hypothesis. This is presented schematically below, where $R_{t/s}$ represents the ratio of the bioavailability of the test formulation to that of the standard.

$$H_0 : R_{t/s} \in [0.8, 1.2]$$

$$H_a : R_{t/s} \notin [0.8, 1.2]$$

Conclude bioequivalence if H_0 is accepted

The logic for this approach is conventional, in that if the null hypothesis is rejected and the alternative hypothesis is accepted, the two products will be declared not to be bioequivalent.

The Mandallaz and Mau procedure also provides an interesting Bayesian interpretation. They showed that with the assumption of an appropriate noninformative prior, the posterior distribution of the ratio of the two formulation means can be approximated to a degree by the usual t-distribution. Mandallaz and Mau also developed the relative merits of symmetrical and shortest confidence intervals. This approach results in decisions which are more precise than those of the usual confidence interval, but still possesses many of the weaknesses of the confidence interval approach.

6.4 Suggestion of Anderson and Hauck

Later, Anderson and Hauck (1983, 1985) and Hauck and Anderson (1984) suggested a very interesting, nonclassical approach to testing the hypothesis of bioequivalence. As discussed previously, the logic of classical hypothesis testing requires that the hypothesis to be demonstrated is the alternative hypothesis—in this case, inequivalence. Thus the hypothesis of interest, bioequivalence, is really concluded by default rather than by demonstration.

In the procedure suggested by Anderson and Hauck, they construct their hypotheses such that the null hypothesis is that the relative bioavailability of the two products falls outside the accepted bioequivalency range (0.8 to 1.2), and that the alternative hypothesis is that the ratio does fall within this range. Thus the roles of the null and alternative hypotheses are reversed:

$$H_0 : R_{t/s} < 0.8 \quad \text{or} \quad R_{t/s} > 1.2$$
$$H_a : 0.8 < R_{t/s} < 1.2$$

Conclude bioequivalence if H_0 is rejected

They then develop an asymptotic theory for evaluating this hypothesis, such that if the null hypothesis is rejected at the appropriate level, the conclusion is that the two products are bioequivalent. Thus their methodology, while approximate, gives a direct statement concerning the equivalence of two formulations. This is in contrast to the conventional methodology which says only that there is no significant difference between the two formulations.

6.5 Bayesian Procedures

Several authors have suggested that Bayesian procedures might be valuable in the evaluation and interpretation of bioavailability studies (Rodda and Davis, 1980; Selwyn and Hall, 1984, 1985; Selwyn et al., 1981). Many people who favor these procedures feel that they address the clinical situation much more directly than do classical procedures.

A probabilistic expression in the classical setting is this:

$$p - \text{value} = \Pr[\text{more extreme results} \mid \mu_s = \mu_t].$$

In the classical approach, we make the assumption that the two bioavailabilities are identical and then, after reviewing the results, develop a probability statement which describes the likelihood of observing the specific results or more extreme results under the assumption that the null hypothesis is true. This is obviously the wrong direction, and it does not consider the important clinical factors that are the only factors of significance in any clinical trial. A more logical direction is represented as

$$\Pr[\mu_s - \mu_t \geq \text{CSD} \mid \text{results}],$$

where CSD is the clinically significant difference. This direct probability is typical of the Bayesian approach, and it has a much more clinically meaningful interpretation. In this methodology, the determination is of the probability that the true difference (or ratio) in bioavailability exceeds the *clinically* significant difference, *given the results of the study.*

In many cases, the results of statistical tests of bioavailability do not indicate any degree of significance. However, the power to detect a 20% difference in bioavailability is often very small, and the 95% confidence intervals can be very wide. By any conventional approach, including the "75/75 rule" discussed in the next section, a conclusion of bioequivalence may not be made, and the study can be left with the potentially difficult position of having inconclusive results. If a Bayesian approach were used to determine the posterior distribution of the true difference, the question would be to determine the probability that the true difference in bioavailability between the two formulations exceeds 20%, given the results of the study. This analysis allows the conclusion that, given the similarity observed in the study, the chance that there really is a difference that exceeds 20% is less than some well-defined probability. Clearly, the actual posterior distribution can be presented, and depending on the degree of assurance necessary, the probability of a greater or lesser difference can be provided. This type of statement may be all the additional information needed to conclude that two formulations will be similar clinically.

The principal objection to the Bayesian approach is the need for a prior distribution. This is usually an academic criticism, since the likelihood dominates the prior in literally all bioavailability studies, and therefore, the use of a mathematically convenient, noninformative prior should minimize criticism of Bayesian techniques for the evaluation of bioequivalence studies.

The Bayesian approach has received broader discussion recently, and it can be a valuable adjunct to current statistical approaches used in the evaluation of bioavailability studies. Although its utility is not yet broadly accepted, the ability to make positive statements based on small differences is a valuable tool when the objective is to conclude similarity.

6.6 The 75/75 Rule

Between 1977 and 1980, the FDA proposed a number of rules regarding the bioequivalence of specific drug products, including certain anticonvulsants, tricyclic antidepressants, carbonic anhydrase inhibitors, probenecid, quinidine, and phenothiazine (Purich, 1980). In these rules, which were never finalized but were often quoted and employed, criteria were proposed for what would constitute a demonstration of bioequivalence. According to these decision rules, the test drug is deemed to meet the bioequivalence requirements if the following conditions are met:

1. The relative bioavailability of the test product to the standard must be greater than 75% and less than 125% in at least 75% of the subjects.
2. There is no more than 20% difference in the average peak concentration and area under the plasma concentration-time curve (AUC).
3. Analytical and statistical techniques used are of sufficient sensitivity to detect these differences.

The first condition listed above has become known as the 75/75 rule (or, in the case of phenothiazines, the analogous 70/70 rule). Numerous publications have questioned the statistical basis for this rule, and one simulation study (Haynes, 1981) has shown that even in the situation where the mean AUCs for the test and reference products are exactly the same, the rule is particularly sensitive for drugs that have large inter- or intrasubject variability—resulting in a very high rejection of formulations with identical bioavailabilities.

The results published by Haynes demonstrate that the 75/75 rule has very undesirable performance characteristics: primarily, that the rejection probability (alpha level) depends on the variability of the formulations to an inordinate and sometimes paradoxical extent. For example, when a test product's variability is large, the smaller the reference product's variation (i.e., the more divergent the two products), the greater the probability that the rule will accept the test product. The performance of the 75/75 rule in this situation is, therefore, the reverse of what it should be.

The 75/75 rule is also very sensitive when the size of the sample is relatively small. This power, however, is attained at the expense of a very high rejection rate, even when there are no differences between the test and reference product. In another simulation study (Metzler and Huang, 1983), it was shown that when intersubject variability is large and the error standard deviations of both formulations are equal, the 75/75 rule rejected 56.3% of the test product when 16 subjects were used, even though both products were equal in mean and variance. The rejection rate, paradoxically, was even higher when 24 subjects were used. Thus, although the 75/75 rule is well defined and appears in public pronouncements by the FDA, it is not valuable as a scientifically based decision rule.

6.7 Two One-Sided Tests

Schuirmann (1981, 1987) has suggested a new approach in the evaluation of bioequivalence studies which involves testing two one-sided hypotheses. The rationale is that if the difference or ratio of the test and reference bioavailabilities is significantly greater than a lower acceptable limit and is simultaneously significantly less than an upper acceptable limit, the two products are concluded to be bioequivalent.

Schuirmann compared this procedure to some of the more common analytical approaches, and it appears that the procedure may be a useful addition to the methodologies available for the analysis of bioequivalence studies.

6.8 Other Procedures

Drug half-lives in plasma are not ordinarily affected by formulation differences. So if the rate of absorption and the extent of absorption are identical for two formulations of the same product, the shapes of the two plasma concentration-time curves should be very similar. Thus two formulations can be compared by analyzing the configuration of their plasma concentration-time curves. The objective of curve comparison analyses is to determine whether two or more curves have the same amplitude and share a common configuration. If the two curves do not have similar configurations, the techniques used should be able to detect the differences.

There is a variety of univariate and multivariate procedures that might be used. For example, considering the multiple plasma concentrations for each subject, a repeated measures analysis of variance might be used (Cole and Grizzle, 1966). There are a number of assumptions associated with this that may or may not be appropriate in a particular case, and perhaps a more appropriate procedure might be some truly multivariate technique, such as principal components analysis (Redman, 1968; Snee, 1972). This has been suggested as one means of comparing plasma concentration curves but has not received (and probably will not receive) significant attention, either in practice or in the literature, because of the difficulty in interpreting the results.

7 OTHER CONSIDERATIONS

7.1 Transformations

There are two schools of thought concerning transformations. One group holds that any transformation of data reduces the information content of the data, and the other group feels that we often measure variables on a convenient scale rather than on the most appropriate scale, and thus transformations often make more biological sense. The question is: Should results of bioavailability studies be routinely transformed, and if they should, what transformations should be used? Should we use logarithms; should we rank the data; and what are the advantages and disadvantages of various transformations?

Often biological data are lognormally distributed rather than normally distributed, which makes logarithmic transformations attractive. In the case of using areas for evaluating bioavailability, the relationship between area and the fraction of the dose absorbed is a multiplicative one, and therefore, logarithms of areas may be the most appropriate data to analyze. On the other hand, simply using logarithms only as a mathematical convenience may not be supportable unless the conclusions can also be made when the analysis is performed without transformations.

Ranking and other nonparametric approaches are gaining popularity because of their robustness to violations of various distributional assumptions, which are common and necessary in the evaluation of bioavailability, and in their flexibility and the variety of hypotheses that can be tested using ranks. The basic difficulty with ranking and other transformational approaches is in estimation. Estimation is as important as testing, and nonparametric procedures do not allow estimation of bioavailability characteristics—in particular, variances of bioavailability. Thus, when estimation is a critically important issue, or comparison or characterization of variances is essential, a transformation of the data may not be appropriate.

7.2 Outliers

Another issue that is extremely common in the evaluation of bioequivalence studies and bioavailability studies is the problem of outliers. Outliers are much like weeds; they are very difficult to define and are only called outliers because they are inconsistent with the environment in which they are observed.

Outliers within blood level curves will primarily affect the peak concentration and the absorption rate constant. The area under the curve is less sensitive to individual outliers because it is an average. Unless there are problems with the assay procedure or with the particular sample that was associated with the outlier, the data must be accepted as real.

The outlying *subject*, on the other hand, must always be considered as valid. If outlying subjects were excluded, biased assessments of both bioavailability and variability would result—with potentially misleading conclusions. The inclusion of outliers of all kinds in the analysis is critically important if estimation and comparison of variability between two formulations is a principal objective.

If transformations or ranks are used, the effect of the outliers will probably be less. In any case, the effect of outliers on the estimates of the measures of bioavailability can be substantial. As a general philosophy, perhaps a conservative approach, such as evaluating the hypotheses both with and without the outlier might be best; the truth should lie somewhere between.

8 CONCLUSIONS

The objective in evaluating bioavailability or bioequivalence studies is to make conclusions. The analysis of these studies is but a very important step toward making those conclusions. The following sentence is a paraphrase of a recently published study: "The bioavailability of drug A was significantly reduced, but was still the same as drug B, whether measured by area, peak concentration or time of peak concentration." This is an example of the confusion that arises in evaluating bioavailability studies. It is logically impossible for bioavailability to be significantly reduced and still be equal.

In addition, this statement is not a conclusion; it is a result. Conclusions are inferences to the population of interest; results are descriptions of the sample. A conclusion is concerned with whether or not the sample difference is within the acceptable range. The answer must be yes or no; the only other option is to repeat the study. One of the responsibilities of statisticians is to design studies so that this last alternative will happen infrequently. Studies must have an adequate number of subjects; they must follow the appropriate experimental design; and appropriate statistical techniques must be used so that the ultimate conclusion is not in doubt. If these elements are not satisfied, the statistician has not adequately fulfilled the appropriate role in the investigational process.

The role of statistics in the bioavailability context has increased in importance during the last 15 years. Statisticians are now in a position to offer a much more positive contribution than previously. There are a variety of techniques available for comparing the bioavailability of two or more agents, and by using appropriate experimental designs and statistical methodologies, the roles of statisticians in the design, conduct, evaluation, and interpretation of bioavailability studies will continue to be essential.

REFERENCES

Anderson, S., and W. W. Hauck (1983). A new procedure for testing equivalence in comparative bioavailability and other clinical trials. *Comm. Statist. A12*, 2663–2692.

Anderson, S., and W. W. Hauck (1985). On testing for bioequivalence: letter to the editor. *Biometrics 41*, 563.

Brown, B. W. (1980). The crossover experiment for clinical trials. *Biometrics 36*, 69–79.

Cole, J. W. L., and J. E. Grizzle (1966). Applications of multivariate analysis of variance to related measurements experiments. *Biometrics 22*, 810–828.

Federal Register (1977). 1621–1653.

Fluehler, H., J. Hirtz, and H. A. Moser (1981). An aid to decision-making in bioequivalence assessment. *Pharmacokinet. Biopharm. 9*, 235–243.

Fluehler, H., A. P. Grieve, D. Mandallaz, J. Mau, and H. A. Moser (1983). Bayesian approach to bioequivalence assessment: an example. *J. Pharm. Sci. 72*, 1178–1181.

Food and Drug Administration (1977). The bioavailability protocol guidelines for ANDA and NDA submission. Division of Biopharmaceutics, Drug Monographs Bureau of Drugs, Food and Drug Administration, Washington, D.C.

Gibaldi, M., and D. Perrier (1975). *Pharmacokinetics*. Marcel Dekker, New York.

Grizzle, J. E. (1965). The two-period changeover design and its use in clinical trials. *Biometrics 21*, 467–480.

Hauck, W. W., and S. Anderson (1984). A new statistical procedure for testing equivalence in two group comparative bioavailability trials. *J. Pharmacokinet. Biopharm. 12*, 83–91.

Haynes, J. D. (1981). Statistical simulation study of new proposed uniformity requirement for bioequivalency studies. *J. Pharm. Sci. 70*, 673–675.

Kirkwood, T. B. L., and W. J. Westlake (1981). Bioequivalence testing—need to rethink. *Biometrics 37*, 589.

Levy, G. (1972). Bioavailability limits. *Canad. Med. Assoc. J. 107*, 722–727.

Mandallaz, D., and J. Mau (1981). Comparison of different methods for decision making in bioequivalence assessment. *Biometrics 37*, 213–222.

Mantel, N. (1977). Do we want confidence intervals symmetrical about the null value? *Biometrics 33*, 759–760.

Metzler, C. M. (1974). Bioavailability: a problem in equivalence. *Biometrics 30*, 309–317.

Metzler, C. M., and D. C. Huang (1983). Statistical methods of bioavailability. *Clin. Res. Pract. Drug Regul. Aff. 1*, 109–132.

Purich, E. (1980). *Drug absorption and disposition: statistical considerations* (K. S. Albert, ed.). American Pharmaceutical Association, Academy of Pharmaceutical Sciences, Washington D.C., p. 115.

Redman, C. E. (1968). Biological applications of principal components (abstract). *Biometrics 24*, 235.

Rodda, B. E., and R. L. Davis (1980). Determining the probability of an important difference in bioavailability. *Clin. Pharmacol. Ther. 28*, 247.

Schuirmann, D. L. (1981). On hypothesis testing to determine if the mean of a normal distribution is contained in a known interval (abstract). *Biometrics 37*, 617.

Schuirmann, D. J. (1987). A comparison of the two one-sided tests procedure and the power approach for assessing the equivalence of average bioavailability. *J. Pharmacokinet. Biopharm. 15*, 657–680.

Selwyn, M. R., and N. R. Hall (1984). On Bayesian methods for bioequivalence. *Biometrics 40*, 1103–1108.

Selwyn, M. R., and N. R. Hall (1985). On testing for bioequivalence: letter to the editor. *Biometrics 41*, 561–563.

Selwyn, M. R, A. P. Dempster, and N. R. Hall (1981). A Bayesian approach to bioequivalence for the 2 × 2 changeover design. *Biometrics 37*, 11–21.

Snee, R. D. (1972). On the analysis of response curve data. *Technometrics 14*, 47–62.

Steinijans, V. W., and E. Diletti (1983). Statistical analysis of bioavailability studies: parametric and nonparametric confidence intervals. *European J. Clin. Pharmacol. 24*, 127-136.

Wagner, J. G. (1970). *Biopharmaceutics and Relevant Pharmacokinetics.* Drug Intelligence Publications, Hamilton, p. 180.

Westlake, W. J. (1972). Use of confidence intervals in analysis of comparative bioavailability trials. *J. Pharm. Sci. 61*, 1340–1341.

Westlake, W. J. (1973). Use of statistical methods in the evaluation of *in vivo* performance of dosage forms. *J. Pharm. Sci. 62*, 1579–1589.

Westlake, W. J. (1974). The use of balanced incomplete block designs in comparative bioavailability trials. *Biometrics 30*, 319–327.

Westlake, W. J. (1976). Symmetrical confidence intervals for bioequivalence trials. *Biometrics 32*, 741–744.

Westlake, W. J. (1979a). Design and statistical evaluation of bioequivalence studies in man. *Principles and Perspective in Drug Bioavailability.* S. Karger, Basel, pp. 192–210.

Westlake, W. J. (1979b). Statistical aspects of comparative bioavailability trials. *Biometrics 35*, 273–280.

3

Analysis of Repeated-Measures Designs

GEORGE A. MILLIKEN Kansas State University, Manhattan, Kansas

1 INTRODUCTION

Many experiments involve obtaining several measurements on each subject or animal, such as repeatedly measuring its heart rate at several times after being treated. The experimenter generally wants to compare the effect of different treatments or conditions on the subjects and make inferences concerning the effect the treatments have on the relationship between the measured response and time. By repeatedly measuring each subject at the end of several predetermined time intervals, two sizes of experimental units are generated. The subject, which is randomly assigned to one of the treatments, is the large size of experimental unit. By repeatedly measuring each subject at the end of each of d time intervals, the subject or the subject's time in the experiment is "split" into d parts (time intervals) and the response is measured on each part. The smaller size of experimental unit is the interval of time the subject is exposed to the treatment between measurements.

Because this repeated-measures experiment has two sizes of experimental unit, the model and analysis has two parts, one to compare treatments based on the subjects' responses and one to compare times and the treatment-time interaction based on the responses in the time intervals. The structure and model for the repeated-measures design are similar to those of a split-plot design, except that the two designs operate under different assumptions. The difference between the two designs is that the levels of one or more factors of repeated-measures designs cannot be randomly assigned to their respective sizes of experimental units, whereas the levels of all the factors of split-plot designs can be randomly assigned to their respective sizes of experimental units.

In the above example, the subjects are randomly assigned to the levels of treatment, but the time intervals cannot be randomly assigned to the levels of time. Hence the resulting experimental design is a repeated-measures design. For further discussions concerning the assumptions associated with these two designs, see Chapters 5 and 24 to 28 of Milliken and Johnson (1984).

2 MODEL AND ASSUMPTIONS

For an experiment involving m treatments where each subject is repeatedly measured d times, the model for a response measured at the kth time of the jth subject assigned to the ith treatment is

$$y_{ijk} = \mu + \delta_i + s_{ij} + \tau_k + (\delta\tau)_{ik} + \epsilon_{ijk}$$

or

$$y_{ijk} = \mu_{ik} + s_{ij} + \epsilon_{ijk}, \qquad i = 1, 2, \ldots, m, \quad j = 1, 2, \ldots, n, \quad k = 1, 2, \ldots, d,$$

where

$$\mu_{ik} = \mu + \delta_i + \tau_k + (\delta\tau)_{ik},$$

the s_{ij}'s represent the subject errors, and the ϵ_{ijk}'s represent the time-interval errors. The subject part of the model is $\mu + \delta_i + s_{ij}$ and the time-interval part of the model is $\tau_k + (\delta\tau)_{ik} + \epsilon_{ijk}$. The "usual" assumptions for the model are that $s_{ij} \sim \text{iid}\, N(0, \sigma_s^2)$ and $\epsilon_{ijk} \sim \text{iid}\, N(0, \sigma_\epsilon^2)$, which are the same as the usual assumptions for the split-plot design. The usual split-plot analyses are valid under more general assumptions (Huynh and Feldt, 1970). If the variances of all the ϵ_{ijk} are assumed to be equal, the usual analysis is appropriate when the errors within a subject (ϵ_{ijk}, $k = 1, 2, \ldots, d$) are equally correlated,that is,when the covariance matrix

Table 1 ANOVA Table for a Repeated-Measures Design Where the Expected Mean Squares (EMS) Are Computed from the Usual Assumptions

Source of variation	d.f.	Sum of squares	EMS
Treatment	$m-1$	$dn\sum_{i=1}^{m}(\bar{y}_{i} \ - \bar{y} \ )^2$	$\sigma_\epsilon^2 + d\sigma_s^2 + Q_3^2$
Error(subject)	$m(n-1)$	$d\sum_{i=1}^{m}\sum_{j=1}^{n}(\bar{y}_{ij} - \bar{y}_{i} \ )^2$	$\sigma_\epsilon^2 + d\sigma_s^2$
Time	$d-1$	$mn\sum_{k=1}^{d}(\bar{y}_{k} \ - \bar{y} \ )^2$	$\sigma_\epsilon^2 + Q_2$
Treatment × time	$(m-1)(d-1)$	$n\sum_{i=1}^{m}\sum_{k=1}^{d}(\bar{y}_{ik} - \bar{y}_{i} \ - \bar{y}_{\ k} + \bar{y} \ )^2$	$\sigma_\epsilon^2 + Q_1$
Error(interval)	$m(n-1)(d-1)$	$\sum_{i=1}^{m}\sum_{j=1}^{n}\sum_{k=1}^{d}(y_{ijk} - \bar{y}_{ij} - \bar{y}_{ik} + \bar{y}_{i} \ )^2$	σ_ϵ^2

of the within-subject errors possesses the compound symmetry property. These assumptions may not be reasonable for a repeated-measures design; in particular, it may not be reasonable to assume that the correlation between errors from adjacent time intervals is the same as the correlation between two errors that are 10 time intervals apart. A major assumption is that the within-subjects error covariance matrices are identical for all subjects. Table 1 contains the sums of squares associated with the analysis corresponding to the repeated-measures model above, where

$$\bar{y}_{ij\cdot} = \sum_{k=1}^{d} y_{ijk/d}, \qquad \bar{y}_{i\cdot k} = \sum_{j=1}^{n} y_{ijk/n}, \qquad \bar{y}_{i\cdot\cdot} = \sum_{j=1}^{n}\sum_{k=1}^{d} y_{ijk/nd},$$

$$\bar{y}_{\cdot\cdot k} = \sum_{i=1}^{m}\sum_{j=1}^{n} y_{ijk/mn}, \qquad \bar{y}_{\cdots} = \sum_{i=j}^{m}\sum_{j=1}^{n}\sum_{k=1}^{d} y_{ijk/mnd}.$$

The sums of squares do not depend on the equal-correlation assumption, whereas the expected mean squares are computed under the equal-correlation assumption. The terms Q_1, Q_2, Q_3 denote noncentrality parameters corresponding to the respective effects where the particular Q_i is zero when there is no corresponding effect. The proper error term to compare the treatment effects is Error(subject) and the test statistic is

$$F_{\text{treatment}} = \text{MS Treatment/MS Error(subject)}.$$

The distribution of $F_{\text{treatment}}$ is $F_{(m-1,m(n-1))}$, which does not depend on the equal-correlation assumption. The appropriate error term to compare time and treatment×time effects is Error(interval) and the test statistics are

$$F_{\text{time}} = \text{MS Time/MS Error(interval)}$$

and

$$F_{\text{treatment}\times\text{time}} = \text{MS Treatment} \times \text{Time/MS Error(interval)}.$$

The distributions of F_{time} and $F_{\text{treatment}\times\text{time}}$ are $F_{(d-1,m(n-1)(d-1))}$ and $F_{((m-1)(d-1),m(n-1)(d-1))}$, respectively, if the covariance matrix of the within-subject errors satisfies the equal-correlation assumption or the Huynh-Feldt condition for unequal variances. Alternative procedures to be used when the equal correlation assumption is not appropriate, are discussed in the next sections.

3 EXAMPLE 1. THE EFFECT OF A DRUG ON HEART RATES

The data in Table 2 consist of the heart rate in beats per minute (bpm) measured at seven times on each of 20 men who were randomly assigned to

Table 2 Data for the Example Representing the Heart Rates Measured Every 5 Minutes for Seven Time Intervals

Treatment	Subject	Time 1	Time 2	Time 3	Time 4	Time 5	Time 6	Time 7
1	1	73	74	74	78	79	81	79
1	2	78	77	76	79	84	88	86
1	3	73	73	74	78	81	81	79
1	4	75	72	73	74	79	82	80
1	5	75	74	73	78	82	84	82
2	6	72	74	76	80	81	83	81
2	7	77	77	78	81	85	86	84
2	8	72	74	78	80	84	86	84
2	9	77	80	78	83	85	86	84
2	10	74	75	75	80	84	85	83
3	11	79	80	81	83	83	83	82
3	12	73	76	74	81	79	82	81
3	13	68	68	74	75	76	78	77
3	14	75	77	80	81	85	89	88
3	15	72	74	81	79	82	83	82
4	16	78	82	83	87	91	92	87
4	17	78	81	81	85	89	92	87
4	18	78	80	81	82	87	87	82
4	19	71	75	76	80	85	85	80
4	20	80	83	86	86	90	90	85

one of four drugs so that there were five subjects per treatment. The time periods were 5 minutes long where the first measurement was obtained 5 minutes after administering the drug. The analysis corresponding to the usual assumptions (compound symmetry) is presented in Table 3. The distribution of $F_{\text{treatment}}$, computed from the between-subject analysis, is uneffected by the correlations between the time-interval errors within a subject. But the time-interval level of analysis can be greatly influenced by deviating from the compound symmetry or equal-correlation assumptions.

Box (1954) proposed a conservative procedure for comparing time and treatment × time effects where the computed F-statistics are compared to the percentage points of an F-distribution with 1 and $m(n-1)$ degrees of freedom and $m-1$ and $m(n-1)$ degrees of freedom, respectively. The approach is to divide the degrees of freedom corresponding to sums of squares within the level of analysis where the repeated measure occurs

Table 3 ANOVA Table for the Heart Rate Data Under the Usual Assumptions

Source	d.f.	Sum of squares	F-value	Pr > F
Treatment	3	615.74	4.57	0.0170
Error(subject)	16	718.63		
Time	6	1835.94	149.74	0.0001
Treatment × time	18	115.31	3.14	0.0002
Error(interval)	96	196.17		

by the number of repeated measures minus 1. In this case all degrees of freedom are divided by $d-1=6$. The analysis-of-variance (ANOVA) table with the Box corrected degrees of freedom and recomputed significance levels are given in Table 4.

Box (1954) provided a measure, θ, as to how far the correlations between the repeated measures within a subject deviate from compound symmetry. Let the covariance between time k and time k' be denoted by $\sigma_{kk'}$; then θ is

$$\theta = \frac{d^2(\bar{\sigma}_{kk} - \bar{\sigma}_{..})^2}{(d-1)\left(\sum_{k=1}^{d}\sum_{k'=1}^{d}\sigma_{kk'}^2 - 2d\sum_{k=1}^{d}\bar{\sigma}_{k.}^2 + d^2\bar{\sigma}_{..}^2\right)},$$

where

$$\bar{\sigma}_{..} = \frac{\sum_{k=1}^{d}\sum_{k'=1}^{d}\sigma_{kk'}}{d^2}, \qquad \bar{\sigma}_{k.} = \frac{\sum_{k'=1}^{d}\sigma_{kk'}}{d},$$

and

$$\bar{\sigma}_{kk} = \frac{\sum_{k'=1}^{d}\sigma_{k'k'}}{d}.$$

Table 4 ANOVA Table for the Heart Rate Data with the Box Conservative Correction for Degrees of Freedom

Source	df	Box conservative d.f.	F-value	Pr > F
Treatment	3	no change	4.57	0.0170
Error(subject)	16	no change		
Time	6	1	149.74	0.0001
Treatment × time	18	3	3.14	0.0545
Error(interval)	96	16		

To estimate the value of θ, compute

$$v_{kk'} = \frac{\sum_{i=1}^{m} \sum_{j=1}^{n} \hat{\epsilon}_{ijk} \hat{\epsilon}_{ijk'}}{mn-1}, k, k' = 1, 2, \ldots, d,$$

which is the sample covariance between the residuals of the kth and k'th time intervals computed over all subjects and treatments where

$$\hat{\epsilon}_{ijk} = y_{ijk} - \bar{y}_{i \cdot k} - \bar{y}_{ij \cdot} + \bar{y}_{i \cdot \cdot}, \quad i = 1, 2, \ldots, m, \quad j = 1, 2, \ldots, n, \quad k = 1, 2, \ldots, d.$$

Then compute

$$\hat{\theta} = \frac{d^2 \bar{v}^2}{(d-1) \sum_{k=1}^{d} \sum_{k'=1}^{d} v_{kk'}^2},$$

where

$$\bar{v} = \frac{\sum_{k=1}^{d} v_{kk}}{d},$$

the mean of the time-interval variances. Box showed that for $d \geq 2$, $1/(d-1) \leq \hat{\theta} \leq 1$; $\hat{\theta} = 1$ when the sample correlations are all equal. The corresponding $\hat{\theta}$ adjustment consists of multiplying all degrees of freedom for sums of squares in the repeated measures part of the analysis by $\hat{\theta}$ and then comparing the computed F-statistics to the percentage points of the F-distribution with the resulting degrees of freedom. The matrix of

Table 5 Variances and Covariances of Each Subject's Seven Time-Interval Errors Computed Across All Subjects for the Heart Rate Data[a]

	T1	T2	T3	T4	T5	T6	T7
T1	1.7762	0.9972	−0.1351	−0.1637	−0.5381	−0.9682	−0.9682
T2	0.9972	1.3762	−0.3983	0.5837	−0.5591	−0.9998	−0.9998
T3	−0.1351	−0.3983	2.1852	−0.1802	0.0769	−0.7742	−0.7742
T4	−0.1637	0.5837	−0.1802	1.3491	−0.1938	−0.6975	−0.6975
T5	−0.5381	−0.5592	0.0769	−0.1938	0.5371	0.3386	0.3386
T6	−0.9682	−0.9998	−0.7742	−0.6975	0.3386	1.5506	1.5506
T7	−0.9682	−0.9998	−0.7742	−0.6975	0.3386	1.5506	1.5506

$$\bar{v} = 1.474974, \quad \sum_{k=1}^{7} \sum_{m=1}^{7} v_{km}^2 = 38.533660, \quad \hat{\theta} = 0.461077$$

[a]Computations are included for estimating θ to be used in adjusting the degrees of freedom.

Table 6 ANOVA Table for the Heart Rate Data with the $\hat{\theta}$ Adjusted Degrees of Freedom where $\hat{\theta} = 0.461077$

Source	d.f.	$\hat{\theta}$ adjusted d.f.	F-value	Pr > F
Treatment	3	no change	4.57	0.0170
Error(subject)	16	no change		
Time	6	2.8	149.74	0.0001
Treatment × time	18	8.3	3.14	0.0063
Error(interval)	96	44.3		

sample covariances of the time-interval residuals is shown in Table 5 along with the quantities necessary to compute $\hat{\theta}$. The ANOVA table for the $\hat{\theta}$ adjusted degrees of freedom is given in Table 6, where the value used is $\hat{\theta} = 0.461077$.

There is no change in the decisions one could make about the effect of time when using the unadjusted, $\hat{\theta}$, or Box conservative degrees of freedom. But the usual and $\hat{\theta}$-adjusted analyses show a strong time × treatment interaction while the Box conservative analysis does not. This example shows the importance of being able to use the appropriate adjustment in degrees of freedom to account for the case when the correlations are unequal. Any further analyses of the heart rate data should be conducted assuming that there is an important treatment × time interaction effect.

4 DETERMINING DIFFERENCES BETWEEN TREATMENTS

Once it has been determined that there are differences between the treatments and/or differences between the responses of treatments over time, one needs to determine which treatments or time intervals are different. Since there are two sizes of experimental unit, the variance of each contrast could be different since they could involve different functions of the respective error terms. There are several types of comparisons that can be used to investigate the relationships between the treatments. The variances of each type of comparison must be determined to be able to make a proper judgment about the importance of the observed values of the comparisons.

One type of comparison is to compare treatment × time means. If the levels of the treatment assigned to the subjects and/or the levels of the treatment assigned to the time intervals (which in our example are times) are quantitative, differences between the treatments can be investigated via modeling the response as a function of the levels of the treatment.

Methods for comparing the treatment $\times$ time means are discussed next, after which techniques to utilize the quantitative levels in comparing the treatments are presented. In comparing the treatment $\times$ time means, there are two types of two comparisons where only one type of comparison is appropriate for a given experiment. If there is no treatment $\times$ time interaction, the comparisons are made between the treatment means and between the time means. One would conclude that there is not treatment $\times$ time interaction if the significance level for the test for no interaction is greater than or equal to the desired significance level used to judge the treatment effects and the time effects. For example, if treatment comparisons are to be made at $\alpha = 0.05$, the interaction would be judged to be important if it is significant at an $\alpha \leq 0.05$, such as 0.05 or 0.01.

The evaluation of the variance of a comparison between time means is expedited by using the time mean model,

$$\bar{y}_{..k} = \bar{\mu}_{.k} + \bar{s}_{..} + \bar{\epsilon}_{..k}.$$

The model for the difference between the two time means, say, time 1 and time 2, is

$$\bar{y}_{..1} - \bar{y}_{..2} = \bar{\mu}_{.1} - \bar{\mu}_{.2} + \bar{\epsilon}_{..1} - \bar{\epsilon}_{..2},$$

which depends on the time-interval errors but does not depend on the subject errors. If the covariance matrix of the within-subject time-interval errors satisfy the equal correlation assumptions, the variance of the difference between two time means is $\text{var}(\bar{y}_{..1} - \bar{y}_{..2}) = 2\sigma_\epsilon^2/mn$ and the standard error of the difference is

$$\text{SE}(\bar{y}_{..1} - \bar{y}_{..2}) = \sqrt{\frac{\text{2MS Error(interval)}}{mn}}.$$

A least-significant-differences multiple comparison can be constructed to compare all time means as

$$\text{LSD}_\alpha = \text{SE}(\bar{y}_{..1} - \bar{y}_{..2})t_{\alpha/2,v},$$

where $v = m(n-1)(d-1)$ for the equal-correlation assumption, $v = \hat{\theta}m(n-1)(d-1)$ if one uses the $\hat{\theta}$ adjusted degrees of freedom, and $v = m(n-1)$ if one uses Box's conservative degrees of freedom. The notation $t_{\alpha/2,v}$ denotes the upper $\alpha/2$ percentage point of a Student's t distribution based on v degrees of freedom. The results for comparing the time heart rate means are summarized in Table 7. Since there is a significant treatment $\times$ time interaction, these comparisons would not be used.

Table 7 The Time Heart Rate Means with LSD Computations for the Equal Correlation Assumption (No Adjustment in the Degrees of Freedom)[a]

Time	N	Heart Rate
1	20	74.90
2	20	76.30
3	20	77.60
4	20	80.50
5	20	83.55
6	20	85.15
7	20	82.65

[a]Since there is a significant treatment × time interaction, these comparisons would not be used.

$$\text{LSD}_{0.05} = 1.983\sqrt{\frac{2(196.2/96)}{20}} = 0.896$$

The second method for comparing two time means is to compute $z_{ij} = y_{ij1} - y_{ij2}$, the difference between the two times for each subject and then compute the mean and the within-treatment variance of the z_{ijk}'s, that is,

$$\bar{z} = \frac{\sum_{i=1}^{m} \sum_{j=1}^{n} z_{ij}}{mn}$$

and

$$S_z^2 = \frac{\sum_{i=1}^{m} \sum_{j=1}^{n} (z_{ij} - \bar{z}_{i\cdot})^2}{m(n-1)}.$$

If one computes the variance between the z_{ij}'s without taking out the treatment effect, the resulting variance will be contaminated by an element of the treatment × time interaction. The two time means are judged to be statistically different if $|\bar{z}|/\sqrt{S_z^2/mn} > t_{\alpha/2,m(n-1)}$, where the value of $\bar{z}$ is $\bar{y}_{\cdot\cdot 1} - \bar{y}_{\cdot\cdot 2}$. The distribution of this statistic for comparing two time means computed from the differences between the times within each subject does not depend on any particular assumptions about the structure of the within-subject time-interval correlations.

In general, the experimenter can look at contrasts between the time means as

$$c_T = c_1\bar{\mu}_{\cdot 1} + c_2\bar{\mu}_{\cdot 2} + \cdots + c_d\bar{\mu}_{\cdot d},$$

where $c_1 + c_2 + \cdots + c_d = 0$. The estimate of c_T is

$$\hat{c}_T = c_1\bar{y}_{\cdot\cdot 1} + c_2\bar{y}_{\cdot\cdot 2} + \cdots + c_d\bar{y}_{\cdot\cdot d}.$$

If the usual assumption of equal-correlations is satisfied, the estimated standard error of $\hat{c}_T$ is

$$\text{SE}(\hat{c}_T) = \sqrt{\frac{\text{MS Error(interval)}}{mn}(c_1^2 + c_2^2 + \cdots + c_d^2)}.$$

A statistic to test H_0: $c_T = 0$ versus H_a: $c_T \neq 0$ is

$$t_c = \frac{|\hat{c}_T|}{\text{SE}(\hat{c}_T)},$$

which is compared to $t_{\alpha/2,m(n-1)(d-1)}$ and a $(1-\alpha)100\%$ confidence interval about c_T has endpoints

$$\hat{c}_T \pm t_{\alpha/2,v}\text{SE}(\hat{c}_T),$$

where $v = m(n-1)(d-1)$.

When the equal-correlation assumption does not hold, the t_c can be compared to $t_{\alpha/2,\hat{\theta}m(n-1)(d-1)}$ and the confidence interval would be computed as above but with $v = \hat{\theta}m(n-1)(d-1)$. The other procedure is to compute $z_{ij} = c_1y_{ij1} + c_2y_{ij2} + \cdots + c_dy_{ijd}$ for each subject and compute the mean and within-treatment variance of the z_{ij} as

$$\bar{z} = \frac{\sum_{i=1}^m \sum_{j=1}^n z_{ij}}{mn} \quad \text{and} \quad S_z^2 = \frac{\sum_{i=1}^m \sum_{j=1}^n (z_{ij} - \bar{z}_{i\cdot})^2}{m(n-1)}.$$

The value of $\bar{z}$ is $\hat{c}_T$ and the statistic to test H_0: $c_T = 0$ versus H_a: $c_T \neq 0$ is $t_c = \bar{z}/\text{SE}(\bar{z})$, where $\text{SE}(\bar{z}) = \sqrt{S_z^2/mn}$, which is compared to $t_{\alpha/2,v}$. A $(1-\alpha)100\%$ confidence interval about c has endpoints

$$\bar{z} \pm t_{\alpha/2,v}\text{SE}(\bar{z}),$$

where $v = m(n-1)$.

The variance of a comparison between treatment means is obtained from the model

$$\bar{y}_{i\cdot\cdot} = \bar{\mu}_{i\cdot} + \bar{s}_{i\cdot} + \bar{\epsilon}_{i\cdot\cdot}.$$

The model for the difference between two treatment means, say treatment 1 and treatment 2, is

$$\bar{y}_{1\cdot\cdot} - \bar{y}_{2\cdot\cdot} = \bar{\mu}_{1\cdot} - \bar{\mu}_{2\cdot} + \bar{s}_{1\cdot} - \bar{s}_{2\cdot} + \bar{\epsilon}_{1\cdot\cdot} - \bar{\epsilon}_{2\cdot\cdot}.$$

This model shows that the difference between two treatment means depends on the subject errors as well as the time-interval errors. The variance of $\bar{y}_{1..} - \bar{y}_{2..}$ is

$$\operatorname{var}(\bar{y}_{1..} - \bar{y}_{2..}) = \frac{2(\sigma_\epsilon^2 + d\sigma_s^2)}{nd}$$

and the standard error the difference is

$$\operatorname{SE}(\bar{y}_{1..} - \bar{y}_{2..}) = \sqrt{\frac{2\text{MS Error(subject)}}{nd}}.$$

An LSD multiple comparison can be computed as

$$\text{LSD}_\alpha = t_{\alpha/2,v}\text{SE}(\bar{y}_{1..} - \bar{y}_{2..})$$

and a $(1-\alpha)100\%$ confidence interval about $\bar{\mu}_{1.} - \bar{\mu}_{2.}$ has endpoints

$$\bar{y}_{1..} - \bar{y}_{2..} \pm t_{\alpha/2,v}\text{SE}(\bar{y}_{1..} - y_{2..}),$$

where $v = m(n-1)$. Fortunately, the distributions associated with these statistics are unaffected by deviations from the equal-correlation assumption for the within-subject time-interval errors. Table 8 contains the LSD computations for comparing the treatments in the heart rate example. Since there is a significant treatment $\times$ time interaction, these comparisons would not be used.

In general, a contrast between the treatment means is

$$c_{\text{treatment}} = c_1\bar{\mu}_{1.} + \cdots + c_m\bar{\mu}_{m.},$$

where $c_1 + c_2 + \cdots + c_m = 0$ and $c_{\text{treatment}}$ is estimated by

$$\hat{c}_{\text{treatment}} = c_1\bar{y}_{1..} + c_2\bar{y}_{2..} + \cdots + c_m\bar{y}_{m..}.$$

Table 8 Treatment Heart Rate Means with the LSD Computations[a]

Treatment	Means N	Heart rate
1	35	77.94
2	35	80.06
3	35	78.89
4	35	83.49

$$\text{LSD}_{0.05} = 2.12\sqrt{\frac{2(718.6/16)}{35}} = 3.396$$

[a] Since there is a significant treatment × time interaction, these comparisons would not be used.

The standard error of $\hat{c}_{\text{treatment}}$ is

$$\text{SE}(\hat{c}_{\text{treatment}}) = \sqrt{\frac{\text{MS Error(subject)}}{nd}(c_1^2 + c_2^2 + \cdots + c_m^2)}.$$

A statistic to test H_0: $c_{\text{treatment}} = 0$ versus H_a: $c_{\text{treatment}} \neq 0$ is

$$t_c = \frac{|\hat{c}_{\text{treatment}}|}{\text{SE}(\hat{c}_{\text{treatment}})},$$

which is compared to $t_{\alpha/2,v}$, where $v = m(n-1)$. A $(1-\alpha)100\%$ confidence interval about $c_{\text{treatment}}$ has endpoints

$$\hat{c}_{\text{treatment}} \pm t_{\alpha/2,v}\text{SE}(\hat{c}_{\text{treatment}}).$$

If there is a treatment × time interaction as determined by $F_{\text{treatment}\times\text{time}}$ from the analysis of variance, the needed comparisons must be made by using the treatment × time cell means.

There are two types of comparisons of interest: comparing time means within treatments and comparing treatment means within and across times. For each type of comparison, the appropriate variance must be determined. The cell mean model is

$$\bar{y}_{i\cdot k} = \mu_{ik} + \bar{s}_{i\cdot} + \bar{\epsilon}_{i\cdot k}.$$

The model to compare two time means at the same treatment, say times 1 and 2 at treatment 1, is

$$\bar{y}_{1\cdot 1} - \bar{y}_{1\cdot 2} = \mu_{11} - \mu_{12} + \bar{\epsilon}_{1\cdot 1} - \bar{\epsilon}_{1\cdot 2},$$

which does not depend on the subject errors. The standard error of this difference is

$$\text{SE}(\bar{y}_{1\cdot 1} - \bar{y}_{1\cdot 2}) = \sqrt{\frac{2\text{MS Error(interval)}}{n}}.$$

An LSD multiple comparison for comparing time means at the same treatment is

$$\text{LSD}_\alpha = t_{\alpha/2,v}\text{SE}(\bar{y}_{1\cdot 1} - \bar{y}_{1\cdot 2}),$$

where $v = m(n-1)(d-1)$. The treatment × time heart rate means are given in Table 9, where the $\text{LSD}_{0.05} = 1.793$ is used to compare time means within a given treatment.

In general, a contrast between time means within the same level of treatment, say treatment 1, is $g_1 = c_1\mu_{11} + c_2\mu_{12} + \cdots + c_d\mu_{1d}$, where $c_1 + c_2 + \cdots + c_d = 0$. The estimate of g_1 and the estimate of the standard error of $\hat{g}_1$ are

$$\hat{g}_1 = c_1\hat{y}_{1\cdot 1} + c_2\hat{y}_{1\cdot 2} + \cdots + c_d\hat{y}_{1\cdot d}$$

Table 9 The Treatment × Time Heart Rate Means with the LSD Computations for the Equal Correlation Assumption (No Adjustment in the Degrees of Freedom)

Time	N	Treatment 1	Treatment 2	Treatment 3	Treatment 4
1	5	74.8	74.4	73.4	77.0
2	5	74.0	76.0	75.0	80.2
3	5	74.0	77.0	78.0	81.4
4	5	77.4	80.8	79.8	84.0
5	5	81.0	83.8	81.0	88.4
6	5	83.2	85.2	83.0	89.2
7	5	81.2	83.2	82.0	84.2

To compare times within a given treatment: $\text{LSD}_{0.05} = 1.983\sqrt{2(196.2/96)/5} = 1.793$

To compare treatments at the same or different times: $\text{LSD}_{0.05} = 3.779$, where

$$\hat{m} = \frac{(718.6/16) + 6(196.2/96)}{7} = 8.1678$$

$$\text{SE} = \sqrt{\frac{2\hat{m}}{5}} = 1.808$$

$$t^* = \frac{2.12(718.6/16) + 1.983(6)(196.2/96)}{7(8.1678)} = 2.090$$

and

$$\text{SE}(\hat{g}_1) = \sqrt{\frac{\text{MS Error(interval)}}{n}(c_1^2 + c_2^2 + \cdots + c_d^2)}.$$

The statistic to test H_0: $g_1 = 0$ versus H_a: $g_1 \neq 0$ is

$$t_c = \frac{|\hat{g}_1|}{\text{SE}(\hat{g}_1)}$$

which is compared to $t_{\alpha/2,v}$. A $(1-\alpha)100\%$ confidence interval about g_1 has endpoints

$$\hat{g}_1 \pm t_{\alpha/2,v}\text{SE}(\hat{g}_1),$$

where $v = m(n-1)(d-1)$. The LSD value, t-test, and confidence interval above are appropriate when the time-interval errors satisfy the equal-correlation assumption, but may not be appropriate when the assumption is not satisfied. The degrees of freedom can be adjusted by $\hat{\theta}$ when $\hat{\theta}$ is less than 1. It is often of interest to compare the same contrast of the times between two levels of the treatment. The statistic is $t_c = (\hat{g}_1 - \hat{g}_2)/[\text{SE}(\hat{g})\sqrt{2}]$, which is compared to the appropriate t-distribution.

Another procedure to compare two time means at the same treatment, say time 1 and time 2 at treatment 1, is to compute $z_{1j} = y_{1j1} - y_{1j2}$, $j = 1, 2, \ldots, n$ and the mean and variance of the z_{1j} as $\bar{z}_{1\cdot}$, and

$$S^2_{(1,2)1} = \sum_{j=1}^{n} \frac{(z_{1j} - \bar{z}_{1\cdot})^2}{n-1}.$$

Under the assumption that the within-subject time-interval correlation structure is the same for all subjects, then $S^2_{(1,2)i}$, $i = 1, 2, \ldots, m$, computed for each treatment, are estimating the same variance and can be pooled to obtain $S^2_{(1,2)} = \sum_{i=j}^{m} \sum_{j=1}^{n} (z_{ij} - \bar{z}_{i\cdot})^2/m(n-1)$. An LSD for comparing time 1 to time 2 at each level of the treatment is

$$\text{LSD}_\alpha = t_{\alpha/2,v} \sqrt{\frac{2S^2_{(1,2)}}{n}} = t_{\alpha/2,v}\text{SE}(z_{12})$$

and a $(1-\alpha)100\%$ confidence interval on the difference of two time means at the ith treatment has endpoints

$$\bar{z}_{i\cdot} \pm t_{\alpha/2,v}\text{SE}(z_{12}),$$

where $v = m(n-1)$. The LSD and confidence intervals above are appropriate for any type of common correlation structure between the time-interval errors, but the variances must be computed for each pair of times to be compared. In general, a contrast of the times within each level of treatment can be investigated, where the particular contrast is computed for each subject and then compared as described above for $\mu_{11} - \mu_{12}$.

The next step in the analysis is to compare the levels of treatment at the same or different times. The model for comparing two treatment means at the same time, say, comparing treatment 1 and treatment 2 at time 1, is

$$\bar{y}_{1\cdot 1} - \bar{y}_{2\cdot 1} = \mu_{11} - \mu_{21} + \bar{s}_{1\cdot} - \bar{s}_{2\cdot} + \bar{\epsilon}_{1\cdot 1} - \bar{\epsilon}_{2\cdot 1},$$

whose variance depends on the subject errors and the time-interval errors. The variance of the difference between the two levels of treatment is

$$\text{var}(\bar{y}_{1\cdot 1} - \bar{y}_{2\cdot 1}) = \frac{2(\sigma^2_\epsilon + \sigma^2_s)}{n} = \frac{2w}{n}.$$

The estimate of $\sigma^2_\epsilon + \sigma^2_s$ is obtained by combining the two error mean squares as

$$\hat{w} = \frac{\text{MS Error(subject)} + (d-1)\text{MS Error(interval)}}{d}.$$

An LSD multiple comparison is

$$\text{LSD}_\alpha = t^*_{\alpha/2}\sqrt{\frac{2\hat{w}}{n}}.$$

The value of $t^*_{\alpha/2}$ is a weighted average of the two t-values corresponding to the degrees of freedom of the two error mean squares as

$$t^*_{\alpha/2} = \frac{t_1\text{MS Error(subject)} + t_2(d-1)\text{MS Error(interval)}}{\text{MS Error(subject)} + (d-1)\text{MS Error(interval)}},$$

where $t_1 = t_{\alpha/2,m(n-1)}$ and $t_2 = t_{\alpha/2,m(n-1)(d-1)}$. The LSD above is appropriate when the within-subject time interval errors are equally correlated. When the within-subject time interval errors are not equally correlated, the value of $t^*_{\alpha/2}$ needs to be recomputed with $t_2 = t_{\alpha/2,\hat{\theta}m(n-1)(d-1)}$.

To investigate a contrast of the levels of treatment at a given level of time, estimate the parameter $u = c_1\mu_{11} + c_2\mu_{21} + \cdots + c_m\mu_{m1}$, where $c_1 + c_2 + \cdots + c_m = 0$ as $\hat{u} = c_1\bar{y}_{1\cdot 1} + c_2\bar{y}_{2\cdot 1} + \cdots + c_m\bar{y}_{m\cdot 1}$, which has standard error

$$\text{SE}(\hat{u}) = \sqrt{\frac{\hat{w}}{n}(c_1^2 + c_2^2 + \cdots + c_m^2)}.$$

An approximate LSD multiple comparison procedure is

$$\text{LSD}_\alpha = t^*_{\alpha/2}\text{SE}(\hat{u})$$

and an approximate $(1-\alpha)100\%$ confidence interval about u has endpoints

$$\hat{u} \pm t^*_{\alpha/2}\text{SE}(\hat{u}).$$

Table 10 LSD Values for Comparing the Means in Table 7 Using the $\hat{\theta}$ Degrees of Freedom

Treatment means: unchanged

Times means: $\text{LSD}_{0.05} = 2.104\sqrt{\frac{2(196.2/96)}{20}} = 1.805$

Compare times within a treatment: $\text{LSD}_{0.05} = 2.104\sqrt{\frac{2(196.2/96)}{5}} = 1.821$

Compare treatment means at same or different times: $\text{LSD}_{0.05} = (2.097)(1.808) = 3.792$, where

$$t^* = \frac{2.12(718.6/16) + 2.014(6)(196.2/96)}{7(8.1678)} = 2.097$$

The LSD computations for comparing the treatment means at a given time or for different times for the heart rate data are presented in Table 9, where there are no adjustments in the degrees of freedom.

The $\hat{\theta}$ adjusted degrees of freedom LSD values for the heart rate data are presented in Table 10. Again only the interaction comparisons are of interest. The use of the $\hat{\theta}$ adjusted degrees of freedom provides slightly larger LSD values.

5 MODELING THE RESPONSE OF EACH TREATMENT AS A FUNCTION OF TIME

Another procedure that can be used to compare the treatments over time is to express the response as a linear model over time for each treatment and then compare the treatments by comparing characteristics of the models. This method is appropriate without the assumption of equal correlations between time-interval errors. To start, assume that the relationship between the response and time can be expressed as a simple linear regression for each treatment:

$$y_{ijk} = \alpha_{ij} + \beta_{ij}T_k + s_{ij} + \epsilon_{ijk},$$

where $i = 1, 2, \ldots, m$, $j = 1, 2, \ldots, n$, $k = 1, 2, \ldots, d$, T_k denotes the kth time, s_{ij} denotes the subject errors, ϵ_{ijk} denotes the time-interval errors, and α_{ij} and β_{ij} denote the intercept and slope of the regression line for the jth subject of the ith treatment. The procedure is to use ordinary least squares to fit the model above to the data from each subject to obtain $(\hat{\alpha}_{ij}, \hat{\beta}_{ij})$, $i = 1, 2, \ldots, m$, $j = 1, 2, \ldots, n$. A one-way analysis of variance can be used to compare the intercepts and compare the slopes through the models

$$\hat{\alpha}_{ij} = \phi_i + e_{ij} \qquad \text{and} \qquad \hat{\beta}_{ij} = \pi_i + r_{ij},$$

where the variances of the e_{ij}'s are equal and the variances of the r_{ij}'s are equal. A test of H_0: $\pi_1 = \pi_2 = \cdots = \pi_m$ versus H_a: (not H_0) is a test of the hypothesis of no treatment $\times$ time interaction, given that the relationship between the response and the time is linear. If the lines are parallel (i.e., if the slopes are equal), a test of H_0: $\phi_1 = \phi_2 = \cdots = \phi_m$ versus H_a: (not H_0) is a test of equal treatment effects.

Any linear model can be used to describe the relationship between the response and time where the model is fit to the data for each subject and then the estimates of the parameters are compared through a one-way ANOVA model in order to compare the treatments (Allen, 1983; Allen et al., 1983). The important points to remember are: (1) for this method to be effective the same functional form of the linear model must adequately describe the relationship between the response and time for all treatments, and (2) this method is appropriate without the equal-correlation assumption on the within-subject interval errors. A plot of the heart rate data treatment $\times$ time means is provided in Figure 1.

For the heart rate data, a cubic polynomial function of time is adequate to describe the heart rates for each subject. The model is

$$y_{ijk} = \alpha_{ij} + \beta_{1ij}T_k + \beta_{2ij}T_k^2 + \beta_{3ij}T_k^3 + s_{ij} + \epsilon_{ijk}.$$

The ordinary least squares estimates of the parameters are obtained for each subject and one-way ANOVA models are used to compare the treat-

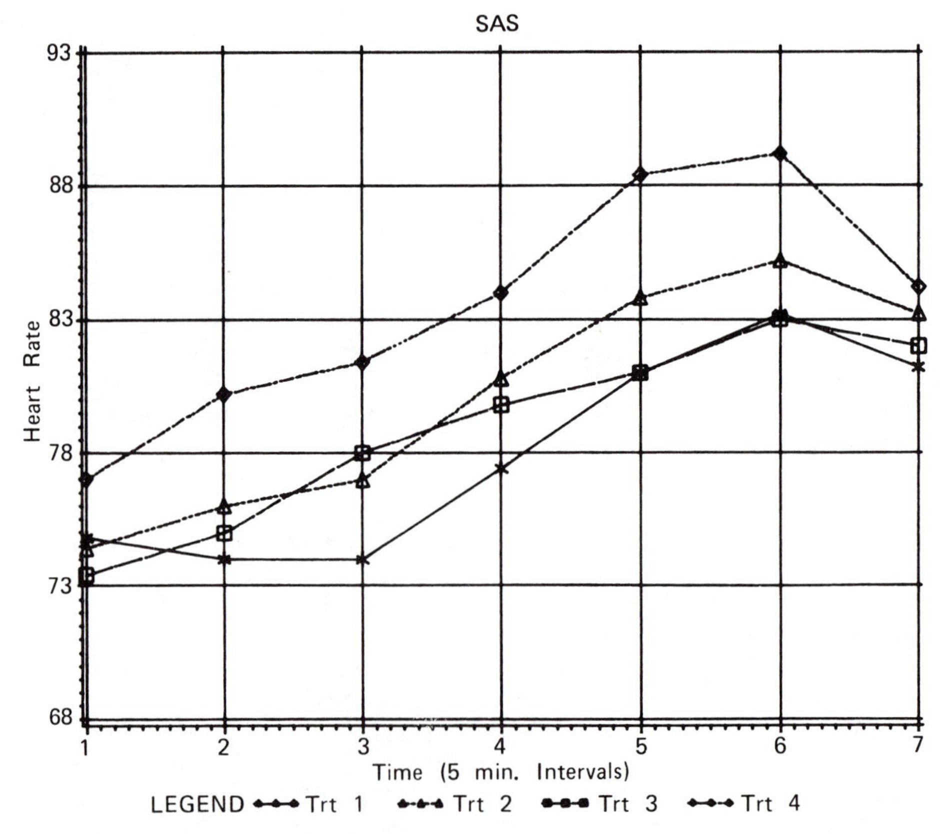

Figure 1 Treatment effect on heart rate over time.

ments, for example,

$$\hat{\alpha}_{ij} = \phi_i + e_{ij}, \qquad \text{where } e_{ij} \sim \text{iid}\, N(0, \sigma_e^2),$$

$$\hat{\beta}_{1ij} = \pi_{1i} + r_{1ij}, \qquad \text{where } r_{1ij} \sim \text{iid}\, N(0, \sigma_{r_1}^2),$$

$$\hat{\beta}_{2ij} = \pi_{2i} + r_{2ij}, \qquad \text{where } r_{2ij} \sim \text{iid}\, N(0, \sigma_{r_2}^2),$$

$$\hat{\beta}_{3ij} = \pi_{3i} + r_{3ij}, \qquad \text{where } r_{3ij} \sim \text{iid}\, N(0, \sigma_{r_3}^2).$$

Figure 2 provides a plot of the estimated cubic polynomial regression model for the four treatments of the heart rate example.

The treatment × time interaction is partitioned into three parts as

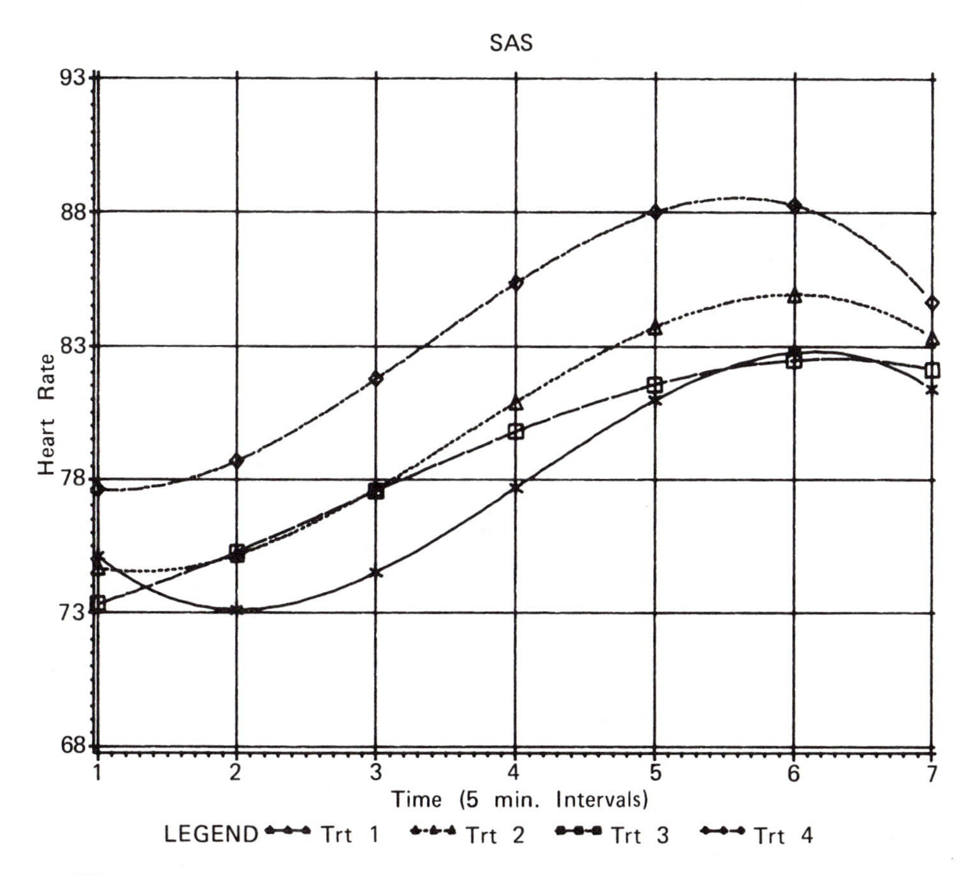

Figure 2 Estimated cubic polynomial models for the treatments.

a. H_{01}: $\pi_{11} = \pi_{12} = \cdots = \pi_{1m}$ versus H_{a1}: (not H_{01})
b. H_{02}: $\pi_{21} = \pi_{22} = \cdots = \pi_{2m}$ versus H_{a2}: (not H_{02})
c. H_{03}: $\pi_{31} = \pi_{32} = \cdots = \pi_{3m}$ versus H_{a3}: (not H_{03})

There is no treatment × time interaction given that the cubic relationship is adequate if H_{01}, H_{02}, and H_{03} are true. The usefulness of this modeling procedure is that the form of the relationship between time and the response can be modeled and interpreted. This method could provide more meaningful interpretations than the methods using multiple comparisons at each time interval.

The cubic polynomial regression model was fit to each subject's data and the ordinary least squares estimates of the model's parameters are given in Table 11, where intercept denotes the $\hat{\alpha}_{ij}$'s, time 1 denotes the $\hat{\beta}_{1ij}$'s, time 2 denotes the $\hat{\beta}_{2ij}$'s, and time 3 denotes the $\hat{\beta}_{3ij}$'s. These estimated parameters were analyzed to compare the treatments via the

Table 11 Estimates of the Parameters of the Cubic Model Fit to Each Subject's Heart Rate Data

Treatment	Subject	Time 1	Time 2	Time 3	Intercept
1	1	−4.464	1.86905	−0.16667	76.0000
1	2	−12.885	3.95238	−0.30556	87.8571
1	3	−7.167	2.79762	−0.25000	77.7143
1	4	−13.254	3.94048	−0.30556	84.8571
1	5	−12.643	4.09524	−0.33333	84.2857
2	1	−1.433	1.35714	−0.13889	72.2857
2	2	−7.845	2.90476	−0.25000	82.4286
2	3	−2.000	1.69048	−0.16667	72.5714
2	4	−3.881	1.80952	−0.16667	79.8571
2	5	−8.246	3.19048	−0.27778	79.7143
3	1	0.139	0.44048	−0.05556	78.4286
3	2	−0.714	0.84524	−0.08333	73.2857
3	3	0.714	0.70238	−0.08333	66.1429
3	4	−1.746	1.28571	−0.11111	75.8571
3	5	5.083	−0.41667	−0.00000	67.0000
4	1	−4.000	2.46429	−0.25000	80.4286
4	2	−6.972	3.03571	−0.27778	83.0000
4	3	−6.060	2.61905	−0.25000	82.2857
4	4	−4.817	2.76190	−0.27778	74.0000
4	5	−1.179	1.44048	−0.16667	80.2857

Table 12 ANOVA Table to Compare Treatments for the Coefficients of the Cubic Polynomial Regression Models

Source	d.f.	Sum of squares	F-value	Pr > F
		Dependent variable: intercept		
Treatment	3	279.16	4.19	0.0229
Error	16	355.66		
		Dependent variable: time 1		
Treatment	3	290.43	10.12	0.0006
Error	16	153.02		
		Dependent variable: time 2		
Treatment	3	19.93	11.25	0.0003
Error	16	9.45		
		Dependent variable: time 3		
Treatment	3	0.1245	13.97	0.0001
Error	16	0.0475		0.0030

one-way ANOVA model and the results are presented in Table 12. The intercept is a comparison of the treatments, but instead of comparing them at the average time, it is a comparison at time = 0. These effects are compared via the LSD multiple comparison procedure and the results are shown in Table 13. The time 1, time 2, and time 3 effects are part of the treatment × time interaction comparisons.

To be complete, the final method involves comparing the treatments through any meaningful linear combination of the time means within a treatment, as $\phi_i = a_1\mu_{i1} + a_2\mu_{i2} + \cdots + a_d\mu_{id}$. The procedure is to compute the linear combination of the observations of each subject and compare those values via a one-way ANOVA model. Let

$$x_{ij} = a_1 y_{ij1} + a_2 y_{ij2} + \cdots + a_d y_{ijd}, \qquad i = 1, 2, \cdots, m, \quad j = 1, 2, \cdots, n.$$

The one-way ANOVA model is

$$x_{ij} = \phi_i + u_{ij},$$

Table 13 Treatment Multiple Comparisons for the Intercept, Linear, Quadratic, and Cubic Coefficients of the Cubic Polynomial Regression Models Fit to the Heart Rate Data

Grouping			Mean[a]	N	Treatment
LSD for the intercept: $\alpha = 0.05$, d.f. = 16, MSE = 22.2286, LSD = 6.32124					
		A	82.143	5	1
		A	80.000	5	4
	B	A	77.371	5	2
	B		72.143	5	3
LSD for coefficients of time 1: $\alpha = 0.05$, d.f. = 16, MSE = 9.56366, LSD = 4.14628					
		A	0.695	5	3
	B		−4.606	5	4
	B		−4.681	5	2
C			−10.083	5	1
LSD for coefficients of time 2: $\alpha = 0.05$, d.f. = 16, MSE = 0.590391, LSD = 1.03019					
		A	3.3310	5	1
	B	A	2.4643	5	4
	B		2.1905	5	2
C			0.5714	5	3
LSD for coefficients of time 3: $\alpha = 0.05$, d.f. = 16, MSE = 0.0029707, LSD = 0.0730759					
		A	−0.06667	5	3
	B		−0.20000	5	2
	B		−0.24444	5	4
	B		−0.27222	5	1

[a]Means with the same letter are not significantly different.

Table 14 Sum, Linear, Quadratic, and Cubic Orthogonal Polynomials Computed for Each Subject Within Each Treatment for the Heart Rate Example

Treatment	Subject	Sum	Linear	Quad	Cubic
1	1	538	37	−11	−6
1	2	568	54	24	−11
1	3	539	41	−17	−9
1	4	535	41	23	−11
1	5	548	50	8	−12
2	6	547	50	−26	−5
2	7	568	46	−8	−9
2	8	558	66	−26	−6
2	9	573	40	−16	−6
2	10	556	56	−12	−10
3	11	571	17	−19	−2
3	12	546	41	−13	−3
3	13	516	49	−25	−3
3	14	575	68	−4	−4
3	15	553	49	−35	0
4	16	600	55	−45	−9
4	17	593	57	−25	−10
4	18	577	32	−32	−9
4	19	552	56	−48	−10
4	20	600	33	−47	−6

where the variances of the u_{ij}'s are equal. If the a_k's are such that $a_1 + a_2 + \cdots + a_k = 0$, analysis of the ϕ_i's is a comparison of the treatment × time interaction effects.

To demonstrate this procedure, the linear combinations corresponding to the (1) sum, (2) linear, (3) quadratic, and (4) cubic orthogonal polynomials for the seven equally spaced time intervals were computed for each subject and analyzed via a one-way ANOVA model.

The values the orthogonal polynomials computed from the data of each subject are shown in Table 14. The orthogonal polynomial values were analyzed via a one-way ANOVA procedure and the analyses are summarized in Table 15. The analysis on sum is equivalent to the comparison

Table 15 ANOVA Tables to Compare Treatments for the Sum, Linear, Quadratic, and Cubic Orthogonal Polynimial Effects for the Heart Rate Example

Source	d.f.	Sum of squares	F-value	Pr > F
		Dependent variable: sum		
Treatment	3	4310.15	4.57	0.0170
Error	16	5030.40		
		Dependent variable: linear		
Treatment	3	159.40	0.32	0.8078
Error	16	2622.40		
		Dependent variable: quad		
Treatment	3	5033.80	10.02	0.0006
Error	16	2678.40		
		Dependent variable: cubic		
Treatment	3	161.35	13.97	0.0001
Error	16	61.60		

of treatments and the analyses on the linear, quad, and cubic variables investigates the treatment × time interaction. These effects are compared via the LSD multiple comparison procedure and the results are given in Table 16. Again, these comparisons are valid even if the equal correlation assumption between time intervals is violated. Analyses of time 1 and time 2 from the polynomial regression model provide results different from those of analyses of linear and quad since the linear and quad effects are computed sequentially whereas time 1 and time 2 are adjusted for all effects in the model. The analyses of time 3 and cubic are identical.

Table 16 Treatment Multiple Comparisons for the Sum, Linear, Quadratic, and Cubic Orthogonal Polynomial Effects for the Heart Rate Example

Grouping	Mean[a]	N	Treatment
LSD for sum: $\alpha = 0.05$, d.f. $= 16$, MSE $= 314.4$, LSD $= 23.7732$			
A	584.4	5	4
B	560.4	5	2
B	552.2	5	3
B	545.6	5	1
LSD for linear: $\alpha = 0.05$, d.f. $= 16$, MSE $= 163.9$, LSD $= 17.1647$			
A	51.6	5	2
A	46.6	5	4
A	44.8	5	3
A	44.6	5	1
LSD for quad: $\alpha = 0.05$, d.f. $= 16$, MSE $= 167.4$, LSD $= 17.347$			
A	5.4	5	1
B	−17.6	5	2
B	−19.2	5	3
C	−39.4	5	4
LSD for cubic: $\alpha = 0.05$, d.f. $= 16$, MSE $= 3.85$, LSD $= 2.63073$			
A	−2.4	5	3
B	−7.2	5	2
B	−8.8	5	4
B	−9.8	5	1

[a]Means with the same letter are not significantly different.

6 EXAMPLE 2. GROWING COOKIES

The process of cookie development during baking is influenced by the type of flour and sweetener used to make the cookie dough (Doescher, 1986). The cookie gradually grows in diameter during baking until it reaches its maximum diameter. The rates the cookies grow were of interest in this study. The data in Table 17 represent the measured growth of three cookies per product, where the diameter of each cookie was measured every minute starting at zero time for 6 minutes. Each cookie of each product was independently formulated (i.e., the three cookies were not from the same batch). But the measurements over time are repeated measures on the same cookies.

Table 18 is the analysis of variance for the usual assumptions where Table 19 is the analysis using the Box conservative degrees of freedom. In Table 19, only those sources of variation associated with the repeated measures were divided by 6, the number of repeated measures minus one.

Table 20 is the matrix of variances and covariances of the within-cookie time-interval error which were used to compute $\hat{\theta} = 0.496769$. Table 21 is the analysis of variance based on the $\hat{\theta}$ adjusted degrees of freedom. Since there is a significant product × time interaction, the multiple comparisons in Table 22 were computed using the $\hat{\theta}$ adjusted degrees of freedom. The time and product means are included for completeness, but the multiple comparison would not be used because of the significant interaction.

The multiple comparisons in Table 22 are interesting, but they do not answer directly the question associated with comparing rates of growth. On plotting the data, one sees that the growth of the cookies in the interval 0 to 6 minutes is quite linear. Figure 3 contains the plot of the time means for each treatment. Thus one would want to compare the slopes of the growth lines. Since the data involve repeated measures, a simple linear regression model was fit to the data for each cookie where the ordinary least squares estimates of the slope and intercept of each line were obtained. Table 23 contain the respective slopes and intercepts. Figure 4 is a graph of the estimated regression lines for each product.

Proceeding as in the preceding section, these slopes and intercepts were subjected to one-way analyses of variance which are summarized in Table 24.

The analyses indicate that there are no significant differences between the intercepts (at $\alpha = 0.05$, i.e., the technician was successful in making the cookies the same size) but that there are significant differences between the slopes or rates of cookie growth.

Table 25 contains the product means for the slopes and intercepts with the corresponding LSD computations. Since there is no significant differ-

Table 17 Diameters (mm) for the Growing Cookie Experiment[a]

Run	Time 0	Time 1	Time 2	Time 3	Time 4	Time 5	Time 6
			Product = Control				
1	62.10	63.08	66.99	72.86	76.28	80.68	85.57
2	61.72	62.21	67.31	72.90	76.79	79.95	84.08
3	61.98	63.19	67.59	74.18	78.08	81.74	85.89
			Product = Fructose syrup				
1	59.41	63.78	67.66	72.51	77.36	79.78	80.75
2	60.62	62.31	66.65	72.21	76.79	79.93	82.11
3	60.62	62.31	67.39	72.69	78.00	81.14	82.83
			Product = Glucose syrup				
1	59.65	62.08	65.47	70.81	76.14	80.02	81.96
2	61.34	63.27	66.17	70.76	76.55	80.90	82.35
3	61.23	62.92	68.00	74.29	78.89	82.04	83.97
			Product = Hard wheat				
1	60.61	62.05	65.42	70.71	74.79	76.96	78.40
2	60.94	62.62	65.49	71.19	74.57	77.44	79.35
3	61.74	63.21	67.13	72.52	76.19	79.13	81.83
			Product = Sucrose syrup				
1	62.02	63.19	68.07	72.96	78.81	83.94	87.59
2	60.98	61.47	64.85	71.15	77.20	82.28	87.36
3	60.11	61.79	65.14	71.13	76.88	81.91	85.50

[a] "Run" denotes an independent observation of the product, which is a cookie, and "time i" denotes the diameter at time i = minutes of baking.

Table 18 ANOVA Table of the Cookie Diameters for the Repeated-Measures Model and the Equal Correlation Between the Time-Interval Assumptions

Source	Unadjusted d.f.	Sum of squares	F-value	$\Pr > F$
Product	4	57.78	2.78	0.0867
Error(cookie)	10	52.03		
Time	6	6926.92	3513.28	0.0001
Product × time	24	97.25	12.33	0.0001
Error(interval)	60	19.72		

Table 19 ANOVA Table of the Cookie Diameters for the Repeated-Measures Model and the Box Conservative Correction on the Degrees of Freedom

Source	Box adjusted d.f.	Sum of squares	F-value	Pr > F
Product	4	57.78	2.78	0.0867
Error(cookie)	10	52.03		
Time	1	6926.92	3513.28	0.0001
Product × time	4	97.25	12.33	0.0007
Error(interval)	10	19.72		

Table 20 Between Time-Interval Variances and Covariances with the Computation of $\hat{\theta}$ for the Cookie Diameter Data

	R0	R1	R2	R3	R4	R5	R6
R0	0.2153	0.0595	−0.0777	−0.1434	−0.0919	−0.00316	0.0415
R1	0.0595	0.3387	0.0332	−0.1141	−0.0819	−0.0495	−0.1860
R2	−0.0777	0.0332	0.1668	0.0530	0.0374	−0.0419	−0.1708
R3	−0.1435	−0.1141	0.0530	0.1844	0.0934	−0.0279	−0.0455
R4	−0.0919	−0.0819	0.0374	0.0934	0.1051	−0.0016	−0.0605
R5	−0.0032	−0.0495	−0.0419	−0.0279	−0.0016	0.0504	0.0738
R6	0.0415	−0.1860	−0.1708	−0.0455	−0.0605	0.0738	0.3476

$$\bar{v} = 0.201188, \qquad \sum_{k=1}^{7}\sum_{k'=1}^{7} v_{kk'}^2 = 0.665418, \qquad \hat{\theta} = 0.496769$$

Table 21 ANOVA Table of the Cookie Diameter Data for the Repeated-Measures Model and the $\hat{\theta}$ Adjusted Degrees of Freedom where $\hat{\theta} = 0.497$

Source	$\hat{\theta}$ adjusted d.f.	Sum of squares	F-value	Pr > F
Product	4	57.78	2.78	0.0867
Error(cookie)	10	52.03		
Time	2.98	6926.92	3513.28	0.0001
Product × time	11.92	97.25	12.33	0.0001
Error(interval)	29.81	19.72		

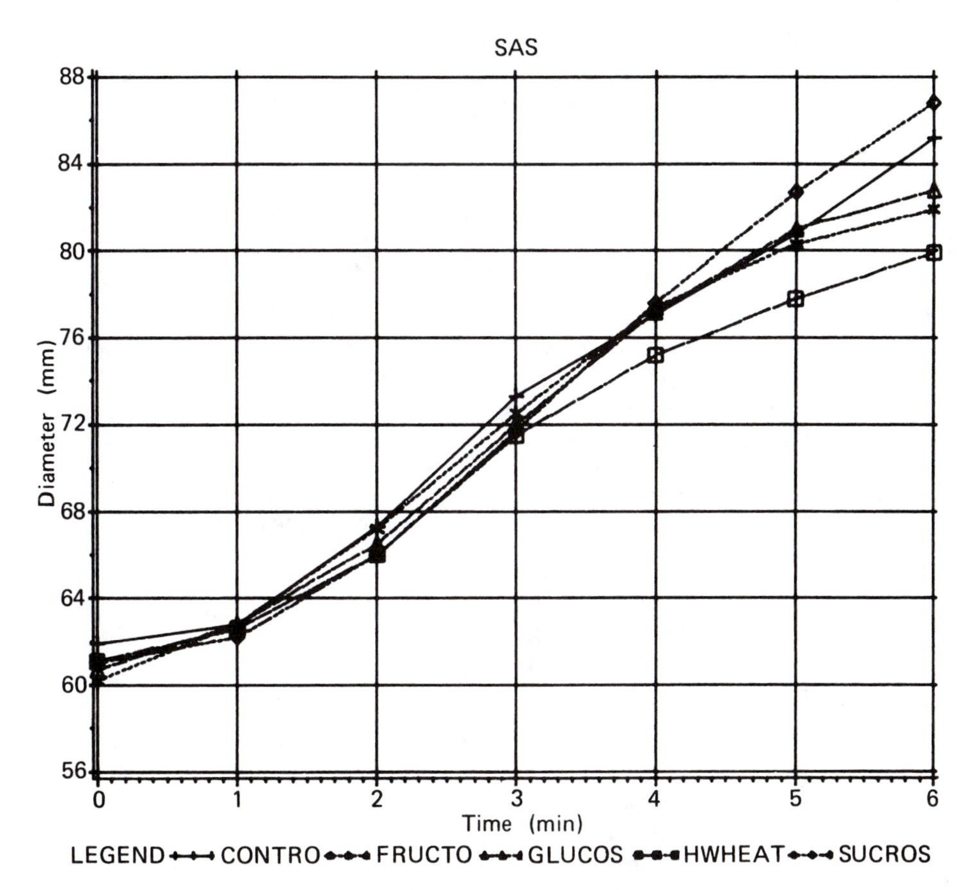

Figure 3 Product effect on diameter over time.

Table 22 Product and Time Means with the LSD Computations[a]

Grouping							Mean[b]	N	Product
LSD for cookie diameter: $\alpha = 0.05$, d.f. = 10, MSE = 5.20311, LSD = 1.56848									
						A	72.627	21	Control
						A	72.587	21	Sucrose syrup
					B	A	71.848	21	Glucose syrup
					B	A	71.755	21	Fructose syrup
					B		70.585	21	Hard wheat

Grouping							Mean[b]	N	Product
LSD for cookie diameter: $\alpha = 0.05$, d.f. = 29.8, MSE = 0.328607, LSD = 0.427426									
						A	83.303	15	6
					B		80.523	15	5
				C			76.888	15	4
			D				72.191	15	3
		E					66.622	15	2
	F						62.632	15	1
G							61.005	15	0

[a]The product and the time LSD comparisons are included for completeness, but they are not be to used because of the presence of product × time interaction.
[b]Means with the same letter are not significantly different.
Compare two time means at the same product $LSD_{0.05} = 2.042\sqrt{2(19.7164/60)/3} = 0.95575$.
To compare two product means at the same or different times:

$$\hat{w} = \frac{52.03/10 + 6(19.7164)/60}{7} = 1.0249$$

$$t^* = \frac{(2.228)(52.03)/10 + 2.042(6)(19.7164)/60}{7.17464} = 2.177$$

$$LSD_{0.05} = 2.177\sqrt{\frac{2(1.0249)}{3}} = 1.799$$

Table 22 (*Continued*)

Cell Means

		Product				
Time	N	Control	Fructose syrup	Glucose syrup	Hard wheat	Sucrose syrup
0	3	61.933	60.217	60.740	61.097	61.037
1	3	62.827	62.800	62.757	62.627	62.150
2	3	67.297	67.233	66.547	66.013	66.020
3	3	73.313	72.470	71.953	71.473	71.747
4	3	77.050	77.383	77.193	75.183	77.630
5	3	80.790	80.283	80.987	77.843	82.710
6	3	85.180	81.897	82.760	79.860	86.817

Table 23 Ordinary Least Squares Estimates of the Parameters of the Linear Regression Model Fit to Each Cookie (Run) of Each Product

Product	Run	Slope	Intercept
Control	1	4.10357	60.1979
	2	4.00143	60.1329
	3	4.26143	60.4514
Fructose syrup	1	3.77571	60.2800
	2	3.92321	59.7475
	3	4.10357	59.8293
Glucose syrup	1	4.05286	58.7171
	2	3.88107	59.9768
	3	4.19107	60.4754
Hard wheat	1	3.30571	59.9314
	2	3.35536	60.1625
	3	3.61321	60.8389
Sucrose syrup	1	4.60536	59.9811
	2	4.75393	57.9225
	3	4.57679	58.0496

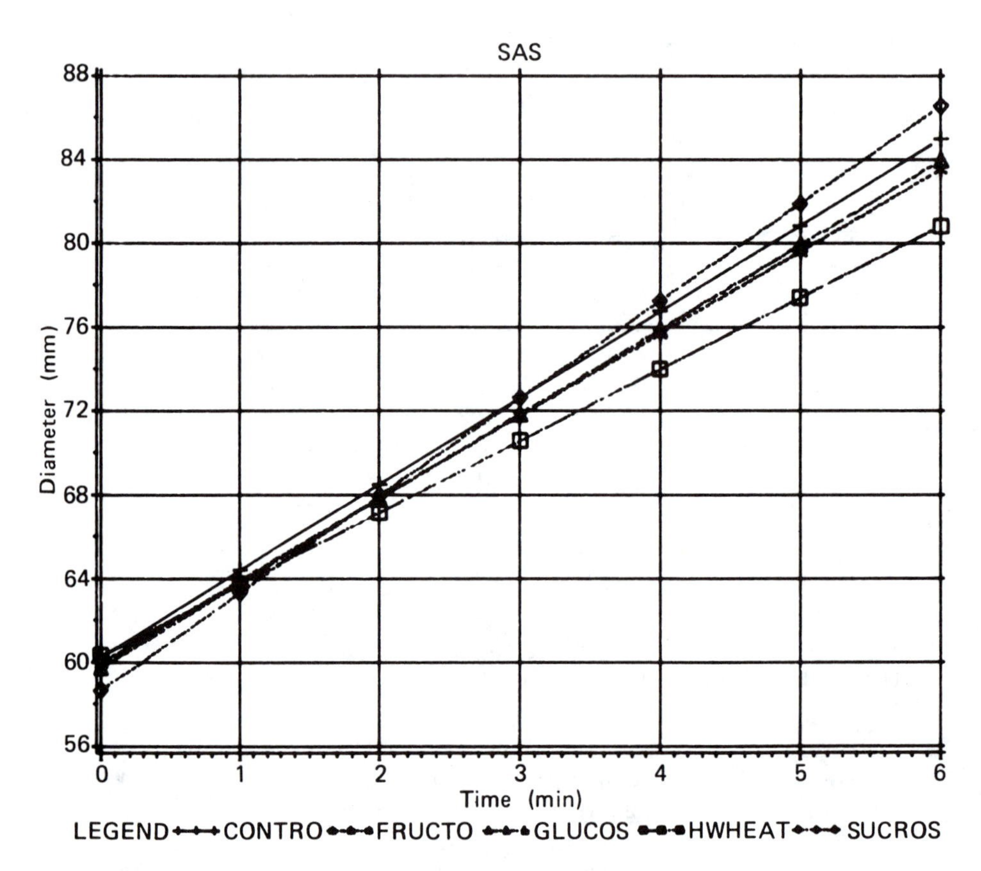

Figure 4 Estimated regression lines for the cookie products.

Table 24 ANOVA Tables for Comparing the Slopes and Intercepts of the Products

Source	d.f.	Sum of squares	F-value	Pr > F
		Dependent variable: slope		
Product	4	2.288	27.36	0.0001
Error	10	0.209		
		Dependent variable: intercept		
Product	4	5.461	2.75	0.0888
Error	10	4.970		

Table 25 Multiple Comparisons of the Products for the Slopes and Intercepts

Grouping	Mean[a]	N	Product
LSD for the slopes: $\alpha = 0.05$, d.f. = 10, MSE = .0209074, LSD = 0.263055			
A	4.6454	3	Sucrose syrup
B	4.1221	3	Control
B	4.0417	3	Glucose syrup
B	3.9342	3	Fructose syrup
C	3.4248	3	Hard wheat
LSD for the intercepts: $\alpha = 0.05$, d.f. = 10, MSE = 0.49696, LSD = 1.2825			
A	60.311	3	Hard wheat
A	60.261	3	Control
A	59.952	3	Fructose syrup
B A	59.723	3	Glucose syrup
B	58.651	3	Sucrose syrup

[a]Means with the same letter are not significantly different.

ence between the products for intercepts, the intercept LSD would not be used for multiple comparisons [see Milliken and Johnson (1984), Chap. 3)].

REFERENCES

Allen, O. B. (1983). A guide to the analysis of growth curve data with special reference to SAS. *Comput. Biomed. Res. 16*, 101.

Allen, O. B., J. H. Burton, and J. D. Holt (1983). Analysis of repeated measurements from animal experiments using polynomial regression. *J. Anim. Sci. 57*, 765–770.

Box, G. E. P. (1954). Some theorems on quadratic forms applied in the study of analysis of variance problems. *Ann. Math. Statist. 25*, 290–302.

Doescher, L. (1986). Ph.D dissertation. Department of Grain Science and Industry, Kansas State University, Manhattan.

Huynh, H., and L. S. Feldt (1970). Conditions under which mean square ratios in repeated measures designs have exact F-distributions. *J. Amer. Statist. Assoc. 65*, 1582–1589.

Milliken, G. A., and D. E. Johnson (1984). *Analysis of Messy Data, Vol. I: Designed Experiments.* Van Nostrand Reinhold, New York.

4

Dose-Response: Relating Doses and Plasma Levels to Efficacy and Adverse Experiences

BRUCE P. EKHOLM and TERRANCE L. FOX 3M/Riker, 3M Health Care, St. Paul, Minnesota

JAMES A. BOLOGNESE Merck Sharp & Dohme Research Laboratories, Rahway, New Jersey

1 INTRODUCTION

A physician prescribing a drug for a particular patient must know how much the patient should take, how often, and for how long. Regulatory agencies properly insist that pharmaceutical companies study exhaustively the efficacy and safety aspects of various dosing regimens. The company must answer these questions, among others:

1. What type of response (safety and efficacy) can be expected as a function of dose?
2. What dose and dosing frequency is recommended?
3. How do the answers to these questions depend on the patient's characteristics (age, sex, weight, severity of disease, etc.)?

As indicated in Chapter 1, these questions are addressed during the entire clinical development of a drug. But these questions must be, at least tentatively, answered early in the process so that the rest of the development can proceed.

In this chapter we focus on phase 1 and 2 dose-response studies. Of special interest are the range of doses that are required to achieve a desired effect, and the range of doses associated with limiting side effects. Obviously, the closer these ranges are to each other, the more difficult it will be to use the drug and the less attractive the drug will be.

Interpreting and analyzing dose-response data are made difficult by small sample sizes, inefficient designs, missing data, multiple observations per patient, and outlying observations. We do not address all of these issues—some are discussed in other chapters. We focus on experimental design and on some methods of analysis and display of dose-response data.

2 DESIGNS OF DOSE-RESPONSE STUDIES

Dose-response studies must be designed to minimize the variability due to different patient and disease characteristics. Also, ethical considerations, such as not exposing patients to high doses of an untested drug, must be taken into account.

In early clinical studies, the choice of doses is based on animal models on a milligram per kilogram basis. Usually, a placebo is included as well as at least one dose that is believed to be too low to be effective. At the other extreme, at least one dose that is believed to be too high to add any further efficacy is included, although ethical considerations must be taken into account. If the dose-response is believed to be additive, the doses studied should increase arithmetically, such as 0, 100, 200, 300. If the response is believed to be multiplicative, the doses studied should increase geometrically, such as 0, 10, 20, 40, 80, and 160. These are equally spaced on a log scale.

2.1 Fixed-Sequence Rising-Dose Design

In a fixed-sequence rising-dose design, each patient receives all doses in sequence (Table 1). Placebo is often inserted in sequences, and ideally should be balanced with period. Washout between dosing periods must be long enough for any comparisons between doses to be valid. This design is frequently used early in the clinical program, especially when ethical considerations prohibit giving patients a high dose of a drug when it is not known whether they can tolerate lower doses. A disadvantage of this design is that dose effect is confounded with period effect.

Table 1 Example of a Fixed-Sequence Rising-Dose Design

Patient	Period 1	Period 2	Period 3	Period 4	Period 5
1	Dose 1	Placebo	Dose 2	Dose 3	Dose 4
2	Dose 1	Dose 2	Dose 3	Placebo	Dose 4
3	Placebo	Dose 1	Dose 2	Dose 3	Dose 4
4	Dose 1	Dose 2	Dose 3	Dose 4	Placebo
5	Dose 1	Dose 2	Placebo	Dose 3	Dose 4
6	Dose 1	Placebo	Dose 2	Dose 3	Dose 4
7	Dose 1	Dose 2	Dose 3	Dose 4	Placebo
8	Dose 1	Dose 2	Placebo	Dose 3	Dose 4
9	Dose 1	Dose 2	Dose 3	Placebo	Dose 4
10	Placebo	Dose 1	Dose 2	Dose 3	Dose 4

2.2 Rising-Dose Titration Design

In a titration design, patients start with a fixed low dose and are then titrated upward until a specified response is obtained. This design is closer to actual clinical practice. This type of design may also be able to include a broader range of doses. However, one must guard against overinterpretation of the data derived from these studies because of the confounding with time. Also, because they are not usually blinded, some investigators cannot resist the temptation to ignore or change the dose titration rules rather than follow the protocol.

In the example in Table 2, patient 4 responded at dose 1; patient 1 at dose 2; patients 2, 3, and 9 at dose 3; patients 5, 7, and 8 at dose 4; and patients 6 and 10 either did not respond at any dose or responded at dose 5. For the duration of the trial, the patients are kept at the same dose at which they responded. This gives information about reproducibility and guards against the regression effect (see Chapter 1).

2.3 Crossover Designs

Crossover dose-response studies are usually Latin square or balanced incomplete block designs; Table 3 gives an example of the former, balanced for carryover effects. If the assumptions underlying a crossover design can be met (see Chapter 8), these designs are usually the most powerful for estimating dose-response characteristics.

Table 2 Example of a Titration Design

Patient	Period 1	Period 2	Period 3	Period 4	Period 5
1	Dose 1	Dose 2	Dose 2	Dose 2	Dose 2
2	Dose 1	Dose 2	Dose 3	Dose 3	Dose 3
3	Dose 1	Dose 2	Dose 3	Dose 3	Dose 3
4	Dose 1	Dose 1	Dose 1	Dose 1	Dose 1
5	Dose 1	Dose 2	Dose 3	Dose 4	Dose 4
6	Dose 1	Dose 2	Dose 3	Dose 4	Dose 5
7	Dose 1	Dose 2	Dose 3	Dose 4	Dose 4
8	Dose 1	Dose 2	Dose 3	Dose 4	Dose 4
9	Dose 1	Dose 2	Dose 3	Dose 3	Dose 3
10	Dose 1	Dose 2	Dose 3	Dose 4	Dose 5

2.4 Parallel Designs

If the underlying disease state is not present long enough for a multiperiod study, a parallel design must be used. In the usual parallel design, equal numbers of patients are randomized to each of the dose groups being studied.

Table 3 Example of a Latin Square Crossover Design Balanced for Carryover Effects

Patient	Period 1	Period 2	Period 3	Period 4	Period 5	Period 6
1	Dose 6	Dose 5	Dose 4	Dose 3	Dose 2	Dose 1
2	Dose 2	Dose 4	Dose 6	Dose 1	Dose 3	Dose 5
3	Dose 4	Dose 1	Dose 5	Dose 2	Dose 6	Dose 3
4	Dose 2	Dose 4	Dose 6	Dose 1	Dose 3	Dose 5
5	Dose 6	Dose 5	Dose 4	Dose 3	Dose 2	Dose 1
6	Dose 1	Dose 2	Dose 3	Dose 4	Dose 5	Dose 6
7	Dose 3	Dose 6	Dose 2	Dose 5	Dose 1	Dose 4
8	Dose 5	Dose 3	Dose 1	Dose 6	Dose 4	Dose 2
9	Dose 3	Dose 6	Dose 2	Dose 5	Dose 1	Dose 4
10	Dose 5	Dose 3	Dose 1	Dose 6	Dose 4	Dose 2
11	Dose 1	Dose 2	Dose 3	Dose 4	Dose 5	Dose 6
12	Dose 4	Dose 1	Dose 5	Dose 2	Dose 6	Dose 3

Table 4 Example of a Parallel Design with Several Hypotheses

Dose group	Period 0 (baseline)	Period 1 (parallel dose-response)	Period 2	Period 3	Within-group objective
1	Placebo	Placebo	40 mg QPM[a]	20 mg BID[b]	QPM vs. BID vs. placebo
2	Placebo	5 mg BID	40 mg QPM	20 mg QPM	20 vs. 40 mg once a day
3	Placebo	10 mg BID	20 mg BID	40 mg BID	Dose-response
4	Placebo	20 mg BID	20 mg BID	20 mg BID	Multiple dose effect of 20 mg BID
5	Placebo	40 mg BID	Placebo	20 mg QPM	Rebound (drug withdrawal effect)

[a]QPM indicates "quaque post meridiam" (once daily with the evening meal).
[b]BID indicates "bis in die" (twice a day).

Designs with parallel aspects can be used to test multiple hypotheses within the same study. For example, Table 4 (Lovastatin Study Group II) uses a parallel design to compare the effects of placebo, 5 mg BID, 10 mg BID, 20 mg BID, and 40 mg BID in period 1. Each dose group is also used to test a different hypothesis using the results from periods 1, 2, and 3.

2.5 Up-and-Down Designs

The up-and-down design is a sequential type of design that assigns each patient's dose based on the previous patient's dose and response. The dose is increased one level if the previous patient did not respond. The dose is decreased one level if the previous patient did respond. The usual increment (decrement) is a twofold increase (decrease) from one dose to the next (Bolognese, 1983).

2.6 Separate Studies in Different Classes of Patients

Patient characteristics may modify the effect of a drug. Some characteristics, such as a drug allergy or a serious adverse experience, may preclude safe use of a drug in such patients. Other factors may produce changes in the usual effects of the drug which can be offset by a dosage adjustment. For example, elderly patients often have an impaired ability to process a drug, while children may be more sensitive to a drug than adults. Therefore, it is important to carry out different studies in various subgroups of the target population (cf. Chapter 1).

3 EVALUATION OF DOSE-RESPONSE DATA

After the data have been collected, the statistician should describe a dose-response curve. The statistician should compare the dose groups with an appropriate analysis. Finally, the statistician should make recommendations regarding effective doses, frequency of dosing, and the possible need for future dose-response studies.

3.1 Characterizing a Dose-Response Curve

Physicians must understand the relationship between dose and effect. Such a relationship can usually be described using a dose-response curve. This curve may be linear, concave upward, concave downward, or sigmoid; further, the effect need not be monotonic. Figure 1 is an example of a very common dose-response curve with a sigmoid shape. This curve could represent a single patient or the mean of a group of patients.

Goodman and Gilman (1985) characterize a dose-response curve with four parameters. Two of these, maximum effect and variability, are generally considered the most important. Maximum effect is the upper limit of the dose-response curve. Variability is influenced by many factors, such as patient age, weight, sex, and drug interactions. A range of doses may be needed to produce a given effect in a group of patients. Also, a range of effects may be produced by a given dose.

The two least important parameters are slope and potency. The slope refers to the linear portion of the dose-response curve. A steep slope describes a drug for which small increments of the dose produce vastly different effects. Potency is the range of the dose that produces an effect. This may be important if the effective dose is so large that it is difficult to administer.

In addition to these four parameters, we also want to determine the minimum and maximum effective doses. The minimum effective dose is the lowest dose that produces a clinically meaningful response. The maximum effective dose is the lowest dose that produces the maximum effect.

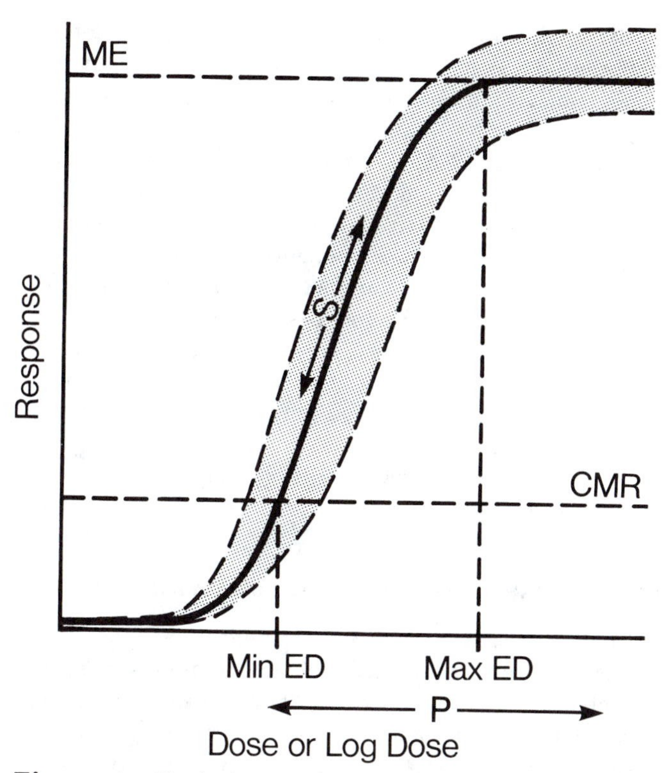

Figure 1 Typical sigmoid dose-response curve with confidence limits (shading) illustrating maximum effect (ME), slope (S), clinically meaningful response (CMR), minimum effective dose (MinED), maximum effective dose (MaxED), and potency (P).

3.2 Analysis of Dose-Response Data

Dose-response data can be either quantal (success/failure), ordered categorical (poor, fair, good, very good), or continuous (blood pressure). For quantal data, the most appropriate test, if the data come from a randomized complete block design, is the Cochran test (Conover, 1980, p. 199). Plotting the proportion of successes versus dose group characterizes the dose-response. For ordered categorical data, appropriate tests are linear model methods (Grizzle et al., 1969) or the Friedman test (Conover, 1980, p. 299). Collapsing the ordered categories into quantal responses may be necessary to plot the dose-response relationship, although the method of collapsing should be decided in advance of collecting the data.

For continuous data, parametric analysis-of-variance ANOVA models are usually the most powerful if assumptions are satisfied. If the assumption of normality is not satisfied, a rank transformation can be used (Conover and Iman, 1981). If the homogeneity-of-variance assumption is not met, continuous monotonic transformations such as logs or square roots can be used.

If parametric ANOVA models are used, orthogonal polynomial contrasts can be used to assess the shape of the dose-response curve. Depending on the number of dose groups, one can partition the dose group sum of squares into linear, quadratic, cubic, and so on, components. Of principal interest is the linear contrast, since it can indicate an increasing or decreasing dose-response relationship. If the dose groups (or logs of the dose groups) are equally spaced, tables for coefficients of these polynomial contrasts given in Pearson and Hartley (1958) can be used. If the dose groups are not equally spaced, a method for constructing orthogonal polynomial contrasts given in Robson (1959) can be used.

These methods are appropriate for characterizing a single dose-response curve. For comparing two dose-response curves, see Chapter 6.

3.3 Example of a Dose-Response Characterization

To consider the effect of the dose of a H_2 receptor antagonist on gastric pH, a Latin square crossover design was carried out on six patients using five active doses and placebo. The five active doses (10, 20, 40, 80, and 160 mg) were chosen based on animal studies and early phase 1 rising-dose studies. No serious, irreversible adverse experiences were observed on any of these five active doses in previous trials. To assure that the previous dose had been eliminated from the patients' bodies, there was a full week washout period between doses. The dose groups were assigned using a Latin square design balanced for carryover effects (Table 5).

Because the gastric pH data seemed to be reasonably normally distributed with approximately equal variances, we compared the dose groups

Table 5 Latin Square Randomization of Dose Groups

Patient	Period 1	Period 2	Period 3	Period 4	Period 5	Period 6
1	Placebo	10 mg	20 mg	40 mg	80 mg	160 mg
2	160 mg	80 mg	40 mg	20 mg	10 mg	Placebo
3	10 mg	40 mg	160 mg	Placebo	20 mg	80 mg
4	20 mg	160 mg	10 mg	80 mg	Placebo	40 mg
5	40 mg	Placebo	80 mg	10 mg	160 mg	20 mg
6	80 mg	20 mg	Placebo	160 mg	40 mg	10 mg

using an analysis of variance with patients, dose groups, and periods as factors in the model. For each dose, gastric pH was measured at hours 0 (immediately prior to taking drug), 2, 4, 6, 8, 10, and 12. In the investigator's opinion, a clinically meaningful response would be raising the gastric pH over 3 for at least two consecutive readings. This was decided before the study was run. Table 6 lists the efficacy data. No adverse experiences were observed for 0, 10, 20, 40, and 80 mg, but patients 1, 2, 4, 5, and 6 reported intolerable diarrhea or abdominal cramps at 160 mg.

First, the mean responses were plotted over time for each dose group (Figure 2). The horizontal line drawn at 3 represents the investigator's definition of a clinically meaningful response. From this figure, it is clear that only the doses of 40, 80, and 160 mg produced a clinically meaningful response on the average. This would suggest that the minimum effective dose was between 20 and 40 mg and the maximum effective dose was no greater than 80 mg.

To test whether the patients were generally similar prior to each test drug, an analysis of variance was done on the hour 0 data, with patients, dose groups, and periods as factors in the model (Table 7). Because this was not significant, it was unlikely to have much effect on the hour 2 to 12 data. However, one might consider change from baseline or include baseline as a covariate in any ANOVA models. We have omitted this for the sake of simplicity.

The peak effect was compared between the six dose groups using an analysis of variance with patients, dose groups, and periods as factors in the model (Table 8). The dose-response relationship was tested using orthogonal contrasts (linear, quadratic, cubic, quartic) of the dose group means. The linear and cubic contrasts were significant. The significance of the linear component indicates an increasing dose-response. The significance of the cubic contrast indicates flatness of the dose-response curve at the low and high pairs of doses. Besides considering peak effect, we could have considered areas under the pH curve or a repeated-measures analysis (see Chapter 3).

The mean peak responses for each dose group are plotted in Figure 3. An estimate of the minimum dose at which the peak gastric pH exceeds 3 would be between 20 and 40 mg. Also, no further efficacy was gained in increasing the dose from 80 mg to 160 mg. However, without any information on doses between 80 and 160 mg, it is possible that additional efficacy could be gained from some doses in this region.

Another question that can be answered from these data is the duration of effect. For each patient and each dose, the duration of effect can be defined as the time the gastric pH is above the clinically meaningful level of 3. The exact time at which this occurs is not known for any patient

Table 6 Gastric pH by Hour and Dose with Means and Standard Deviations

Patient	Dose	Period	pH0	pH2	pH4	pH6	pH8	pH10	pH12
1	0	1	1.4	1.8	1.8	1.4	1.4	1.2	1.1
	10	2	2.6	1.6	1.4	2.6	1.0	1.3	1.5
	20	3	2.5	1.9	1.4	1.9	1.0	1.4	1.9
	40	4	1.4	1.0	2.9	2.7	3.1	2.3	1.5
	80	5	1.0	2.4	4.8	5.3	5.4	3.2	1.5
	160	6	1.0	2.3	5.0	5.4	4.2	3.7	3.4
2	0	6	1.0	2.0	1.4	2.2	1.0	1.0	1.0
	10	5	1.6	1.0	1.0	1.7	1.0	1.3	1.6
	20	4	1.4	1.5	1.0	1.9	2.7	1.8	1.0
	40	3	1.0	2.2	3.4	2.3	3.3	1.7	1.0
	80	2	1.9	1.9	5.5	4.9	4.0	2.5	1.4
	160	1	1.0	1.0	5.9	6.1	3.2	2.5	2.4
3	0	4	1.6	2.4	1.0	1.3	1.3	1.6	2.5
	10	1	1.0	3.3	1.0	1.0	2.0	1.8	1.6
	20	5	1.4	1.5	3.1	2.6	3.5	2.2	1.0
	40	2	1.0	1.2	3.8	4.0	2.5	1.7	1.0
	80	6	1.6	2.5	5.0	5.3	4.7	3.4	2.5
	160	3	1.3	2.4	5.0	3.4	3.8	2.2	1.0
4	0	5	2.0	1.0	1.0	1.0	1.0	1.0	1.0
	10	3	2.2	1.2	1.5	1.6	1.0	1.3	1.6
	20	1	1.3	1.0	1.0	1.0	2.2	2.5	2.9
	40	6	1.0	1.9	4.3	3.4	2.2	2.6	3.2
	80	4	1.0	4.0	6.4	6.4	3.7	2.8	2.4
	160	2	1.7	1.3	5.1	4.5	3.6	2.6	1.8
5	0	2	2.6	1.0	1.0	2.3	1.0	1.0	1.0
	10	4	1.7	2.1	1.0	1.0	1.9	1.4	1.0
	20	6	1.8	1.4	2.3	2.3	2.0	1.6	1.3
	40	1	2.6	1.9	2.2	4.0	2.1	1.5	1.0
	80	3	1.0	2.6	5.6	5.1	3.8	3.0	2.7
	160	5	1.2	2.7	5.0	4.9	5.8	3.1	1.0
6	0	3	1.0	1.7	1.3	1.0	1.3	1.2	1.0
	10	6	1.8	1.0	1.4	3.2	1.7	1.3	1.0
	20	2	1.0	1.1	1.8	1.8	2.1	2.2	2.2
	40	5	1.0	2.0	3.6	2.7	4.4	3.0	1.7
	80	1	1.0	2.1	5.1	4.5	3.9	2.7	1.4
	160	4	1.0	3.7	4.5	5.1	4.6	2.8	1.8

Table 6 *(Continued)*

Patient	Dose	Period	pH0	pH2	pH4	pH6	pH8	pH10	pH12
Mean	0		1.6	1.6	1.2	1.5	1.2	1.2	1.3
	10		1.8	1.7	1.2	1.8	1.4	1.4	1.4
	20		1.6	1.4	1.8	1.9	2.2	2.0	1.7
	40		1.3	1.7	3.4	3.2	2.9	2.1	1.6
	80		1.2	2.6	5.4	5.2	4.2	2.9	2.0
	160		1.2	2.2	5.1	4.9	4.2	2.8	1.9
SD	0		0.6	0.6	0.3	0.6	0.2	0.2	0.6
	10		0.5	0.9	0.2	0.9	0.5	0.2	0.3
	20		0.5	0.3	0.8	0.5	0.8	0.4	0.8
	40		0.6	0.5	0.7	0.7	0.9	0.6	0.9
	80		0.4	0.7	0.6	0.6	0.7	0.3	0.6
	160		0.3	1.0	0.5	0.9	0.9	0.5	0.9

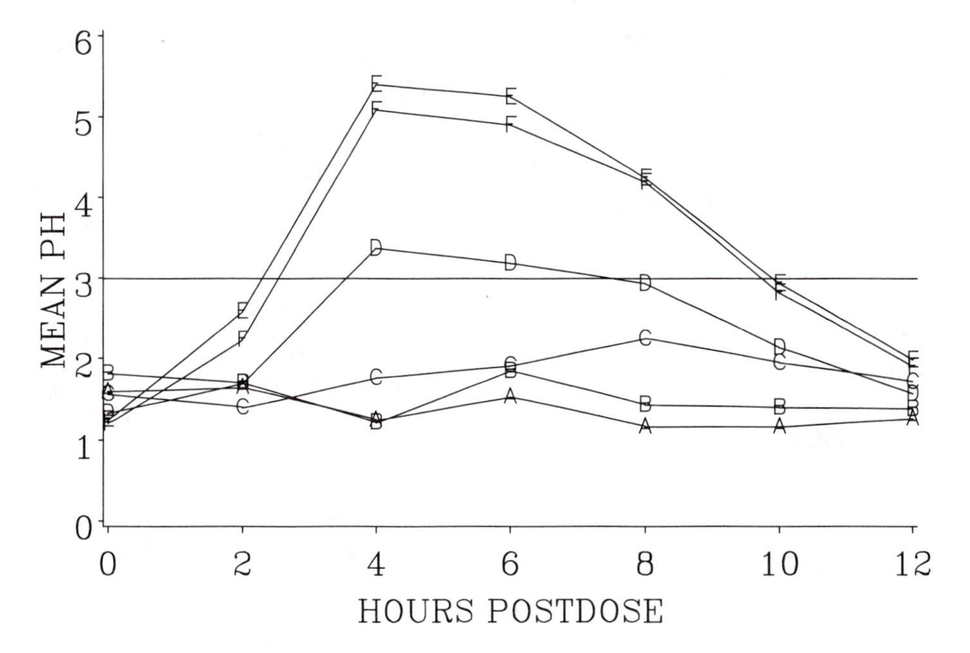

Figure 2 Mean gastric pH versus hours postdose by dose group.

Table 7 Analysis of Variance on Time 0 pH Data: General Linear Models Procedure (SAS, 1985)

DEPENDENT VARIABLE: PHO

SOURCE	DF	SUM OF SQUARES
MODEL	15	4.53000000
ERROR	20	5.19555556
CORRECTED TOTAL	35	9.72555556
SOURCE	DF	TYPE III SS
PATIENT	5	1.89888889
PERIOD	5	0.91555556
DOSE	5	1.71555556

Table 8 Analysis of Variance on Peak Effect: General Linear Models Procedure (SAS, 1985)

DEPENDENT VARIABLE: PEAK

SOURCE	DF	SUM OF SQUARES
MODEL	15	69.38333333
ERROR	20	5.47555556
CORRECTED TOTAL	35	74.85888889
SOURCE	DF	TYPE III SS
PATIENT	5	0.84222222
PERIOD	5	0.82888889
DOSE	5	67.71222222
CONTRAST	DF	SS
LINEAR DOSE-RESPONSE	1	45.06666667
QUAD DOSE-RESPONSE	1	0.00428571
CUBIC DOSE-RESPONSE	1	4.81666667
QUART DOSE-RESPONSE	1	0.27771429

MEAN SQUARE	F VALUE	PR > F	R-SQUARE	C.V.
0.30200000	1.16	0.3701	0.465783	34.8833
0.25977778		ROOT MSE		PHO MEAN
		0.50968400		1.46111111

F VALUE	PR > F
1.46	0.2461
0.70	0.6265
1.32	0.2954

MEAN SQUARE	F VALUE	PR > F	R-SQUARE	C.V.
4.62555556	16.90	0.0001	0.926855	14.1628
0.27377778		ROOT MSE		PEAK MEAN
		0.52323778		3.69444444

F VALUE	PR > F
0.62	0.6895
0.61	0.6965
49.47	0.0001

F VALUE	PR > F
164.61	0.0001
0.02	0.9017
17.59	0.0004
1.01	0.3259

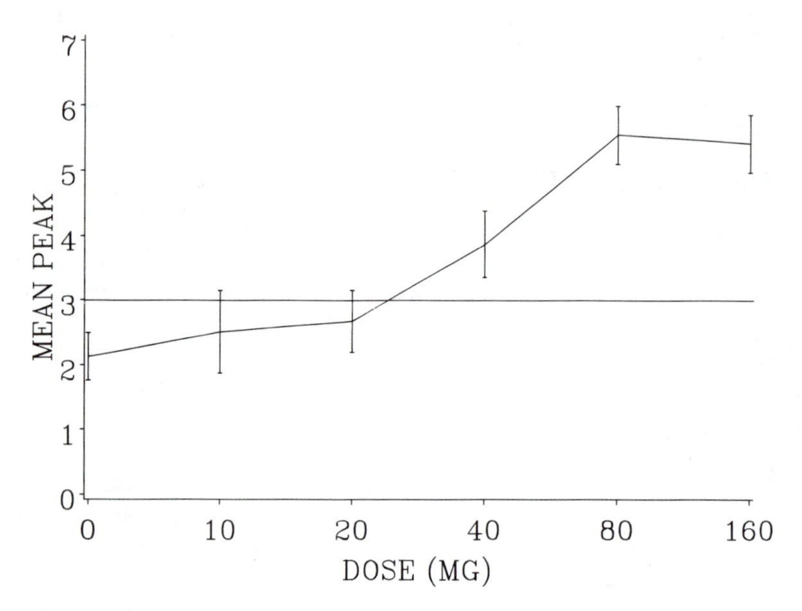

Figure 3 Mean peak effect ($\pm$ one standard deviation) versus dose.

because we do not have continual measurements over time, but it can be estimated by assuming that the change in gastric pH between two time intervals is linear [more generally, a curve could be fit (see Chapters 3 and 6)]. For example, for patient 1, 80 mg, the pH at 2 hours was 2.4 and the pH at 4 hours was 4.8, suggesting that the pH rose above 3 at some time in this interval. If we assume that the pH increases linearly in this interval, an estimate of the time that the pH rises above 3 would be at 2.5 hours. Similarly, we can estimate the time at which the pH will drop below 3. Table 9 lists these estimates.

We can do the same analysis for duration of effect as we did for peak effect. The ANOVA results are shown in Table 10, and a plot of the mean duration of effect versus dose is shown in Figure 4. Thus the mean duration of effect with the 80-mg dose was about four times that of the 40-mg dose, and the duration of effect for the 160-mg dose was not much greater than that of the 80-mg dose. The mean duration of effect for an 80-mg single dose was 7.6 hours.

Table 9 Estimates of Duration of Effect

Dose[a]	Patient	Period	Estimate of hour at which gastric pH rises above 3	Estimate of hour at which gastric pH falls below 3	Duration of effect (hours)
40	1	4	[b]	[b]	0
	2	3	[b]	[b]	0
	3	2	3.4	7.3	3.9
	4	6	2.9	6.7	3.8
	5	1	[b]	[b]	0
	6	5	6.4	10.0	3.6
Mean			2.1	4.0	1.9
SD			2.6	4.5	2.1
80	1	5	2.5	10.2	7.7
	2	2	2.6	9.3	6.7
	3	6	2.4	10.9	8.5
	4	4	1.3	9.6	8.3
	5	3	2.3	10.0	7.7
	6	1	2.6	9.5	6.9
Mean			2.3	9.9	7.6
SD			0.5	0.6	0.7
160	1	6	2.5	14.7	12.2
	2	1	2.8	8.6	5.8
	3	3	2.5	9.0	6.5
	4	2	2.9	9.2	6.3
	5	5	2.3	10.1	7.8
	6	4	1.5	9.8	8.3
Mean			2.4	10.2	7.8
SD			0.5	2.3	2.3

[a]No patients in the placebo group, the 10-mg group, or the 20-mg group had a gastric pH above 3 for two consecutive periods.
[b]No effect was observed for this patient at this dose. These were treated as zero for the calculation of means.

Table 10 Analysis of Variance on Duration of Effect: General Linear Models Procedure (SAS, 1985)

DEPENDENT VARIABLE: DURATION

SOURCE	DF	SUM OF SQUARES
MODEL	15	457.97000000
ERROR	20	30.56555556
CORRECTED TOTAL	35	488.53555556
SOURCE	DF	TYPE III SS
PATIENT	5	6.50888889
PERIOD	5	14.41555556
DOSE	5	437.04555556
CONTRAST	DF	SS
LINEAR DOSE-RESPONSE	1	324.80266667
QUAD DOSE-RESPONSE	1	7.68047619
CUBIC DOSE-RESPONSE	1	33.30150000
QUART DOSE-RESPONSE	1	11.17202381

These data were also be examined by using a quantal approach, where success was defined as raising the gastric pH over 3 for at least two consecutive readings. For doses of 0, 10, and 20 mg, no patients were considered successes, whereas there were three successes for 40 mg and six successes for both 80 and 160 mg (Figure 5).

The following recommendations about dosing can be made using these data:

1. The minimum effective dose is likely to be between 20 and 40 mg.
2. The maximum effective dose is about 80 mg; this is estimated to increase the mean peak gastric pH to a level of approximately 5.6.
3. The dose-response curve seems to be increasing and linear (versus log dose) in the range 20 to 80 mg, and flat in the ranges 10 to 20 mg and 80 to 160 mg.
4. The mean duration of effect for the 80-mg dose is about 7.6 hours. This suggests that dosing three times a day should be investigated in multiple-dose studies. However, knowledge of the steady-state pharmacokinetics of this drug should be considered before deciding on any dosing schedule.

MEAN SQUARE	F VALUE	PR > F	R-SQUARE	C.V.
30.53133333	19.98	0.0001	0.937434	42.7928
1.52827778		ROOT MSE		DURATION MEAN
		1.23623532		2.88888889

F VALUE	PR > F
0.85	0.5297
1.89	0.1418
57.19	0.0001

F VALUE	PR > F
212.53	0.0001
5.03	0.0365
21.79	0.0001
7.31	0.0137

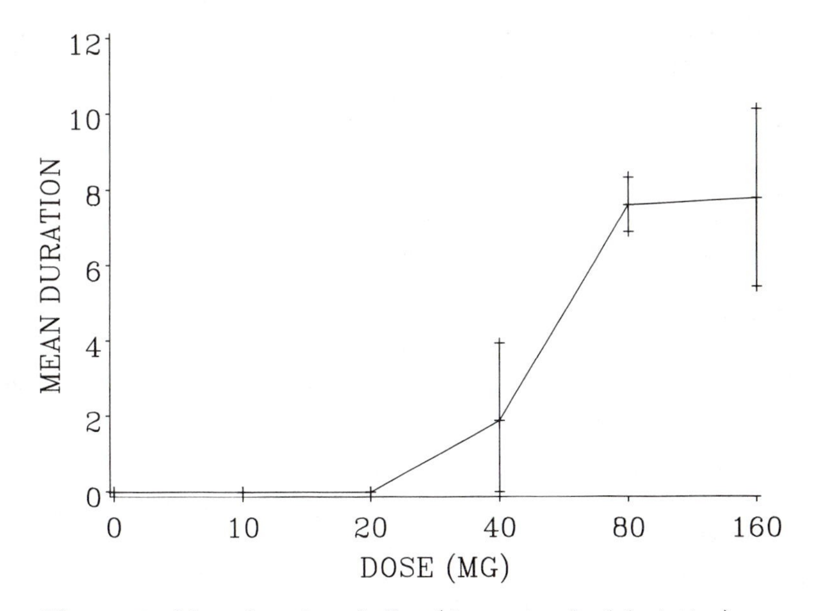

Figure 4 Mean duration of effect (± one standard deviation) versus dose.

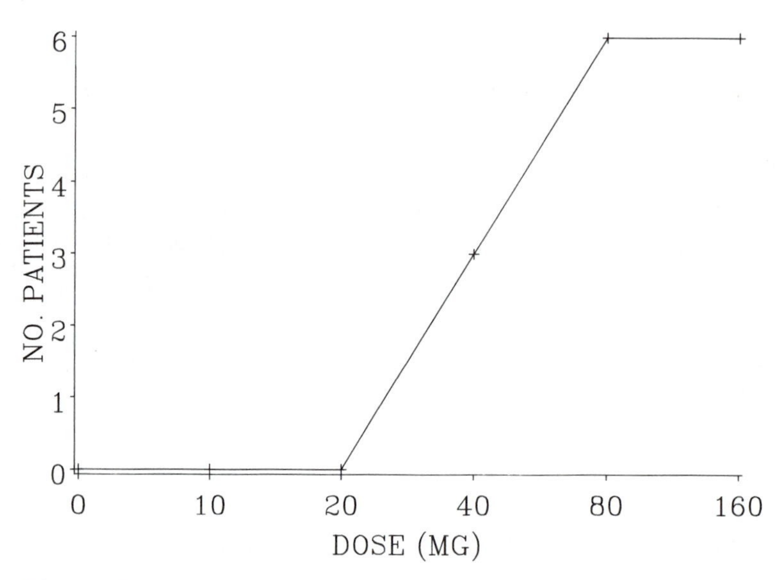

Figure 5 Number of patients with gastric pH over 3 for at least two consecutive readings versus dose.

4 THERAPEUTIC WINDOW

A physician prescribing a drug also needs to know the therapeutically useful dosage range—the "therapeutic window" in which the drug is both effective and reasonably safe. The lower endpoint of this window is the minimum effective dose, the lowest dose for which clinically useful efficacy is demonstrated. The upper endpoint of the window is the maximum tolerated dose, the largest dose for which there are no clinically important adverse experiences. This range can vary between patients and over time within the same patient.

If the maximum tolerated dose is much larger than the minimum effective dose, the window is large. If the maximum tolerated dose is close to the minimum effective dose, the window is narrow and the physician must be cautious with the dosing. If the maximum tolerated dose is similar to or lower than the minimum effective dose, the drug will not be therapeutically useful for that specific effect unless the benefit to the patient exceeds the risk of intolerance.

In our example in the preceding section, the minimum observed effective dose was 40 mg. Because five of the six patients reported intolerable diarrhea and abdominal cramps at 160 mg, the maximum tolerated dose tested was 80 mg. Therefore, the therapeutic window was 40 to 80 mg. It is possible that testing doses between 80 and 160 would help us determine the exact maximum tolerated dose.

It is important to recognize that therapeutic windows can be quite variable between patients. Some patients may have a large therapeutic window, and some patients may have none. In the preceding example, patient 3 had a window of 40 to 160 mg, while for all others it was 40 to 80 mg.

Because patients absorb the same dosage differently, it may be important to consider the effect of drug plasma levels, if obtainable. (Some drugs, in particular some drugs given by the aerosol route, may not have detectable plasma levels.) The bioavailability and pharmacokinetics of the drug will have an effect on the response and are usually different from patient to patient. Further, for some especially toxic drugs, the FDA may require plasma level monitoring in each patient. Therefore, we could apply the same analysis techniques to plasma response as we applied to dose-response. We could also apply the population-based models described in Chapter 5.

4.1 Example of Therapeutic Window Using Plasma Levels

Flecainide acetate, a drug to control ventricular arrhythmias, was studied in 43 patients to determine how efficacy and adverse experiences correlate with plasma levels (Salerno et al., 1986). To ensure that each patient reached steady-state plasma levels, blood samples were drawn after at least 2 days of stable flecainide dosing. Dosing was adjusted to maximize efficacy and to minimize adverse experiences. Efficacy was measured as a quantal response, where a success was defined as achieving at least 90% suppression of ventricular ectopic depolarizations (VED), a measure of ventricular arrhythmia. Adverse experiences were also measured as quantal responses by the presence or absence of cardiac adverse experiences such as death, left or right bundle branch block, congestive heart failure, ventricular tachycardia, bradycardia, and syncope.

Multiple plasma levels were obtained for each patient. For estimating the relationship between plasma levels and efficacy, the lowest level of flecainide for each patient who achieved 90% suppression was used. For those patients who did not reach this level, the highest plasma level reached was used in the analysis. For estimating the relationship between plasma levels and safety, the lowest plasma level for each patient with a cardiac adverse experience was used. If no adverse experience occurred for a given patient, the highest plasma level obtained was used.

Graphs of the Kaplan-Meier product limit estimator were used to illustrate the relationship of efficacy and adverse experiences to plasma levels

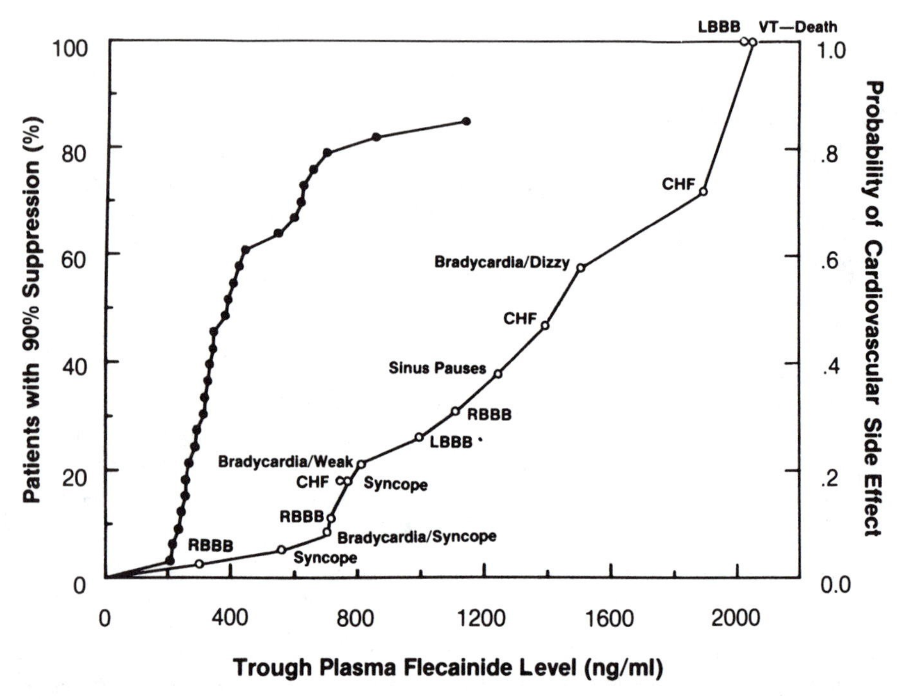

Figure 6 The probability of a cardiovascular side effect occurring is compared with the flecainide plasma level, by use of the Kaplan–Meier product limit estimator, for all 43 patients (o). The efficacy/plasma concentration curve for 90% suppression of VEDs is also shown for those 33 patients with available data for both efficacy and flecainide levels (•). Twenty-eight of the 33 patients achieved at least 90% suppression of VEDs. *RBBB* = Right bundle branch block; *CHF* = congestive heart failure; *LBBB* = left bundle branch block; *VT* = ventricular tachycardia.

(Kaplan and Meier, 1958). This method estimates the cumulative likelihood of a quantal response (such as 90% suppression of VEDs or occurrence of a cardiac adverse experience) as a function of some variable (such as flecainide plasma levels). Figure 6 shows these estimates for both 90% suppression and occurrence of cardiac adverse experiences on the same plot. From this picture we see that the minimum effective plasma level was approximately 200 ng/ml and no further improvement in efficacy was achieved after approximately 1000 ng/ml with more than 80% of the patients treated successfully. The cumulative likelihood of a cardiac adverse experience was 50% at approximately 1500 ng/ml, and increased to 100% at 2000 ng/ml.

Such a picture also helps a physician determine the benefit-to-risk ratio of increasing plasma levels to achieve greater efficacy.

5 SUMMARY

A physician prescribing a drug needs to know as much as possible about the relationship between dose or plasma levels and efficacy and safety. To provide this information for an adequate benefit-to-risk assessment, pharmaceutical companies carry out a program of dose-response studies. Statisticians must ensure that these studies are both scientifically and ethically valid. These studies should be analyzed using the most powerful statistical techniques, which are usually analysis of variance (possibly on transformed data) for continuous data. Estimating the therapeutic window, and presenting it in an easily understood picture provides both the FDA and prescribing physicians with clear estimates of the benefit-to-risk ratio.

REFERENCES

Bolognese, J. A. (1983) A monte carlo comparison of three up-and-down designs for dose-ranging. *Controlled Clin. Trials 4*, 187–196.

Conover, W. J. (1980) *Practical Nonparametric Statistics*, 2nd ed. Wiley, New York.

Conover, W. J., and R. L. Iman (1981). Rank transformations as a bridge between parametric and nonparametric statistics. *Amer. Statist. 35*, 124–133.

Goodman, L. S., and A. Gilman, eds. (1985). *The Pharmacological Basis of Therapeutics*, 7th ed. Macmillan, New York.

Grizzle, J. E., C. F. Starmer, and G. G. Koch (1969). Analysis of categorical data by linear models. *Biometrics 25*, 489–504.

Kaplan, E. L., and P. Meier (1958). Nonparametric estimation from incomplete observations. *J. Amer. Statist. Assoc. 53*, 457–481.

Lovastatin Study Group II (1986). Therapeutic response to lovastatin (mevinolin) in nonfamilial hypercholersterolemia. *J. Amer. Med. Assoc. 256*, 2829–2834.

Pearson, E. S., and H. O. Hartley (1958). *Biometrika Tables for Statisticians*, Vol. 1. Cambridge University Press, Cambridge.

Robson, D. S. (1959). A simple method for constructing orthogonal polynomials when the independent variable is unequally spaced. *Biometrics 15*, 187–191.

Salerno, D. M., G. Granrud, P. Sharkey, J. Krejci, T. Larson, D. Erlien, D. Berry, and M. Hodges (1986). Pharmacodynamics and side effects of flecainide acetate. *Clin. Pharmacol. Ther. 40*, 101–107.

SAS Institute, Inc. (1985). *SAS User's Guide; Statistics Version 5th ed.* SAS Institute, Cary, N.C.

5

Population Models

AMY RACINE-POON CIBA-GEIGY AG, Basel, Switzerland

ADRIAN F. M. SMITH University of Nottingham, University Park, Nottingham, England

1 INTRODUCTION

The following general structure is typical of many of the studies undertaken in the pharmaceutical sciences. For each of a collection of *individual* subjects (e.g., clinical patients or experimental animals), measurements of a response of interest have been made at several selected, or observed, values of a related variable (a so-called covariate). For example, in toxicity growth-curve studies the response would be size or weight and the covariate would be time from birth; in pharmacokinetic studies the response would be plasma concentration of a drug and the covariate would be time from administration; in pharmacodynamic studies the response would be therapeutic effect and the covariate would be plasma concentration.

The individuals are then assumed to be a representative sample of a *population* of such individuals, all of whose responses are related to the covariate in a basically similar way (e.g., all having a linear growth pattern) but with some degree of variation from individual to individual (e.g., different straight-line growth trajectories for each individual).

From a statistical inference perspective, information from all the individuals collectively then provides the basis for learning about some form of mean underlying population response profile; conversely, knowledge about the population provides additional information about an individual profile beyond that provided by the (often limited) direct measurement data on that individual. From a modeling perspective, therefore, whether the main interest in the study is in the individual or the population (or both), it is important to incorporate both a model for the measurement process on individual profiles and also a model of the variation of these individual profiles around a mean population profile. The two examples that follow will serve to illustrate the problems we consider in this chapter.

EXAMPLE 1 In a series of growth-curve studies conducted by CIBA-GEIGY, young rats (between 1 and 2 weeks old) were assigned randomly into a control and a treatment group. A substance (placebo in the control group, test preparation in the treatment group) was then administered daily to each animal as part of its diet. Each animal was then regularly weighed at certain predetermined times. Figures 1 and 2 provide a graphical presentation (with superimposed straight-line profiles of the data from two such studies (study A and study B). In study A, all the animals (15 in

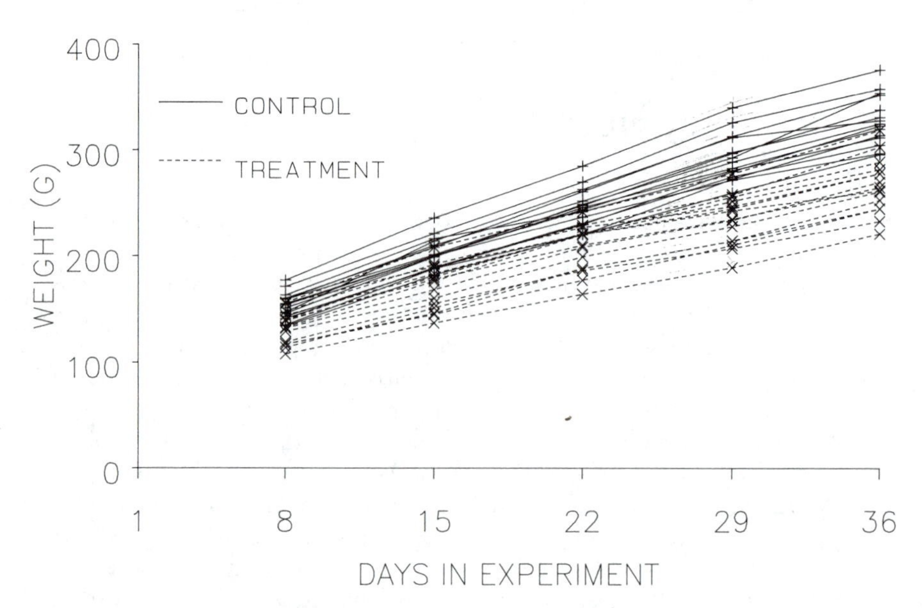

Figure 1 Data of Example 1, study A.

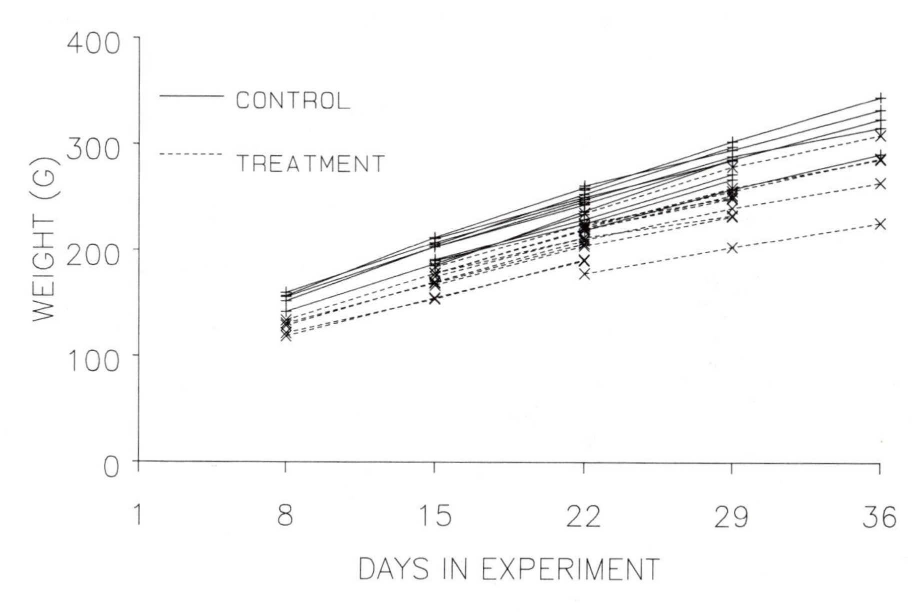

Figure 2 Data of Example 1, study B.

each of the control and treatment groups) were weighed at weekly intervals for five consecutive weeks following the start of the experiment. In study B, five rats in each group were weighed only for the first 3 weeks, five were weighed only for the middle 3 weeks, and five were weighed only in the final 3 weeks. The objective of these studies was to discover whether the test substance had an effect on the growth profile of the rats.

EXAMPLE 2 In a pharmacokinetic study conducted by CIBA-GEIGY, plasma concentration profiles of German heart failure patients were observed following the administration of a single dose of 30 mg of the drug Cadralazine. Figure 3 provides a graphical presentation (with superimposed nonlinear profiles) of the data on 10 such patients, 8 of whom were observed at 2, 4, 6, 8, 10, and 24 hours after the drug was administered, and 2 of whom were, in addition, observed at 28 and 32 hours after administration. There were several objectives in this study. On the one hand, there was interest in learning about the individual kinetic profiles (absorption, elimination, and distribution) with a view to providing guidance on dose levels and dosing time intervals for future patients; on the other hand, there was interest in learning about the mean profile for the population (of heart failure patients), with a view to making comparisons with other pop-

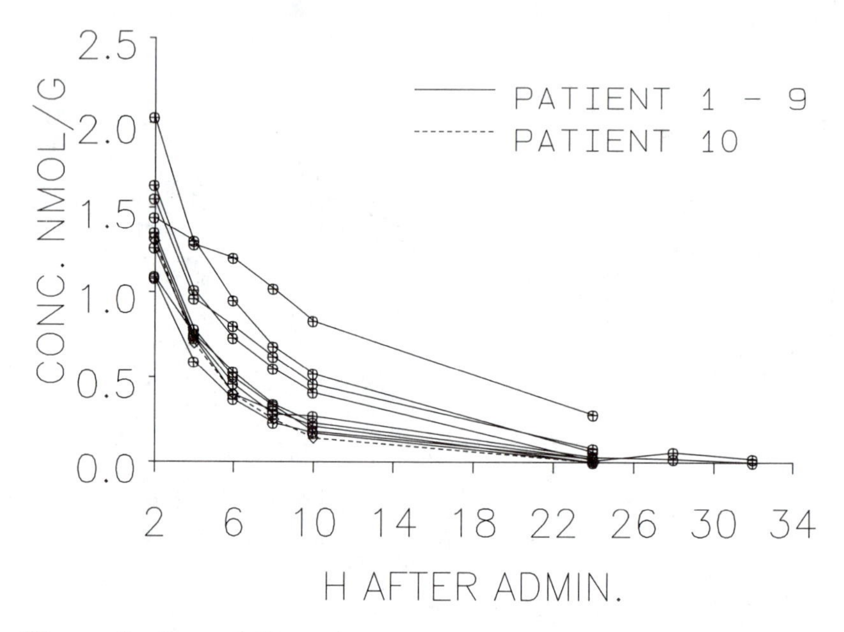

Figure 3 Data of Example 2.

ulations (e.g., healthy volunteers, hypertensive patients, elderly patients, or patients with renal impairment).

In the next section we discuss a general modeling strategy for studies having the type of general structure described above. A review is then given of some possible methods of statistical analysis for such models and illustrative analyses are presented. A final section provides a summary recommendation, together with comments on issues such as data transformation and model checking.

2 MODELING

2.1 Notation

In formulating population models, we shall use the following notation. The observed response corresponding to a covariate value x_{ij} will be denoted by y_{ij}. The number of individuals sampled from the population will be denoted by k (so that $i = 1, \ldots, k$) and the number of observations made on individual i will be denoted by n_i (so that $j = 1, \ldots, n_i$). In general, the number and values of the covariate will differ from individual to individual, but in those cases where the same sample design is used for each individual, and there are no missing observations, n_i and x_{ij} will not require the subscript i.

2.2 Individual Measurement Models

It is often reasonable to assume, perhaps following suitable transformation of the data, that the relationship between y_{ij} and x_{ij} takes the form

$$y_{ij} = f(\boldsymbol{\theta}_i, x_{ij}) + \epsilon_{ij},$$

where

$f(\boldsymbol{\theta}, x)$ = parametrized curve, describing, as a function of x for given parameter vector $\boldsymbol{\theta}$, the expected value of the response at the different covariate values

$\boldsymbol{\theta}_i$ = parameter vector identifying the specific form of the functional relationship in the case of individual i

ϵ_{ij} = zero-mean measurement error, typically assumed independent from observation to observation, whose variance might either be assumed constant for all observations [so that $V(\epsilon_{ij}) = \sigma^2$], or constant within individuals but differing across individuals [$V(\epsilon_{ij}) = \sigma_i^2$], or functionally related to the mean value $f(\boldsymbol{\theta}_i, x_{ij})$ [e.g., $V(\epsilon_{ij}) = \sigma^2 f(\boldsymbol{\theta}_i, x_{ij})$], the appropriate choice depending, of course, on the nature of the measurement process

2.3 Population Structure Models

For a sample of individuals identified as being from the same population, the same general *form* of functional relationship, f, is assumed to hold between the expected response and the covariate for each individual, but the parameters, $\boldsymbol{\theta}_i$, determining the precise *shape* of profile for each individual are assumed to vary across the population in the manner of a random sample. It is then often reasonable to assume, possibly following suitable reparametrization of the individual components of the parameter vector, that

$$\boldsymbol{\theta}_i = \boldsymbol{\theta} + \boldsymbol{\nu}_i,$$

where $\boldsymbol{\theta}$ can be interpreted as a mean population parameter, defining a mean population profile, and the zero-mean random vectors $\boldsymbol{\nu}_i$, assumed independent across individuals, represent variation of the individual parameter vectors (and hence individual profiles) around the population parameter vector (and hence mean population profile), the elements of the covariance matrix, $V(\boldsymbol{\nu}_i) = \boldsymbol{\Sigma}$, reflecting the magnitudes and interrelationships of this variation.

2.4 Illustrative Models

Model for Example 1

In each of the two growth-curve studies described in the introduction, there are two population samples: the subjects in the control groups (+) and the subjects in the treatment groups (×). Let us first focus attention on the control groups. For the time period covered in this study, it turns out to be reasonable to assume individual *straight-line* growth curves, so that

$$y_{ij} = \alpha_i + \beta_i x_{ij} + \epsilon_{ij}.$$

The nature of the measurement process in this case is such that it is reasonable to assume that

$$\epsilon_{ij} \sim N(0, \sigma^2),$$

so that

$$y_{ij} \sim N(\alpha_i + \beta_i x_{ij}, \sigma^2)$$

provides the full measurement model. In both the control groups there are $k = 15$ subjects; in study A, $n_i = 5$, and in study B, $n_i = 3$ (and in the latter case the design points are not the same for all subjects).

The population structure can be modeled in this case by assuming that

$$\begin{bmatrix} \alpha_i \\ \beta_i \end{bmatrix} \sim N \left[\begin{bmatrix} \alpha_C \\ \beta_C \end{bmatrix}, \boldsymbol{\Sigma}_C \right],$$

so that the underlying individual straight-line growth curves, $\alpha_i + \beta_i x$, are regarded as a random sample varying around a mean population straight-line growth curve, $\alpha_C + \beta_C x$. (Since the β_i are positive in this case, it might be more reasonable to assume $\log \beta_i$ to be normally distributed. We shall not consider this further here, but will illustrate the possibility with the model for Example 2.)

An analogous modeling framework holds for the treatment groups, except that the population model now takes the form

$$\begin{bmatrix} \alpha_i \\ \beta_i \end{bmatrix} \sim N \left[\begin{bmatrix} \alpha_T \\ \beta_T \end{bmatrix}, \boldsymbol{\Sigma}_T \right],$$

allowing for a possible difference in the mean population straight-line growth curve from that in the control group, as well as a possibly different pattern of variation about the population curve.

In these particular studies, the main interest was in inference about the population differences $\alpha_C - \alpha_T$ and $\beta_C - \beta_T$. We shall return to a full analysis of this example in Section 4.

Model for Example 2

In the case of the pharmacokinetic study described in the introduction, there is a single population sample whose individual response profiles may be assumed to be well described by modeling the ith individual response curve by the nonlinear form

$$C\alpha_i^{*-1} \exp(-\beta_i^* x_{ij}),$$

where C is a fixed, dose-related, constant, α_i^* defines the initial response of individual i immediately following drug administration, and β_i^* defines the rate at which the drug is eliminated from the system. However, in this form of representation of the profile the parameters α_i^* and β_i^* are necessarily positive and this is rather inconvenient when it comes to modeling the population distribution. In this case, therefore, it is appropriate to perform a suitable reparametrization to obtain real-valued parametric components whose population distribution could more reasonably be regarded as normal. Writing

$$\alpha_i = \log \alpha_i^*, \qquad \beta_i = \log \beta_i^*,$$

the measurement and population models in this case are assumed to be

$$y_{ij} \sim N\left\{C[\exp(\alpha_i)]^{-1} \exp[-\exp(\beta_i)x_{ij}], \sigma^2\right\},$$

$$\begin{bmatrix} \alpha_i \\ \beta_i \end{bmatrix} \sim N\left[\begin{bmatrix} \alpha \\ \beta \end{bmatrix}, \mathbf{\Sigma}\right],$$

with $i = 10$ and $n_i = 6$ for $i = 1, \ldots, 8$, $n_i = 8$ for $i = 9, 10$.

3 STATISTICAL METHODS

3.1 Overview

A variety of methods have been proposed for making inferences about the unknown parameters in models that combine individual and population components. In this section we give a brief account of a selection of these methods, together with a more detailed account of one specific approach, which provides a framework within which to obtain an overview of many of the aspects of the other approaches and which has performed most efficiently in a number of applied and simulated comparative case studies.

3.2 The Naive Pooled Data Approach

If interest if focused entirely on the estimation of population parameters, it is perhaps tempting to pool all the data together, ignoring the subscript i that identifies particular individuals, and to regard all observations, reindexed as y_l, say, where $l = 1, \ldots, \sum_{i=1}^{k} n_i = N$, as coming from the model

$$y_l = f(\boldsymbol{\theta}, x_l) + \epsilon_l,$$

where $\boldsymbol{\theta}$ denotes the mean population parameters and ϵ_l is some form of zero-mean random deviation of the observations from the expected mean population response. Applying a standard linear or nonlinear least squares estimation procedure (depending on the nature of f), the estimate of $\boldsymbol{\theta}$ is then obtained by minimizing the sum of squares

$$S(\boldsymbol{\theta}) = \sum_{l=1}^{N} [y_l - f(\boldsymbol{\theta}, x_l)]^2.$$

Clearly, such a procedure ignores the rather complex combination of intra- and inter-individual variation implicit in the assumed model and is not to be recommended.

3.3 The NONMEM Approach

NONMEM is an acronym for the analysis of *nonlinear mixed effects models* and refers to a procedure introduced by Sheiner and Beal (1979). The NONMEM approach first linearizes the individual profiles by taking a first-order Taylor expansion around the population parameter value and then proceeds by maximum likelihood estimation. The linearization leads to the approximation

$$\begin{aligned} y_{ij} &= f(\boldsymbol{\theta}_i, x_{ij}) + \epsilon_{ij} \\ &\approx f(\boldsymbol{\theta}, x_{ij}) + [\nabla f(\boldsymbol{\theta}, x_{ij})]^T (\boldsymbol{\theta}_i - \boldsymbol{\theta}) + \epsilon_{ij}, \end{aligned}$$

where the $\boldsymbol{\theta}_i$ have independent multivariate normal distributions with mean $\boldsymbol{\theta}$ and covariance matrix $\boldsymbol{\Sigma}$, and the ϵ_{ij}, have independent zero-mean normal distributions with an appropriate form of variance (see the discussion at the end of Section 2.3). The maximum likelihood estimates of $\boldsymbol{\theta}$, $\boldsymbol{\Sigma}$ and the individual variance components are then found by means of an iterative algorithm, and approximate asymptotic normality is invoked for making inferences.

There are several potential problems with this approach. First, when the interindividual variation is high (which is often the case with population kinetic problems), the linear approximation used by NONMEM may be inadequate. Second, as we shall mention again briefly in our concluding section, population models involve a lot of assumptions both about the forms of individual profiles and the choices of parametrization that make the assumed population distribution and the adequacy of asymptotic approximations reasonable. Model checking and diagnostic procedures are therefore particularly important for these kinds of population models. Most such checks and diagnostics are based on residuals, but in the case of the NONMEM procedure, these are a confounding of intra and interindividual variation, as well as the errors produced by the global linearization. Unless interindividual variation is fairly low and a good parametrization is chosen, the NONMEM approach will often run into numerical difficulties.

3.4 Two-Stage Approaches

A more reasonable approach, particularly if there is interest in estimating individual profile parameters as well as population parameters, might be first to obtain estimates of the individual $\boldsymbol{\theta}_i$ and then to combine these in some manner to form an estimate of $\boldsymbol{\theta}$.

If least squares is used as a basis of the estimation procedure (or, equivalently, maximum likelihood under the assumption of normal measurement error distributions), we obtain estimates of the $\boldsymbol{\theta}_i$ by minimizing

$$S(\boldsymbol{\theta}_i) = \sum_{j=1}^{n_i} [y_{ij} - f(\boldsymbol{\theta}_i, x_{ij})]^2.$$

If the resulting estimates of the $\boldsymbol{\theta}_i$ are given by $\hat{\boldsymbol{\theta}}_i$, $i = 1, \ldots, k$, these might then be combined into an estimate $\hat{\boldsymbol{\theta}}$ of $\boldsymbol{\theta}$ by some form of "mean," such as

$$\hat{\boldsymbol{\theta}} = \begin{cases} k^{-1} \sum_{i=1}^{k} \hat{\boldsymbol{\theta}}_i & \text{(arithmetic)} \\ \left(\prod_{i=1}^{k} \hat{\boldsymbol{\theta}}_i \right)^{1/k} & \text{(geometric)} \\ \sum_{i=1}^{k} w_i \hat{\boldsymbol{\theta}}_i & \text{(weighted)} \end{cases}$$

where, in the latter case, the weights $(w_i \geq 0, w_1 + \cdots + w_k = 1)$ reflect the relative uncertainty attached to the individual parameter vector estimates. Although standard linear or nonlinear least squares fitting programs will return suitable values of $\hat{\boldsymbol{\theta}}_i$, together with standard error estimates from which individual confidence intervals can be formed, there are clearly some difficulties with this approach. First, there is an unsatisfactory ad hoc flavor to the rather arbitrary choice of a form of "mean." Second, one of the features of population modeling, as we remarked earlier in the introduction, is that knowledge about the population profile should help to improve estimates of individual profiles, so that, intuitively, $\hat{\boldsymbol{\theta}}$ should somehow be combined with $\hat{\boldsymbol{\theta}}_i$ to form an estimate of $\boldsymbol{\theta}_i$ which "improves" on $\hat{\boldsymbol{\theta}}_i$. These two problems have led to attempts to develop more refined two-stage approaches.

Steimer et al. (1984) have reviewed two such procedures: the general two-stage (GTS) and the iterative two-stage (ITS) procedures (originally proposed by Prévost). Both of these procedures start with $\hat{\boldsymbol{\theta}}_i$, the maximum likelihood estimate, and $\mathbf{V}_i$, the asymptotic covariance matrix of $\boldsymbol{\theta}_i$, and then proceed to refine estimates of $\boldsymbol{\theta}_i$ and $\boldsymbol{\theta}$ by an iterative process. The lth step of the GTS procedure consists of

$$\boldsymbol{\theta}_i^{(l)} = (\mathbf{V}_i^{-1} + \boldsymbol{\Sigma}^{(l-1)^{-1}})^{-1}(\mathbf{V}_i^{-1}\hat{\boldsymbol{\theta}}_i + \boldsymbol{\Sigma}^{(l-1)^{-1}}\boldsymbol{\theta}^{(l-1)})$$

$$\boldsymbol{\theta}^{(l)} = \frac{\sum_{i=1}^{k} \boldsymbol{\theta}_i^{(l)}}{k},$$

where $\boldsymbol{\theta}_i^{(j)}$, $\boldsymbol{\theta}^{(j)}$, and $\boldsymbol{\Sigma}^{(j)}$ denote the estimates of $\boldsymbol{\theta}_i$, $\boldsymbol{\theta}$, and $\boldsymbol{\Sigma}$ at the jth step, and the iterative estimate of $\boldsymbol{\Sigma}$ is defined by

$$\boldsymbol{\Sigma}^{(l)} = \frac{\sum_{i=1}^{k}(\boldsymbol{\theta}_i^{(l)} - \boldsymbol{\theta}^{(l)})(\boldsymbol{\theta}_i^{(l)} - \boldsymbol{\theta}^{(l)})^T}{k} + \frac{\sum_{i=1}^{k}(\mathbf{V}_i^{-1} + \boldsymbol{\Sigma}^{(l-1)^{-1}})^{-1}}{k}.$$

The first term of $\boldsymbol{\Sigma}^{(l)}$ is the maximum likelihood estimate of $\boldsymbol{\Sigma}$ assuming $\boldsymbol{\theta}_i^{(l)}$ to be the known value of $\boldsymbol{\theta}_i$; the second term is an approximation to the additional uncertainty arising from the fact that the $\boldsymbol{\theta}_i^{(l)}$'s are only estimates of the $\boldsymbol{\theta}_i$'s.

The computation of the ITS is considerably more complicated. Its lth step consists of evaluating $\boldsymbol{\theta}_i^{(l)}$ and $\mathbf{V}_i^{(l)}$ to be the posterior mode and the posterior covariance matrix of $\boldsymbol{\theta}_i$ from a Bayesian analysis that uses $N(\boldsymbol{\theta}^{(l-1)}, \boldsymbol{\Sigma}^{(l-1)})$ as the prior distribution for $\boldsymbol{\theta}_i$, where $\boldsymbol{\theta}^{(l)}$ and $\boldsymbol{\Sigma}^{(l)}$ are defined recursively by

$$\boldsymbol{\theta}^{(l)} = \frac{\Sigma \boldsymbol{\theta}_i^{(l)}}{k},$$

$$\boldsymbol{\Sigma}^{(l)} = \frac{\sum_{i=1}^{k}(\boldsymbol{\theta}_i^{(l)} - \boldsymbol{\theta}^{(l)})(\boldsymbol{\theta}_i^{(l)} - \boldsymbol{\theta}^{(l)})^T}{k} + \frac{\sum_{i=1}^{k} \mathbf{V}_i^{(l)}}{k}.$$

The interpretation of $\boldsymbol{\Sigma}^{(l)}$ here is similar to that of GTS.

3.5 The Bayes/Empirical Bayes Approach

As an introduction to the flavor of the Bayesian approach to individual and population analysis, we shall reconsider the straight-line growth-curve study discussed in Example 1 and Section 2. Considering just the control group for study A, where $i = 15$, $n_i = 5$, $x_{i1} = 8$, $x_{i2} = 15$, $x_{i3} = 22$, $x_{i4} = 29$, and $x_{i5} = 36$, we recall that the measurement model for individual i has the form

$$\mathbf{y}_i = \begin{bmatrix} y_{i1} \\ y_{i2} \\ y_{i3} \\ y_{i4} \\ y_{i5} \end{bmatrix} \sim N\left\{ \begin{bmatrix} 1 & 8 \\ 1 & 15 \\ 1 & 22 \\ 1 & 29 \\ 1 & 36 \end{bmatrix} \begin{bmatrix} \alpha_i \\ \beta_i \end{bmatrix}, \quad \sigma_i^2 \begin{bmatrix} 1 & & & & \\ & 1 & & 0 & \\ & & 1 & & \\ & 0 & & 1 & \\ & & & & 1 \end{bmatrix} \right\},$$

which can be written more compactly as

$$\mathbf{y}_i \sim N[\mathbf{X}_i \boldsymbol{\theta}_i, \sigma_i^2 \mathbf{I}].$$

Defining

$$\mathbf{y} = \begin{bmatrix} \mathbf{y}_1 \\ \vdots \\ \mathbf{y}_{15} \end{bmatrix}, \qquad \mathbf{X} = \begin{bmatrix} \mathbf{X}_1 & & 0 \\ & \ddots & \\ 0 & & \mathbf{X}_{15} \end{bmatrix},$$

$$\boldsymbol{\phi} = \begin{bmatrix} \boldsymbol{\theta}_1 \\ \vdots \\ \boldsymbol{\theta}_{15} \end{bmatrix}, \qquad \boldsymbol{\Omega} = \begin{bmatrix} \sigma_1^2 \mathbf{I} & & 0 \\ & \ddots & \\ 0 & & \sigma_{15}^2 \mathbf{I} \end{bmatrix},$$

the complete measurement model for all individuals can be written even more compactly in the form

$$\mathbf{y} \sim N(\mathbf{X}\boldsymbol{\phi}, \boldsymbol{\Omega}).$$

Similarly, the assumption that the $\boldsymbol{\theta}_i$ form a random sample distributed around a mean population parameter $\boldsymbol{\theta}$ can be reformulated compactly as

$$\boldsymbol{\phi} \sim N(\mathbf{Z}\boldsymbol{\theta}, \boldsymbol{\Lambda})$$

where

$$\mathbf{Z} = \begin{bmatrix} \mathbf{I} \\ \vdots \\ \mathbf{I} \end{bmatrix} \quad \text{and} \quad \boldsymbol{\Lambda} = \begin{bmatrix} \boldsymbol{\Sigma} & & 0 \\ & \ddots & \\ 0 & & \boldsymbol{\Sigma} \end{bmatrix}.$$

Throughout, $\mathbf{I}$ is to be understood as the identity matrix, of appropriate dimension.

Assuming for the present that $\boldsymbol{\Omega}$ and $\boldsymbol{\Lambda}$ are known, so that interest centers on the unknown parameters $\boldsymbol{\phi}$ (i.e., $\boldsymbol{\theta}_1, \ldots, \boldsymbol{\theta}_{15}$) and $\boldsymbol{\theta}$, the implementation of the Bayesian inference procedure for $\boldsymbol{\phi}$ and $\boldsymbol{\theta}$ requires specification of a prior distribution for $\boldsymbol{\theta}$. We shall assume in this exposition that prior knowledge about the mean population parameter vector $\boldsymbol{\theta}$ is vague, compared with the information about $\boldsymbol{\theta}$ to be provided by the study. We shall assume further that this vague prior knowledge is specified mathematically by taking the density for $\boldsymbol{\theta}$ to be a constant.

The full model for the Bayesian analysis is then seen to be the hierarchical form

$$\begin{cases} \mathbf{y} \sim N(\mathbf{X}\boldsymbol{\phi}, \boldsymbol{\Omega}) \\ \boldsymbol{\phi} \sim N(\mathbf{Z}\boldsymbol{\theta}, \boldsymbol{\Lambda}) \\ \boldsymbol{\theta} \sim \text{vague.} \end{cases}$$

Such hierarchical structures have been studied extensively [see, e.g., Lindley and Smith (1972)] and the following general algebraic results have been established (conditional throughout, for the moment, on $\boldsymbol{\Omega}$ and $\boldsymbol{\Lambda}$).

The Bayes estimate (i.e., the posterior mean) for $\boldsymbol{\phi}$ is given by

$$\boldsymbol{\phi}^* = (\mathbf{X}^T\boldsymbol{\Omega}^{-1}\mathbf{X} + \boldsymbol{\Lambda}^{-1})^{-1}(\mathbf{X}^T\boldsymbol{\Omega}^{-1}\mathbf{X}\hat{\boldsymbol{\phi}} + \boldsymbol{\Lambda}^{-1}\mathbf{Z}\hat{\boldsymbol{\theta}}),$$

where

$$\hat{\boldsymbol{\phi}} = (\mathbf{X}^T\boldsymbol{\Omega}^{-1}\mathbf{X})^{-1}\mathbf{X}^T\boldsymbol{\Omega}^{-1}\mathbf{y}$$

and

$$\hat{\boldsymbol{\theta}} = [\mathbf{Z}^T\mathbf{X}^T(\boldsymbol{\Omega} + \mathbf{X}\boldsymbol{\Lambda}\mathbf{X}^T)^{-1}\mathbf{X}\mathbf{Z}]^{-1}\mathbf{Z}^T\mathbf{X}^T(\boldsymbol{\Omega} + \mathbf{X}\boldsymbol{\Lambda}\mathbf{X}^T)^{-1}\mathbf{y}$$

are the least squares estimates of $\boldsymbol{\phi}$ (i.e., the individual parameter vectors) and $\boldsymbol{\theta}$ (the mean population parameter), respectively, $\hat{\boldsymbol{\theta}}$ also turning out to be the Bayes estimate of $\boldsymbol{\theta}$.

After straightforward algebraic manipulation, it is easily seen that

$$\boldsymbol{\theta}_i^* = \mathbf{W}_i\hat{\boldsymbol{\theta}}_i + (\mathbf{I} - \mathbf{W}_i)\hat{\boldsymbol{\theta}},$$

$$\hat{\boldsymbol{\theta}} = \left(\sum_{i=1}^{k}\mathbf{W}_i\right)^{-1}\sum_{i=1}^{k}\mathbf{W}_i\hat{\boldsymbol{\theta}}_i,$$

and

$$\mathbf{W}_i = (\sigma_i^{-2}\mathbf{X}_i^T\mathbf{X}_i + \boldsymbol{\Sigma}^{-1})^{-1}\sigma_i^{-2}\mathbf{X}_i^T\mathbf{X}_i.$$

Qualitatively, therefore—and subject to the current assumption that $\boldsymbol{\Omega}$ and $\boldsymbol{\Lambda}$ are known—we see that the estimate of the ith individual parameter vector is a pooling between $\hat{\boldsymbol{\theta}}_i$, the direct (generalized/weighted) least squares estimate, derived from data on the ith individual only, and $\hat{\boldsymbol{\theta}}$, the (generalized/weighted) least squares estimate of the mean population parameter $\boldsymbol{\theta}$ derived from combining

$$\mathbf{y} \sim N(\mathbf{X}\boldsymbol{\phi}, \boldsymbol{\Omega}) \qquad \text{and} \qquad \boldsymbol{\phi} \sim N(\mathbf{Z}\boldsymbol{\theta}, \boldsymbol{\Lambda})$$

into

$$\mathbf{y} \sim N(\mathbf{X}\mathbf{Z}\boldsymbol{\theta}, \boldsymbol{\Omega} + \mathbf{X}\boldsymbol{\Lambda}\mathbf{X}^T).$$

The estimate $\hat{\boldsymbol{\theta}}$ is itself seen to be a complicated weighted average of the individual $\hat{\boldsymbol{\theta}}_i$. Comparing this weighted form with Section 3.4, we see the potential naivete of some of the simple intuitive ways in which one might seek to combine the individual estimates into a mean population estimate and the need for an appropriate form of matrix weighted average. However, if, in fact, the $\mathbf{X}_i$ are identical for all individuals, and the measurement variances σ_i^2 are also equal for all individuals, we see that

$$\hat{\boldsymbol{\theta}} = k^{-1} \sum_{i=1}^{k} \hat{\boldsymbol{\theta}}_i,$$

so that the "naive" two-stage procedure of individual parameter estimation followed by straightforward averaging coincides, in this special case, with the Bayes estimate of the mean population parameter.

The posterior covariance matrix for $\boldsymbol{\phi}$ is given by

$$[\mathbf{X}^T\boldsymbol{\Omega}^{-1}\mathbf{X} + \boldsymbol{\Lambda}^{-1} - \boldsymbol{\Lambda}^{-1}\mathbf{Z}(\mathbf{Z}^T\boldsymbol{\Lambda}^{-1}\mathbf{Z})^{-1}\mathbf{Z}^T\boldsymbol{\Lambda}^{-1}]^{-1}$$

and for $\boldsymbol{\theta}$ is given by

$$[\mathbf{Z}^T\mathbf{X}^T(\boldsymbol{\Omega} + \mathbf{X}\boldsymbol{\Lambda}\mathbf{X}^T)^{-1}\mathbf{X}\mathbf{Z}]^{-1}.$$

The analysis above was structured around the straight-line growth-curve example. However, the general hierarchical form

$$\mathbf{y} \sim N(\mathbf{X}\boldsymbol{\phi}, \boldsymbol{\Omega})$$
$$\boldsymbol{\phi} \sim N(\mathbf{Z}\boldsymbol{\theta}, \boldsymbol{\Lambda})$$
$$\boldsymbol{\theta} \sim \text{vague}$$

in fact serves to represent *any* linear model representation of individual response relationships, simply by replacing the specific forms of $\mathbf{X}_i$ and $\boldsymbol{\theta}_i$ defining the straight-line case by a general design matrix and vector of individual regression coefficients. The weighted-average forms of estimates and the general forms of the covariance matrices are unchanged.

As a first step toward the analysis of nonlinear individual response forms, we note that the analysis of the hierarchical model is unchanged if the individual measurement models

$$\mathbf{y}_i \sim N(\mathbf{X}_i\boldsymbol{\theta}_i, \sigma_i^2\mathbf{I})$$

are replaced by the induced distribution for the sufficient statistic

$$\hat{\boldsymbol{\theta}}_i \sim N(\boldsymbol{\theta}_i, \sigma_i^2(\mathbf{X}_i^T\mathbf{X}_i)^{-1}).$$

Moreover, if σ_i^2 is unknown, it might not be too unreasonable to assume that, approximately,

$$\hat{\boldsymbol{\theta}}_i \sim N(\boldsymbol{\theta}_i, \hat{\sigma}_i^2(\mathbf{X}_i^T\mathbf{X}_i)^{-1}),$$

where $\hat{\sigma}_i^2$ is a suitable estimate of σ_i^2.

This then suggests that in the very general case of

$$\mathbf{y}_i \sim N(f(\boldsymbol{\theta}_i, x_{ij}), \sigma_i^2 g[f(\boldsymbol{\theta}_i, x_{ij})]),$$

where g allows for the possible functional dependence of the variance on the mean of the response, we might reasonably use the approximate assumption, following a maximum likelihood (or nonlinear least squares) fitting procedure, that

$$\hat{\boldsymbol{\theta}}_i \sim N(\boldsymbol{\theta}_i, \mathbf{V}_i),$$

where $\hat{\boldsymbol{\theta}}_i$ is the maximum likelihood estimate and $\mathbf{V}_i$ is the asymptotic covariance matrix. This enables us then to write

$$\hat{\boldsymbol{\phi}} = \begin{bmatrix} \hat{\boldsymbol{\theta}}_i \\ \vdots \\ \hat{\boldsymbol{\theta}}_k \end{bmatrix} \sim N\left\{ \begin{bmatrix} \boldsymbol{\theta}_1 \\ \vdots \\ \boldsymbol{\theta}_k \end{bmatrix}, \begin{bmatrix} \mathbf{V}_1 & & \mathbf{0} \\ & \ddots & \\ \mathbf{0} & & \mathbf{V}_k \end{bmatrix} \right\} \equiv N(\boldsymbol{\phi}, \mathbf{V}),$$

which leads to the hierarchical model formulation

$$\begin{cases} \hat{\boldsymbol{\phi}} \sim N(\boldsymbol{\phi}, \mathbf{V}) \\ \boldsymbol{\phi} \sim N(\mathbf{Z}\boldsymbol{\theta}, \boldsymbol{\Lambda}) \\ \boldsymbol{\theta} \sim \text{vague.} \end{cases}$$

The required estimates and covariance matrices, for known $\boldsymbol{\Lambda}$, are then given by the previous formulas with $\mathbf{y}$ replaced by $\hat{\boldsymbol{\phi}}$, $\mathbf{X}$ by $\mathbf{I}$, and $\boldsymbol{\Omega}$ by $\mathbf{V}$.

In applications, $\boldsymbol{\Sigma}$ will, of course, be unknown, and completion of the Bayesian analysis requires the assignment of a prior distribution to $\boldsymbol{\Sigma}$, or, equivalently, $\boldsymbol{\Sigma}^{-1}$. If the latter is assigned a Wishart distribution with degrees of freedom ρ and matrix $\mathbf{R}$ (so that $\rho^{-1}\mathbf{R}$ plays the role of a prior estimate of $\boldsymbol{\Sigma}$), it can easily be shown that the joint posterior density for

ϕ and Σ^{-1}, given $\hat{\phi}$, is proportional to

$$\prod_{i=1}^{k} |\mathbf{V}_i|^{-1/2} \exp\left[-\frac{1}{2}\sum_{i=1}^{k}(\hat{\boldsymbol{\theta}}_i - \boldsymbol{\theta}_i)^T \mathbf{V}_i^{-1}(\hat{\boldsymbol{\theta}}_i - \boldsymbol{\theta}_i)\right] |\boldsymbol{\Sigma}|^{-(k+\rho-p-2)/2}$$
$$\times \exp\left\{-\frac{1}{2}\operatorname{tr}\boldsymbol{\Sigma}^{-1}\left[\mathbf{R} + \sum_{i=1}^{k}(\boldsymbol{\theta}_i - \bar{\boldsymbol{\theta}}_0)(\boldsymbol{\theta}_i - \bar{\boldsymbol{\theta}}_0)^T\right]\right\}, \quad (1)$$

where $\bar{\boldsymbol{\theta}}_0 = k^{-1}\sum_{i=1}^{k}\boldsymbol{\theta}_i$ and p is the dimension of the individual parameter vectors $\boldsymbol{\theta}_i$.

Reexpressing the general forms given earlier, we see that the posterior distribution for $\boldsymbol{\theta}$, given $\hat{\boldsymbol{\theta}}_1, \ldots, \hat{\boldsymbol{\theta}}_k$ and $\boldsymbol{\Sigma}$, is p-variate normal with mean $\boldsymbol{\theta}^*$ and covariance matrix $\mathbf{D}$, where

$$\boldsymbol{\theta}^* = \mathbf{D}\sum_{i=1}^{k}[(\mathbf{V}_i + \boldsymbol{\Sigma})^{-1}\hat{\boldsymbol{\theta}}_i]$$

and (2)

$$\mathbf{D} = \left[\sum_{i=1}^{k}(\mathbf{V}_i + \boldsymbol{\Sigma})^{-1}\right]^{-1}.$$

We also see that the posterior distributions for $\boldsymbol{\theta}_1, \ldots, \boldsymbol{\theta}_k$, given $\hat{\boldsymbol{\theta}}_1, \ldots, \hat{\boldsymbol{\theta}}_k$, $\boldsymbol{\theta}$ and $\boldsymbol{\Sigma}$ are independently p-variate normals with means $\boldsymbol{\theta}_i^*$ and covariance matrices $\mathbf{D}_i$, where

$$\boldsymbol{\theta}_i^* = \mathbf{D}_i(\mathbf{V}_i^{-1}\hat{\boldsymbol{\theta}}_i + \boldsymbol{\Sigma}^{-1}\boldsymbol{\theta})$$

and (3)

$$\mathbf{D}_i = (\mathbf{V}_i^{-1} + \boldsymbol{\Sigma}^{-1})^{-1}.$$

From (1) to (3), we can produce an effective EM-type iterative algorithm [see, also, Racine (1985)] for the estimation of $\boldsymbol{\theta}_i^*$, $\boldsymbol{\theta}$ and $\boldsymbol{\Sigma}$. At the lth iteration, $\boldsymbol{\theta}_i^{(l-1)}$, $\boldsymbol{\theta}^{(l-1)}$, and $\boldsymbol{\Sigma}^{(l-1)}$ will denote the current approximations to $\boldsymbol{\theta}_i$, $\boldsymbol{\theta}$, and $\boldsymbol{\Sigma}$.

E-Step

We approximate $\boldsymbol{\Sigma}$ in (2) by $\boldsymbol{\Sigma}^{(l-1)}$, obtaining

$$\boldsymbol{\theta}^{(l)} = \mathbf{D}^{(l)}\sum_{i=1}^{k}(\mathbf{V}_i + \boldsymbol{\Sigma}^{(l-1)})^{-1}\hat{\boldsymbol{\theta}}_i$$

and

$$\mathbf{D}^{(l)} = \left[\sum_{i-1}^{k}(\mathbf{V}_i + \mathbf{\Sigma}^{(l-1)})^{-1}\right]^{-1}.$$

Conditioning now on $\boldsymbol{\theta} = \boldsymbol{\theta}^{(l)}$ and $\mathbf{\Sigma} = \mathbf{\Sigma}^{(l-1)}$ in (3), we obtain

$$\boldsymbol{\theta}_i^{(l)} = (\mathbf{V}_i^{-1} + \mathbf{\Sigma}^{(l-1)})^{-1}(\mathbf{V}_i^{-1}\hat{\boldsymbol{\theta}}_i + \mathbf{\Sigma}^{(l-1)-1}\boldsymbol{\theta}^{(l)}).$$

M-Step

Conditioning on $\boldsymbol{\theta}_i = \boldsymbol{\theta}_i^{(l)}$, the conditional posterior mode of (1) is given by

$$\mathbf{\Sigma}^{(l)} = \frac{\mathbf{R} + \sum_{i=1}^{k}(\boldsymbol{\theta}_i^{(l)} - \boldsymbol{\theta}_0^{(l)})(\boldsymbol{\theta}_i^{(l)} - \boldsymbol{\theta}_0^{(l)})^T}{k + \rho - p - 2}.$$

The E and M steps are repeated until $\mathbf{\Sigma}^{(l)}$ converges. A reasonable set of starting values are given by

$$\boldsymbol{\theta}^{(0)} = k^{-1}\sum_{i=1}^{k}\hat{\boldsymbol{\theta}}_i$$

and

$$\mathbf{\Sigma}^{(0)} = \frac{\mathbf{R} + \sum_{i=1}^{k}(\hat{\boldsymbol{\theta}}_i - \boldsymbol{\theta}^{(0)})(\hat{\boldsymbol{\theta}}_i - \boldsymbol{\theta}^{(0)})^T}{k + \rho - p - 2}.$$

4 APPLIED AND SIMULATED CASE STUDIES

4.1 The Bayes/Empirical Bayes Approach

For the two illustrative examples introduced earlier, the intra-individual error variances are assumed to be equal, an assumption that is quite reasonable in these cases as a consequence of the form of the measurement procedures. (For an estimation of the population parameters, this assumption is not necessary. However, if one wishes to predict a new individual's profile, information about the error variance for that individual would need to be available, either from the sample population or from some other source.)

The individual parameters $\boldsymbol{\theta}_i$ were first estimated using standard least squares methods and the residual sum of squares based on the estimates $\hat{\boldsymbol{\theta}}_i$ were then pooled to evaluate $\hat{\sigma}^2$, the posterior mode of σ^2. In these examples, the pooled degrees of freedom for estimating σ^2 are quite large, so that σ^2 can reasonably be regarded as known and equal to $\hat{\sigma}^2$.

In Example 1, the covariance matrix $\mathbf{V}_i$ for individual i is then given by

$$\hat{\sigma}^2(\mathbf{X}_i\mathbf{X}_i^T)^{-1},$$

where $\mathbf{X}_i$ is the corresponding design matrix. In Example 2, $\mathbf{V}_i$ is given by

$$\hat{\sigma}^2 \left\{ [\nabla f(\hat{\boldsymbol{\theta}}_i)][\nabla f(\hat{\boldsymbol{\theta}}_i)]^T \right\}^{-1},$$

where $\nabla f(\boldsymbol{\theta}_i)$ denotes the $2 \times n_i$ vector of partial derivatives of $f(\boldsymbol{\theta}, x_{ij})$, $j = 1, \ldots, n_i$ evaluated at $\hat{\boldsymbol{\theta}}_i$.

The prior specification for the population covariance matrix [see the discussion preceding equation (1) in Section 3.5] was in both cases taken to be $\rho = 2$, $\mathbf{R} = 0.1\mathbf{I}$, reflecting very vague prior information about the population covariance matrix. The EM algorithm was then applied (as detailed in Section 3.5) to approximate $\boldsymbol{\theta}^*$, $\mathbf{D}^*$, and $\boldsymbol{\Sigma}^*$, the posterior mean and covariance matrix of $\boldsymbol{\theta}$, and the marginal posterior mode of $\boldsymbol{\Sigma}$, respectively.

4.2 Analysis of Example 1

To summarize inferences about the effect of the treatment on the initial weight (weight at day 0) and the growth rate, the bivariate posterior contours for $\alpha_C - \alpha_T$ and $\beta_C - \beta_T$ corresponding to 0.50, 0.90, and 0.95 posterior regions for $\boldsymbol{\theta}_C - \boldsymbol{\theta}_T$, are plotted in Figure 4 (study A) and Figure 5

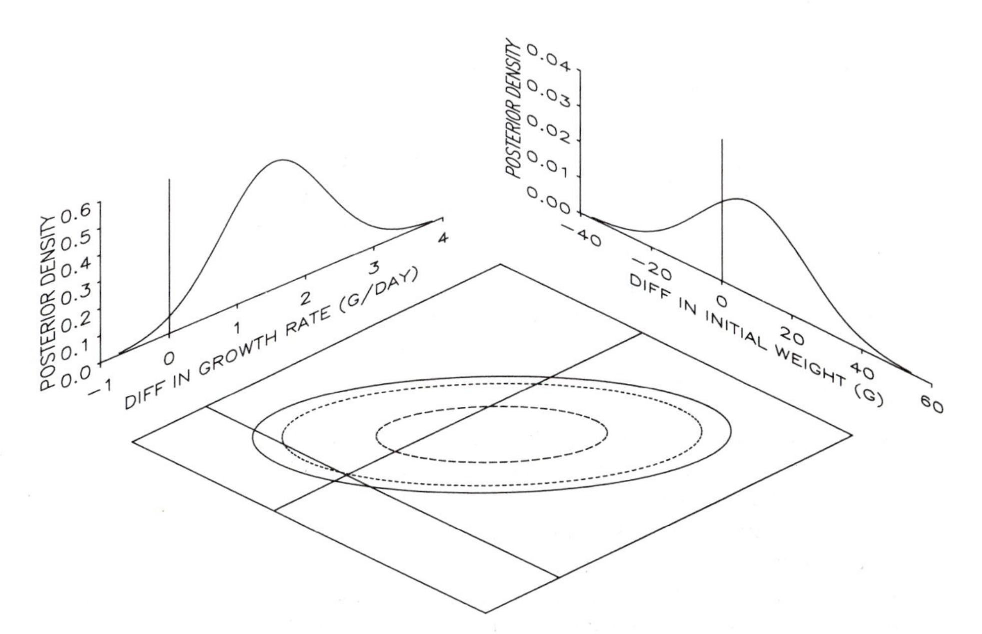

Figure 4 Inference for Example 1, study A.

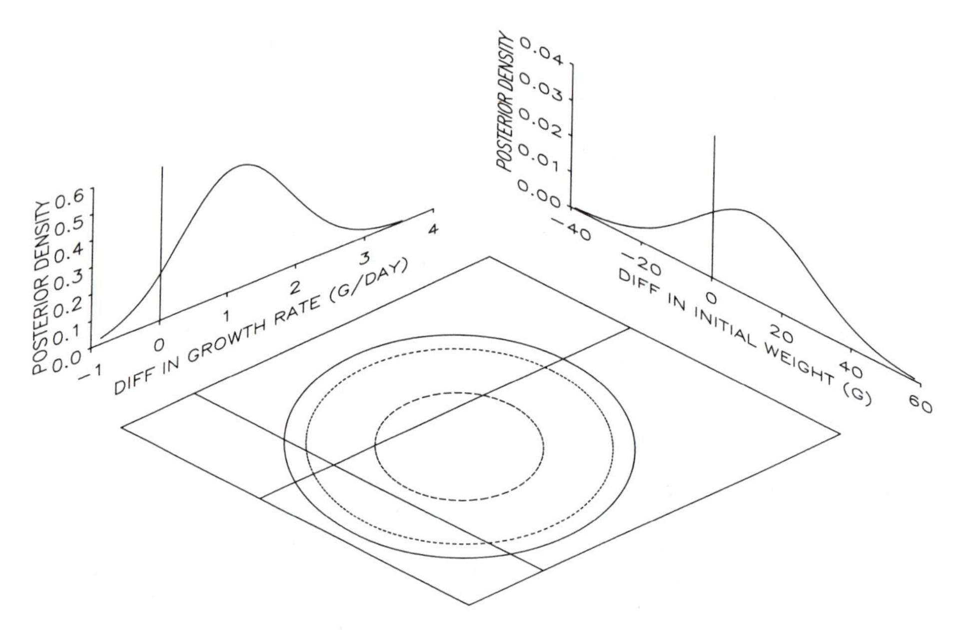

Figure 5 Inference for Example 1, study B.

(study B), along with the marginal posterior densities for $\alpha_C - \alpha_T$ (the difference in initial weight) and $\beta_C - \beta_T$ (the difference in growth rate). These posterior summaries reveal good agreement between the two studies, even though they have very different designs (reflected in somewhat greater uncertainty in study B). Inspecting the marginal densities, one can conclude that the treatment reduced the growth rate of the animals, but that (as expected since the animals were randomly assigned to control and treated groups at the beginning of the experiments) there is no real evidence of treatment effect on the initial weights of the animals.

4.3 Analysis of Example 2

To illustrate the predictive aspect of population modeling, patients 1 to 9 in this study have been taken to be the "original" sample population and patient 10 has been taken to be a new patient. Figure 6, based on the data from patients 1 to 9, shows the 95% highest joint posterior region for the population parameters $\log \alpha$ and $\log \beta$, together with the marginal posterior densities. Figure 7 shows the 95% highest joint posterior region and the corresponding marginal posterior densities of $\log \alpha_{10}$ and $\log \beta_{10}$, the individual parameters for patient 10, based (a) on only the 2-and 6-hour

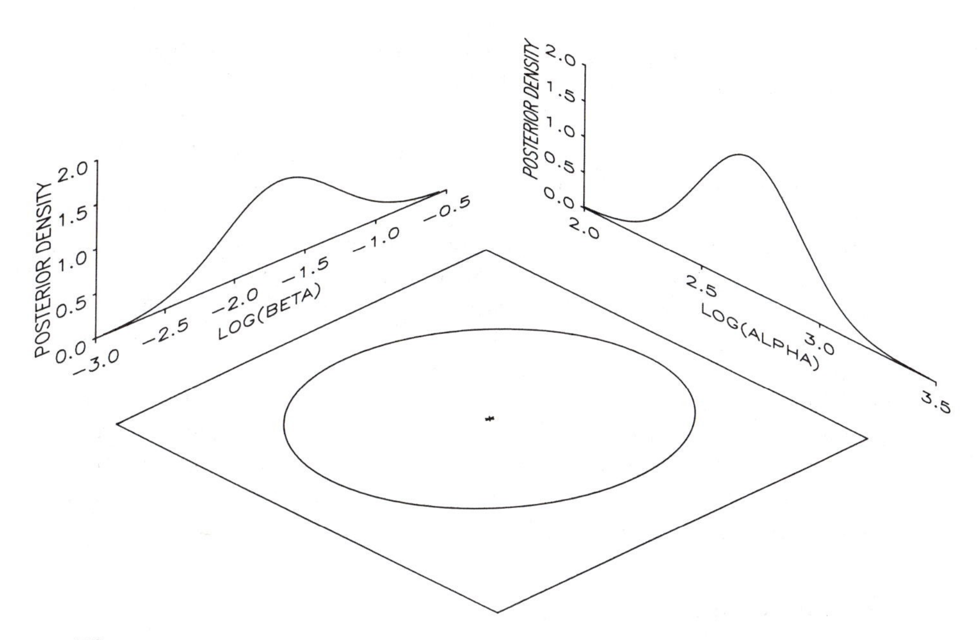

Figure 6 Inference for Example 2, population parameters.

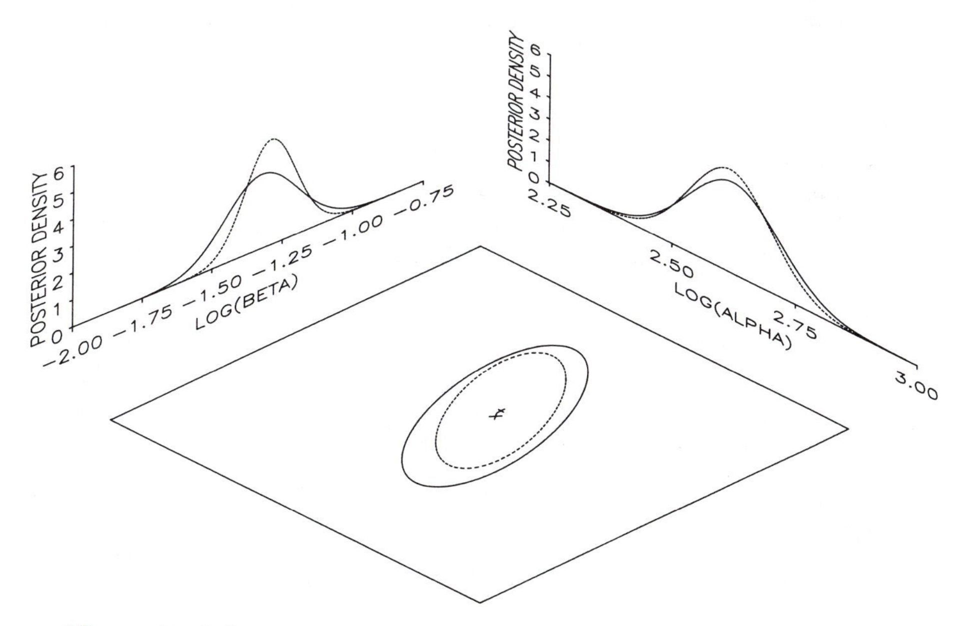

Figure 7 Inference for Example 2, patient 10.

samples for that patient, together with the data from sample population (indicated by the solid line), and (b) on all the data from all the patients (indicated by the dashed line). Comparative studies such as these can help to reveal which are the more informative sampling times. Here, comparing Figures 6 and 7, we note that just two observations (at 2 and 6 hours) from individual 10 have sharpened up the inferences considerably beyond the general population summary (compare the solid-line inferences in Figure 7 with those of Figure 6), and that although the additional four observations on individual 10 provide some further sharpening of the inferences (compare the dashed and solid lines in Figure 7), much of the information is already contained in the 2-and 6-hour data. Systematic studies of this type can lead to substantial improvements in the treatment of new patients when only limited initial observations on the latter are possible. Figure 8 shows that 90% predictable profile regions for patient 10, (a) just based on the sample population (solid lines) and (b) based on the sample population together with the new patient's 2-and 6-hour data (dashed lines).

4.4 Other Numerical Studies

Racine-Poon (1985) studied the performance of the EM algorithm for three simulated cases, and the results from one of these cases, the one-compartment model, are presented here to illustrate the conclusions

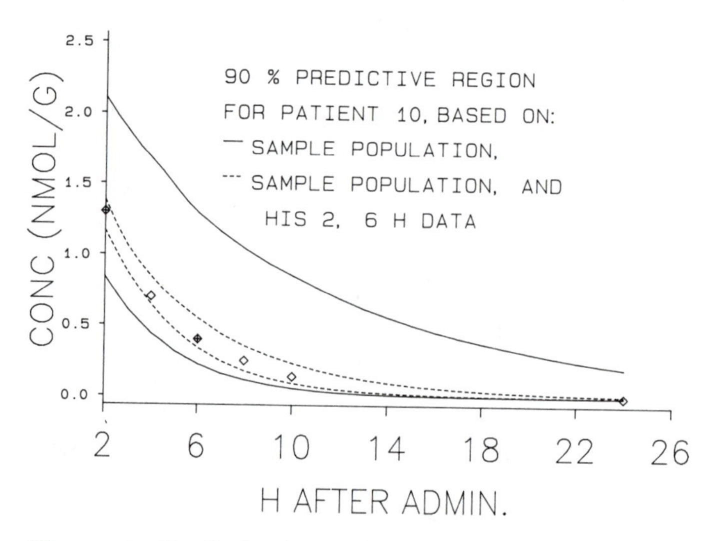

Figure 8 Predictive intervals for patient 10.

reached by Racine-Poon. The model is given by

$$y_i = \frac{\text{dose} \cdot k_{a_i}}{v_i(k_{a_i} - k_{e_i})}[\exp(-k_{a_i} x_{ij}) - \exp(-k_{e_i} x_{ij})] + \epsilon_{ij},$$

where k_{a_i}, k_{e_i}, and v_i are the individual's absorption rate, elimination rate, and the volume of distribution in the central compartment. This model is commonly used to describe the plasma profile when the drug is administered orally in tablet form. Twenty individual profiles were simulated at time points 0.5, 1, 2, 4, 6, 8, 12, 18, and 24 hours after administration of an assumed unit dose.

The population mean and covariance matrix were, respectively,

$$\boldsymbol{\theta} = \begin{bmatrix} \log k_a \\ \log k_e \\ \log v \end{bmatrix} = \begin{bmatrix} -0.06411 \\ -2.2926 \\ 1.79 \end{bmatrix}$$

and

$$\boldsymbol{\Sigma} = \begin{bmatrix} 0.09 & -0.045 & 0.072 \\ & 0.09 & 0.036 \\ & & 0.16 \end{bmatrix}.$$

Such large magnitudes of variation among individual parameters are very commonly encountered in applications, even for seemingly rather "homogeneous" populations. The errors, ϵ_{ij}, are assumed to be normally distributed, with the standard deviations of the errors proportional to the underlying response, so that

$$\epsilon_{ij} \sim N(0, \sigma_i^2[f(\boldsymbol{\theta}_i, x_{ij})]^2).$$

Sixteen of the 20 subjects were assumed to have a 10% error ($\sigma_i = 0.1$), whereas the other 4 were assumed to have a 40% error ($\sigma_i = 0.4$).

The averaged results from 10 simulations are shown in Table 1 and indicate, in this as in the other cases studied by Racine-Poon, that the iteration algorithm performs very well, even though four of the subjects in this case display rather high intrasubject variation.

Experience with the NONMEM approach (Section 3.3) has proved far less satisfactory across a range of models, although positive results have been reported for specific models by Sheiner and Beal (1980, 1981, 1983). Racine et al. (1986) give an outline report on simulations of a one-compartment model where the Bayes/empirical Bayes EM algorithm in general outperformed the NONMEM procedure. The results of the simulations were measured by the accuracy and precision of the methods: the former measured by the average percentage bias of the estimates, the latter by the sample standard deviation of the percentage bias. In several cases,

Table 1 Mean and Standard Deviation (SD) of the Posterior Mean of $\boldsymbol{\theta}$ and the Model Approximation of $\boldsymbol{\Sigma}$ from 10 Simulations

Parameter	True value	Mean	SD
$\log k_a$	−0.6411	−0.6150	0.0802
$\log k_e$	−2.2926	−2.3346	0.0742
$\log v$	1.79	1.7927	0.1123
$\boldsymbol{\Sigma}_{11}$	0.09	0.0832	0.0599
$\boldsymbol{\Sigma}_{12}$	−0.045	−0.0450	0.0488
$\boldsymbol{\Sigma}_{13}$	0.073	0.0623	0.0397
$\boldsymbol{\Sigma}_{22}$	0.09	0.0922	0.0347
$\boldsymbol{\Sigma}_{23}$	0.036	0.0486	0.0499
$\boldsymbol{\Sigma}_{33}$	0.16	0.1692	0.0468

the NONMEM procedure failed to converge. In cases where convergence was obtained in estimating the population mean and covariance parameters, NONMEM proved from two to six and from two to ten times less accurate, respectively, and from three to four times less precise.

Steimer et al. (1984) also carried out simulation studies to compare NONMEM with the GTS and ITS two-stage procedures (Section 3.4). Using the same measures of accuracy and precision, the performances of GTS and ITS were found to be rather similar, and in estimating the population covariance matrix, NONMEM was found to be about four to five times less accurate and two to three times less precise. The GTS method tends to underestimate the covariance matrix, and despite its greatly increased computational overhead, the ITS method provides only marginal improvement.

5 SUMMARY AND RECOMMENDATIONS

Population models involve complex covariance structures and, particularly in the case of nonlinear profiles, present a difficult challenge in terms of both estimation and model checking. Naive approaches are likely to be extremely misleading and there is a need for considerable care in the choice of models, parametrizations, and estimation algorithms. Whatever estimation procedure is followed, a substantial amount of diagnostic and cross-validating checking has to be performed to investigate the appropriateness of the choice of profile function, error variance form, distributional assumptions, and approximations invoked in the inference procedure. Response and parameter transformations may be required as well as the evaluation of measures of nonlinearity [see, e.g., Beale (1960)] to verify that the assumed model and parametrization are adequate to ensure satisfactory performance of the iterative algorithm.

As far as estimation procedures are concerned, the general procedures that currently appear to be available and of most interest are NONMEM (Section 3.3), GTS and ITS (Section 3.4), and the Bayesian EM algorithm (Section 3.5). NONMEM is by far the most expensive computationally and appears to be the least satisfactory in practice, although it has the advantage that it does not need estimates of the individual profiles to be available. GTS tends to underestimate the population covariance matrix, and ITS, despite the greatly increased computational overhead, provides only a marginal improvement. At present, the balance of advantage seems to lie with the Bayesian EM algorithm. It has proved effective in a number of applied and simulated studies, and is very easy and cheap to implement.

All the calculations reported here using the Bayesian EM algorithm were performed using SAS. Estimation of the $\boldsymbol{\theta}_i$ and $\mathbf{V}_i$ for individual profiles was carried out using PROC GLM (for linear profiles) and PROC NLIN (for nonlinear profiles). A list of the EM algorithm written in PROC IML is available from the first author on request.

REFERENCES

Beale, E. M. L. (1960). Confidence regions in nonlinear estimation (with discussion). *J. Roy. Statist. Soc. B 22*, 1–41.

Lindley, D. V., and A. F. M. Smith (1972). Bayes estimates for the linear model (with discussion). *J. Roy. Statist. Soc. B 34*, 1–42.

Racine, A., A. P. Grieve, H. Flühler and A. F. M. Smith (1986). Bayesian methods in practice: experiences in the pharmaceutical industry (with discussion). *Appl. Statist. 35*, 93–150.

Racine-Poon, A. (1985). A Bayesian approach to nonlinear random effects models. *Biometrics 41*, 1015–1024.

Sheiner, L. B., and S. L. Beal (1979). *NONMEM Users Guide—Part 1: Users Basic Guide*. Division of Clinical Pharmacology, University of California, San Francisco.

Sheiner, L. B., and S. L. Beal (1980). Evaluation of methods of estimating pharmacokinetic parameters: I. Michaelis-Menten model: routine clinical pharmacokinetic data. *J. Pharmacokinet. Biopharm. 8*, 553–571.

Sheiner, L. B., and S. L. Beal (1981). Evaluation of methods of estimating pharmacokinetic parameters: II. Biexponential model and experimental pharmacokinetic data. *J. Pharmacokinet. Biopharm. 9*, 635–651.

Sheiner, L. B., and S. L. Beal (1983). Evaluation of methods of estimating pharmacokinetic parameters: III. Monoexponential model: routine clinical pharmacokinetic data. *J. Pharmacokinet. Biopharm. 11*, 303–319.

Steimer, J., A. Mallet, J. Golmard, and J. Boisieux (1984). Alternative approaches to estimation of population pharmacokinetic parameters: comparison with the nonlinear mixed effect model. *Drug Metab. Rev. 15*, 265–292.

6

Linear and Nonlinear Regression

R. DENNIS COOK and SANFORD WEISBERG University of Minnesota, St. Paul, Minnesota

Fitting curves to data is called regression analysis. The purpose of this chapter is to provide an introduction to this important area of statistics by studying dose-response relationships for different drugs or treatments as dosage is varied. We shall use both linear and nonlinear models. Our emphasis is on summarization of results, basic methods for inference, and considerations for the design of such experiments. Throughout most of this chapter, we consider a particular experiment, which we now describe. Although the setting involves poultry diets, the methods apply directly to many other problems that arise in the pharmaceutical industry.

Corn and soybean meal are the basic ingredients of poultry diets used in most Western countries. It is well known, however, that such basal diets are deficient in an essential amino acid, methionine. Birds grown under methionine-deficient diets are obviously smaller and less healthy than are birds grown under diets with supplemented methionine. Consequently, evaluation of the bioefficacy of available methionine is an important problem in the poultry industry.

Although added methionine is known to improve growth, neither the dose-response relationship nor the differences between sources of methionine are exactly known. To study this relationship, and to make these comparisons, Noll, Waibel, Cook, and Witmer (Noll et al., 1984) conducted a series of experiments, and we shall use data from an experiment similar to the ones they describe.

From 1 to 7 days of age, all the male poults in the experiment were fed a common diet. At 7 days of age, they were weighed and divided at random into pens of 15. Each pen was then randomly assigned to receive a supplemental amount of methionine from one of three sources. We call the three sources, S, $M1$, and $M2$. Source S is difficult and expensive to produce, and was included as a laboratory standard against which the two experimental sources $M1$ and $M2$ would be compared. In all, 50 pens of 15 animals were used in the study, allocated to six different levels of supplementation ranging from 0 to 0.44% of the total diet. The animals were weighed at 56 days when the experiment ended, and the average weight gain for each pen was computed. Since all animals in the same pen were treated alike, the unit of analysis in this and in may other animal experiments is the pen, not the individual animal. The pen averages are the raw data.

Dose-response curves are generally nonlinear, perhaps exhibiting a shape similar to that of the two curves shown in Figure 1. In this figure we see

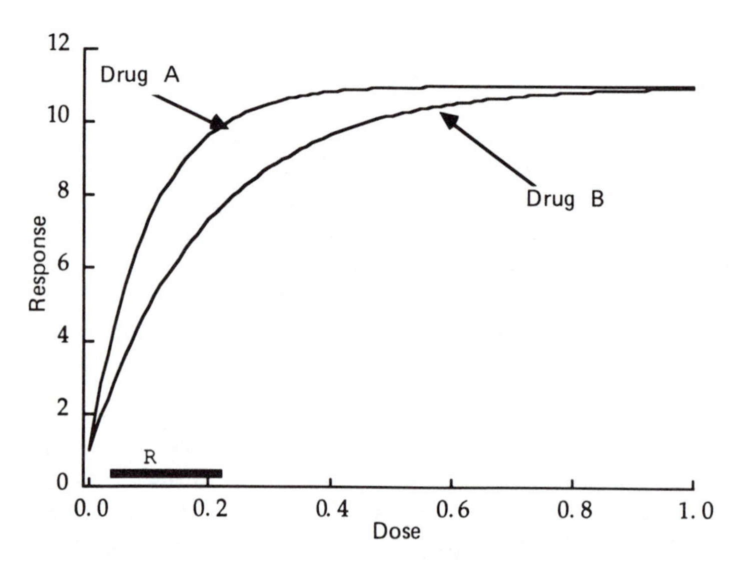

Figure 1 Schematic dose-response curves.

that the rate of change in response is larger for small doses than it is for large doses, and that for very large doses, the rate of change may be zero, implying that there is a maximum response that is the same for any large dose. The latter feature of Figure 1 may be little more than a practical idealization, since may drugs that show a beneficial positive response for reasonable doses may be lethal for a sufficiently large dose (cf. Chapter 4 Ekholm, Fox, Bolognese). Often, the shape of the curve in the region marked R in Figure 1 is of greatest interest, and sometimes in this region a linear approximation may be adequate. In the figure the response for drug B seems to be approximately linear over R, while that for drug A is less well approximated by a line. The effects of the two drugs are compared by comparing their response curves, or if the curves are assumed to be in a parametric family, by comparing parameters. As shown in the figure, both drugs have the same maximum and minimum response. But drug A has a higher response over region R. If higher response is beneficial, and if cost per unit dose is the same for each drug, drug A might be preferred.

If the doses in a particular experiment are confined to a range where the response curve is approximately linear, simple regression models may be useful. However, the parameters of the approximating linear model, the slope and the intercept, may have little physical meaning since if the range of doses in the experiment were changed, the values of these parameters would change as well.

1 LINEAR MODELS

Consider fitting a single straight line to data generated from experimental units with varying amounts of a single drug. We let x_i be the ith dose used in the experiment, $i = 1, \ldots, k$, and let y_{ij} be the responses of the units receiving that dose, $j = 1, 2, \ldots, n_i$. The total number of units in the experiment is $N = \sum n_i$. The linear model stipulates that

$$y_{ij} = \beta_0 + \beta_1 x_i + \epsilon_{ij}, \qquad j = 1, \ldots, n_i, \quad i = 1, 2, \ldots, k, \tag{1}$$

where β_0 and β_1 are the unknown intercept and slope parameters of the straight line, and the ϵ_{ij} are random errors, which are included in the model to recognize that the y_{ij} will surely not be determined exactly by the x_i, and to recognize that several patients, animals, or units treated with the same dose will not give exactly the same response. For simplicity of notation in the following, we will suppress one or both of the subscripts on data y and errors ϵ whenever the presence of the subscripts will tend to make presentations appear more difficult.

To proceed, it is necessary to make assumptions concerning the random errors. The first assumption we make is that of unbiasedness: $E(\epsilon) = 0$. This is unlikely to be true in this approximating framework, as it requires that the response curve be *exactly* linear in the region under study. However, this assumption may be acceptable if the deviations from linearity are small relative to the variation of the ϵ. We will provide a diagnostic test of lack of fit of the model as a check on this assumption.

Next, we assume the errors to be independent. This assumption is reasonable in our example since each observation is taken on a separate, randomly assigned pen of animals. In experiments with each subject measured at several different doses, as in a repeated measures experiment, a different methodology may be required (see Chapter 3). Next, we need to make assumptions concerning the variability of the errors. The simplest assumption is that $\text{var}(\epsilon_{ij}) = \sigma^2$, an unknown positive number, for all i and j, but the same methodology can be applied if $\text{var}(\epsilon_{ij}) = \sigma^2/w_{ij}$, for $w_{ij} > 0$ known.

Finally, we consider distributional assumptions concerning the errors. Although explicit assumptions are not required for least-squares estimation, we will assume that errors are normally distributed. It is a pleasant fact that maximum likelihood estimates with normal errors are essentially the same as least squares estimates, but the likelihood framework allows for more general results, and this assumption will help us later in making inferences and in finding good experimental designs.

Most computer packages include routines for linear regression based on the foregoing assumptions, and most elementary statistics books will present the usual estimates and other related statistics [see, e.g., Draper and Smith (1981) or Weisberg (1985)]. We will suppose that such a statistical package has been used, resulting in least squares estimates $\hat{\beta}_0$ and $\hat{\beta}_1$ of the intercept and slope; residuals $e = y - \hat{\beta}_0 - \hat{\beta}_1 x$; residual sum of squares $\text{RSS} = \sum e^2$; and the total sum of squares, $\text{TSS} = \sum (y - \bar{y})^2$. The residual degrees of freedom is equal to $n - p$, where p is the number of β's in the model; for simple regression, $p = 2$, but in many problems $p > 2$. Most other regression summaries are functions of these basic statistics: the regression sum of squares is $\text{SSreg} = \text{TSS} - \text{RSS}$, the squared multiple correlation $R^2 = 1 - \text{RSS}/\text{TSS}$, the overall test statistic that all β's except for the intercept equal zero is given by $F = R^2(n-p)/[p(1-R^2)]$, and the estimate of σ^2, the residual mean square, is $\hat{\sigma}^2 = \text{RSS}/(n-p)$.

Table 1 gives the average response for the 10 pens with the standard supplement S. We have $k = 4$ levels of dose between 0.04 and 0.28%, with samples sizes $n_1 = n_3 = n_4 = 2$, and $n_2 = 4$, so the total number of units is $N = \sum n = 10$.

Table 1 Average Weights of Animals in Pens Receiving Standard Supplement S

Dose (%)	Average weight (g)
0.04	2368
0.04	2468
0.10	2723
0.10	2873
0.10	2453
0.10	2418
0.16	3074
0.16	2739
0.28	2836
0.28	3296

We begin the analysis by plotting response versus dose, as shown in Figure 2. A straight line is plausible. Because the same levels of supplement were applied to several pens, the plot also gives a visual impression of the variability between pens treated alike and hence of the assumed constant σ; this will provide the basis for a test of lack of fit of the model. Since the spread of points within each group is similar, the assumption of constant variance seems reasonable.

Most computer programs will fit model (1) to the data in Table 1 by treating the columns in Table 1 as variables with length 10, and then using a regression routine. Table 2, column (a), presents some usual computer output, suggesting that the change in response for a change in dose of 0.1% is about 274 g ($= 0.1\hat{\beta}_1$). The large t-value for dose, which is the ratio of the estimate to its standard error, or $2739/809 = 3.39$ with d.f. $= 8$ (p-value $= 0.005$), suggests strongly that response increases with dose, a fact that seems clear from Figure 2.

The RSS for this regression can be written as a sum of two terms,

$$\begin{aligned} \text{RSS} &= \sum n_i(\bar{y}_{i+} - \hat{\beta}_0 - \hat{\beta}_1 x_i)^2 + \sum (n_i - 1)\text{SD}_i^2 \\ &= \text{SS(lof)} + \text{SS(pe)}, \end{aligned} \tag{2}$$

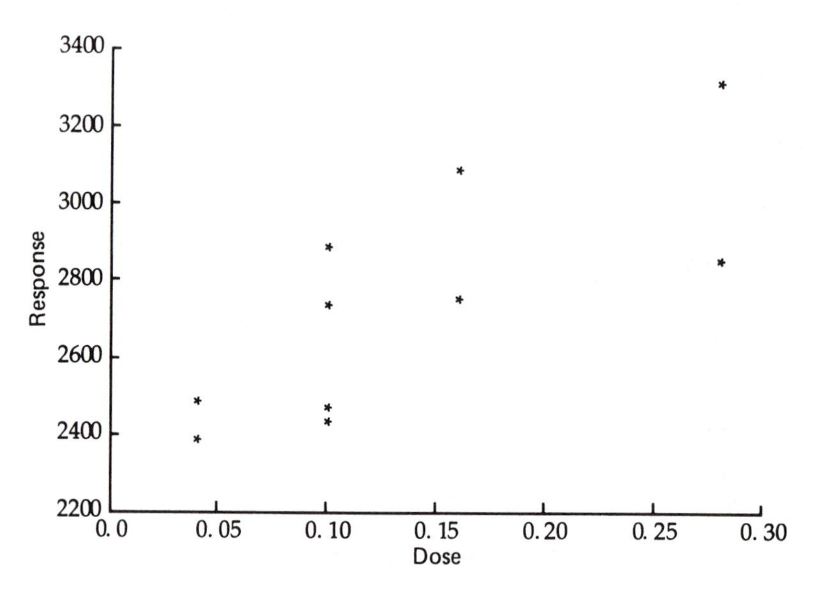

Figure 2 Weight gain versus dose for supplement S.

where $\bar{y}_{i+}$ and SD_i are, respectively, the average and standard deviation of the response for all units given dose x_i. The first term on the right side in (2), which we call the sum of squares for lack of fit, SS(lof), is a weighted sum of the squared deviations of the dose averages ($\bar{y}_{i+}$) from the fitted line ($\hat{\beta}_0 + \hat{\beta}_1 x_i$). If the straight-line model is appropriate, this estimates a multiple of σ^2, but if the model is not appropriate, it estimates a larger quantity ($\sigma^2 + \text{bias}^2$). The latter term on the right of (2), which we call

Table 2 Regression Estimates[a]

Quantity	(a) Eq. (1)	(b) Eq. (4)
$\hat{\beta}_0$	2,352 (128)	2,352 (83)
$\hat{\beta}_1$	2,739 (809)	2,739 (527)
$\hat{\sigma}^2$	43,368	18,381
d.f.	8	2
R^2	0.59	0.96

[a]Values in parentheses are standard errors.

the sum of squares for pure error, SS(pe), is a weighted sum of within-dose standard deviations, and $\tilde{\sigma}^2 = \text{SS(pe)}/\sum(n_i - 1)$ is an appropriate estimate of σ^2 whether or not the model is correct. Comparison of these two estimates of σ^2 provides the basis for a lack-of-fit test for the straight-line model: compute

$$F = \frac{\text{SS(lof)}/(k-p)}{\tilde{\sigma}^2} = \frac{[\text{RSS} - \text{SS(pe)}]/(k-p)}{\tilde{\sigma}^2}. \tag{3}$$

To get a p-value for the test, the value of (3) is compared to the percentage points of an F distribution with $k-p$ and $\sum(n_i - 1) = N - k$ degrees of freedom. Our notation for this F distribution is $F(k-p, N-k)$. For the example, the within-group standard deviations are 70.7, 218.5, 236.9, and 325.3, respectively, and SS(pe) $= 310{,}181.2$, $\tilde{\sigma}^2 = 51{,}696.9$. Thus SS(lof) $= 346{,}944.0 - 310{,}181.2 = 36{,}762.8$, and $F = (36{,}762.8/2)/51{,}696.9 = 0.36$. Since F is so small, the p-value is large, suggesting little evidence against the straight-line approximation over this region.

Alternatively, the estimates of β_0 and β_1 and the sum of squares for lack of fit can be obtained directly from the fit of a single regression equation obtained by averaging both sides of (1) over the second subscript (averaging all cases with the same level of dose),

$$\bar{y}_{i+} = \beta_0 + \beta_1 x_i + \bar{\epsilon}_{i+}, \qquad i = 1, \ldots, k. \tag{4}$$

Since ϵ_{ij} has been replaced by $\bar{\epsilon}_{i+}$, so that $\text{var}(\bar{\epsilon}_{i+}) = \sigma^2/n_i$, we should use weighted least squares, with weights given by the sample sizes n_i, when performing regressions based on (4). The results from fitting (4) are summarized in Table 2, column (b). While the estimates in columns (a) and (b) are the same, any quantity that depends on a computation of the residual sum of squares is different in the two approaches. In column (b) of Table 2, the RSS consists solely of SS(lof), and this provides a check on the earlier calculation. Thus, if the n_i and the within-group standard deviations SD_i are computed and saved, all regression calculations can be made using the weighted regression of the within-dose averages on the level of dose, with the n_i as weights. The resulting RSS is the sum of squares for lack of fit.

The previous comment also suggests that the usual standard errors of estimates given in both columns of Table 2 may not be appropriate since they both use the RSS for that particular regression to estimate σ^2. Since $\tilde{\sigma}^2$ estimates the variance of the errors whether or not the model is appropriate, an alternative estimate of standard error, to be used in testing and confidence procedures for coefficients, is $\text{se}(\hat{\beta}_j)\hat{\sigma}/\tilde{\sigma}$, where $\text{se}(\hat{\beta}_j)$ and $\hat{\sigma}^2$ are the estimates printed by the computer program.

1.1 Comparing Groups

Table 3 gives the source, within-dose sample size, average response, and SD for all three sources used in the experiment; for the moment, we will concentrate on doses between 0.04 and 0.28%. Over this range, the groups or sources can be compared by fitting a sequence of linear models. The most general model, which we will call model 1, allows each source to have its own slope and intercept, as illustrated by the upper left plot in Figure 3. We can then imagine a sequence of more restrictive models, also illustrated in Figure 3: model 2, slopes are equal but intercepts are different; model 3, slopes differ but the intercept is common; and model 4, all groups have the identical regression line. These models can then, assuming normality of errors, be compared by using F-tests.

Table 3 Averages ($\bar{y}$) and Standard Deviations (SD) for All 15 Conditions Used in the Turkey Growth Experiment

X	Source	n	$\bar{y}$	SD
0.00	—	5	2142	162.535
0.04	S	2	2418	70.7107
0.10	S	4	2616.75	218.532
0.16	S	2	2906.5	236.881
0.28	S	2	3066	325.269
0.44	S	5	3139.8	101.09
0.04	$M1$	2	2484	91.9239
0.10	$M1$	4	2572.75	141.394
0.16	$M1$	2	2818	77.7817
0.28	$M1$	2	2899	106.066
0.44	$M1$	5	3040.4	51.1596
0.04	$M2$	2	2236	254.558
0.10	$M2$	4	2608.75	139.172
0.16	$M2$	2	2720	26.8701
0.28	$M2$	2	2822.5	34.6482
0.44	$M2$	5	2863	197.756

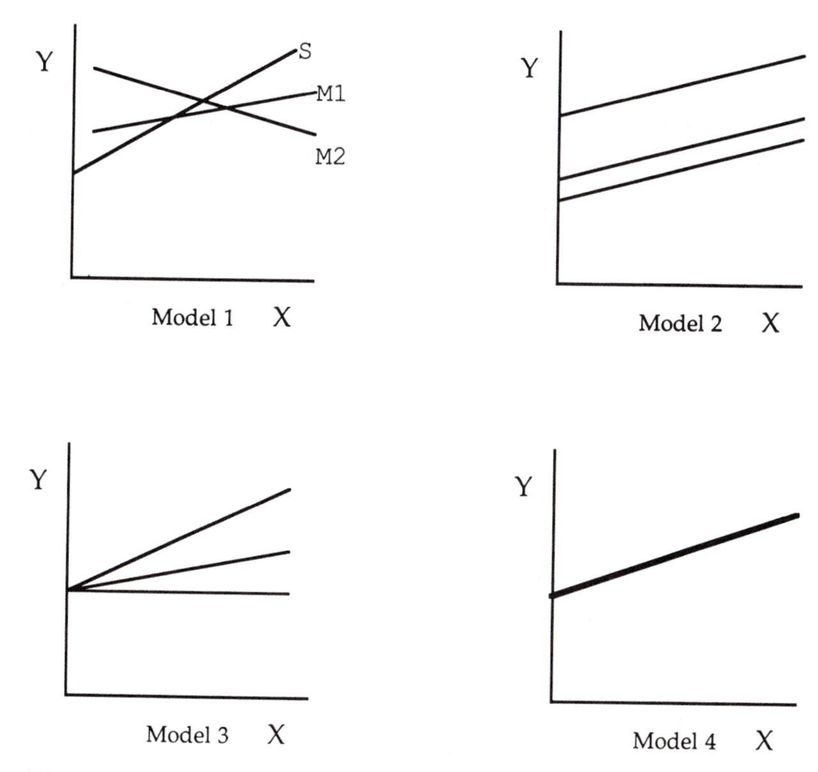

Figure 3 Four models for comparing three groups of data (X, Y).

To facilitate the tests, it is helpful to define three group indicator variables:

$G_1 = 1$ for units given source S, 0 otherwise

$G_2 = 1$ for units given source $M1$, 0 otherwise

$G_3 = 1$ for units given source $M2$, 0 otherwise.

We now define dose variables x_1, x_2, and x_3 for each of the three sources by multiplying each of the group indicators by the value of the dose, x. For example, $x_2 = G_2 \times x$ has the value of the dose for pens that received $M1$, but has the value 0 for pens that received some other source. Elegant computer programs, such as GLIM (Payne, 1985), create indicator variables and products internally, releasing the user from this tedious task.

Model 1

This is the least restrictive model shown in Figure 3. It requires estimation of six parameters, a slope and intercept for each group. The most straightforward parametrization for this model is

$$y = \beta_{01}G_1 + \beta_{02}G_2 + \beta_{03}G_3 + \beta_{11}x_1 + \beta_{12}x_2 + \beta_{13}x_3 + \epsilon. \tag{5}$$

The results of this fit are shown in Table 4. Standard errors can be obtained by computing the estimate $\tilde{\sigma}^2$ from the SD_i as outlined previously. For the example, $\tilde{\sigma}^2 = 28,930$ with 18 d.f. Since the regressions in Table 4 were done on dose averages, the values shown for $\hat{\sigma}^2$ are the mean squares for lack of fit.

Model 2

This is the model of parallel regressions, requiring one slope parameter and three intercept parameters. One common parameterization is

$$y = \beta_0 + \beta_1 x + \beta_{02}G_2 + \beta_{03}G_3 + \epsilon_{ij}. \tag{6}$$

The estimates of the coefficients for (6) are given in Table 4. Alternatively, one could fit a model that uses any three of the four terms for the intercept, G_1, G_2, and G_3. These models will give identical residuals and summary statistics such as R^2 and $\hat{\sigma}^2$, but the parameters will have somewhat differing interpretations. In the parameterization given by (6), $\hat{\beta}_0$ is

Table 4 Weighted Regression Estimates[a]

Variable	Model 1	Model 2	Model 3	Model 4
Intercept		2422 (69)	2361 (60)	2361 (60)
X		2228 (352)		2228 (382)
G_1	2352 (105)			
G_2	2417 (105)	−56 (76)		
G_3	2315 (105)	−127 (76)		
X_1	2739 (661)		2689 (472)	
X_2	1853 (661)		2155 (472)	
X_3	2090 (661)		1838 (472)	
$\hat{\sigma}^2$	28,095	24,554	22,839	27,567
d.f.	6	8	8	10
R^2	0.87	0.84	0.85	0.78

[a]Values in parentheses are standard errors.

the estimated intercept for source S, while the intercept for source $M1$ is estimated by $\hat{\beta}_0 + \hat{\beta}_{02}$. In the parameterization

$$y = \beta_{01}G_1 + \beta_{02}G_2 + \beta_{03}G_3 + \beta_1 x + \epsilon$$

the intercepts for the three groups are given directly by β_{0j}, $j = 1, 2, 3$. The latter parameterization, although less frequently used in practice, is often the most convenient for interpretation.

Model 3

This model requires that all sources share a common intercept but have different slopes. The most convenient parameterization is

$$y = \beta_0 + \beta_{11}x_1 + \beta_{12}x_2 + \beta_{13}x_3 + \epsilon. \qquad (7)$$

If the lines are required to be concurrent at some point other than the origin, say at dose $x = x^*$, merely define a new version of the predictor to be $X = x - x^*$ and proceed as if this were the dose variable.

Model 4

This most restrictive model is fit by ignoring group effects entirely, fitting the simple regression of y on x, and estimating one slope and one intercept. The results for the methionine data are given in Table 4.

Comparison of Nested Models

Two models are *nested* if the smaller can be obtained from the larger by setting some of the parameters equal to known values, typically setting them to be zero. In the sequence of models above, all of models 2, 3, and 4 are nested in model 1, and model 4 is nested in both 2 and 3. However, models 2 and 3 are not nested within one another. Comparison of nested models is done via an F-test, assuming that errors are normally distributed. Let RSS(full) and df(full) be the residual sum of squares and residual degrees of freedom for the larger model, and RSS(restricted) and df(restricted) be the residual sum of squares and degrees of freedom for a smaller model obtained from the larger by setting selected parameters equal to zero. Then the F-statistic for comparing H_0: full model versus H_a: restricted model is given by

$$F = \frac{[\text{RSS(restricted)} - \text{RSS(full)}]/[\text{df(restricted)} - \text{df(full)}]}{\tilde{\sigma}^2} \qquad (8)$$

where $\tilde{\sigma}^2$ is the estimate of σ^2 from pure error. If no pure error is available or if df(pe) is small, use the estimate of σ^2 from the full model in (8). To get a p-value, compare F to the F-distribution with [df(restricted) − df(full), df in $\tilde{\sigma}^2$] degrees of freedom. For example, Table 5 gives the RSS and df for each of the models, along with the F-statistics for comparing models. Since the p-values computed from these F-statistics are all large, there is no real reason to prefer any of the models, and the smallest one is plausible: over the range of doses in the data, the response is similar for the three sources of drug.

1.2 Adding the Rest of the Data

Now we consider fitting models for the entire range of doses given in Table 3. This includes data at dose $x = 0$ and at $x = 0.44$. Inclusion of a zero dose gives data about growth that would occur without supplementation. The fact that a dose of zero of one source is necessarily the same as a dose of zero of any other source leads us to reconsider the four models suggested in Section 1.1. The intercepts for all the dose-response curves must be the same; hence only models 3 and 4 (Figure 3) make sense. In the example without $x = 0$, we could justify fitting separate intercepts because each straight line used is intended only to approximate a curved surface over a limited range that does not include zero.

Fitting model 3 can now be done as follows. First, we add the observations for $x = 0$ to the data set, and set $G_1 = G_2 = G_3 = x_1 = x_2 = x_3 = 0$ for those units. We again use weighted least squares for fitting with weights equal to the number of units at each dose. We then fit the regression of y on x_1, x_2, and x_3, allowing a separate slope in each group, but one intercept; for $x = 0$ the model gives $E(y) = \beta_0$. We then compute the test for lack of fit to decide if the straight-line approximation is appropriate for these data; $F(\text{lof}) = 2.58$, with $(12, 34)$ d.f., giving a p-value of 0.015, suggesting that the straight-line approximation is inadequate over the whole range of the experiment. The data are replotted in Figure 4 to include the entire

Table 5 Summary of Tests for Comparing Models 2, 3, and 4 to Model 1

Model	DF	RSS	F (vs. model 1)
1	6	168,570	
2	8	196,435	0.48
3	8	182,711	0.24
4	10	275,667	0.93
Pure error	18	520,737	

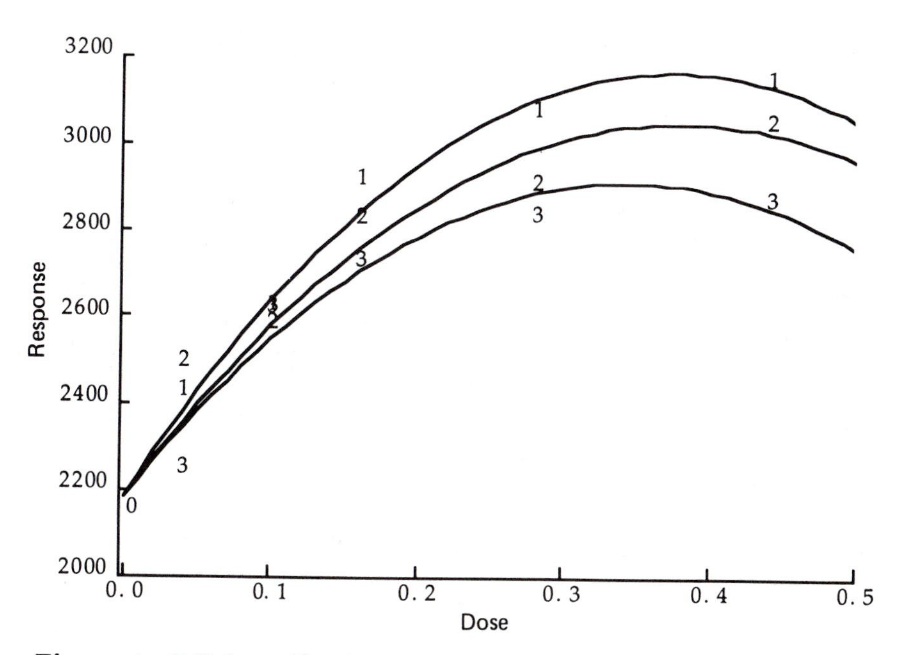

Figure 4 Full data. Numbers on the plot indicate groups: 1, S; 2, $M1$; 3, $M2$.

range of doses in the experiment (the curves will be discussed shortly). The figure shows the reason for the lack of fit: the regression surface is curved.

The simplest next step is to try adding a quadratic term to account for the curvature. This is done by creating new variables x_j^2, $j = 1, 2, 3$, and then fitting the expanded version of model 3,

$$y = \beta_0 + \beta_1 x_1 + \beta_2 x_2 + \beta_3 x_3 + \beta_{11} x_1^2 + \beta_{22} x_2^2 + \beta_{33} x_3^2 + \epsilon. \tag{9}$$

The F for lack of fit can be shown to be 0.58, with corresponding p-value larger than 0.05, suggesting that the quadratic model provides an adequate approximation to the response curve. We now compare model 3 (separate dose-response curves with common intercept) to model 4 (identical dose-response curves) by fitting model 4; we find that $F = 2.91$, which, when compared to $F(4, 34)$, gives a p-value of 0.036. Thus there is some evidence that the response curves differ over the entire range of the experiment. The separate response curves for the three sources are given in Figure 4.

The fitted curves in Figure 4 are disappointing since the fitted model suggests that the response decreases for doses greater than about 0.35%, a finding that is biologically unreasonable and at odds with the data. The quadratic model will often fail to provide a meaningful summary of results, even if the model apparently provides an adequate fit to the data. We are therefore led to consider alternative approaches.

1.3 Additional Comments

In most situations where dose-response curves are to be compared, linear models provide an *approximate* solution. Curvature in the response function is provided either by adding polynomial terms, as was done here, or by transforming the response or perhaps the dose to a nonlinear scale. The former method rarely has a theoretical foundation; and the latter approach, through transformations, can exactly match only a limited range of functions. Yet each of these can have great power and utility in describing the local behavior of a dose-response curve.

Our emphasis in this section has been on modeling and on basic inference, with only minor attention given to the problems of model verification. These methods, which generally go under the title of *regression diagnostics*, provide a whole range of methods for checking assumptions, such as constant variance or normal errors; choosing transformations, either to obtain a linear model or normal errors; finding outlying observations; and discovering influential observations. These topics are covered in some detail for linear models by Atkinson (1985), Weisberg (1985, Chaps. 5, 6), and at a more advanced level, by Cook and Weisberg (1982).

2 NONLINEAR MODELS

The approach used in Section 1.2 is a form of empirical modeling that involves continued expansion of the model until a satisfactory fit is obtained. Empirical modeling is most useful in situations where a concrete theory connecting the response and independent variables is lacking. When such a theory is available, it should generally be used to enhance scientific relevance of the results. This is the view we now pursue for the methionine study.

Parks (1982) describes a theory of animal growth that results in a definite connection between weight and level of supplementation. Specifically, for a single source of supplementation, the theory holds that pen weight will be related to level of supplementation x through the model

$$y = \theta_1 + \theta_2[1 - \exp(-\theta_3 x)] + \epsilon, \tag{10}$$

where θ_1, θ_2, and θ_3 are unknown parameters with the restriction that $\theta_3 \geq 0$, and the errors ϵ are assumed to be uncorrelated and to have mean zero and constant variance σ^2 (as in Section 1, we shall suppress subscripts on the y's, x's, and ϵ's unless they are specifically needed for clarity). We again assume that the errors are normally distributed when tests and confidence regions are required. In contrast to the linear models of the previous sections, the expected response from (10), $E(y) = \theta_1 + \theta_2[1 - \exp(-\theta_3 x)]$, is nonlinear in the θ's and is thus called a *nonlinear model.*

At the basal diet $x = 0$, $E(y) = \theta_1$. Thus θ_1 is simply the mean weight in the absence of supplementation. As the level of supplementation increases, the expected response also increases and tends to $\theta_1 + \theta_2$. The parameter θ_2 can be interpreted as the maximal increase in weight possible from supplementation. The parameter θ_3 controls the rate at which the expected response approaches the asymptote $\theta_1 + \theta_2$, with larger values producing faster rates. Figure 1 was constructed to illustrate the behavior of model (10): for drug A, $\theta_1 = 1$, $\theta_2 = 10$, and $\theta_3 = 10$, while for drug B, $\theta_1 = 1$, $\theta_2 = 10$, and $\theta_3 = 8$.

Unlike the modeling in Section 1, the approach based on model (10) provides a definite connection between the parameters of the model and scientific literature. For example, from Figure 4 we see that the quadratic model predicts that weight will begin to decrease somewhere between the highest two levels of supplementation, a conclusion that is at odds with prior information.

Estimates, tests, and confidence regions for nonlinear models are a bit more difficult to obtain than those for linear models. Our discussion of these topics will be phrased in terms of the generic nonlinear model

$$y_i = f(x_i, \theta) + \epsilon_i, \qquad i = 1, \ldots, N, \tag{11}$$

where y, x, and ϵ are as defined previously, θ is a $p \times 1$ vector of unknown parameters, and f is a known function that is assumed to be twice continuously differentiable in θ. The ordinary least squares estimate $\hat{\theta}$ of θ, which is the same as the maximum likelihood estimate under normal theory, is obtained by minimizing the least squares objective function

$$\mathrm{RSS}(\theta) = \sum_{i=1}^{n} [y_i - f(x_i, \theta)]^2. \tag{12}$$

Particular methods for minimizing RSS(θ), choice of starting value, and other computational issues are discussed in several texts, including Gallant (1987), Kennedy and Gentle (1980), and Ratkowsky (1983). We assume that a standard program such as BMDP, SPSS, or SAS is available.

2.1 Starting Values

Most programs require an initial guess or starting values for the parameters in the model, and in some problems good starting values, especially for parameters that enter nonlinearly, may be crucial for the computer algorithm to find the global minimum. In model (10), for example, once θ_3 has been selected, the remaining two linear parameters, θ_1 and θ_2, can be determined by ordinary least squares, and hence a good initial guess at θ_3 may be important. The selection of starting values is mostly an ad hoc process. The following four alternative methods may be helpful to determine starting values.

1. Select p distinct data points and attempt to solve the resulting p equations $y_j = f(x_j, \theta)$, $j = 1, \ldots, p$, for θ. Since there are p equations and p unknowns, the hope is that an exact solution will exist and be easy to find. If so, this solution forms the starting values. Selecting data points that are diverse often works well.
2. Form an approximating linear model by expanding $f(x, \theta)$. In model (10), $\theta_1 + \theta_2[1 - \exp(-\theta_3 x)] \approx \theta_1 + \theta_2\theta_3 x - \theta_2\theta_3^2 x^2/2$ for small values of $\theta_3 x$. Thus, after fitting the linear model $y = \beta_1 + \beta_2 x + \beta_3 x^2 + \epsilon$ at data points corresponding to small values of x, a starting value for θ_3 may be obtained from $-2\hat{\beta}_3/\hat{\beta}_2$.
3. If possible, transform to an approximately linear model that can be solved for starting values. If our model is $y_i = \theta_1 \exp(\theta_2 x_i) + \epsilon_i$, we should be able to get reasonable starting values for $\log(\theta_1)$ and θ_2 as the slope and intercept from the ordinary least squares regression of $\log y_i$ on x_i.
4. If nothing else works, try a grid search over values of the parameters that enter the model nonlinearly, with the grid point having the smallest RSS being used as the starting value.

Once $\text{RSS}(\theta)$ has been minimized, the maximum likelihood estimate of σ^2 is $\hat{\sigma}^2 = \text{RSS}(\hat{\theta})/N$. Some programs give $\hat{\sigma}^2$, while others give a direct analogy with linear regression, $s^2 = \text{RSS}(\hat{\theta})/(N - p)$. When N is large relative to p, the distinction between $\hat{\sigma}^2$ and s^2 is unimportant.

In normal linear regression, the distribution of $\hat{\beta}$ and the level of tests and confidence regions are all known exactly. This is not so in nonlinear regression, where it is often necessary to rely on approximations suggested by asymptotic theory. There are several ways in which such approximations can be constructed. Here we discuss only two: Wald procedures and methods based on the likelihood. Our discussion is strongly methodological; relevant theoretical details can be found in Gallant (1987) and the references cited therein.

2.2 Wald Procedures

Let θ^* denote the true value of the unknown parameter θ and let V^* denote the $N \times p$ matrix with elements

$$v_{ij}^* = \frac{\partial f(x_i, \theta)}{\partial \theta_j} \mid \theta = \theta^*, \qquad i = 1, \ldots, N; \quad j = 1, \ldots, p. \tag{13}$$

In the case of model (10), for example, $v_{23}^* = \theta_2^* x_2 \exp(-x_2 \theta_3^*)$. With certain regularity conditions and in sufficiently large samples, $\hat{\theta}$ is approximately normally distributed with mean θ^* and covariance matrix

$$\text{var}(\hat{\theta}) = (V^{*T} V^*)^{-1} \sigma^2. \tag{14}$$

Of course, in practice θ^* is unknown, so that it is necessary to replace θ^* with $\hat{\theta}$ to obtain usable results. Accordingly, we let V denote the $N \times p$ matrix as defined in (13) with the derivatives evaluated at $\hat{\theta}$ rather than θ^*. The estimated covariance matrix of $\hat{\theta}$ is now

$$\widehat{\text{var}}(\hat{\theta}) = (V^T V)^{-1} s^2. \tag{15}$$

The standard error of $\hat{\theta}_j$, $\text{se}(\hat{\theta}_j)$, is the square root of the jth diagonal element of (15), and most computer programs report this statistic.

With these results the *Wald test* for a null hypothesis involving a single parameter is easily formed. The test statistic for the hypothesis that θ_j, the jth component of θ, is equal to a specified value θ_j^0 is simply

$$t = \frac{\hat{\theta}_j - \theta_j^0}{\text{se}(\hat{\theta}_j)}. \tag{16}$$

Under the null hypothesis, this statistic is distributed approximately as a Student's t random variable with $N - p$ degrees of freedom. Thus the hypothesis is rejected if $|t| > t_{\alpha/2}(N - p)$, where $t_{\alpha/2}(N - p)$ is the upper $\alpha/2$ percentage point of a t-distribution with $N - p$ degrees of freedom. Similarly, an approximate $(1 - \alpha)100\%$ confidence region for θ_j is

$$\hat{\theta}_j \pm t_{\alpha/2}(N - p)\text{se}(\hat{\theta}_j). \tag{17}$$

Here, as in most methods for nonlinear regression, justification comes from large-sample arguments, but such arguments are of little help since it is usually unclear if N is large enough to ensure accurate inferences. Depending on the problem, (16) and (17) can have true levels that are far from the nominal values. For example Donaldson and Schnabel (1987) report simulation studies in which a nominal 95% region based on (17) has an actual coverage rate that is close to 75%.

The results in (16) and (17) for a single parameter can be extended to multiple parameters, but the accuracy of inferences based on these extensions deteriorates as number of parameters involved in the hypothesis or confidence region increases. In some multiple-parameter situations, Donaldson and Schnabel (1987) obtain coverage rates as low as 25% for nominal 95% confidence regions. For these reasons it seems wise to restrict use of the Wald tests (16) and confidence intervals (17) to situations involving a single parameter.

2.3 Likelihood-Based Inference

Wald tests and the associated confidence regions have the distinct advantage of being easy to construct from standard regression output. On the other hand, simulation studies reported by Donaldson and Schnabel (1987) and Gallant (1987) give a clear indication that inferences based directly on the likelihood ratio will be more accurate. In Donaldson and Schnabel's studies, the true level of likelihood-based confidence regions was always within a few percentage points of the nominal value regardless of the number of parameters involved. Likelihood ratio tests can be constructed from any program that gives $\text{RSS}(\hat{\theta})$, but constructing likelihood-based confidence regions is more difficult. We next consider likelihood ratio tests and later turn attention to the corresponding confidence regions.

Partition the parameter vector as $\theta^T = (\theta_1^T, \theta_2^T)$, where the dimension of θ_1 is $p - q$ and the dimension of θ_2 is q. The hypothesis of interest is $\theta_2 = \theta_2^0$. Let $\text{RSS}(\hat{\theta})$ denote the residual sum of squares from the fit of the full model and let $\text{RSS}(\hat{\theta}_1 \mid \theta_2 = \theta_2^0)$ denote the residual sum of squares from the fit under the hypothesis that $\theta_2 = \theta_2^0$. Then under the null hypothesis $\theta_2 = \theta_2^0$ the test statistic

$$\begin{aligned} F &= \frac{(N-p)[\text{RSS}(\hat{\theta}_1 \mid \theta_2 = \theta_2^0) - \text{RSS}(\hat{\theta})]}{q\text{RSS}(\hat{\theta})} \\ &= \frac{[\text{RSS}(\hat{\theta}_1 \mid \theta_2 = \theta_2^0) - \text{RSS}(\hat{\theta})]}{qs^2} \end{aligned} \tag{18}$$

is distributed approximately as an F random variable with q and $N - p$ degrees of freedom. Comparing the calculated value of F to the percentage points of the corresponding F distribution provides the test, with large values indicating evidence against the null hypothesis. Once the sums of squares for the competing models are available, this statistic is constructed exactly as the corresponding statistic (7) for linear regression. In particular, if sufficient degrees of freedom are available, s^2 can be replaced by the pure error estimate of σ^2.

In well-behaved situations with $q = 1$, the Wald test (16) and the likelihood ratio test (18) will give essentially the same results, $t^2 \approx F$, but there is no guarantee that this will always happen. The Wald test has the advantage of being easier to obtain since it can be constructed from the output of a single run of most regression programs. In contrast, the likelihood ratio test requires two computer fits, one to obtain $\text{RSS}(\hat{\theta})$ and one to obtain $\text{RSS}(\hat{\theta}_1 \mid \theta_2 = \theta_2^0)$. On the other hand, inference based on the likelihood ratio will generally be more accurate in the sense that the actual levels of tests and confidence regions will generally be closer to the nominal levels than to those for the Wald procedures.

To construct a confidence region for θ_2, let $F(\theta_2^0)$ denote the value of the F statistic (18) for the hypothesis $\theta_2 = \theta_2^0$. Then an approximate $(1-\alpha)100\%$ likelihood-based confidence region for θ_2 is

$$\{\theta_2^0 \mid F(\theta_2^0) \le F_\alpha(q, N-p)\}, \tag{19}$$

where $F_\alpha(q, N-p)$ is the upper α percentage point of an F-distribution with q and $N-p$ degrees of freedom. Unfortunately, these likelihood-based confidence regions are not obtained easily from standard programs [Gallant (1987) gives a method for computing these regions for $q = 1$ by quadratic interpolation]. In contrast to Wald intervals (17), confidence regions for a single parameter ($q = 1$) based on (19) will generally not be symmetric about $\hat{\theta}_2$, and in higher dimensions ($q > 1$) these regions can take on unusual shapes. In fact, likelihood-based regions can be unbounded or disjoint, although such occurrences are unusual in practice. These regions are most useful when $q = 1$ or 2, so that they can be drawn and visually inspected.

To illustrate the difference between Wald and likelihood confidence regions, consider a sample of size N from each of two normal populations, $N(\mu_1, \sigma^2)$ and $N(\mu_2, \sigma^2)$, with known variance σ^2. The nonlinear model for inference on the pair of parameters $\theta_1 = \mu_1$ and $\theta_2 = \mu_2/\mu_1$ can be written as

$$y_i = \theta_1 x_i + \theta_1\theta_2(1 - x_i) + \epsilon_i, \qquad i = 1, \ldots, 2N, \tag{20}$$

where x_i is an indicator variable that takes values 1 and 0 for populations 1 and 2, respectively. By using (18) and after a little algebra, a $(1-\alpha)100\%$ confidence region for (θ_1^*, θ_2^*) can be expressed as the following region centered at $(\hat{\theta}_1, \hat{\theta}_2)$:

$$\{(k_1, k_2) \mid k_1^2 + (\hat{\theta}_2 k_1 + \hat{\theta}_1 k_2 + k_1 k_2)^2 \le c\}, \tag{21}$$

where $k_1 = \theta_1 - \hat{\theta}_1$ and $k_2 = \theta_2 - \hat{\theta}_2$ and $c = \sigma^2\chi_\alpha^2(2)/N$. Since σ^2 is assumed known for simplicity, we have used the upper α percentage point of a chi-squared distribution with 2 degrees of freedom $\chi^2_\alpha(2)$ rather than corresponding percentage point from an F distribution.

The corresponding Wald region for (θ_1^*, θ_2^*) is obtained by deleting the term $k_1 k_2$ that occurs in (21),

$$\{(k_1, k_2) \mid k_1^2 + (\hat{\theta}_2 k_1 + \hat{\theta}_1 k_2)^2 \leq c\}. \tag{22}$$

These regions are displayed in Figure 5 for $(\hat{\theta}_1, \hat{\theta}_2) = (3, 0)$ and $\alpha = 0.05$. Since the true coverage rate for the likelihood region (21) is exactly 95%, the Wald region (22) does not seem to be a good approximation in this example. A Wald or likelihood confidence regions for either θ_1^* or θ_2^* can be obtained by projecting the joint regions in Figure 5 onto the k_1-or k_2-axis, respectively. When this is done for θ_1^* we see that the Wald and likelihood regions are identical, and this makes sense because θ_1 is just the mean of a normal population. However, when projecting onto the k_2-axis, we see that the Wald interval for θ_2^* is substantially shorter than the corresponding likelihood interval.

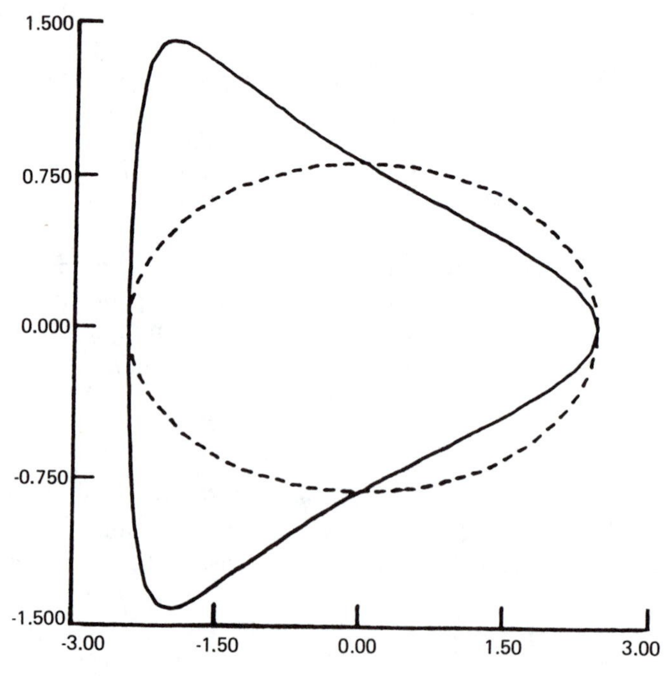

Figure 5 95% confidence regions (22) and (23). Solid line, likelihood; dashed line, Wald.

The point of this example is to reinforce the notion that while Wald procedures can give useful results, likelihood-based inferences are generally more accurate.

Pure Error

As in linear regression, replication allows for an omnibus goodness-of-fit test of a model. Let $\tilde{\sigma}^2 = \text{SS(pe)}/(N-k)$ denote the estimate of σ^2 from replication, as defined for linear regression. Then the test statistic for lack of fit of a chosen model is

$$F = \frac{\text{RSS}(\hat{\theta}) - \text{SS(pe)}}{(k-p)\tilde{\sigma}^2}. \tag{23}$$

This statistic is compared to the percentage points of an F-distribution with $k-p$ and $N-k$ degrees of freedom, with large values indicating lack of fit.

2.4 Regularity Conditions

The results for nonlinear regression above are justified by large-sample arguments. As the sample size increases, the approximations used to construct tests and confidence regions become more accurate. Regularity conditions are imposed to ensure that the sampling process is well behaved as the sample size increases. Many of these conditions have little relevance in practice, but one seems to be particularly important: when testing a hypothesis, the matrix V^* defined at (13) must have full column rank under the null and alternative hypotheses. Situations when V^* is less than full rank are difficult to handle theoretically and simulation may be the only practically useful approach for obtaining p-values.

2.5 Methionine Study Again

With these general results, we now return to our analysis of the methionine study. Equation (10) provides the basic model for a single source of supplementation. As a first step we could fit model (10) separately to each of the three sources, but this does not make much sense in view of the structure of the experiment. The basal diet $x = 0$ is common to all sources so that the models should share a common value for θ_1. There are still several possible models that include all three sources. The first is model (10), which provides a common fit for all the data; it is the counterpart of model 4 in the linear regression treatment of the data. The second model restricts the sources to have the same mean basal response θ_1 and the same asymptote $\theta_1 + \theta_2$, but allows for different values of the rate parameter θ_3:

$$y = \theta_1 + \theta_2 \{1 - \exp[-(\theta_{31}x_1 + \theta_{32}x_2 + \theta_{33}x_3)]\} + \epsilon. \tag{24}$$

The most general model restricts the sources to have the same mean basal response θ_1, but allows for different asymptotes and different rate parameters,

$$y = \theta_1 + \theta_{21}[1 - \exp(-\theta_{31}x_1)] + \theta_{22}[1 - \exp(-\theta_{32}x_2)] + \theta_{23}[1 - \exp(-\theta_{33}x_3)] + \epsilon. \tag{25}$$

Other models are possible depending on the restrictions placed on the asymptote and rate parameters.

Since model (25) is the largest model that we entertain, we first assess its goodness of fit by using the test associated with (23). As discussed previously, the estimate of σ^2 based on pure error is $\tilde{\sigma}^2 = \text{SS(pe)}/\sum(n_i - 1) = 24,535$ with 34 degrees of freedom. From Table 6 the residual sum of squares for model (25) is RSS $= 930,933$ with 43 degrees of freedom. Thus $F = [930,933 - 834,183]/[(43 - 34)\tilde{\sigma}^2] = 0.44$. Clearly, there is no reason to question the fit of the full model.

As mentioned previously, source S is difficult and expensive to produce and was included as a laboratory standard against which the other two sources would be compared. Sources with a notably smaller asymptote than the laboratory standard are generally deemed inferior regardless of the value of the rate parameter. On the other hand, if there is no firm evidence that the asymptotes for the three sources differ, the rate parameters form the basis for comparison, with larger rates being preferred. With this in mind, a statistical comparison of models (24) and (25) is a useful way to proceed.

The residual sum of squares for models (24) and (25) are available in Table 6. The test statistic (18) for comparing these models has the value $[(1,056,860 - 930,933)/2]/21,649.6 = 2.91$, which is compared to the percentage points of an F distribution with 2 and 43 degrees of freedom to yield a p-value of 0.065. Thus there is some indication that the asymptotes differ, although it is certainly not strong. Since the situation is somewhat ambiguous, we next carry out separate comparisons of the asymptotes for sources $M1$ and $M2$ with the asymptote for the standard S.

To compare the asymptotes for S and $M2$, we calculate the F statistic for comparing the model (25) with the model

$$y = \theta_1 + \theta_{21}[1 - \exp(-\theta_{31}x_1 - \theta_{33}x_3)] + \theta_{22}[1 - \exp(-\theta_{32}x_2)] + \epsilon, \tag{26}$$

which restricts S and $M2$ to have equal asymptotes $\theta_1 + \theta_{21}$. The sum of squares for model (26) is available in Table 6 and the F-statistic has the value $(1,053,150 - 930,933)/21,649.6 = 5.64$. Since models (25) and (26)

Table 6 Summary of Fits for Various Nonlinear Models in the Methonine Study

Parameter	Model (10)	Model (24)	Model (25)	Model (26)	Model (28)	Model (29)
Intercept: θ_1	2138.52	2176.56	2138.95	2177.24	2146.66	2139.32
Increases: θ_2	910.82	937.11				
θ_{21}			1064.32	956.64	1005.97	995.95
θ_{22}			927.73	902.30		
θ_{23}			747.88		741.22	747.56
Rates: θ_3	7.48					
θ_{31}		7.82	6.77	7.49	7.46	6.98
θ_{32}		6.21	7.24	6.56	5.82	
θ_{33}		4.22	8.72	4.01	8.59	8.71
$RSS(\hat{\theta})$	1,212,840	1,056,860	930,933	1,053,150	953,313	986,095
d.f.	47	45	43	44	44	45

differ by only one parameter, we compare this value to an F distribution with 1 and 43 degrees of freedom, giving a p-value of 0.024 and thus a reasonable indication that the asymptote for $M2$ is less than that for the standard. A similar calculation for comparing the S and $M1$ asymptotes yields $F = 2.38$, again with 1 and 43 degrees of freedom. In summary, there is evidence to indicate that the asymptote for $M2$ is less than that for S, but we have been unable to detect a clear difference between the S and $M1$ asymptotes.

Before turning to a comparison of rate parameters, it may be instructive to see how the asymptotes for S and $M2$ can be compared by using the Wald test (16). To this end it is helpful to reparameterize model (25) in the form

$$\begin{aligned} y = \theta_1 &+ \theta_{21}[1 - \exp(-\theta_{31}x_1)] + \theta_{22}[1 - \exp(-\theta_{32}x_2)] \\ &+ (\theta_{21} + \delta)[1 - \exp(-\theta_{33}x_3)] + \epsilon, \end{aligned} \tag{27}$$

where $\delta = \theta_{23} - \theta_{21}$. The hypothesis of interest is now $\delta = 0$. Standard programs applied to model (27) will give $\hat{\delta}$ and its standard error: $\hat{\delta} = -316.343$, $\text{se}(\hat{\delta}) = 120.966$. The Wald statistic for $\delta = 0$ is now $t = -316.343/120.966 = -2.615$, which should be compared to the t distribution with 43 degrees of freedom. As described above, the square of the Wald statistic will be approximately equal to the corresponding likelihood ratio statistic in well-behaved situations. In our example, $t^2 = 6.84$ but $F = 5.64$. Thus, although the statistics give the same general indication, their difference is large enough to indicate the potential problems that can arise when using Wald procedures.

If we adopt the conclusion that any difference between the asymptotes for S and $M1$ is not large enough to be scientifically relevant, we may restrict attention to the reduced model

$$\begin{aligned} y &= \theta_1 + \theta_{21}[1 - \exp(-\theta_{31}x_1)] + \theta_{21}[1 - \exp(-\theta_{32}x_2)] \\ &\quad + \theta_{23}[1 - \exp(-\theta_{33}x_3)] + \epsilon \\ &= \theta_1 + \theta_{21}[1 - \exp(-\theta_{31}x_1 - \theta_{32}x_2)] + \theta_{23}[1 - \exp(-\theta_{33}x_3)] + \epsilon \\ &= \theta_1 + \theta_{21}\{1 - \exp[-\theta_{31}(x_1 + \rho_{12}x_2)]\} \\ &\quad + \theta_{23}[1 - \exp(-\theta_{33}x_3)] + \epsilon. \end{aligned} \tag{28}$$

The third parameterization of the model is the most useful since, when the asymptotes are regarded as equal, the ratio $\rho_{12} = \theta_{32}/\theta_{31}$ of the rate parameters is often of interest. In particular, is there evidence to indicate that $\rho_{12} \neq 1$? Using the Wald test for $\rho_{12} = 1$ we find that $\hat{\rho}_{12} = 0.78$, $\text{se}(\hat{\rho}_{12}) = 0.153$, and $t = (0.78 - 1)/0.153 = -1.44$, indicating that the data provide no firm evidence to suggest that $\rho_{12}^* \neq 1$. The likelihood ratio test comes to the same conclusion: from model (28) $\text{RSS}(\hat{\theta}, \hat{\rho}_{12}) = 953{,}313$, $\text{RSS}(\hat{\theta} \mid \rho_{12} = 1) = 986{,}095$, and thus $F = 1.51$ with 1 and 44 degrees of freedom.

Our analysis to this point indicates that the data from the methionine study can be described reasonably by the model

$$y = \theta_1 + \theta_{21}\{1 - \exp[-\theta_{31}(x_1 + x_2)]\} + \theta_{23}[1 - \exp(-\theta_{33}x_3)] + \epsilon. \quad (29)$$

The general conclusion reflected by this model is that based on these data, source $M1$ cannot be distinguished statistically from the laboratory standard S, while $M2$ appears to be inferior due to its lower asymptote. The fitted version of model (29), along with the data observed, is plotted in Figure 6. Depending on specific interests, there are various ways in which the basic techniques described above might be used for further analysis. However, rather than continue illustrating these techniques, we turn to a new topic: experimental design.

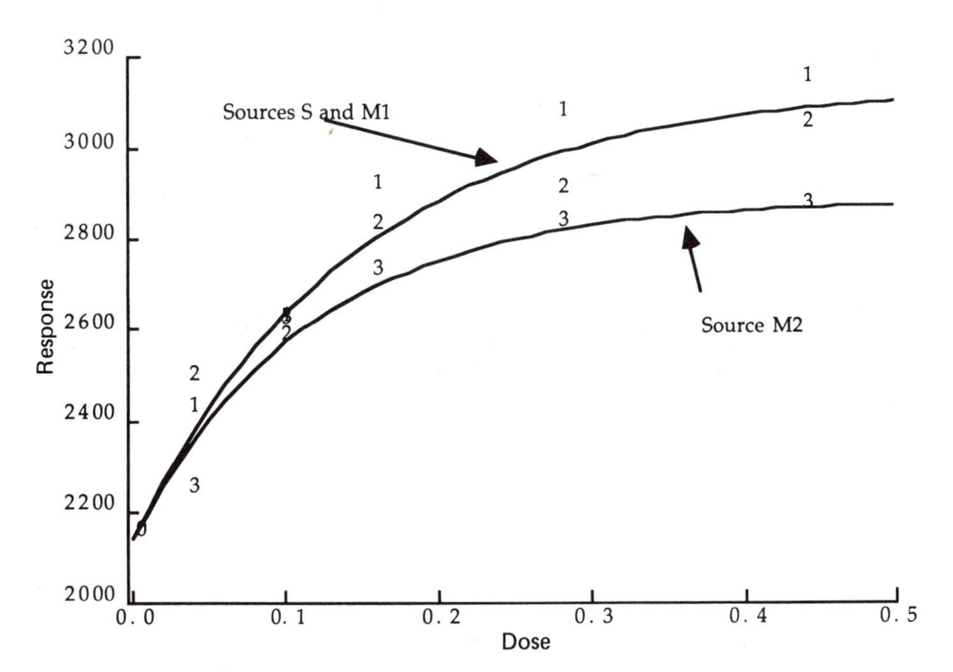

Figure 6 Nonlinear model. Numbers on the plot refer to sources: 1, S; 2, $M1$; 3, $M2$.

3 EXPERIMENTAL DESIGNS

When planning an experiment, an investigator must decide on the number of subjects to use, the number of drugs or treatment combinations, the dosage levels of the drugs, and a plan assigning drugs to subjects. Taken together, these four items are called an experimental design, and in the remainder of this chapter we discuss some issues of design. Our emphasis is on the choice of dosage levels and the number of subjects to receive each dosage. Poor choice of dosages and assignment of subjects can markedly degrade the quality of an experiment. Our goal here is to present some of the important ideas of *optimal experimental design* as they relate to the problem of comparing dose-response curves from animal experiments of the types discussed earlier in this chapter.

Consider first an experiment with only one drug. Suppose that the number N of experimental units is fixed, so the design consists of choosing the dosage x_i to be assigned to the ith unit. In the methionine study described previously, the experimental unit is a pen of 15 poults. Since dosages can always be scaled, we assume that x_i is between 0 and 1. Consider using one of the three following designs:

$D1$. Spread the N points uniformly over the design region (0,1).
$D2$. Put N/2 points at 0 and N/2 points at 1.
$D3$. Put N/3 points at each of 0, 1/2, and 1.

To compare designs, we must specify a criterion function. Most criteria, and there are many, would order one design over another if the first design has a smaller variance, in some sense, than does the second. To compute a variance, we need a model. Suppose that the correct dose-response model is $y_i = \beta_0 + \beta_1 x_i + \epsilon_i$, and that we agree to compare designs by comparing var($\hat{\beta}_1$ | design). If observations are to be taken independently and are assumed to have a common error variance σ^2, and least-squares estimates are to be used, we can easily compute this variance, $\text{var}(\hat{\beta}_1 \mid \text{design}) = \sigma^2/\sum(x_i - \bar{x})^2$. For our three designs, we find that

$$\text{var}(\hat{\beta}_1 \mid D1) \approx \sigma^2 12/N,$$
$$\text{var}(\hat{\beta}_1 \mid D2) = \sigma^2 4/N,$$
$$\text{var}(\hat{\beta}_1 \mid D3) = \sigma^2 6/N.$$

The variances for $D2$ and $D3$ are exact calculations, while that for $D1$ is appropriate as N grows large. Using this criterion and the simple regression model, design $D2$ is to be preferred. Indeed, if $D1$ is used in place of $D2$, about three times as many observations are required for $D1$ to have the same precision for $\hat{\beta}_1$. We can define the *efficiency* of design $D1$ relative to $D2$ to be $\mathrm{var}(\hat{\beta}_1 \mid D2)/\mathrm{var}(\hat{\beta}_1 \mid D1) = 0.33$ in this case.

If the correct model is quadratic regression, $y_i = \beta_0 + \beta_1 x_i + \beta_2 x_i^2 + \epsilon_i$, both the choice of the design, and the criterion to be used, are different. Since there are now coefficients for the linear and quadratic terms, a criterion function that just looks at the variance of one coefficient estimate is less appealing. There are several ways to generalize variance to handle several coefficients. One useful method is to choose a design to minimize the determinant of the covariance matrix of the estimated coefficients. If errors are normally distributed, this is equivalent to minimizing the volume of the confidence ellipsoid for the coefficients. This criterion is called *D-optimality.*

We want to compute the determinant for each of the three designs; however, design $D2$, the preferred design for the simple regression problem, is unacceptable because it specifies collection of data at only two points, so we cannot estimate a coefficient for the quadratic component of the model. For design $D1$, the determinant of the inverse of the cross product matrix, for large n, is approximately $2880/N^3$; for models with p parameters, it is usual to take the pth root of this quantity, which is $14.228/N$ for $D1$. For $D3$, the determinant is $576/N^3$, and its cube root is $8.320/N$. Design $D3$ dominates $D1$ on this criterion, and design $D1$ would require $14.228/8.320 = 1.71$ times as many observations as would $D3$ to achieve the same precision.

This elementary example displays all the essential ingredients of the optimal design problem. The investigator must choose the model and a criterion for comparing models. Different models may lead to different designs. Similarly, if we were to consider other design criteria, we may again get different designs. The best design for one model may be unusable if that model is incorrect. Thus a secondary consideration is one of robustness of the design: a design should be reasonably good even if the model used is incorrect.

We have made no claim that any of $D1$, $D2$, or $D3$ would be the optimal design, and all comparisons have been made just among these three designs (however, one can show that $D2$ is D-optimal for simple linear regression and $D3$ is D-optimal for quadratic regression). Finding D-optimal designs is generally a complicated computational problem that requires relatively sophisticated software. Fortunately, the necessary software is quickly becoming available, both for microcomputers and for mainframes [see Nachtsheim (1987) for a comprehensive comparison of software currently available]. These programs require the user to input the sample size N, the model, and a list of candidate levels or dosages that can be used in an experiment. The program will then produce a listing of the number of observations that should be taken at each possible dosage of each drug (these will mostly be zeros, as only a few dosage/drug combinations will be needed for most models). Except in problems where the total number of observations N is small, the calculation of an exact D-optimal design is nearly impossible since the determinant objective function can have many local minima, and this requires essentially exhaustive search over all possible designs to ensure that the final design is in fact D-optimal. Because of this computational complexity, most programs rely on clever algorithms that can produce good but possibly less than optimal designs.

We have used the program ACED (Welch, 1985).* This program permits the user to specify almost any set of design points, and will find optimal designs using several different algorithms and several different criteria. We will use exclusively the D-optimality criterion in combination with the "excursion" algorithm, which is a generalization of Mitchell's (1974) method called DETMAX. This program may find several nearly D-optimal designs, from which the user can make the final selection, perhaps incorporating concerns that are not adequately reflected by D-optimality.

We now consider finding the optimal design for comparing three drugs by using the quadratic regression model,

$$y_i = \beta_0 + \sum_{j=1}^{3}(\beta_{1j}x_{ij} + \beta_{2j}x_{ij}^2) + \epsilon_i, \tag{30}$$

where x_{ij} is nonzero only if the ith unit received a dose of drug $j(x_{i1} = x_{i2} = x_{i3} = 0$ for units receiving the basal dose). This model specifies a common intercept for the three groups, but different slopes. To use ACED, we must prepare two files. The first is the set of candidate values for (x_{i1}, x_{i2}, x_{i3}). We will suppose that the candidate doses are in the range 0 to 0.50, corresponding to the range of doses in the experiment discussed earlier in the chapter. Appendix Table 1 gives the 31 candidate settings we will consider for the experiment. For most experiments, a rough grid is adequate. Next, we need to specify a model, via a Fortran subroutine called *xtof* that computes one row of the matrix of derivatives V^* given at (14), which is used by the program to compute the determinant of the covariance matrix of the estimates. For linear models, V^* is not a function of the parameters, but for nonlinear models V^* does depend on

*Available from William J. Welch, Department of Statistics, University of Waterloo, Waterloo, Ontario, Canada N2L 3G1. ACED is available in Fortran 77 source code, and should therefore run on most computer systems that have a Fortran 77 compiler. We used a VAX 11/750 running Berkeley Unix 4.3.

the unknown parameters. This complication is discussed a bit later. For now, we examine the linear model (30).

The ith row of V^* for the model function (30) is

$$v_i^* = \begin{pmatrix} 1 & x_{1j} & x_{2j} & x_{3j} & x_{1j}^2 & x_{2j}^2 & x_{3j}^2 \end{pmatrix}.$$

The routine *xtof* simply returns the value of v_i^*, and is given in Appendix Table 2.

Appendix Table 3 gives the relevant parts of the ACED session for finding the D-optimal design for model (30). User responses to questions are shown in boldface. In question A, we specify three "explanatory variables," corresponding to the dose for each of the three sources. In question B, we specify input of a list of candidate design points rather than using the default of a factorial arrangement of points. The list of candidate points in Table 1, preceded by the number of candidates, here 31, was supplied to the program in a file called "can2." The routine *xtof* has previously been supplied to the program; the method for doing this is dependent on the computer. ACED permits first-order and full quadratic models [which differ from (30) by allowing interactions and separate intercepts] by default. Since we use neither of these, we select the user-supplied model, given by the routine *xtof*, in question D. ACED has several computing algorithms that can be selected in question E; we used the exchange algorithm, given by *ex*, and choose three different starting values (question F), as each starting value may lead to a different design. The starting values are chosen at random, and question G essentially controls the random mechanism; we have used the default. In question H, we choose D-optimality as our criterion of interest, and specify 21 observations in the design in question I. The sample size of 21 was a fortuitous choice, since it gives an exact D-optimal design, with three observations each at candidate points 5, 10, 15, 20, 25, 30, and 31 which correspond to three points at the basal dose (candidate 31), and three at the midpoint and end of the range for each drug. If the sample size had been, say, 20, the three designs might differ slightly, with the number of replications at one of the midpoints reduced to 2.

There are some interesting observations to make about the design chosen. First, the number of basal observations is the same as the number of observations at any other dosage for a given drug. Most experimenters would probably believe that more basal replication is desirable because these observations are used in fitting all three curves, but this leads to inefficient experimentation if model (30) is appropriate. Second, for each drug there are only three points in the design (including basal), so if the model were not quadratic (say, a cubic were needed for fitting), we could not estimate the cubic component, nor could we test for lack of fit of the quadratic. Finally, the design would be the same for fitting any number of drugs over any range. For example, if we increased the range of acceptable dosages to 0 to 1 rather than 0 to 0.5, the optimal design for each drug would place equal numbers of observations at 0, 0.5, and 1.0 rather than at 0, 0.25, and 0.5. Thus the choice of the acceptable range of dosages is crucial.

3.1 Nonlinear Design

We now turn to the problem of designing an optimal experiment with a nonlinear response function. Consider first designing an experiment for a single group, using model (10),

$$y = \theta_1 + \theta_2[1 - \exp(-\theta_3 x)] + \epsilon. \tag{31}$$

The concepts are the same for the nonlinear model as they are of the linear model: we still wish to minimize the determinant of the covariance matrix of the estimates, given by (14). The complicating factor here is that the matrix V^* in (14) is a function of the unknown θ's, so to design an experiment optimally to estimate the θ's, we must know them in advance!

For this particular model, however, it is possible to compute the optimal design exactly by finding the determinant of $V^{*T}V^*$, and minimizing it analytically as a function of the θ's; as it happens, the design is only a function of θ_3, and we find the following design. If the region of acceptable doses is from 0 to M, put

$n/3$ observations at $x = 0$,

$n/3$ observations at $x = M$,

$n/3$ observations at $x = \dfrac{1}{\theta_3}\left[1 - \dfrac{\theta_3 M \exp(-\theta_3 M)}{1 - \exp(-\theta_3 M)}\right].$

The optimal design will always put one-third of the observations at each of the endpoints, but the placement of the remaining third will depend on θ_3. If $M = 0.5$, and θ_3 is near zero, the middle third will be put at $x = 0.25$. As θ_3 increases, the third design point moves toward the origin; at $\theta_3 = 1$, $x = 0.21$; at $\theta_3 = 5$, $x = 0.09$; and at $\theta_3 = 10$, $x = 0.05$. Given the range of rates θ_3 observed in the experiment discussed earlier in this chapter, one may consider designs with the third design point near 0.05 or 0.10.

An instructive result of this last example is that although the design is nonlinear, the optimal design depends on only one of the three parameters, the rate θ_3. Simplifications like this are common but by no means universal. For example, we now consider (25), which has three drugs, one intercept, but separate slopes and asymptotes. One can show that the optimal design is independent of θ_1, and definitely depends on the rate parameters θ_{3j}. The situation for the θ_{2j} is more complicated, and the design will depend on these parameters for some values of θ_{3j}, but not for others.

If we have reasonable guesses for the θ's, ACED can again be used to find optimal (or nearly optimal) designs given those θ's. For model (25), we need only supply a new function *xtof* that computes rows of the matrix V^* with elements defined by (13). The required routine is given in Appendix Table 4, and edited output from a session using the program is given in Appendix Table 5. The questions asked by the program are a bit different now, as an additional question is asked in the routine *xtof* to allow the user to specify values for the θ's. We have set the θ's equal to their MLEs from the fit of (25) in Section 2. The optimal design places three points at 0.15 and 0.50 for source S; one point at 0.10, two at 0.15, and three at 0.50 for source $M1$; and three at 0.10 and 0.50 for source $M2$. In addition, the basal diet is replicated three times to complete the design.

Since the θ's are only estimated, ACED should be rerun with a grid of values for the θ's. For values of the rate parameters in the interval 1 to 20, the optimal designs are independent of the asymptote parameters, so we need consider varying only the rate parameters. The optimal design (for $N = 21$) will allocate three subjects to the basal diet, and six to each of the drugs. Within a drug, the six subjects will be divided into two groups of three, one group getting the maximal dose of 0.5 and the other group getting an intermediate dose. The larger the value of the rate parameter for that group, the smaller the intermediate dose. For example, at $\theta_{31} = 1$, the intermediate dose is 0.25; when $\theta_{31} = 5$, the intermediate dose is 0.15; and at $\theta_{31} = 10$, the intermediate dose is 0.10. Thus a reasonable design for this experiment would replicate equally: the basal diet, the maximum dose for each drug, and an intermediate value for each drug, between 0.10 and 0.15. If the sample size ($N = 21$) is judged inadequate, perhaps on the basis of a power calculation, the size of the experiment can be increased by replicating the design points chosen.

The ideas on nonlinear design above reflect how the methionine study was actually designed. Model (25) was used for the initial design, which was based on parameter estimates from previous experiments. The initial design was then compared to other optimal designs obtained by varying both the parameter values used for design construction and the model. The alternative models were all nested within (25). The resulting efficiencies of the initial design were judged to be acceptably high over a reasonable range of parameter values and models. This turns out to be the case in many applications: The efficiencies of designs obtained by imposing modest modifications on a D-optimal design are usually high. This type of design robustness enables the user to modify a D-optimal design, and thus satisfy requirements that are not reflected by D-optimality, while maintaining a high efficiency. In the methionine study the initial design was modified to allow for a check on the model.

Alternatively, one can systematically include any prior information concerning the θ's in the determination of the design by modifying the criterion function. Suppose that $G(\theta)$ is a function of the θ's that represents our current state of belief concerning the θ's; perhaps $G(\theta)$ is the likelihood function for θ from an experiment completed previously. Then we could choose a design that minimizes some function of the average determinant, perhaps just

$$\int \det[V(\theta)^T V(\theta)] G(\theta) d\theta. \tag{32}$$

Computation of this function can be very complex, as the integral may be in many dimensions, but it does use all available information to select a model. For a discussion of related approaches, see Cook and Nachtsheim (1982) and the references cited therein.

REFERENCES

Atkinson, A. C. (1985). *Plots, Residuals and Regression.* Oxford University Press, Oxford.

Cook, R. D., and C. J. Nachtsheim (1982). Model robust, linear-optimal design. *Technometrics 24*, 49–54.

Cook, R. D., and S. Weisberg (1982). *Residuals and Influence in Regression.* Chapman & Hall, London.

Donaldson, J. R., and R. B. Schnabel (1987). Computational experiences with confidence regions and confidence intervals in nonlinear least squares. *Technometrics 29*, 67–82.

Draper, N., and H. Smith (1981). *Applied Regression Analysis*, 2nd ed. Wiley, New York.

Gallant, A. R. (1987). *Nonlinear Statistical Models.* Wiley, New York.

Kennedy, W., and J. Gentle (1980). *Statistical Computing.* Marcel Dekker, New York.

Mitchell, T. J. (1974). An algorithm for the construction of D-optimal experimental designs. *Technometrics 16*, 203–211.

Nachtsheim, C. J. (1987). Tools for computer-aided design of experiments: review and comment. *J. Qual. Technol. 17*, 132–160.

Noll, S. L., P. E. Waibel, R. D. Cook, and J. A. Witmer (1984). Biopotency of methionine sources for young turkeys. *Poult. Sci. 63*, 2458–2470.

Parks, J. R. (1982). *A Theory of Feeding and Growth of Animals.* Springer-Verlag, New York.

Payne, C. D. (1985). *The GLIM System Release 3.77 Manual.* Numerical Algorithms Group, Oxford.
Ratkowsky, D. (1983). *Nonlinear Regression Modeling.* Marcel Dekker, New York.
Weisberg, S. (1985). *Applied Linear Regression*, 2nd ed. Wiley, New York.
Welch, B. L. (1985). *ACED: Algorithms for the Construction of Experimental Designs. User's Guide Version 1.61.* Faculty of Commerce and Business Administration, University of British Columbia, Vancouver.

APPENDIX TABLES

Appendix Table 1 Candidate Design Points for the Experiment Comparing Three Drugs

ID	x_1	x_2	x_3	ID	x_1	x_2	x_3
1	0.05	0	0	17	0	0.35	0
2	0.10	0	0	18	0	0.40	0
3	0.15	0	0	19	0	0.45	0
4	0.20	0	0	20	0	0.50	0
5	0.25	0	0	21	0	0	0.05
6	0.30	0	0	22	0	0	0.10
7	0.35	0	0	23	0	0	0.15
8	0.40	0	0	24	0	0	0.20
9	0.45	0	0	25	0	0	0.25
10	0.50	0	0	26	0	0	0.30
11	0	0.05	0	27	0	0	0.35
12	0	0.10	0	28	0	0	0.40
13	0	0.15	0	29	0	0	0.45
14	0	0.20	0	30	0	0	0.50
15	0	0.25	0	31	0	0	0
16	0	0.30	0				

Appendix Table 2 Subroutine to Compute the ith Row of F for the Quadratic Regression Model Using ACED[a]

```
      subroutine xtof (x, nv, mix, nmix, f, maxk, k)
c
c        user-supplied subroutine to define linear model.
c        fits quadratic model with common intercept and no interactions
c
c        nv     on entry nv is the number of explanatory variables.
c        x      on entry x of dimension nv contains the values of the nv
c               variables for an arbitrary candidate point.
c        mix    on entry mix(i) = 1 if explanatory variable i is
c               a mixture variable, 0 otherwise (i = 1, nv). (not used here)
c        nmix   on entry nmix is the number of mixture variables.
c        maxk   on entry maxk is the maximum number of parameters for
c               which aced has been compiled.
c        ***    none of the above parameters should be          ***
c        ***    changed on exit.                                ***
c        k      on exit the actual number of parameters.
c        f      on exit f of dimension maxk will contain the k
c               functions of x comprising the model in the first k
c               positions.
c
      double precision x(nv), f(maxk)
      integer mix(nv)
c
c        intercept and linear terms
c
   10 f(1) = 1.0d0
      do 12 j = 1, nv
   12 f(j + 1) = x(j)
c
c        quadratic terms
c
      k = nv + 1
      do 24 i = 1, nv
c
c
      k = k + 1
      f(k) = x(i)  **2
   24 continue
      return
      end
```

[a]Code in the box is specific to model (30).

Appendix Table 3 ACED Output for Quadratic Regression

```
*************************************************
aced (algorithms for construction of experimental designs)
version 1.6.1
*************************************************
```

A. Number of explanatory variables (max 8)? **3**
B. Factorial arrangement or miscellaneous list of design candidates (f or m)? **m**
C. File name for candidates (file name in single quotes or 'term')? **'can2'**
D. Model: first-order, second-order, or user-supplied? **user supplied**
The model has 7 parameters.
E. Algorithm (ap, ex, br, nu, or help)? **ex**
F. Number of attempts from different starting designs (max 100)? **3**
G. The number of random observations in the starting design is uniformly distributed between a and b. Type 2 integers for a and b (2 zeros for default). **0 0**
H. Criterion (do, av, mv, am, or help)? **do**
I. Number of observations (max 50)? **21**

input summary

candidates	31	variables	3	model	u	parameters	7
algorithm	ex	criterion	do	obs	21	protected	0
limit a	0	b	0				

design properties

design ref	itera- tions	det**(1/7) covariance matrix	maximum variance	average variance	max e-val covariance matrix	trace covariance matrix
1	59	0.1365e+03	0.7000e+01	0.5712e+01	0.4745e+04	0.1026e+05
2	56	0.1365e+03	0.7000e+01	0.5712e+01	0.4745e+04	0.1026e+05
3	58	0.1365e+03	0.7000e+01	0.5712e+01	0.4745e+04	0.1026e+05

design points

design ref	candidate (replication)						
1	5 (3)	10 (3)	15 (3)	20 (3)	25 (3)	30 (3)	31 (3)
2	5 (3)	10 (3)	15 (3)	20 (3)	25 (3)	30 (3)	31 (3)
3	5 (3)	10 (3)	15 (3)	20 (3)	25 (3)	30 (3)	31 (3)

Appendix Table 4 Subroutine to Compute ith Row of V^* for Model (26)

Replace the code in the box in Appendix Table 2 by the following code:

```
          double precision x(nv), f(maxk),theta(10)
          integer mix(nv),j ,nv,nmix,maxk,k
c
          data theta(1)/-99.d10/
          save theta
c
c      on first call to routine, user types values of thetas
c
          if (theta(1) .le. -99.d10) then
              write(*,*)' no. of groups =',nv
              write(*,*)' type values for all ranges, then all rates'
              read(*,*)(theta(j), j=1,2*nv)
              k = 2*nv+1
            endif
c
c      compute derivatives
c
c   with respect to theta(1)
            f(1)=1.0d0
            do 3 j=1,nv
c   with respect to asymptote parameters
            f(2*j)=1.-exp(-theta(nv+j)*x(j))
c   with respect to rate parameters
  3         f(2*j+1)=theta(j)*x(j)*exp(-theta(nv+j)*x(j))
            return
          end
```

Appendix Table 5 ACED Session for Model (26)

```
************************************************
aced (algorithms for construction of experimental designs)
version 1.6.1
************************************************
```

Number of explanatory variables (max 8)? **3**
Is this a mixture-variables experiment (y, n, or help)? **n**
Factorial arrangement or miscellaneous list of design candidates (f or m)? **m**
File of candidates (file name in single quotes or 'term')? **'../can2'**
Model: first-order, second-order, or user-supplied subroutine (f, s, or u)? **u**
No. of groups = **3**
Type values for all ranges, then all rates
1064 928 748 6.77 7.24 8.72
The model has 7 parameters.
Algorithm (ap, ex, br, nu, or help)? **ex**
Number of attempts from different starting designs (max 100)? **2**
The number of random observations in the starting design is uniformly distributed between a and b. Type 2 integers for a and b (2 zeros for default). **0 0**
Criterion (do, av, mv, am, or help)? **do**
Number of observations (max 50)? **21**

input summary

candidates	31	variables	3	model	u	parameters	7
algorithm	ex	criterion	do	obs	21	protected	0
limit a	0	b	0				

design properties

design ref	itera- tions	det**(1/ 7) covariance matrix	maximum variance	average variance	max e-val covariance matrix	trace covariance matrix
1	65	0.3239e+00	0.7112e+01	0.5744e+01	0.3322e+02	0.5776e+02
2	60	0.3239e+00	0.7112e+01	0.5744e+01	0.3322e+02	0.5776e+02

design points

design ref	candidate (replication)							
1	3 (3)	10 (3)	12 (1)	13 (2)	20 (3)	22 (3)	30 (3)	31 (3)
2	3 (3)	10 (3)	12 (1)	13 (2)	20 (3)	22 (3)	30 (3)	31 (3)

7

Design and Analysis of Multicenter Trials

JUDITH D. GOLDBERG and KENNETH J. KOURY Lederle Laboratories, American Cyanamid Company, Pearl River, New York

1 INTRODUCTION

A multicenter clinical trial is a trial conducted at more than one distinct site. Such a trial provides replication and generalizability of results to a variety of patients and treatment settings. The design and analysis of such a trial involve ideas and methods that are fundamental to statistical thinking and scientific inference. In the application of a new treatment and the study of its effects, it is desirable to replicate the setting as well as the individuals tested within a specific setting. Therefore, the multicenter trial with site or center as a blocking variable provides a useful approach.

The issues that pertain to the design and analysis of a single-center trial must be considered for a multicenter trial. The particular difficulties in the conduct and implementation of a multicenter trial require attention to additional issues. In this chapter we discuss various types of multicenter trials, their uses and limitations, and approaches to the analysis and interpretation of the data resulting from such a trial.

1.1 Definition

In the design of a clinical trial, we want to evaluate the efficacy and safety of some intervention, either treatment or prevention, in a defined population. The simplest kind of trial is one that is carried out at a single site or center. This center should be able to provide adequate numbers of relatively homogeneous participants treated in a common manner in a uniform setting. There may, however, be some characteristic, possibly unknown, associated with this center that is uniquely related to the treatment effect at the center. Effects unique to any one center can be identified if the experiment is repeated at other centers.

When the trial is carried out at more than one site or center, we define it to be a *multicenter trial*. Implicit in this definition is that the identical study protocol is used at each center.

1.2 Examples

Let us illustrate with some examples of the kinds of diseases for which multicenter trials are appropriate or necessary.

EXAMPLE 1. CHRONIC DISEASE: POLYCYTHEMIA VERA Polycythemia vera is a relatively rare chronic disease characterized by an elevated hematocrit [described in Berk et al. (1981)] which has as natural consequences, stroke, hemorrhage, leukemia, and death. In the late 1960s, several therapeutic avenues were available, each of which had its proponents. No serious randomized trials had yet been undertaken to evaluate the alternatives. An additional complication was that diagnostic criteria were ill defined.

In 1967, the Polycythemia Vera Study Group was formed with funding from the National Cancer Institute to conduct clinical studies of this rare disease. The major study conducted by this group was PVSG-01, a randomized, controlled multicenter trial to compare treatment of these patients with phlebotomy (blood letting or bleeding), chlorambucil (a chemotherapeutic agent), and ^{32}P (radioactive phosphorus which is injected into the bloodstream). A total of 478 patients, of whom 431 were eligible, were entered into this study from 1967 to 1974. The study involved over 40 institutions in four countries. Some patients are still being followed on treatments for long-term complications of the disease and for survival.

EXAMPLE 2. RELATIVELY SHORT-TERM OUTCOME ASSESSMENT: HYPERTENSION In clinical trials to evaluate therapy for mild-to-moderate hypertension the primary objective is to assess the reduction in blood pressure during a defined period of therapy. Generally, patients are required to have a specified level of hypertension prior to randomization. Although this disease is relatively well defined, there are numerous difficulties in establishing an accurate diagnosis (see Chapter 1 for discussion). Goldberg et al. (1986) described a design for a complex multicenter trial of a new antihypertensive agent in which the methods for standardization of entry criteria were incorporated into the protocol. Patients were to be randomized to three treatments (new drug, standard therapy, or placebo) following a 3-week placebo run-in period. During this period, repeated blood pressure readings were made at each weekly visit to produce an average for each visit. These weekly readings were then averaged to establish the baseline level. Only those patients who met study criteria for disease were randomized. The protocol specified similar requirements for response (measured as change from baseline), explicit rules for removal of patients from therapy if the disease worsened, and definitions of "failures."

The trial was further complicated by the addition of a second therapy following evaluation in the initial period. During this second stage, the new drug or the standard was to be added to supplement the previously assigned treatment to ascertain the improvement in response rates associated with combination therapy. Randomization to the stage 1 and 2 treatments (considered a regimen) was carried out within center. That is, patients were randomized to six regimens. For example, patients could be randomized to the new drug in stage 1 with the addition of the standard therapy in stage 2 for failures, or to the new drug in stage 1 followed by the addition of placebo in stage 2 for failures. Similarly, the other regimens were standard/new, standard/placebo, placebo/new, and placebo/standard.

Each of 15 to 20 centers was to enroll 24 to 30 patients. This would enable a comparison of the initial three treatment groups with adequate power to detect a difference of at least 6 mmHg in mean diastolic blood pressure; this difference is regarded as clinically significant. In addition, the treatment $\times$ center interaction could be assessed at the end of the first stage. Secondary comparisons of the added treatments were possible at the end of the second stage of the study, but not with the same precision as that of the primary comparisons and with limited ability to assess treatment $\times$ center interaction.

EXAMPLE 3. MORTALITY TRIALS: BETA-BLOCKER HEART ATTACK TRIAL A multicenter randomized clinical trial to evaluate the use of therapy with beta-blockers in patients with acute myocardial infarction was initiated in 1977 (Beta-Blocker Heart Attack Trial Research Group, 1982). A total of 3827 patients were randomized to therapy with propranolol or placebo at each of 31 centers with 134 participating hospitals during a 27-month period. This trial was designed to be of adequate size and power to detect a difference in mortality of patients on active treatment compared with patients treated with placebo allowing for noncompliance [for details of the method of sample size estimation, see Wu et al. (1980)]. This large-scale trial was sponsored by the National Heart, Lung and Blood Institute. It was terminated 9 months ahead of schedule when it showed a reduction in total mortality for patients treated with propranolol (7.2%) compared with placebo (9.8%), as well as in mortality from arteriosclerotic heart disease and sudden coronary death.

As a result, beta-blockers are considered to have a beneficial effect on mortality. Trials of new beta-blockers for regulatory approval are unlikely to confirm these mortality results. Pharmaceutical companies are more likely to run trials to establish claims for nonmortality endpoints.

EXAMPLE 4. CORONARY ARTERY SURGERY STUDY The Coronary Artery Surgery Study (CASS, 1983) includes a multicenter patient registry and a randomized controlled clinical trial at 11 of the 15 study sites to assess the effect of coronary artery bypass surgery on mortality and selected nonfatal endpoints. During a 4-year period, 780 patients with ischemic heart disease were randomized in strata defined by clinical site, number of diseased vessels, left ventricular ejection fraction (proportion of blood in the heart pumped by a single beat), and presence of angina. They received surgical or nonsurgical (medical) treatment. The average annual mortality rate (over 5 years of follow-up) was 1.1% for surgery compared with 1.6% for medical treatment (not statistically significant).

When the study was designed, available data suggested that the average annual mortality rate for these patients was 4%. Therefore, the study was planned to be able to detect a 50% decrease in the mortality rate for surgery from 4% to 2%. With the observed nonsurgery rate of 1.6%, a 50% reduction in mortality would be detectable with a probability of 0.65 with the given study size. A sample size greater than 4600 would have been required to detect the observed 30% reduction in mortality given a 1.6% nonsurgical rate with 90% power. The results of CASS suggest that an advantage may exist for surgery for some patients. The size in this multicenter trial is inadequate to rule out the possibility of a large improvement due to surgery.

2 RATIONALE

Multiple centers yield results applicable to a wider range of centers or patient groups than would a trial at a single site. The multicenter trial should permit estimation of overall treatment differences in the patient populations under study at the various sites.

Multicenter trials can also be expedient; that is, the desired number of patients can be accrued more rapidly than in a single-center trial. The particular usefulness of the multicenter trial in the pharmaceutical industry is the ability to conduct a trial quickly with relatively large numbers of patients. The results can be generalized across a range of patient groups and centers.

The polycythemia vera trial discussed in Example 1 could not have been carried out in a single center. Polycythemia is a rather rare disease. Since each institution can provide very few patients for study, only through the mechanisms of a multicenter trial can such a trial be undertaken. Even with 40 participating centers, 7 years were required to enroll 478 patients in PVSG-01.

The need for the multicenter trial is also apparent for the study of relatively rare endpoints even for a relatively common disease (e.g., mortality in the acute myocardial infarction trial described in Example 3). Thousands of patients must be entered in a relatively limited time to observe a reasonable difference in death rates between the treatment and control groups. Moreover, the trial should be carried out during a period of relatively unchanging patient management and supportive care.

Additional reasons for the choice of a multicenter trial are as follows. They include the availability of highly specialized equipment or laboratory tests located at selected sites to all centers. They allow small centers to participate in the trial. They encourage cooperation and collaboration among investigators interested in similar diseases. Multicenter trials can also take advantage of centralized data management and data analysis facilities (Machin et al., 1979).

There are further distinctions between multicenter trials for chronic and acute diseases. Acute diseases, even if they are rare, require only a short-term commitment from the participating centers. In contrast, chronic diseases such as polycythemia vera with distant endpoints require a long-term commitment. There are additional difficulties in the management of multicenter trials for chronic disease. Both patients and investigators tend to lose interest with time. This and protocol violations result in increased numbers of patients lost to follow-up; both can differ greatly by institution as well as by treatment. Moreover, there may be time trends in patient entry characteristics and accrual rates as well as changes in patient management.

3 DESIGN OF MULTICENTER TRIALS

3.1 Requirements of Randomized Clinical Trials with Particular Reference to Many Centers

A successful clinical trial must meet several requirements (see Chapter 1). These requirements become even more stringent for a multicenter trial. In particular, the objectives of the study must be clear, preferably simple, and the multiple investigators must agree that these are indeed the trial objectives.

The information that the trial will provide must be specified in advance and, again, all participants must agree. A careful design and protocol are requirements of any trial. The need for agreement of all participants in a multicenter trial makes it even more important that the design and procedures be kept as simple and focused as possible. On the other hand, the ability to obtain relatively large numbers of patients for study lends itself to the use of more complex designs to answer a variety of questions from the same trial. In the hypertension study described in Example 2, a compromise between the primary and secondary goals was possible: in the first stage, the new therapy was compared with standard treatment and with placebo, while the second stage was designed to collect information for planning definitive future studies of combination therapies.

The choice of treatments under study also requires agreement. If the investigators are not fully committed to studying the treatments involved (and the specific regimens), the uniformity of the trial across centers may be compromised. The investigators must agree with the choice of the control group (active or placebo or both), as well as with the choice of the specific population for study (limited disease or extensive disease in cancer trials; mild, moderate, or severe hypertension; etc.). Although it may appear reasonable to use different control groups at different centers, this really means that there are *multiple studies* rather than multiple centers in the one study. Similarly, the investigators must agree on the key endpoints for analysis as well as the evaluation times for these endpoints.

In summary, all involved must agree to the objectives and procedures to be used in the trial.

3.2 Determining Numbers of Patients and Centers

The usual guidelines for determining sample size for a randomized trial are appropriate in the design considerations for a multicenter trial. Several additional aspects, however, enter the determination of sample size.

We indicated in Section 2 that a primary reason for such trials is to obtain adequate numbers of patients for study. The distinction that arises in trials sponsored by a pharmaceutical company is the regulatory requirement for marketing approval that the new agent must be shown to be active. This requirement is most simply met by comparing the new drug to placebo. When there is an available treatment that is recognized as being effective, a placebo controlled trial may be unethical. In this case a trial with an active control may be undertaken. The usual goal is to show that the new drug is as good or better than the reference drug. Such a trial must, of course, be larger than a placebo-controlled trial. Even when a placebo control is feasible, pharmaceutical companies try to develop comparative information if there is a currently available effective therapy. Such trials will tend to have three or more treatment groups, and the sample size requirements increase correspondingly.

Fixed Versus Sequential Trials

The decision to conduct a trial with a fixed sample size versus a sequential or group sequential trial depends on the nature of the disease under study, the endpoint(s) for analysis, the time frame of the study, and the procedures for data collection. Fixed sample size and group sequential designs are possible in multicenter studies. Although when cases occur infrequently, the endpoint can be observed quickly, and the results can be communicated rapidly, a completely sequential design might be useful, the logistics of a multicenter trial make it unlikely that such a trial could be carried out successfully.

A group sequential design can be useful for the study of endpoints that require long-term follow-up. With appropriate data collection mechanisms, results can be made available at specified times to allow for early decisions. Such designs are useful for chronic disease trials. These designs are discussed in Chapter 10.

Fixed Sample Size

The simplest trials have fixed sample sizes. These trials are most useful when patient follow-up is relatively short and when patients are rapidly accrued. Hypertension and arthritis drug trials would usually be conducted as fixed-sample-size studies with a 6-to 12-week observation period for each patient and with the completion of total study accrual within one year.

The power considerations for a multicenter trial are similar to those of any other clinical trial: the desired detectable difference is specified along with the significance level (e.g., $\alpha = 0.05$, two-sided) and power (e.g., $1 - \beta = 80\%, 95\%$). Since the multicenter trial is usually meant to be definitive, the size and power should be adequate to meet that goal.

In the design of a multicenter trial, we generally consider the center or institution to be a stratification variable. The total sample size requirement of the trial and the available numbers of patients at each center usually dictate the number of centers. For ease of analysis and interpretation, it is desirable to have similar precision for the estimates of response in each center (Yates and Cochran, 1938). We would like to have "adequate" numbers of patients and centers to test for treatment by center interaction, which is required by the regulatory guidelines (Food and Drug Administration, 1988). Cochran (1937) suggests that fewer than 20 degrees of freedom for the error estimate in an individual center (i.e., fewer than 20 patients/center) would make interaction tests difficult to carry out in a two-group comparison. Further, it is helpful to have approximately equal numbers of patients at each center.

Machin, Staquet, and Sylvester (Machin et al., 1979) discuss the optimal number of centers in a multicenter trial to compare two treatments with n patients per treatment in each of m centers with nm fixed. Based on the analysis of Chakravorti and Grizzle (1975), which assumes that centers are randomly selected, Machin et al. show that for a trial with $nm = 200$ patients, the optimal design in terms of minimizing costs is one with 10 patients per treatment at each of ten centers. For 20 or 25 centers, costs are not very different from optimal, but the designs become more inefficient as the number of patients per center per treatment decreases because it is more difficult to obtain a meaningful assessment of treatment $\times$ center interaction.

Very small numbers of patients per center are often the case in trials of relatively rare diseases such as polycythemia vera (Example 1) or metastatic breast cancer. In such cases, with few patients per center, the center is typically ignored in the analysis. Alternatively, while the center can be treated as random (Chakravorti and Grizzle, 1975), this is seldom done in practice.

The choice of sample size for multicenter trials is further complicated by the need to incorporate, in the baseline stratification, other important variables that may be associated with outcome to treatment. For example, randomization is usually carried out with stratification for performance status and estrogen receptor status for metastatic breast cancer trials or race for hypertension studies (blacks tend to respond more favorably to diuretic therapy than do nonblacks).

Imbalances between treatments groups within a center with regard to baseline variables can confound subsequent analyses. For example, we can have four patients at center A, three on the new treatment with estrogen receptor status positive and one patient on the standard treatment with estrogen receptor status negative, while the reverse is true at center B.

Thus we are faced with trying to strike some balance based on what we can control and what we cannot.

3.3 Randomization

If we consider the center as a stratification variable, the usual choice of a randomization scheme for a randomized trial must be made: to balance treatment assignments within strata or across strata. It is generally agreed that treatment allocations should be balanced within center. We address this question in the next section.

Procedures for Balancing Treatment Allocation

Randomized permuted blocks (Zelen, 1974) can be used to balance treatment within centers. The basic idea of this approach is to ensure that the difference between treatment totals within each center is controlled and is smaller than some randomly chosen value d (usually, $1 < d < 3$). If the difference is greater than d, the next treatment assignment is used, and the rejected assignment is used later or simply ignored. Generally, the size of the random permuted blocks in practice is twice the number of treatments (Pocock and Lagakos, 1982).

Alternative methods include adaptive allocation schemes. Adaptive methods and randomized permuted blocks permit a balance of treatment groups within levels of any stratification variables. With relatively few stratification variables other than center, randomization can be carried out within strata within center. This is simplest to implement because the allocation scheme is completely predetermined at the start of the study. (The predetermined scheme, however, is not known to the investigators.)

It is also possible to use unrestricted randomization, ignoring center. The danger is that the treatment and center may be at least partially confounded. Even with small numbers of patients per center, it is preferable to use procedures to balance treatment assignments within centers.

Mechanisms for Randomization

The choice of a randomization procedure is, in part, related to the mechanism to be used. Randomization can be carried out at a centralized location by telephone or computer, or it can be carried out at each site.

Centralized randomization by telephone to an individual or computer system in a multicenter trial has many advantages. Patient eligibility can be verified at the central site prior to randomization. This reduces the number of ineligible patients entered and assures that the protocol entry criteria are adhered to at each participating center. Balanced randomization schema such as randomized permuted blocks (Zelen, 1974) or some adaptive allocation procedures that require dynamic balancing are easier to manage. Finally, a record of the patient entry is obtained centrally at the time of randomization.

The alternative is to provide the randomization schedule to each center prior to the start of the trial. This can be done by placing the assignment in sealed opaque envelopes for the center coordinator or by providing randomization schedules to the dispensing pharmacist at the center. When it is feasible, the most convenient implementation of randomization at the center is accomplished by providing prepackaged, blinded drug supplies for each patient (identified only by patient number). This becomes more difficult to implement, however, as the number of stratification variables (in addition to center) increase. A verification is sent to the central site after a patient is randomized. It is easier for unblinding to occur in certain on-site approaches. On the other hand, there are some situations in which centralized randomization is not always feasible: international trials, and trials with 24-hour patient accession requiring immediate randomization. With the increased use of computer facilities, however, centralized randomization becomes a reasonable possibility in these circumstances as well.

3.4 Feasibility

The decision to undertake a multicenter trial must consider feasibility. Will the design proposed for the trial work? The trial will be possible if the investigators have agreed to the protocol and if procedures are in place to carry it out. Furthermore, the trial should be adequate to assess, for interpretation as well as for regulatory requirements, treatment × center interaction. The sample size should, therefore, be sufficiently large in each center to permit assessment of the consistency of treatment differences with approximately equal precision. Circumstances can impose constraints. For example, if a study must be completed within a year and no centers will be able to randomize more than six patients in the year, it may be difficult to provide any assessment of treatment × center interaction.

4 CONDUCT AND IMPLEMENTATION OF THE MULTICENTER TRIAL

The successful completion of the multicenter trial depends on its conduct and implementation.

4.1 Protocol Development

The importance of a clear, well-thought-out protocol is of paramount importance. A protocol for such a study should be developed with input from the participating investigators and should serve to document the study objectives as well as to standardize definitions and procedures across centers. In addition to specifying the study objectives, the protocol should include:

Requirements for patient accrual from each center
Criteria for patient entry and randomization
Details of patient management procedures
Details of the drug regimens under study and how to implement them
Criteria for evaluation of the patient as well as criteria for altering the management of the patient
Definitions of response and endpoints and specifications for documentation

The protocol must be accompanied by case report forms or "flow sheets" to record data. A manual of procedures should be available to provide detailed specifications of the test and evaluation procedures to be used as well as detailed instructions for the uniform recording of observations.

4.2 Methods to Ensure Consistency Across Centers

The importance of ensuring uniformity in all centers cannot be overestimated, and considerable effort should be devoted to accomplishing this. Training is provided for participating investigators at meetings to discuss interpretation and implementation of the protocol. Data are monitored on a routine basis by blinded personnel to identify and correct problems as they occur. This monitoring takes place at each center, as well as centrally by clinical, data processing, and statistical staff.

Consistency in a multicenter trial is aided by centralized data processing and statistical analysis. In addition, the use of a single laboratory removes center-to-center laboratory variation. Blinded central and/or "expert" review of patient eligibility, evaluability, and outcome also ensure that consistent interpretations are given to the study protocol.

EXAMPLE 1 (REVISITED) The PVSG held regular group meetings twice each year to review the progress of the study described above. The investigators jointly reviewed patient accrual, patient eligibility, and outcome. In addition to this review, a quality control committee reviewed data quality and completeness, problem cases, all cases with complications, and all deaths; required bone marrow studies were reviewed centrally by experts in pathology and cytogenetics.

One of the problems in this study was that the entry criteria permitted patients to be randomized based on the technology available at each institution. This quirk led to entry criteria that differed by institution. Furthermore, the duration of the disease at entry could vary up to 4 years from diagnosis; the only requirement was that there be no prior treatment. Because of the variability in the locations and types of institutions ranging from primary to tertiary care hospitals in the United States to national centers abroad, the numbers and types of patients accrued varied widely by institution and geographic region (from 1 to 174 in a region). Ineligibility rates were different by treatment and institution. Loss-to-follow-up rates differed by region and treatment group as well. As the trial continued, investigators and patients grew less interested. Evaluation of protocol adherence became almost meaningless; almost all long-term survivors under follow-up were violators by the criteria of the original protocol. In addition, patient characteristics and entry changed over the course of the study because interim results were reported and investigators became more comfortable entering sicker patients.

5 ANALYSIS AND INTERPRETATION

5.1 Baseline Characteristics and Conduct of Study

As in any analysis of the results of a randomized clinical trial, the characteristics of the patients randomized to the treatment groups at baseline or at the time of randomization should be compared. This is done both within center and across centers to identify imbalances that could confound the analysis and interpretation of the effects of treatment on the outcome of interest. In particular, the comparison of characteristics across centers allows the description of differences in patient groups at the different centers so that some of those factors that might be associated with centers can be isolated. "Center" may, in fact, serve as a surrogate for an unknown constellation of demographic-illness variables. Factors of concern, in addition to center, can also be identified for further exploratory analyses of treatment effects.

Further, as described in the PVSG-01 study, many other factors may be associated with "center." To assess the conduct of the trial and to aid in interpretation, treatment groups should be compared with respect to eligibility rates, patient management, protocol adherence, withdrawal, and loss-to-follow-up rates within centers as well as across centers. Within-center comparisons of these factors will identify some possibly treatment-related center differences, while comparisons across centers will identify center-associated differences in protocol compliance and patient management.

EXAMPLE 1 (AGAIN) In this study, the ineligibility rates differed by treatment group (14% on phlebotomy, 9% on chlorambucil, and 6% on radioactive phosphorus) and by region (from 4% of patients in the United States to 18% in the largest foreign region). Further, the early loss-to-follow-up rates differed by treatment, and, in particular, were largest for patients treated on phlebotomy, who were randomized in the same foreign region (23%) that also had the highest ineligibility rate. Thus subsequent analyses of treatment effects had to take into account these center-related differences.

Many authors have addressed the problems of evaluating the quality of the contributions of an individual center to a multicenter trial. Evaluation is generally based on eligibility rate, protocol adherence rate, completeness and quality of the data submitted, and the numbers of patients entered [see for discussion Sylvester et al. (1981)]. There is usually a requirement to enter a minimal number of patients. Canner et al. (1981) describe slippage and outlier tests to identify those institutions that are really different with respect to outcomes and adherence in multicenter trials. Wermuth and Cochran (1979) suggest that systematic errors often occur in multiclinic data. The examination of the measurement processes and univariate as well as joint frequency distributions of variables of interest can help identify and lead to corrections of sources of bias.

Judgment is required to assess the comparability of treatment groups with regard to patient characteristics and conduct of trial and to evaluate the potential impact of lack of comparability on the results of the trial.

5.2 Estimating Overall Treatment Differences

The primary goal of the analysis of a clinical trial is to estimate overall treatment effects in the patient population under study. These estimates are used to draw inferences concerning the efficacy (placebo-controlled trials) or relative efficacy (active-controlled trials) of one or more treatments.

As noted in Section 5.1, center is an important stratification variable. It is confounded with any special characteristics of the patient population at that center. There may be center-specific variations in the many factors that affect the response to treatment. When a rating scale is used, for example, the investigator's overall level of efficacy scores may differ by center. Trial procedures and equipment may be implemented differently, and equipment may be calibrated differently. It is not surprising, therefore, that substantial center-to-center variation is often seen in the overall (across treatment group) levels of the response variables. It is for this reason that center is usually regarded as a stratification variable. The overall (across-center) estimates of treatment effect are adjusted for center; that is, the estimates are adjusted for any treatment group imbalances within and across centers.

When center is used as a stratification variable, the fundamental quantities to be estimated are the population means and mean treatment differences:

μ_{ij} = population or true mean response for patients receiving treatment i at center j; $i = 1, \ldots, t$ and $j = 1, \ldots, c$,

$\mu_{ij} - \mu_{i'j}$ = difference between the population means for treatment groups i and i' at center j; $i, i' = 1, \ldots, t$ and $j = 1, \ldots, c$.

Overall estimators of the mean response for treatment group i are

$$\hat{\mu}_{i\cdot} = \frac{\sum_{j=1}^{c} w_j \hat{\mu}_{ij}}{\sum_{j=1}^{c} w_j}.$$

The corresponding estimators of the overall mean treatment differences are

$$\hat{\mu}_{i\cdot} - \hat{\mu}_{i'\cdot} = \frac{\sum_{j=1}^{c} w_j (\hat{\mu}_{ij} - \hat{\mu}_{i'j})}{\sum_{j=1}^{c} w_j},$$

for $i, i' = 1, 2, \ldots, t$. These overall estimators are weighted averages of the center-specific estimators. The choice of weights, w_j, depends on the corresponding population quantity being estimated and precision considerations for the overall estimator. When there is no reason to consider any one center as more important than any other center, the overall population treatment means and mean differences are obtained by using $w_j = 1$:

$$\mu_{i\cdot} = \frac{1}{c} \sum_{j=1}^{c} \mu_{ij}, \qquad i = 1, \ldots, t,$$

$$\mu_{i\cdot} - \mu_{i'\cdot} = \frac{1}{c} \sum_{j=1}^{c} (\mu_{ij} - \mu_{i'j}), \qquad i, i' = 1, \ldots, t.$$

If it can be ascertained that the population at center j is typical of a proportion p_j of some general population of interest, it is natural to use $w_j = p_j$. When centers are pooled under the assumption of no center effect, w_j is the number of patients at center j.

The statistical analysis of a multicenter trial usually focuses on the estimation of the overall or average population treatment differences defined above for each pair of treatment groups (i, i'). In general, these population quantities are estimated by

$$\hat{\mu}_{i\cdot} - \hat{\mu}_{i'\cdot} = \frac{1}{c}\sum_{j=1}^{c}(\hat{\mu}_{ij} - \hat{\mu}_{i'j}).$$

However, if the population treatment differences are uniform across centers, that is, if

$$\mu_{ij} - \mu_{i'j} = d_{ii'} \qquad \text{for all } j = 1, \ldots, c,$$

the average population treatment differences can be written as

$$\mu_{i\cdot} - \mu_{i'\cdot} = d_{ii'} = \frac{1}{c}\sum_{j=1}^{c} d_{ii'} = \frac{\sum_{j=1}^{c} w_j d_{ii'}}{\sum_{j=1}^{c} w_j}$$

for any choice of w_j.

In this case, if $\hat{\mu}_{ij}$ and $\hat{\mu}_{i'j}$ are unbiased estimators, then

$$\frac{\sum_{j=1}^{c} w_j(\hat{\mu}_{ij} - \hat{\mu}_{i'j})}{\sum_{j=1}^{c} w_j}$$

is an unbiased estimator of the average population treatment difference. It is natural to choose w_j to reduce the variance of this overall estimator. For example, the weighting function

$$w_j = [\text{var}(\hat{\mu}_{ij} - \hat{\mu}_{i'j})]^{-1}$$

gives greater weight to centers with larger sample sizes.

5.3 Assessment of Center Effects

Before we can draw any inferences with respect to the overall (average) population treatment difference, it is necessary to examine the consistency of the observed treatment differences across centers. The goals are to determine whether a single overall summary statistic is adequate to describe the trial results and to identify that statistic. When the treatment differences vary across centers, we say that there is a *treatment* × *center interaction.*

Consider any two treatments, i and i'. With the notation of Section 5.2, there is no treatment × center interaction when

$$\mu_{ij} - \mu_{i'j} = d_{ii'}$$

for all $j = 1, \ldots, c$. That is, $d_{ii'}$ is constant. This condition can be expressed as

$$(\mu_{ij} - \mu_{i'j}) - (\mu_{ij'} - \mu_{i'j'}) = 0$$

for each pair of centers (j, j').

When there is no treatment × center interaction, the overall treatment effect or difference is usually called a main effect rather than an average effect, since the population treatment differences are uniform from center to center. The main effect, when it exists, is equal to the average effect, but it implies a very specific type of consistency across centers. In this ideal situation, there is no question that an overall estimate of treatment differences provides a reasonable, interpretable summary of trial results, and the specific estimator used should be chosen on the basis of its precision.

5.4 Tests for Treatment × Center Interaction

To justify pooling results across centers, most regulatory agencies require or strongly suggest that a preliminary test for treatment × center interaction be carried out (Food and Drug Administration, 1988). Classical linear models provide formal tests to assess the significance of this interaction. Of course, failure to reject the null hypothesis of no interaction at $\alpha = 0.10$, say, or some other specified level of significance does not mean that there is no interaction. A nonsignificant test result, however, is often accepted as reasonable evidence that the treatment differences are sufficiently consistent to justify pooling results across centers.

On the other hand, the presence of a statistically significant treatment × center interaction does not mean that an overall estimate of treatment effect is inappropriate. Any differences in the patient populations or trial procedures across centers are likely to result in center-to-center differences in the magnitude of the treatment differences. The traditional test for treatment × center interaction can be viewed as a convenient mathematical tool. The lack of an interaction is a sufficient but certainly not necessary condition to justify pooling results across centers.

When a significant interaction is identified, for example, with a test for interaction at $p \leq 0.10$, exploratory analyses to ascertain reasons for the interaction and its possible effect on the study conclusions are useful. Sylvester et al. (1981), Overall (1979), and Canner et al. (1981a, 1981b) provide approaches to identifying and removing aberrant centers. Possible sources of treatment × center interaction include eligibility rates and dropout rates that vary by treatment and center, such as in Example 1.

When the treatment × center interaction is substantial, it is also helpful to characterize the nature of the interaction as either quantitative or qualitative (Gail and Simon, 1985). In *quantitative* interactions the treatment differences are in the same direction across centers but differ in magnitude from center to center. This type of interaction does not invalidate a pooled analysis. An overall estimate of the average treatment difference is well defined and provides a meaningful, reasonable summary of the trial results that is easy to interpret.

Qualitative or crossover interactions, on the other hand, are characterized by substantial treatment differences that occur in different directions in different centers. In this case, an overall or average summary statistic may be considered inadequate and misleading. It is preferable simply to describe the nature of the interaction and to indicate those centers at which treatment i was better than treatment i'. These centers may be similar in ways that shed light on the interaction. The average treatment effect or difference is well defined even in this case. In particular, it may still be of interest to test the hypothesis that the average population treatment difference is 0.

5.5 ANOVA Models

In this section we discuss basic methods to obtain overall estimates of treatment differences and to test the null hypothesis that the population or true average treatment difference is 0.

Classical linear models using least squares estimation procedures are powerful analytical tools—for alternatives, see Chapter 12. In particular, two-way analysis-of-variance (ANOVA) models, both with and without interaction, are extensively used to analyze multicenter trials. The model with interaction is more general and is sometimes called a *cell means model* since the expected value of an observation from a patient in treatment group i at center j is simply the population "cell mean," μ_{ij}. This model can be written as

$$y_{ijk} = \mu_{ij} + \epsilon_{ijk}$$

for $i = 1, \ldots, t$, $j = 1, \ldots, c$, and $k = 1, \ldots, n_{ij}$; here y_{ijk} denotes the value of the response variable for patient k on treatment i at center j, n_{ij} is the number of patients on treatment i at center j, and the ϵ_{ijk} denote random errors assumed to be independent and identically distributed $N(0, \sigma^2)$ variables. Using traditional ANOVA notation, this model is equivalently written as

$$y_{ijk} = \mu + \alpha_i + \beta_j + \alpha\beta_{ij} + \epsilon_{ijk},$$

where μ is the overall mean of population means (across treatments and centers), α_i is the effect of treatment i, β_j is the effect of center j, and $\alpha\beta_{ij}$ is the effect of the interaction of treatment i with center j.

This model is quite general since it places no restrictions on the manner in which the treatment differences vary from center to center. Least squares estimators of the population quantities of interest are given by

Population cell means:

$$\hat{\mu}_{ij} = \bar{y}_{ij}$$
$$= \frac{1}{n_{ij}} \sum_{k=1}^{n_{ij}} y_{ijk}, \qquad i = 1, \ldots, t, \quad j = 1, \ldots, c$$

Average population treatment means:

$$\hat{\mu}_{i\cdot} = \frac{1}{c} \sum_{j=1}^{c} \bar{y}_{ij}, \qquad i = 1, \ldots, t$$

Average population treatment differences:

$$\hat{\mu}_{i\cdot} - \hat{\mu}_{i'\cdot} = \frac{1}{c} \sum_{j=1}^{c} (\bar{y}_{ij} - \bar{y}_{i'j}), \qquad i, i' = 1, \ldots, t.$$

Standard errors of these estimators are obtained by using the mean square error from the ANOVA to estimate $\sigma^2 = \text{var}(y_{ijk})$.

The two-way analysis of variance model without interaction, the *main effects model*, is characterized by expressing the population mean for treatment i at center j as the sum of a grand mean, a constant effect due to treatment i, and a constant effect due to center j:

$$\mu_{ij} = E(y_{ijk}) = \mu + \alpha_i + \beta_j.$$

Since the effects of treatment and center are assumed to be additive and no interaction effects are included in the model, it follows that the population treatment differences are identical across centers. Specifically, for each pair of treatments (i, i'),

$$\mu_{ij} - \mu_{i'j} = \alpha_i - \alpha_{i'} \qquad \text{for all } j = 1, \ldots, c.$$

The average population treatment difference is also given by

$$\mu_{i\cdot} - \mu_{i'\cdot} = \frac{1}{c} \sum_{j=1}^{c} (\alpha_i - \alpha_{i'}) = \alpha_i - \alpha_{i'}.$$

Least squares estimates for the model parameters are obtained, in general, by solving the corresponding normal equations. These estimates are used to calculate the least squares estimates of the population cell means and treatment differences:

$$\hat{\mu}_{ij} = \hat{\mu} + \hat{\alpha}_i + \hat{\beta}_j,$$
$$\hat{\mu}_{ij} - \hat{\mu}_{i'j} = \hat{\mu}_{i\cdot} - \hat{\mu}_{i'\cdot} = \hat{\alpha}_i - \hat{\alpha}_{i'}.$$

In practice, these quantities and their standard errors are estimated by fitting the model using linear models procedures available in statistical computing packages.

When the treatment × center interaction is zero or negligible, the main effects model accurately describes the true relationship between the response variable and the effects of treatment and center. In this case the least squares estimators of the population cell means and the average population treatment differences are more precise than the corresponding least squares estimators based on the more general cell means model (although both sets of estimators are unbiased). This results directly from the theory of linear models since adding unnecessary terms to a linear model (e.g., an interaction term) does not bias the least squares estimators but increases their variances.

Least squares estimators are the best linear unbiased estimators regardless of the distribution of the underlying errors. These estimators are also asymptotically normally distributed under mild regularity conditions. These properties, along with their flexibility and relative computational simplicity, justify the extensive use of classical linear models in clinical trials and other applications. Nevertheless, improved estimators are available in certain cases, particularly when the underlying distribution has long or thick tails. These alternative approaches are described in Chapter 12.

EXAMPLE 5 A small pilot study was conducted at three centers to evaluate a new antihypertensive drug in patients with mild to moderate hypertension. Patients were enrolled in a clinical facility for 7 days. The response variable calculated for each patient is the change from baseline in sitting diastolic blood pressure (mmHg) averaged over the 7-day treatment. A negative response corresponds to a decrease from baseline, that is, an improvement in the patient's hypertension. Individual patient data and the observed cell means are presented in Table 1. Treatment 1 is active (A); treatment 2 is placebo (P).

Although the treatment differences are in the same direction (favoring the active treatment) in each center, the sample sizes are too small to assess comfortably the consistency of the results across centers. To illustrate the method, however, we analyzed the data by fitting ANOVA models with and without interaction using the general linear models procedure of the

Table 1 Change from Baseline in Sitting Diastolic Blood Pressure by Treatment Group and Center

Treatment	Center I	Center II	Center III
1 Active (A)	+3.7	+2.3	−9.4
	−6.7	−7.9	−10.4
	−10.5	−8.9	−10.9
	−6.1	−4.5	−9.3
	−17.6	−7.7	−16.7
			−7.2
	$\bar{y}_{11} = -7.44$	$\bar{y}_{12} = -5.34$	$\bar{y}_{13} = -10.65$
2 Placebo (P)	−0.7	+0.2	−2.3
	−2.2	−7.4	+1.8
		−1.0	−11.7
		−3.1	+2.3
	$\bar{y}_{21} = -1.45$	$\bar{y}_{22} = -2.83$	$\bar{y}_{23} = -2.48$

Statistical Analysis System [PROC GLM in SAS (1985)]. Table 2 displays the SAS code that generated the output shown in Tables 3a and 3b.

Table 4 displays the least squares estimates of the relevant population means (referred to as LSMEANS in SAS terminology) and their standard errors based on each model.

The least squares estimates of the population cell means, μ_{ij}, based on the cell means model can be obtained directly from the SAS LSMEANS option for the treatment × center interaction effect. For the main effects model, however, SAS does not provide LSMEANS for this effect because it is not included in the model statement; instead, appropriate ESTIMATE statements shown in Table 5 are used. For both models, the LSMEANS option for the treatment effect provides the estimates for the average population treatment means, $\mu_{1.}$ and $\mu_{2.}$, while the estimate of the average population treatment difference, $\mu_{1.} - \mu_{2.}$, is obtained using an estimate statement.

Table 6 lists the null hypotheses of interest and the associated p-values based on the two ANOVA models. The p-values for testing these null hypotheses are obtained from the type III sums of squares for the appropriate effect calculated by PROC GLM for each model. Since there are only two treatment groups in this study, a test of the null hypothesis that the average population treatment means are equal (i.e., H_0: $\mu_{1.} = \mu_{2.}$) is also provided by the estimate statement for the average population treatment

Table 2 SAS Code for ANOVA Models

```
PROC GLM; CLASSES TRT CENTER;
MODEL CHANGE = TRT CENTER TRT*CENTER;
ESTIMATE 'AVG TRT DIFF A–P' TRT 3 –3 TRT*CENTER 1 1 1 –1 –1 –1 /DIVISOR=3;
MEANS TRT CENTER TRT*CENTER;
LSMEANS TRT CENTER TRT*CENTER / STDERR PDIFF;
TITLE 'CELL MEANS MODEL FOR BLOOD PRESSURE EXAMPLE';

PROC GLM; CLASSES TRT CENTER;
MODEL CHANGE = TRT CENTER ;
ESTIMATE 'CELL MEAN A,I   ' INTERCEPT 1 TRT 1 0 CENTER 1 0 0;
ESTIMATE 'CELL MEAN A,II  ' INTERCEPT 1 TRT 1 0 CENTER 0 1 0;
ESTIMATE 'CELL MEAN A,III ' INTERCEPT 1 TRT 1 0 CENTER 0 0 1;
ESTIMATE 'CELL MEAN P,I   ' INTERCEPT 1 TRT 0 1 CENTER 1 0 0;
ESTIMATE 'CELL MEAN P,II  ' INTERCEPT 1 TRT 0 1 CENTER 0 1 0;
ESTIMATE 'CELL MEAN P,III ' INTERCEPT 1 TRT 0 1 CENTER 0 0 1;
ESTIMATE 'AVG TRT DIFF A–P' TRT 1 –1;
LSMEANS TRT CENTER / STDERR PDIFF;
TITLE 'MAIN EFFECTS MODEL FOR BLOOD PRESSURE EXAMPLE';
```

Table 3a Cell Means Model for Blood Pressure Example: General Linear Models Procedure

DEPENDENT VARIABLE: CHANGE

SOURCE	DF	SUM OF SQUARES	MEAN SQUARE
MODEL	5	273.06446154	54.61289231
ERROR	20	535.73900000	26.78695000
CORRECTED TOTAL	25	808.80346154	

SOURCE	DF	TYPE I SS	F VALUE	PR > F
TRT	1	191.43696154	7.15	0.0146
CENTER	2	44.34964271	0.83	0.4514
TRT*CENTER	2	37.27785729	0.70	0.5103

PARAMETER	ESTIMATE	T FOR HO: PARAMETER=0	PR > !T!
AVG TRT DIFF A−P	−5.56000000	−2.57	0.0181

LEAST SQUARES MEANS

TRT	CHANGE LSMEAN	STD ERR LSMEAN	PROB > !T! HO:LSMEAN=0
ACTIVE	−7.81000000	1.29868616	0.0001
PLACEBO	−2.25000000	1.72520369	0.2070

CENTER	CHANGE LSMEAN	STD ERR LSMEAN	PROB > !T! HO: LSMEAN=0
I	−4.44500000	2.16511345	0.0534
II	−4.08250000	1.73595273	0.0290
III	−6.56250000	1.67042129	0.0008

NOTE: TO ENSURE OVERALL PROTECTION LEVEL, ONLY PROBABILITIES

TRT	CENTER	CHANGE LSMEAN	STD ERR LSMEAN	PROB > !T! HO:LSMEAN=0
ACTIVE	I	−7.4400000	2.3146036	0.0044
ACTIVE	II	−5.3400000	2.3146036	0.0319
ACTIVE	III	−10.6500000	2.1129344	0.0001
PLACEBO	I	−1.4500000	3.6597097	0.6961
PLACEBO	II	−2.8250000	2.5878055	0.2880
PLACEBO	III	−2.4750000	2.5878055	0.3503

NOTE: TO ENSURE OVERALL PROTECTION LEVEL, ONLY PROBABILITIES

F VALUE	PR > F	R-SQUARE	C.V.
2.04	0.1165	0.337615	88.5885
	ROOT MSE		CHANGE MEAN
	5.17561108		−5.84230769

DF	TYPE III SS	F VALUE	PR > F
1	177.58876596	6.63	0.0181
2	32.12295698	0.60	0.5586
2	37.27785729	0.70	0.5103

STD ERROR OF
ESTIMATE

2.15937804

PROB > !T! HO:
LSMEAN1=LSMEAN2

0.0181

PROB > !T! HO: LSMEAN(I)=LSMEAN(J)

I/J	1	2	3
1	.	0.8974	0.4478
2	0.8974	.	0.3156
3	0.4478	0.3156	.

ASSOCIATED WITH PREPLANNED COMPARISONS SHOULD BE USED.

PROB > !T! HO: LSMEAN(I)=LSMEAN(J)

I/J	1	2	3	4	5	6
1	.	0.5285	0.3179	0.1818	0.1987	0.1681
2	0.5285	.	0.1057	0.3797	0.4772	0.4190
3	0.3179	0.1057	.	0.0416	0.0296	0.0238
4	0.1818	0.3797	0.0416	.	0.7622	0.8214
5	0.1987	0.4772	0.0296	0.7622	.	0.9248
6	0.1681	0.4190	0.0238	0.8214	0.9248	.

ASSOCIATED WITH PREPLANNED COMPARISONS SHOULD BE USED.

Table 3b Main Effects Model for Blood Pressure Example: General Linear Models Procedure

DEPENDENT VARIABLE: CHANGE

SOURCE	DF	SUM OF SQUARES	MEAN SQUARE
MODEL	3	235.78660425	78.59553475
ERROR	22	573.01685729	26.04622079
CORRECTED TOTAL	25	808.80346154	

SOURCE	DF	TYPE I SS	F VALUE	PR > F
TRT	1	191.43696154	7.35	0.0128
CENTER	2	44.34964271	0.85	0.4404

PARAMETER	ESTIMATE	T FOR HO: PARAMETER=0	PR > !T!
CELL MEAN A,I	−7.32298006	−3.63	0.0015
CELL MEAN A,II	−6.70241343	−3.46	0.0022
CELL MEAN A,III	−9.61217209	−5.30	0.0001
CELL MEAN P,I	−1.74254984	−0.72	0.4813
CELL MEAN P,II	−1.12198321	−0.55	0.5906
CELL MEAN P,III	−4.03174187	−1.98	0.0606
AVG TRT DIFF A−P	−5.58043022	−2.69	0.0134

LEAST SQUARES MEANS

TRT	CHANGE LSMEAN	STD ERR LSMEAN	PROB > !T! HO:LSMEAN=0
ACTIVE	−7.87918853	1.27878492	0.0001
PLACEBO	−2.29875831	1.64214362	0.1755

CENTER	CHANGE LSMEAN	STD ERR LSMEAN	PROB > !T! HO: LSMEAN=0
I	−4.53276495	1.97953244	0.0320
II	−3.91219832	1.70508367	0.0317
III	−6.82195698	1.62716565	0.0004

NOTE: TO ENSURE OVERALL PROTECTION LEVEL, ONLY PROBABILITIES

F VALUE	PR > F	R-SQUARE	C.V.
3.02	0.0516	0.291525	87.3550
	ROOT MSE		CHANGE MEAN
	5.10354982		−5.84230769

DF	TYPE III SS	F VALUE	PR > F
1	188.42898398	7.23	0.0134
2	44.34964271	0.85	0.4404

STD ERROR OF ESTIMATE
2.01799015
1.93502327
1.81476098
2.43251126
2.05489744
2.03820425
2.07475198

PROB > !T! HO:
LSMEAN1=LSMEAN2

0.0134

PROB > !T! HO: LSMEAN(I)=LSMEAN(J)

I/J	1	2	3
1	.	0.8131	0.3747
2	0.8131	.	0.2281
3	0.3747	0.2281	.

ASSOCIATED WITH PREPLANNED COMPARISONS SHOULD BE USED.

Table 4 Results of ANOVA for Example in Table 1

Population quantity estimated		Cell means model[a] Estimate (SE)	Main effects model[b] Estimate (SE)
Cell mean			
(A,I)	μ_{11}	−7.44 (2.31)	−7.32 (2.02)
(P,I)	μ_{21}	−1.45 (3.66)	−1.74 (2.43)
(A,II)	μ_{12}	−5.34 (2.31)	−6.70 (1.94)
(P,II)	μ_{22}	−2.83 (2.59)	−1.12 (2.05)
(A,III)	μ_{13}	−10.65 (2.11)	−9.61 (1.81)
(P,III)	μ_{23}	−2.48 (2.59)	−4.03 (2.04)
Average treatment mean			
Active	$\mu_{1\cdot}$	−7.81 (1.30)	−7.88 (1.28)
Placebo	$\mu_{2\cdot}$	−2.25 (1.73)	−2.30 (1.64)
Average treatment difference			
A − P	$\mu_{1\cdot} - \mu_{2\cdot}$	−5.56 (2.16)	−5.58 (2.07)

[a] $\mu_{ij} = E(y_{ijk}) = \mu + \alpha_i + \beta_j + \alpha\beta_{ij}$.
[b] $\mu_{ij} = E(y_{ijk}) = \mu + \alpha_i + \beta_j$.

difference, and by the LSMEANS option for the treatment effect, which, as noted above, estimates the average population treatment means.

The estimates of the average population treatment means and their difference are nearly identical under the two models. Since there is little evidence of a treatment × center interaction, it is not surprising that the results are in close agreement. The estimates based on the main effects

Table 5 Estimate Statements Linear Combination to Calculate Estimate

Cell Mean	μ	α_1	α_2	β_1	β_2	β_3
μ_{11}	1	1	0	1	0	0
μ_{12}	1	1	0	0	1	0
μ_{13}	1	1	0	0	0	1
μ_{21}	1	0	1	1	0	0
μ_{22}	1	0	1	0	1	0
μ_{23}	1	0	1	0	0	1

Table 6 Results of Example in Table 1

Null hypothesis of interest	Cell means model	Main effects model
Average population treatment means are equal H_0: $\mu_{1\cdot} = \mu_{2\cdot}$	$p = 0.02$	$p = 0.01$
Average population center means are equal H_0: $\mu_{\cdot 1} = \mu_{\cdot 2} = \mu_{\cdot 3}$	$p = 0.56$	$p = 0.44$
No treatment × center interaction H_0: $(\mu_{11} - \mu_{21}) - (\mu_{12} - \mu_{22}) = 0$ $(\mu_{11} - \mu_{21}) - (\mu_{13} - \mu_{23}) = 0$	$p = 0.51$	Not testable

model are slightly more precise. Both models lead to the conclusion that the average population treatment means are significantly different and that the new drug is efficacious in this patient population.

The choice of a final model requires some judgment. The cell means model is attractive because it is more general and provides unbiased estimates of the average population means and differences, regardless of whether treatment × center interactions exist. Under this model, the estimates of these population quantities give equal weight to each observed cell mean, regardless of sample size. On the other hand, estimators based on the main effects model give more weight to larger centers, but they are not unbiased estimators of the relevant population quantities in the presence of treatment × center interactions. The trade-off associated with choosing between an unbiased estimator and a more precise estimator can be minimized by using a balanced study design with equal numbers of patients in each treatment group at each center.

5.6 Rating Scales and ANOVA

Classical linear models are sometimes used even when the response variable is not normally distributed. This can be justified by the optimum properties of least square estimators (when extreme data points that have excessive influence on the estimates are not present) and their asymptotic distributions. For example, in pharmaceutical trials, efficacy variables are frequently measured on a rating scale. Such a scale might be: 0 = none, 1 = mild, 2 = moderate, 3 = severe. Efficacy data of this type can be summarized for each treatment group at each center as follows:

Efficacy score	0	1	2	3	Total
Number of patients	n_{ij0}	n_{ij1}	n_{ij2}	n_{ij3}	n_{ij}

Here n_{ij} is the number of patients in treatment group i at center j ($i = 1, \ldots, t$ and $j = 1, \ldots, c$). The total number of patients in the trial is $n = \sum\sum_{ij} n_{ij}$.

Clinical researchers often find it convenient to summarize the results further in terms of a mean efficacy score (or mean improvement from baseline), $\bar{y}_{ij}$, and to use this quantity as the basis for treatment comparisons. Let $\mathbf{L}' = (0\ 1\ 2\ 3)$, $\mathbf{n_{ij}} = (n_{ij0}\ n_{ij1}\ n_{ij2}\ n_{ij3})'$, and $\mathbf{p}_{ij} = (1/n_{ij})\mathbf{n_{ij}}$. Then

$$\begin{aligned}\bar{y}_{ij} &= \mathbf{L}' \frac{1}{n_{ij}} \mathbf{n}_{ij} \\ &= \mathbf{L}'\mathbf{p}_{ij}.\end{aligned}$$

Consequently, the weighted least squares (WLS) methods of Grizzle, Starmer, and Koch (GSK) described in Chapter 13 can be applied directly to compare treatments with respect to the mean score, $\bar{y}_{ij}$, or some other function of $\mathbf{p}_{ij}$.

However, in the simple case when the mean score is the response variable of interest, ordinary least squares (OLS) or ANOVA methods provide a popular alternative approach to the more general WLS methods. Let $\boldsymbol{\beta}$ be the $p \times 1$ ($p \leq tc$) vector of model parameters, $\mathbf{X}$ be the $n \times p$ design matrix, and $\mathbf{y}$ be the $n \times 1$ data vector; then the ordinary least squares estimator of $\boldsymbol{\beta}$ is

$$\mathbf{b} = (\mathbf{X}'\mathbf{X})^{-1}\mathbf{X}'\mathbf{y},$$

and its covariance matrix is

$$\text{var}(\mathbf{b}) = (\mathbf{X}'\mathbf{X})^{-1}\sigma^2.$$

The variance of the response variable y, denoted by σ^2, is assumed to be the same for each of the treatment-center subpopulations and is estimated by

$$\hat{\sigma}^2 = \frac{(\mathbf{y} - \mathbf{Xb})'(\mathbf{y} - \mathbf{Xb})}{n - p}.$$

For a $k \times p$ matrix ($k \leq p$) of constants, $\mathbf{C}$, $\mathbf{Cb}$ has an asymptotically normal distribution,

$$\mathbf{Cb} \longrightarrow N(\mathbf{CB}, \sigma^2\mathbf{C}(\mathbf{X}'\mathbf{X})^{-1}\mathbf{C}').$$

Therefore, tests of hypotheses,

$$H_0\colon \mathbf{CB} = \mathbf{0},$$

can be based on the asymptotic distribution of Wald or likelihood ratio statistics:

Wald:

$$\frac{(\mathbf{Cb})'[\mathbf{C}(\mathbf{X}'\mathbf{X})^{-1}\mathbf{C}']^{-1}(\mathbf{Cb})}{\sigma^2} \longrightarrow \chi^2(k).$$

Likelihood ratio:

$$\frac{(\mathbf{Cb})'[\mathbf{C}(\mathbf{X}'\mathbf{X})^{-1}\mathbf{C}']^{-1}(\mathbf{Cb})}{k\hat{\sigma}^2} \longrightarrow F(k, n-p).$$

From the scheme above and the details of the GSK methods provided in Chapter 13, it follows that when the sample mean $\bar{y}_{ij}$ is the function of $\mathbf{p}_{ij}$ which is of interest, the WLS and OLS approaches are quite similar. Both methods are large-sample procedures that use familiar regression techniques with design matrices based on an ANOVA framework. Although these methods give very similar results in most applications, there are some computational differences. In particular, the WLS approach is slightly more general even in this special case since it does not require the variance of the response variable to be homogeneous across the treatment-center subpopulations. This leads to differences in the estimation of the variance of the $\bar{y}_{ij}$. Specifically, GSK uses estimates of σ_{ij}^2 which are functions of the estimated covariance matrices of the $\mathbf{p}_{ij}$, whereas OLS uses the mean square error to estimate the common variance σ^2. In addition, the OLS approach is most conveniently implemented with an ANOVA program for unbalanced data (e.g., PROC GLM in SAS). Therefore, hypothesis testing is based on likelihood ratio statistics for OLS and Wald statistics for WLS. Under the assumption of homogeneous variance, the GSK and (unbalanced) ANOVA procedures are asymptotically equivalent. Although the GSK estimators of $\sigma_{ij}^2 = \sigma^2$ are consistent, they are not unbiased.

EXAMPLE 6. RATING SCALES A randomized double-blind multicenter trial compared an anti-inflammatory agent with placebo in the treatment of patients with osteoarthritis of the knee. The trial was conducted at five centers. The five key efficacy variables were physician and patient overall assessment, pain on active motion, pain at rest, and joint tenderness on palpation. These were measured at baseline and after 2, 4, and 6 weeks of treatment using the following rating scales:

Overall assessments:

$$0 = \text{excellent},\ 1 = \text{good},\ 2 = \text{fair},\ 3 = \text{poor}.$$

Pain on active motion, pain at rest, tenderness:

$$0 = \text{none},\ 1 = \text{mild},\ 2 = \text{moderate},\ 3 = \text{severe}.$$

The distribution of patients by treatment group and center is shown in Table 7.

For each efficacy parameter at each time point, the change from baseline was calculated as

$$\text{change} = \text{baseline value} - \text{value on treatment}.$$

Positive changes reflect an improvement from baseline. These response variables were analyzed by fitting an ANOVA model with sources of variation extracted for treatment, center, and the treatment $\times$ center interaction. Patients who were asymptomatic at baseline (severity score $= 0$) for a given variable were excluded from the analysis of that variable at weeks 2, 4, and 6. These exclusions can introduce bias in the estimates of treatment effects. Since these exclusions occurred in both treatment groups to a similar degree, the comparison of treatment and placebo should be unbiased. Based on this model, the treatment groups were compared with respect to the

Table 7 Number of Eligible[a] Patients by Treatment Group and Center

Center	Treatment 1 (active)	Treatment 2 (placebo)
I	15	15
II	14	9
III	27	27
IV	13	12
V	13	12
Total	82	75

[a]Imbalances between treatments with respect to patient numbers resulted from different eligibility rates by center. Analysis of all randomized patients confirms the results of the analysis presented.

change from baseline in each variable at each time point by testing the hypothesis that the average population treatment means are equal; that is:

$$H_0: \mu_{1\cdot} = \mu_{2\cdot} \quad \text{versus} \quad H_1: \mu_{1\cdot} \neq \mu_{2\cdot}.$$

Repeated measures analyses described in Chapter 3 may also be useful here. Although both approaches are frequently carried out in practice, for ease of presentation the three visits are considered individually. Further, one time point is usually key for efficacy.

Before accepting the estimates of the average treatment differences $(\mu_{1\cdot} - \mu_{2\cdot})$, and the associated tests of significance as a reasonable overall summary of the trial results, it is necessary to assess the consistency of the treatment differences across centers. P-values for testing the significance of the treatment × center interaction are presented in Table 8. Of the 15 models fit, the interaction is significant ($p \leq 0.10$) in four cases—pain on active motion at week 6, tenderness at week 4, and the patient evaluation at week 4 and week 6. In addition, the center-specific treatment differences in mean change from baseline were examined for each variable at each visit. For each of the five variables, the active group showed greater improvement than the placebo group at each time point in each center, with these exceptions: pain on active motion at week 2 for center V, tenderness at weeks 4 and 6 for center IV, and patient evaluation at all three visits for center IV.

The four cases for which treatment × center interaction is significant ($p \leq 0.10$) were examined further to characterize the nature of these interactions. The interaction is quantitative for pain on active motion at week 6 since the results at each center favor the active compound. For each of the remaining three cases, the test for qualitative interaction proposed by Gail and Simon (1985) was performed. To carry out this procedure, an estimate D_j of the true treatment difference and an estimate s_j^2 of the variance of D_j are obtained for each center j. In this example, D_j is an estimate of $\mu_{1j} - \mu_{2j}$, the true treatment difference in mean change from baseline in

Table 8 *p*-Values for the Treatment × Center Interaction, by Efficacy Variable and Visit

Variable	Week 2	Week 4	Week 6
Physician overall	0.49	0.17	0.20
Patient overall	0.12	< 0.01	0.04
Pain on active motion	0.22	0.35	0.10
Pain at rest	0.73	0.64	0.61
Tenderness	0.64	0.08	0.28

the patient population studied at center j; that is,

$$D_j = \bar{y}_{1j} - \bar{y}_{2j},$$

the difference between the observed treatment group mean change at center j. The variance of D_j is estimated by

$$s_j^2 = s_{Dj}^2 = [\mathrm{SE}(\bar{y}_{1j})]^2 + [\mathrm{SE}(\bar{y}_{2j})]^2,$$

where SE denotes standard error. Using these center-specific estimates, the quantities Q^+ and Q^- are calculated as follows:

$$Q^+ = \sum_j \frac{D_j^2}{s_j^2} I(D_j < 0),$$

$$Q^- = \sum_j \frac{D_j^2}{s_j^2} I(D_j > 0),$$

where $I(G) = 1$ if the event G obtains and 0 otherwise. The null hypothesis of no qualitative interaction is rejected if

$$\min(Q^+, Q^-) > c,$$

where c is the appropriate critical value obtained from Table 1 of Gail and Simon (1985). For five centers this table provides the critical values corresponding to the 0.05, 0.10, and 0.20 levels of significance:

α	0.05	0.10	0.20
c	6.50	4.96	3.39

The required calculations and results of the test for qualitative interaction are shown in Table 9 for patient evaluations at week 4 and week 6 and tenderness at week 2. In each case a fairly small treatment difference favoring placebo is seen at center IV, and considerably larger treatment differences favoring the active agent are seen at the other four centers. Consequently, there is little evidence of qualitative interaction ($p > 0.20$).

The discussion presented above indicates that the treatment × center interaction is either small or quantitative for each of the 15 models fit. The center-specific results are therefore sufficiently consistent to justify combining these results across centers to obtain an overall estimate of treatment effect. The estimates of the average population treatment means and the

Table 9 Tests for Qualitative Interaction

Treatment	Center I 1	Center I 2	Center II 1	Center II 2	Center III 1	Center III 2	Center IV 1	Center IV 2	Center V 1	Center V 2
					Patient evaluation, week 4					
Mean change	1.43	0.69	1.50	0.00	1.42	0.64	0.70	1.09	1.27	0.36
SE	0.14	0.33	0.20	0.27	0.10	0.22	0.33	0.25	0.19	0.15
D_j	0.74		1.50		0.78		−0.39		0.91	
s_j^2	0.13		0.11		0.06		0.17		0.06	
D_j^2/s_j^2	4.26		19.93		10.42		0.89		14.13	
Test for qualitative interaction: $Q^+ = 0.89$, $Q^- = 48.74$, $\min(Q^+, Q^-) = 0.89$, $p > 0.20$[a]										
					Patient evaluation, week 6					
Mean change	1.40	0.62	1.45	0.00	1.28	0.78	1.20	1.30	1.15	0.33
SE	0.16	0.31	0.25	0.33	0.12	0.24	0.25	0.15	0.19	0.22
D_j	0.78		1.45		0.50		−0.10		0.82	
s_j^2	0.12		0.17		0.07		0.09		0.08	
D_j^2/s_j^2	5.00		12.23		3.47		0.12		7.96	
Test for qualitative interaction: $Q^+ = 0.12$, $Q^- = 28.66$, $\min(Q^+, Q^-) = 0.12$, $p > 0.20$[a]										
					Tenderness, week 2					
Mean change	1.19	0.92	1.79	0.50	1.28	1.09	1.36	1.44	0.85	0.40
SE	0.25	0.29	0.24	0.26	0.18	0.12	0.28	0.21	0.15	0.10
D_j	0.27		1.29		0.19		−0.08		0.45	
s_j^2	0.15		0.13		0.05		0.12		0.03	
D_j^2/s_j^2	0.50		13.29		0.77		0.05		6.23	
Test for qualitative interaction: $Q^+ = 0.05$, $Q^- = 20.79$, $\min(Q^+, Q^-) = 0.05$, $p > 0.20$[a]										

[a]The test statistic, $\min(Q^+, Q^-)$, is compared to critical values of 3.39 ($\alpha = 0.20$), 4.96 ($\alpha = 0.10$), and 6.50 ($\alpha = 0.05$) obtained from Table 1 of Gail and Simon (1985).

Table 10 Estimate of the Average Population Mean Change and Its Standard Error, by Treatment Group, for Efficacy Variable at Week 6

Variable	Treatment 1 (active) Estimate[a] (SE)	Treatment 2 (placebo) Estimate[b] (SE)	Treatment difference[c]	p-value[d]
Physician evaluation	1.46 (0.16)	0.20 (0.17)	1.23	< 0.01
Patient evaluation	1.30 (0.10)	0.61 (0.11)	0.69	< 0.01
Pain on active motion	2.11 (0.10)	1.34 (0.10)	0.77	< 0.01
Pain at rest	1.74 (0.09)	1.21 (0.10)	0.53	< 0.01
Tenderness	1.36 (0.10)	1.09 (0.11)	0.27	0.08

[a]Estimate $= \hat{\mu}_{1\cdot} = (1/5)\sum \bar{y}_{1j}$, where $\bar{y}_{1j}$ denotes the mean change from baseline for the active group at center j.
[b]Estimate $= \hat{\mu}_{2\cdot}$, defined similarly to $\hat{\mu}_{1\cdot}$ above.
[c]Treatment difference $= \hat{\mu}_{1\cdot} - \hat{\mu}_{2\cdot}$.
[d]p-value for test of H_0: $\mu_{1\cdot} = \mu_{2\cdot}$ vs. H_1: $\mu_{1\cdot} \neq \mu_{2\cdot}$.

p-value for assessing the significance of the difference in these means are presented in Table 10 for each efficacy variable at week 6. (The week 2 and week 4 results are not shown but are similar to those seen at week 6.) These results provide substantial evidence that the anti-inflammatory agent is effective.

5.7 Other Methods

We have given a detailed example for the analysis of a multicenter trial using a classical linear models approach. Other statistical methods that allow adjustment for center using stratification or blocking techniques may be useful for analysis. In particular, log-linear models as developed for the National Halothane Study (Bishop et al., 1975), and the weighted least squares models of Grizzle, Starmer, and Koch may be used in a similar manner for categorical data (see Chapter 13). The Mantel–Haenszel procedure is particularly useful to test the null hypothesis that the overall (standardized) treatment difference adjusted for the effects of stratification variables is zero; its use requires minimal assumptions (see Chapter 13).

The usual methods for the analysis of censored data may also be applied in the same manner. These methods including the log-rank test and its generalizations (Cox proportional hazards model) are discussed in Chapter 11.

6 SUMMARY AND RECOMMENDATIONS

We have described the complexities in the design and implementation of the multicenter trial as well as in the analysis and interpretation of its results. In multicenter trials run by the pharmaceutical industry, regulatory requirements for the approval of a new drug also enter and add to the complexity. Multiple small trials conducted by single investigators for combination at the time of a regulatory submission described by Pocock (1982) have been replaced with large, multicenter trials of the type sponsored by the National Heart Lung and Blood Institute (such as CASS, Beta-Blocker Heart Attack Trial) or the National Cancer Institute Collaborative Groups.

The general principles for the design, conduct, and analysis of experiments have been described by numerous authors [see Cox (1958)]. Clinical trials, with their particular problems have also been discussed extensively [e.g., Pocock (1982); Fleiss (1986b)].

There is considerable controversy in the literature concerning the identification of and the interpretation of the treatment × center interaction. In the United States much of this controversy is generated by the Final Statistical Guidelines (Food and Drug Administration, 1988). This document suggests strongly that treatment × center interaction be examined minimally with ANOVA F-tests for interaction, consistency across investigators assessed, and justification for combining centers provided. As Fleiss (1986a) points out, however, there are no substantive suggestions or guidelines for decision making with regard to the presence or absence of interaction. Furthermore, the emphasis is on hypothesis testing; the primary goal of the analysis should be to estimate the magnitude of the average treatment effect.

Average treatment effects are defined regardless of the presence of interaction (Cox, 1958). Cochran (1937, 1954) and Yates and Cochran (1938) described the problems of combining the results of agricultural experiments. They recommend that whereas the weighted mean is appropriate in the absence of interaction, the unweighted mean or mean with equal weight for each center is appropriate in the presence of interaction. If we use approximately equal sample sizes in each center, the precision of the estimate of the treatment difference in each center is similar. In this case, no single center would have an undue influence as a function of its size. Models with interaction giving equal weight to each center are almost always useful in the setting we have described. If sample sizes are very small in each center, then center should be ignored in the analysis.

The criterion for the identification of a treatment × center interaction is also an issue of controversy. The purpose of a multicenter trial is to provide results generalizable to a wide range of settings. In such a case, some treatment × center interaction is not surprising (Fleiss 1986a). Whether the interaction tests should be performed at $p \leq 0.05$, 0.10, or 0.15 is an issue and depends on the goal of the results of the analysis.

The distinction between quantitative and qualitative interactions (Gail and Simon, 1985) described above provides a useful approach to a coherent interpretation of the results of a multicenter trial. Judgment is required at all stages in the design, conduct, analysis, and interpretation of multicenter trials.

REFERENCES

Berk, P. D., J. D. Goldberg, M. N. Silverstein et al. (1981). Increased incidence of acute leukemia in Polycythemia Vera associated with Chlorambucil therapy. *New England J. Med. 304*, 441–447.

Beta-Blocker Heart Attack Trial Research Group (1982). A randomized trial of propranolol in patients with acute myocardial infarction. *J. Amer. Med. Assoc. 247*, 1701–1714.

Bishop, Y. M. M., S. E. Feinberg, P. W. Holland (1975). *Discrete Multivariate Methods.* MIT Press, Cambridge, Mass.

Canner, P. L., Y. B. Huang, and C. L. Meinert (1981a). On the detection of outlier clinics in medical and surgical trials: I. Practical considerations. *Controlled Clin. Trials 2*, 231–240.

Canner, P. L., Y. B. Huang, and C. L. Meinert (1981b). On the detection of outlier clinicsin medical and surgical trials: II. Theoretical considerations. *Controlled Clin. Trials 2*, 241–253.

CASS. Principal investigators and their associates (1983). Coronary artery surgery study (CASS): a randomized trial of coronary artery bypass surgery: survival data. *Circulation 68*, 939–950.

Chakravorti, S. R., and J. E. Grizzle (1975). Analysis of data from multiclinic experiments. *Biometrics 31*, 325–338.

Cochran, W. G. (1937). Problems arising in the analysis of a series of similar experiments. *J. Roy. Statist. Soc. Suppl. 4(1)*, 102–118.

Cochran, W. G. (1954). The combination of estimates from different experiments. *Biometrics 10*, 101–129.

Cox, D. R. (1958). *Planning of Experiments.* Wiley, New York.

Fleiss, J. L. (1986a). Analysis of data from multiclinic trials. *Controlled Clin. Trials 7*, 267–275.

Fleiss, J. L. (1986b). *The Design and Analysis of Clinical Experiments.* Wiley, New York.

Food and Drug Administration (1988). Guideline for the format and content of the clinical and statistical sections of an application. July, 1988.

Gail, M., and R. Simon (1985). Testing for qualitative interactions between treatment effects and patient subsets. *Biometrics 41*, 361–372.

Goldberg, J. D, A. I. Weiss, and K. J. Koury (1986). Design of clinical trials for chronic diseases: implications for periodontal disease. *J. Clin. Periodontol. 13*, 411–414.

Machin, D., M. J. Staquet, and R. J. Sylvester (1979). Advantages and defects of single center and multicenter trials. In *Controversies in Cancer: Design of Trials and Treatment*, (H. J. Tagnon and M. J. Staquet, eds.). Masson, New York, pp. 7–15.

Overall, J. E. (1979). General linear model analysis of variance. In *Coordinating Clinical Trials in Psychopharmacology: Planning, Documentation, and Analysis.* U.S. Government Printing Office, Washington D.C., pp. 63–86.

Pocock, S. J. (1983). *Clinical Trials: A Practical Approach.* Wiley, New York.

Pocock, S. J., and S. W. Lagakos (1982). Practical experiences of randomization in cancer trials: an international survey. *British J. Cancer 46*, 368–375.

SAS Institute, Inc. (1985). *SAS User's Guide: Statistics Version, 5th ed.* SAS Institute, Cary, N.C.

Sylvester, R. J., H. M. Pinedo, M. Depauw, et al. (1981). Quality of institutional participation in multicenter clinical trials. *New England J. Med. 305*, 852–855.

Wermurth, N., and W. G. Cochran (1979). Detecting systematic errors in multi-clinic observational data. *Biometrics 35*, 683–686.

Wu, M., M. Fisher, and D. DeMets (1980). Sample sizes for long-term medical trials with time-dependent drop-out and event rates. *Controlled Clin. Trials 1*, 109–121.

Yates, F., and W. G. Cochran (1938). The analysis of groups of experiments. *J. Agric. Sci. 28*, 556–580.

Zelen, M. (1974). The randomization and stratification of patients to clinical trials. *J. Chronic Dis. 27*, 365–375.

8

Crossover Versus Parallel Designs

ANDREW P. GRIEVE CIBA-GEIGY Pharmaceuticals, Horsham,
West Sussex, England

1 INTRODUCTION

The essential feature of a crossover design in clinical trials is that each patient receives more than one of the treatments in the study. In the simplest design, the two-treatment two-period crossover, with treatments A and B, patients are randomly allocated to one of the treatment sequences A → B and B → A. Such a design, or similar, more complicated designs with more than two treatments and/or periods, are attractive to clinicians due largely to an intuitive feeling that comparing different treatments on the same patient is likely to be more efficient than comparing the treatments on different patients. This intuitive feeling has essentially two components. First, the patient is his/her own control; this has the effect of increasing the precision of treatment comparisons since these are made within patients rather than between patients. Second, patients can express preferences for one or more treatments. Without doubt the first component is the more important since it has important ethical and economic consequences. Ethical, in that a clinician will wish to minimize the number of patients who receive less efficacious treatments; economic, in that the use of fewer patients will reduce costs. In essence the argument in favor of crossover designs is that to obtain a given treatment-comparison precision, a within-patient comparison will require fewer patients than a between-patient comparison; they are therefore more ethical and less costly.

These or similar arguments in favor of crossover designs would certainly make them the designs of choice in a large number of clinical trials were it not for three disadvantages. First, crossover designs are not applicable in conditions in which either the treatments are expected to effect a cure, or in which the natural course of the condition is such that it would disappear within a short period: for example, the common cold. Second, crossover designs with a large number of treatments, and consequently a large number of periods, may not be advantageous as the number of patients dropping out may be large. Finally, if the effect of a treatment is not confined to the period in which it is applied, or if the effect of a treatment differs from period to period, estimates of treatment effects may be biased.

It is this last possibility that lead the Biometric and Epidemiology Methodology Advisory Committee (BEMAC) of the Food and Drug Administration (FDA) to conclude with respect to the two-period crossover design that it "is not the design of choice in clinical trials, where unequivocal evidence of treatment effect is required." Rather, they recommended that, "in most cases, the completely randomized (or randomized block) design with baseline measurements will be the design of choice because it furnishes unbiased estimates of treatment effects without appeal to any modeling assumptions save those associated with the randomization procedure itself" [Food and Drug Administration (1977); see also O'Neill (1978)].

In this chapter we consider and compare the merits and demerits of the two-period crossover design and the parallel design for comparing two treatments with and without baseline measurements. We restrict attention to the two-period crossover design not because designs with more than two treatments are not important or useful, but simply because most of the recent work and discussions have been focused on the two-period crossover and because all the major problems occur in this design. We will concentrate on normal linear-model theory, but will give references to other assumptions: nonparametric, randomization theory, Poisson-distributed data, and binomial data. In Sections 2 to 5 a straightforward presentation of the models and approaches that have been suggested in the literature is given; a more critical discussion of the alternatives is given in Section 6. To illustrate the various methods, data from Grizzle (1965), Hills and Armitage (1979), Brown (1980), and Racine et al. (1986)—trials 1 and 2—are used; these are denoted Examples 1 to 5 respectively.

2 ANALYSIS OF THE TWO-PERIOD CROSSOVER DESIGN

2.1 Grizzle's Models

The standard, classical approach to the analysis of the two-period crossover design was originally proposed by Grizzle (1965) [see also Grizzle (1974) and Grieve (1982)]. Suppose that patients have been randomized to one of the treatment sequences A $\rightarrow$ B or B $\rightarrow$ A, where A and B are the treatments, and that a *single* observation is made on each patient during each of the two treatment periods, which are separated by a washout period. Assume that the study produces n_1 patients from the first sequence group and n_2 patients from the second treatment group, and let y_{ijk} denote the response of the jth patient in the ith sequence group in the kth period. Under these assumptions, Grizzle (1965) considered the following two statistical models:

$$I. \quad y_{ijk} = \mu + \pi_k + \tau_l + \gamma_{l'} + \eta_{ij} + \epsilon_{ijk} \qquad (i = 1,2; j = 1,\cdots,n_i; k = 1,2; l \neq l' = 1,2).$$

$$II. \quad y_{ijk} = \mu + \pi_k + \tau_l + \eta_{ij} + \epsilon_{ijk} \qquad (i = 1,2; j = 1,\cdots,n_i; k = 1,2; l = 1,2).$$

where μ, π_k, τ_l, $\gamma_{l'}$ are the overall mean, period, direct treatment, and carryover effects (also termed residual effects or period $\times$ treatment interaction), respectively, and η_{ij} and ϵ_{ijk} are the random patient and error effects, which are assumed to be independently normally distributed, with zero means and variances σ_η^2 and σ_ϵ^2, respectively. For convenience, reparametrize models I and II by defining

$$\pi_1 = -\pi_2 = \pi, \qquad \tau_1 = -\tau_2 = \tau, \qquad \gamma_1 = -\gamma_2 = \gamma;$$

that is, consider a cell mean model with means defined as in Table 1. Define $N = n_1 + n_2$, $m = N/(n_1 n_2)$, $\sigma_A^2 = \sigma_\epsilon^2 + 2\sigma_\eta^2$, and $\sigma^2 = \sigma_\epsilon^2 + \sigma_\eta^2$. Model II may be derived from model I by setting $\gamma = 0$. Throughout this chapter "treatment effect" means the difference between the effects of treatments A and B. Similarly, testing for treatment effect means testing of the null hypothesis H_0: $\tau = 0$. These remarks also apply to period and carryover effects.

These parametrizations follow Selwyn et al. (1981), Grieve (1985), and Racine et al. (1986). Selwyn et al. (1981) develop a Bayesian analysis of a balanced two-period crossover, $n_1 = n_2$, for use in bioequivalence testing (see Chapter 2). The latter two papers deal with a Bayesian analysis of the type of design of interest in this chapter. Details of this Bayesian analysis are given in Section 2.5. The cell means model described above is convenient for exposition. However, in model I there are problems of estimability; interested readers should refer to Grizzle (1965) for details.

Table 1 Cell Means for Model I

Sequence group	Period 1	Period 2
$A \to B$	$\mu + \pi + \tau$	$\mu - \pi - \tau + \gamma$
$B \to A$	$\mu + \pi - \tau$	$\mu - \pi + \tau - \gamma$

2.2 Analysis of Variance for Model II

Under model II the standard analysis of variance (ANOVA) is as shown in Table 2 [see Grizzle (1965, 1974) and Grieve (1982)]. Corresponding to the sums of squares for periods and treatments the least squares estimates of the parameters are

$$\hat{\pi} = \frac{1}{4}(\bar{y}_{1\cdot 1} - \bar{y}_{1\cdot 2} + \bar{y}_{2\cdot 1} - \bar{y}_{2\cdot 2}),$$

$$\hat{\tau} = \frac{1}{4}(\bar{y}_{1\cdot 1} - \bar{y}_{1\cdot 2} - \bar{y}_{2\cdot 1} + \bar{y}_{2\cdot 2}).$$

It is clear from Table 2 that a valid test for treatment effect under model II may be made by forming the ratio of the treatment and error mean squares, the latter denoted by FT, which will follow an F-distribution with 1 and $N - 2$ degrees of freedom (d.f.) under the null hypothesis of no treatment effect. The results from the five data sets are given in Table 3, from which it may be seen that under model II three of the five data sets give a significant treatment effect.

Table 2 ANOVA for Model II

Source	d.f.	Sums of squares	Expected mean squares
Patients	$N-1$	$2\sum_i \sum_j \bar{y}^2_{ij\cdot} - 2N\bar{y}^2_{\cdots}$	σ^2_A
Periods	1	$\frac{1}{2m}(\bar{y}_{1\cdot 1} - \bar{y}_{1\cdot 2} + \bar{y}_{2\cdot 1} - \bar{y}_{2\cdot 2})^2$	$\sigma^2_\epsilon + 8\pi^2/m$
Treatments	1	$\frac{1}{2m}(\bar{y}_{1\cdot 1} - \bar{y}_{1\cdot 2} - \bar{y}_{2\cdot 1} + \bar{y}_{2\cdot 2})^2$	$\sigma^2_\epsilon + 8\tau^2/m$
Error	$N-2$	$\text{SSE} = \sum_i \sum_j \sum_k y^2_{ijk} - 2\sum_i \sum_j \bar{y}^2_{ij} - \sum_i n_i \sum_k \bar{y}^2_{i\cdot k} + 2\sum_i n_i \bar{y}^2_{i\cdot\cdot}$	σ^2_ϵ

Table 3 ANOVA for Quoted Examples: Model II[a]

Source	Example 1	Example 2	Example 3	Example 4	Example 5
Patients	16.580 (13)	600.897 (28)	18.551 (62)	5601.000 (26)	3865.120 (24)
Periods	6.243	8.709	0.988	34.490	16.066
Treatments	3.563	58.364	19.094	161.008	164.866
Error	14.944 (12)	145.360 (27)	29.487 (61)	655.325 (25)	1820.654 (23)
$\hat{\pi}$	−0.477	0.393	0.088	0.804	−0.567
$\hat{\tau}$	0.360	1.018	−0.387	1.738	−1.817
FT	2.861	10.841	40.148	6.142	2.083
p-value	0.117	0.0028	< 0.0001	0.020	0.163

[a]Values in parentheses are degrees of freedom.

2.3 Analysis of Model I

Incorporating carryover effect in model I results in a less simple analysis than under model II. Under model I the expectation of $\hat{\tau}$ given above is $\tau - \gamma/2$, and it is therefore no longer an unbiased estimate of the direct treatment effect. On the other hand, an unbiased estimate of γ does exist:

$$\hat{\gamma} = \frac{1}{2}(\bar{y}_{1\cdot 1} + \bar{y}_{1\cdot 2} - \bar{y}_{2\cdot 1} - \bar{y}_{2\cdot 2}).$$

Therefore, under model I an unbiased estimate of τ is

$$\tilde{\tau} = \hat{\tau} + \frac{\hat{\gamma}}{2} = \frac{1}{2}(\bar{y}_{1\cdot 1} - \bar{y}_{2\cdot 1}).$$

The significance of the carryover effect may be tested by noting that

$$\text{var}(\hat{\gamma}) = \frac{m}{2}\sigma_A^2$$

and that the expected value of the sum of squares

$$\text{SSP} = 2\left(\sum_i \sum_j \bar{y}_{ij\cdot}^2 - \sum_i n_i \bar{y}_{i\cdot\cdot}^2\right),$$

is $(N-2)\sigma_A^2$. So since $\hat{\gamma}$ and SSP are independent,

$$\text{FR} = \frac{2(N-2)\hat{\gamma}^2}{m\text{SSP}}$$

follows an F-distribution with 1 and $N-2$ d.f.

It can be shown that

$$\text{var}(\tilde{\tau}) = \frac{m}{4}\sigma^2.$$

Although $\text{E(SSE+SSP)} = 2(N-2)\sigma^2$, SSE+SSP does not have a chi-square distribution [see Grizzle (1965)]. Grizzle suggests that the sum of squares

$$\text{SS1} = \sum_i \sum_j (y_{ij1} - \bar{y}_{i\cdot 1})^2$$

be used for testing the significance of $\tilde{\tau}$ under model I since it has expectation $(N-2)\sigma^2$ and is chi-square distributed, independently of $\tilde{\tau}$. So

$$\text{F1} = \frac{4(N-2)\tilde{\tau}^2}{m\text{SS1}}$$

follows an F-distribution with 1 and $N-2$ d.f.

Grieve (1987b) has also considered the problem of making inferences about τ under model I. He shows that under model I,

$$\text{var}(\hat{\tau}) = \frac{m}{8}\sigma_\epsilon^2, \qquad \text{E}(\hat{\tau}\hat{\gamma}) = 0.$$

Further since $\mathrm{SSE}/\sigma_\epsilon^2 \sim \chi^2_{N-2}$ and $\mathrm{SSP}/\sigma_A^2 \sim \chi^2_{N-2}$ it follows that

$$\frac{[8(N-2)]^{1/2}[\hat{\tau}-(\tau-\gamma/2)]}{(m\mathrm{SSE})^{1/2}} \sim t_{N-2}$$

and

$$\frac{[8(N-2)]^{1/2}[\hat{\gamma}/2-\gamma/2]}{(m\mathrm{SSP})^{1/2}} \sim t_{N-2}.$$

Thus the problem of testing the significance of treatment effects under model I is equivalent to a Behrens-Fisher problem since $(\bar{y}_{1\cdot 1} - \bar{y}_{2\cdot 1})/2$ may be written as the sum of independent t-statistics with differing variances. From a Bayesian point of view this result is given by Grieve (1985). Since no universally acceptable solution to the Behrens-Fisher problem exists, the choice of procedure to be used will be made on the basis of one's belief in the "correctness" of the competing schools of statistical inference: frequency, fiducial, or Bayesian. Grieve (1987b) compares various approximate solutions to the Behrens-Fisher problem as it relates to the two-period crossover. For the moment we consider only Grizzle's original analysis based on first-period data alone, but will return to the Behrens-Fisher aspects in Section 2.5 when dealing with the Bayesian approach.

The results of Grizzle's analysis of model I are shown in Table 4. In this table only two of the examples give p-values less than 5%, and in fact, comparison with Table 3 shows that three of the five examples give different conclusions under the two models. This might have been expected since as we have noted above, the model II estimate of τ is biased if model I is correct. It is clear, therefore, that it is important to be able to distinguish between models I and II, that is, to decide whether a carryover effect is

Table 4 Grizzle's Model I Analysis for Quoted Examples[a]

Source	Example 1	Example 2	Example 3	Example 4	Example 5
$\hat{\gamma}$	0.817	−1.586	0.167	1.725	4.667
$\tilde{\tau}$	0.769	0.225	−0.303	2.600	0.516
SSP	12.007 (12)	565.517 (27)	17.658 (62)	5579.325 (25)	3593.333 (23)
SS1	18.799 (12)	334.431 (27)	30.951 (62)	4182.400 (25)	3169.994 (23)
FFR	4.571	1.689	3.134	0.178	1.740
p-value	0.0538	0.2047	0.0816	0.6769	0.2002
FF1	5.174	0.115	11.748	1.078	0.0482
p-value	0.0421	0.7366	0.0011	0.3092	0.8281

[a]Values in parentheses are degrees of freedom.

real or not, if we wish to make valid inferences concerning the treatment effect. It is, of course, possible to test for carryover effect, FR being the appropriate test statistic. However, in the case of our five examples, none of these tests reaches a nominal 5% significance level.

Based on work by Larson and Bancroft (1963), Grizzle proposes that because the test for carryover is a preliminary test, in that the main interest focuses on the treatment effect, this test should be carried out at a higher significance level than usual, namely 10%. If the hypothesis of no carryover is rejected, model I should be used to test for a treatment effect, using F1; if accepted, model II should be used using FT. Figure 1 summarizes Grizzle's approach to the analysis of the two-period crossover design.

2.4 Hills-Armitage Approach

Grizzle's approach, outlined above, is based on standard linear model theory, with slight modifications in the case of model I. Hills and Armitage (1979) provide a slightly different viewpoint that leads to the same results.

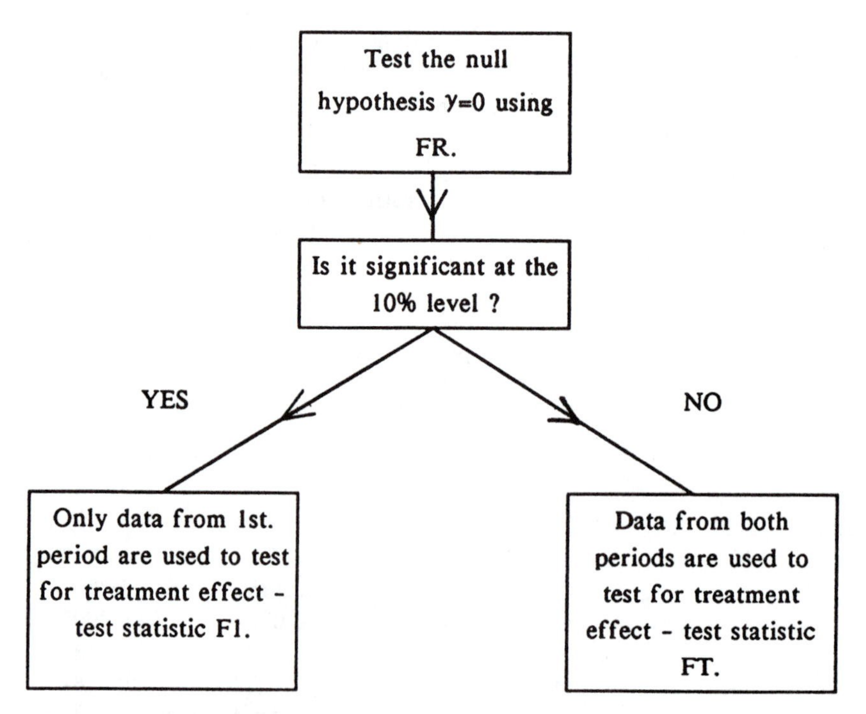

Figure 1 Grizzle's approach to the analysis of the two-period crossover.

Under model II consider the differences

$$d_{1j} = y_{1j1} - y_{1j2}, \qquad d_{2j} = y_{2j1} - y_{2j2}$$

which have expectations

$$2\pi + 2\tau, \qquad -2\pi + 2\tau,$$

respectively, with common variance $2\sigma_\epsilon^2$ (from Table 1 with $\gamma = 0$). It is therefore clear that since d_{1j} and d_{2j} are independent, the sums and differences of the mean d's have expectations,

$$4\tau, \qquad -4\pi,$$

respectively, and have equal variances, which may be shown to be $2\sigma_\epsilon^2(1/n_1 + 1/n_2)$. It is therefore possible under model II to test for both period and treatment effects using simple t-tests, which are the square roots of the corresponding F-tests from Table 2.

Under model I consider the sums

$$s_{1j} = y_{1j1} + y_{1j2}, \qquad s_{2j} = y_{2j1} + y_{2j2},$$

with expectations

$$2\pi + 2\tau + \gamma, \qquad 2\pi + 2\tau - \gamma,$$

respectively. It is clear, therefore, that $\bar{s}_{1.} - \bar{s}_{2.}$ has expectation 2γ and variance $2\sigma_A^2(1/n_1 + 1/n_2)$, so that again a standard t-test, being the square root of FR, may be used to test for a carryover effect.

2.5 A Bayesian Analysis

In this section we consider a Bayesian analysis of the two-period crossover design, studied in detail by Grieve (1985, 1986) and summarized by Racine et al. (1986). This analysis circumvents the problems associated with a preliminary test of significance for the carryover effect to some extent.

Using the same notation as in Section 2.1, and assuming the conventional prior specification,

$$p(\mu, \pi, \tau, \gamma, \sigma_\epsilon^2, \sigma_A^2) \propto \sigma_\epsilon^{-2}\sigma_A^{-2}, \qquad \sigma_\epsilon^2 < \sigma_A^2.$$

A standard Bayesian linear model analysis leads to the following posterior distributions:

$$p(\tau, \gamma \mid Y) = \frac{p^*(\tau, \gamma \mid Y) P(F_{N-1,N-1} < Q_2/Q_1)}{P(F_{N-2,N-2} < \text{SSP}/\text{SSE})},$$

$$p(\gamma \mid Y) = \frac{p^*(\gamma \mid Y) P(F_{N-1,N-2} < (N-2)Q_2/[(N-1)\text{SSE}])}{P(F_{N-2,N-2} < \text{SSP}/\text{SSE})},$$

$$p(\tau \mid \gamma, Y) = \frac{p^*(\tau \mid \gamma, Y) P(F_{N-1,N-1} < Q_2/Q_1)}{P(F_{N-1,N-2} < (N-2)Q_2/[(N-1)\mathrm{SSE}])}, \tag{1}$$

$$p(\tau \mid Y) = \int p(\tau, \gamma \mid Y) d\gamma, \tag{2}$$

where $Q_1 = 8(\tau - \gamma/2 - \hat{\tau})^2/m + \mathrm{SSE}$, $Q2 = 2(\gamma - \hat{\gamma})^2/m + \mathrm{SSP}$, Y denotes the data, and

$$p^*(\tau, \gamma \mid Y) \propto \left(\frac{Q_1 Q_2}{\mathrm{SSESSP}}\right)^{-(N-1)/2}$$

$$p^*(\gamma \mid Y) \propto \left(\frac{Q_2}{\mathrm{SSP}}\right)^{-(N-1)/2}$$

$$p^*(\tau \mid \gamma, Y) \propto \left(\frac{Q_1}{\mathrm{SSE}}\right)^{-(N-1)/2}$$

are the posterior densities that would have been obtained had the constraint on the variance components been omitted from the prior specification. The integral in (2) is not analytically solvable, even in the case when the variance component constraint is ignored. Grieve (1985) shows that the posterior distribution of τ is exactly the Behrens-Fisher distribution discussed in Section 2.3 and provides an approximation to it based on work by Patil (1965) [see also Grieve (1987b)].

The posterior distributions given above provide all the necessary information to make Bayesian inferences about treatment effects under models I and II with the given prior specification. Thus treatment effects may be investigated under model I using (2), and under model II using (1) with γ set to zero.

Figures 2 and 3 display the bivariate posterior distributions of the carryover effect and treatment effect and their marginals under model I and the treatment effect under model II for Examples 2 and 3. Similar analyses for the other examples are given in Grieve (1985) and Racine et al. (1986).

Comparison of Grizzle's analysis with the posterior distributions displayed in these two figures reveals the following. In the case of Example 2, $p(\tau \mid \gamma = 0, Y)$ and $p(\tau \mid Y)$ are markedly different, giving rise to differing conclusions, the former distribution suggesting a definite positive treatment effect, the latter no treatment effect. In the case of Example 3 the two posterior distributions lead to essentially the same conclusions regarding treatment effect. However, whereas for Example 3 the F-test for carryover effect is significant under Grizzle's scheme ($p = 0.082$), suggesting that model I is appropriate, that for Example 2 is not ($p = 0.205$), although $p(\gamma \mid Y)$ in this case suggests the presence of a carryover effect.

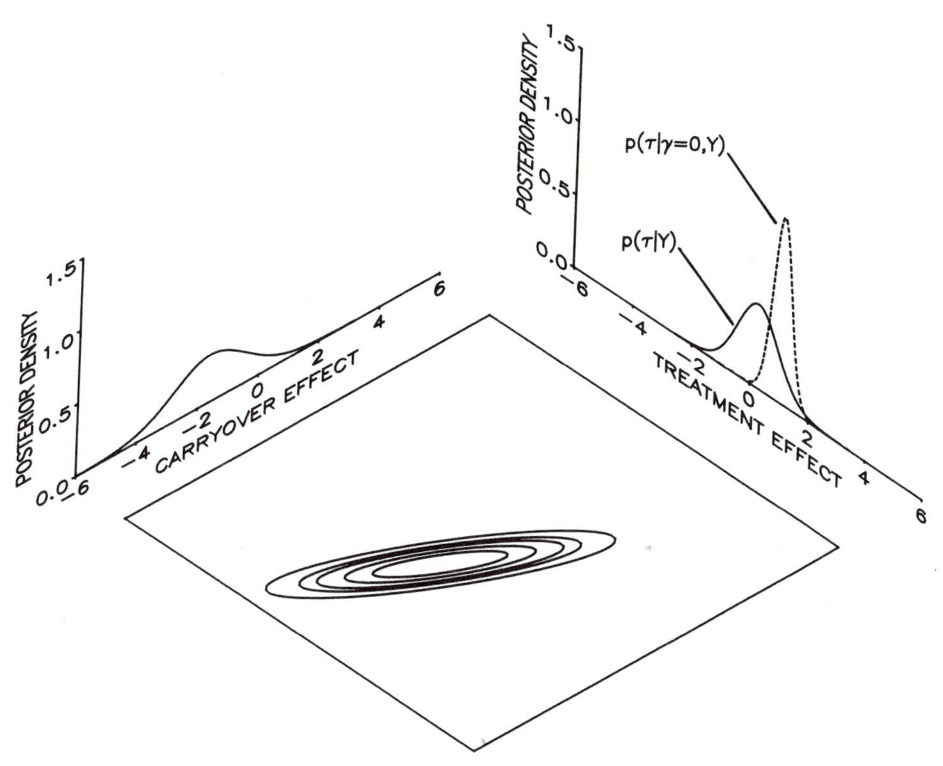

Figure 2 Posterior distributions: Example 2.

The Bayesian approach to the problem of differentiating between models I and II is to seek a form of prior specification that allows one to incorporate directly an assessment of the likelihood of each model. One way to do this is to model the setup as a mixture of the two separate models. Let models I and II be denoted by M_1 and M_0, respectively, and let the prior be

$$p(\mu, \pi, \tau, \gamma, \sigma_\epsilon^2, \sigma_A^2 \mid M_i) \propto \sigma_\epsilon^{-2} \sigma_A^{-2} \qquad (i = 0, 1).$$

Suppose that $\lambda = P(M_0)/P(M_1)$ are the prior odds in favor of model II (i.e., no carryover effect); then the posterior probabilities of the two models are

$$P(M_0 \mid Y) = \frac{\lambda B_{01}}{1 + \lambda B_{01}}, \qquad P(M_1 \mid Y) = \frac{1}{1 + \lambda B_{01}},$$

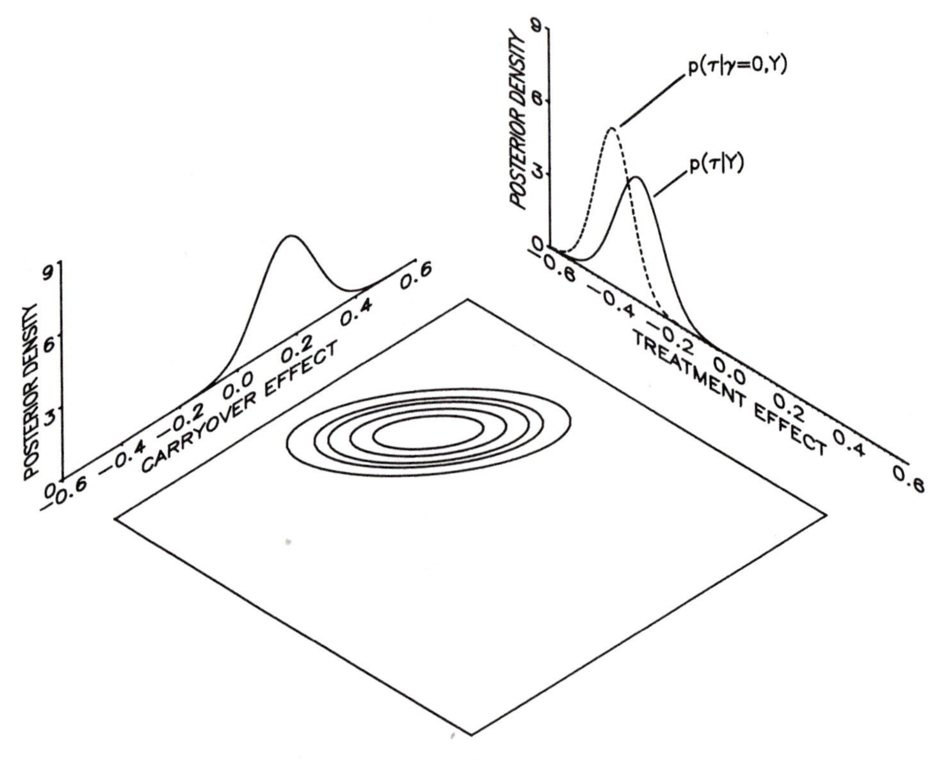

Figure 3 Posterior distributions: Example 3.

where B_{01} is the Bayes factor given by

$$B_{01} = \frac{P(M_0 \mid Y)}{P(M_0)} \frac{P(M_1)}{P(M_1 \mid Y)} = \frac{P(Y \mid M_0)}{P(Y \mid M_1)}.$$

Inferences concerning the treatment effect can be made using

$$p(\tau \mid Y) = \frac{\lambda B_{01}}{1 + \lambda B_{01}} p(\tau \mid Y, M_0) + \frac{1}{1 + \lambda B_{01}} p(\tau \mid Y, M_1) \qquad (3)$$

where $p(\tau \mid Y, M_0)$ is given by (1) with $\gamma = 0$ and $p(\tau \mid M_1)$ is given by (2). Grieve (1985) shows that the Bayes factor has the form

$$B_{01} = \left(\frac{3}{2m}\right)^{1/2} \left(1 + \frac{\text{FR}}{N-2}\right)^{-N/2}.$$

The choice of λ provides a means of introducing a sliding scale of plausibility between the extremes of either assuming no carryover or assuming

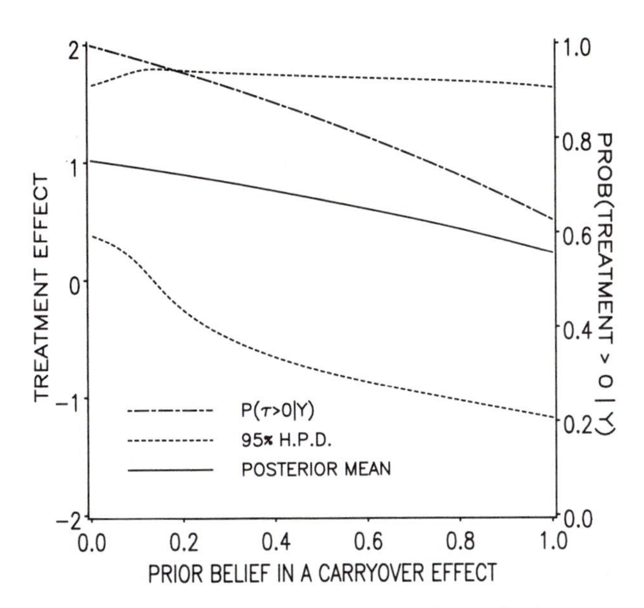

Figure 4 Posterior summaries: Example 2.

carryover which one is forced into in the classical significance testing procedure. Figures 4 and 5 provide posterior summaries of (3) for Examples 2 and 3, respectively, as a function of $P(M_1) = 1/(1+\lambda)$. In these figures the posterior mean of the treatment effect and the 95% highest posterior density (HPD) interval for the treatment effect are plotted against the left vertical axis, and the posterior probability of either a positive treatment effect (Figure 4) or a negative treatment effect (Figure 5) against the right vertical axis.

Figure 4 shows that for Example 2 a dogmatic belief that there is no carryover effect results in very different inferences from those which arise when less dogmatic beliefs are used. In the case of Example 3, Figure 5 shows that very different prior beliefs in the likelihood of a carryover effect have practically no influence on posterior inferences.

2.6 Other Assumptions and Approaches

Grizzle's and Hills and Armitage's approaches to the analysis of the two-period crossover are based on the assumption that the data follow a normal-theory linear model. Clearly, this is a strong assumption and needs to be investigated for each case. One possibility would be to consider the use

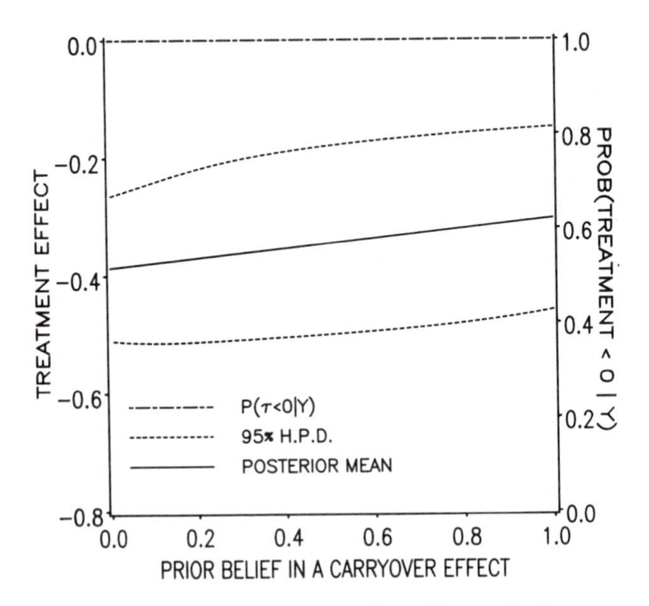

Figure 5 Posterior summaries: Example 3.

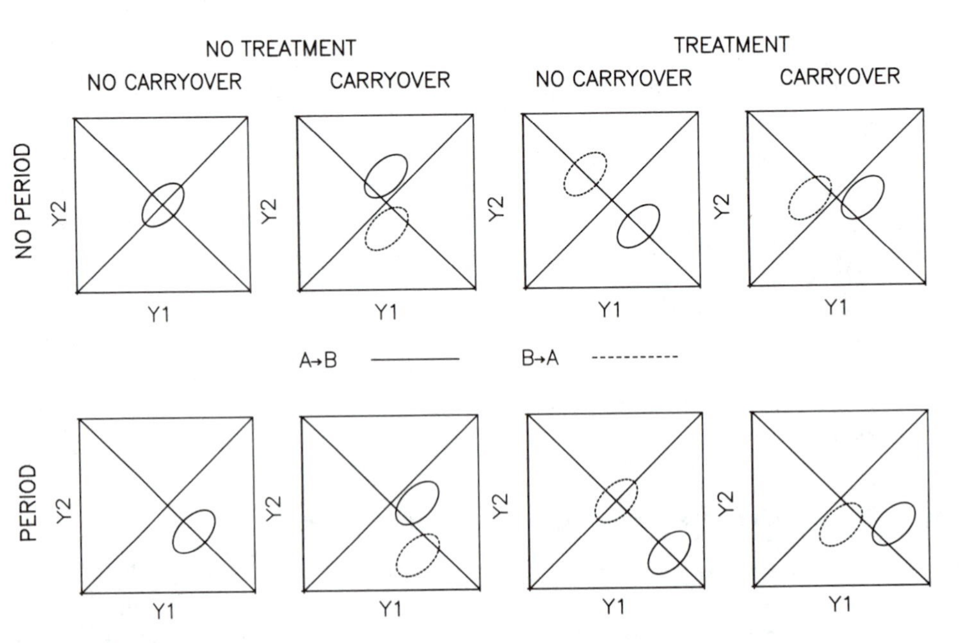

Figure 6 Possible configurations of centroid separations.

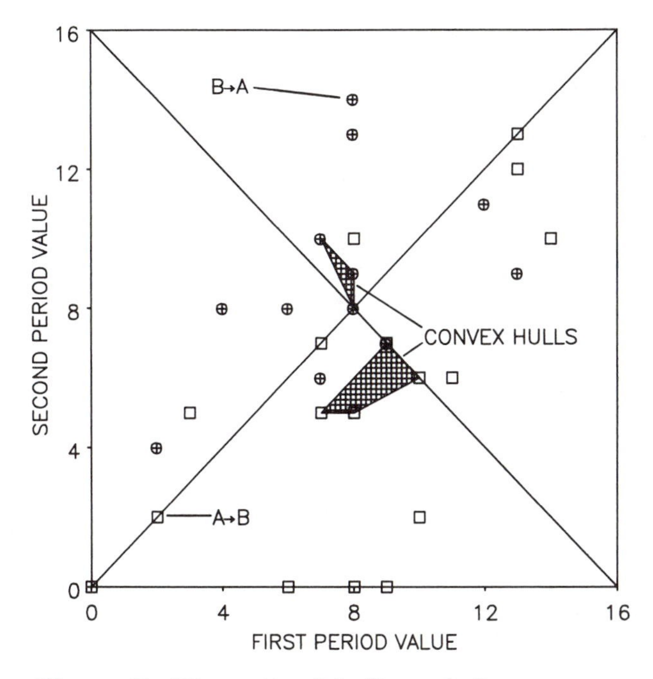

Figure 7 Diagnostic plot: Example 2.

of transformations [see the discussion and reply in Racine et al. (1986)]. Alternative assumptions have been considered by many authors.

Many, for instance, have considered two-period crossovers in which the response variable is binary (Gart, 1969; Zimmermann and Rahlfs, 1978; Hills and Armitage, 1979; Prescott, 1981; Armitage and Hills, 1982; Fidler, 1984; Farewell, 1985; Nagelkerke et al., 1986). The appropriateness of the various tests proposed in these papers is investigated by Kenward and Jones (1987), to which interested readers should refer. Layard and Arvesen (1978) consider the analysis of Poisson-distributed data in a two-period crossover design, basing their test procedures on a conditional analysis following work by Gart (1975) and Hamilton and Bissonnette (1975). Koch (1972) proposes a nonparametric alternative to Grizzle's analysis. In essence Koch's approach is equivalent to replacing the t-tests outlined in Section 2.4 with Wilcoxon tests. Gomez-Marin and McHugh (1984) derive randomization analogs of Grizzle's tests based on a finite permutation model. Zimmermann and Rahlfs (1980) consider a multivariate analysis of the two-period crossover.

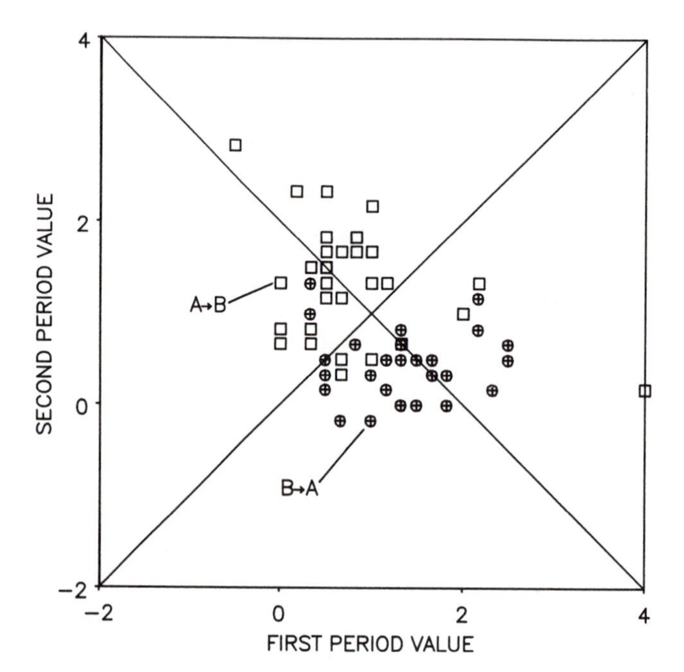

Figure 8 Diagnostic plot: Example 3.

One final approach—more an aid to interpretation than an inferential procedure—is a graphical method proposed by Huitson (1980) and Hews (1981) [see also Barker et al. (1982)]. The graphical procedure is as follows:

1. Plot the period 2 observation (y_2) for each patient against the period 1 observation (y_1), with different identifications for the two sequence groups.
2. Add the lines $y_2 = y_1$ and $y_2 + y_1 = c$, where c is a constant equal to the mean total of periods 1 and 2.
3. Period, treatment, and carryover effects will be noticeable by separation of the centroids of the two groups in different directions.

A schematic representation of the possible separations is shown in Figure 6. Clearly with real data the separation will not be as clear cut as is illustrated in Figure 7, which displays such a plot for Example 2. The convex hull for each group may be used as an aid to identifying the group centroids. In this example the innermost convex hulls are clearly separated about the line $y_2 = y_1$, indicating a treatment effect.

Figure 8, which shows a similar plot for Example 3, clearly indicates a treatment effect without the need to draw the convex hulls. Additionally, the existence of an outlier in the sequence A $\rightarrow$ B is apparent.

3 PARALLEL STUDIES

Suppose that in a simple comparative study, patients have been randomized to one of two treatment groups, A or B. Further suppose that at the study's conclusion *single* measurements on n_1 patients in group A and n_2 patients in group B are available and let y_{ij} denote the response of the jth patient in the ith group. Consider the following statistical model:

$$III. \quad y_{1j} = \mu + \tau + \epsilon_{1j}, j = 1, \cdots, n_1;$$
$$y_{2j} = \mu - \tau + \epsilon_{2j}, j = 1, \cdots, n_2,$$

where μ is the overall mean and τ represents the treatment effect and ϵ_{ij} are iid $N(0, \sigma^2)$. It should be clear that model III corresponds to a simple two-sample comparison so that the null hypothesis of no treatment effect may be tested using the statistic

$$\frac{4(N-2)(\bar{y}_{1\cdot} - \bar{y}_{2\cdot})^2}{m \sum_i \sum_j (y_{ij} - \bar{y}_{i\cdot})^2}$$

which follows an F-distribution with 1 and $N-2$ d.f., where N and m are as before. This test is equivalent to the F1 test of no treatment effect in Grizzle's analysis of model II.

4 THE USE OF BASELINE MEASUREMENTS

The quote from the FDA BEMAC committee given in Section 1 makes it clear that in comparing crossover and parallel studies it is necessary to consider the use of baseline measurements in parallel studies. In this section we consider their use in both parallel and crossover studies.

4.1 Baselines in Parallel Studies

In the case of parallel studies model III may simply be generalized to incorporate baseline measurements in the following way. Suppose that patients are randomly allocated to treatment groups A and B. Further suppose that prior to treatment a single measurement x_{ij} is taken on the jth patient in the ith group, that post treatment a further measurement y_{ij} is taken, and that there are n_i patients in group i. We consider the following statistical model:

$$\begin{aligned} IV.\quad x_{ij} &= \mu_0 + \eta_{ij} + \epsilon_{ij}, & i = 1,2; j = 1,\ldots,n_i; \\ y_{1j} &= \mu + \tau + \eta_{1j} + \epsilon'_{1j}, & j = 1,\ldots,n_1; \\ y_{2j} &= \mu - \tau + \eta_{2j} + \epsilon'_{2j}, & j = 1,\ldots,n_2, \end{aligned}$$

where μ_0 is the pretreatment mean, μ and τ are as in Section 3, and η_{ij}, ϵ_{ij}, and ϵ'_{ij} are the random patient and error effects, which are assumed to be independently, normally distributed with zero means and variances σ^2_η, σ^2_ϵ, and σ^2_ϵ, respectively. The structure of model IV is such that the measurements x_{ij} and y_{ij} are bivariately, normally distributed with covariance matrix

$$\begin{pmatrix} \sigma^2 & \rho\sigma^2 \\ \rho\sigma^2 & \sigma^2 \end{pmatrix} \tag{4}$$

where, as before, $\sigma^2 = \sigma^2_\epsilon + \sigma^2_\eta$ and $\rho = \sigma^2_\eta/(\sigma^2_\epsilon + \sigma^2_\eta)$.

The standard approach to the analysis of model IV [see Chassan (1970)] is to consider the differences $d_{ij} = y_{ij} - x_{ij}$, which may be shown to have means

$$\mu + \tau - \mu_0, \qquad \mu - \tau - \mu_0,$$

for groups 1 and 2, respectively, and common variance $2\sigma^2(1-p)$. Clearly, from the independence of $\bar{d}_{1\cdot}$ and $\bar{d}_{2\cdot}$,

$$\mathrm{E}(\bar{d}_{1\cdot} - \bar{d}_{2\cdot}) = 2\tau$$

with variance $2m\sigma^2(1-\rho) = 2m\sigma^2_\epsilon$. Thus

$$\frac{1}{2}(\bar{d}_{1\cdot} - \bar{d}_{2\cdot}) \sim N(\tau, m\sigma^2_\epsilon/2),$$

from which it follows that

$$\frac{(N-2)(\bar{d}_{1\cdot} - \bar{d}_{2\cdot})^2}{2m\sum_i\sum_j(d_{ij} - \bar{d}_{i\cdot})^2}$$

has an F-distribution with 1 and $N-2$ d.f. under the null hypothesis that there is no treatment effect.

Parallel designs with baseline measurements have found many uses in behavioral research (Lord, 1967), in which they are termed pretest-posttest designs, nutritional studies (Lee, 1980a) as well as in clinical studies. In addition to the two papers mentioned above, there has been a recent resurgence of interest in these designs, particularly into the "correct" form of analysis (Brogan and Kutner, 1980; Lee, 1980b; Schafer, 1981; Laird, 1983). The main focus of interest in this research has been whether the foregoing type of analysis, usually termed a gain-score analysis, is preferable to one in which the pretreatment measurements are used as a covariate to adjust posttreatment values.

Many of the arguments for preferring analysis of covariance (ANCOVA) to a gain-score analysis are irrelevant to clinical studies, since they have to do with nonrandom allocation of subjects to groups. As an example, Lord (1967) highlights an apparent paradox in which one statistician, using the gain-score analysis, concludes that among students at a university there is no evidence of a sex difference with respect to weight gain over the university year, while a second statistician using ANCOVA concludes that the males have a significantly larger weight gain than do females. Clearly, there is no randomization of subjects to groups possible. Both Bock (1975) and Lee (1980b) investigate this paradox and both conclude that ANCOVA is the correct approach, Bock from a randomized perspective, Lee from a nonrandomized. Bock's argument is as follows [see also Hills and Armitage (1979)]: Given that x_{ij} takes the value x, the expected values of y_{1j} and y_{2j} are

$$\mu + \tau + \rho(x - \mu_0), \qquad \mu - \tau + \rho(x - \mu_0),$$

with common variance $\sigma^2(1 - \rho^2)$. It follows that

$$\mathrm{E}\left[\frac{1}{2}(\bar{y}_{1\cdot} - \bar{y}_{2\cdot}) \mid x\right] = \tau, \qquad \mathrm{var}\left[\frac{1}{2}(\bar{y}_{1\cdot} - \bar{y}_{2\cdot}) \mid x\right] = \frac{m}{4}\sigma^2(1 - \rho^2).$$

If we measure the relative efficiency (RE) of the gain-score to that of ANCOVA by the ratio of variances, we have

$$\mathrm{RE} = \frac{m\sigma^2(1-\rho)}{2} \frac{4}{m\sigma^2(1-\rho^2)} = \frac{2}{1+\rho}.$$

From this ratio we see that only when $\rho = 1$ are the analyses equally efficient, and are in this case identical.

Complications can arise in a number of ways in the analysis above:

1. We have assumed in model IV that the pretreatment means in the two groups are equal. This is a reasonable assumption since the randomization of patients to groups should ensure that any difference detected if the groups were to be compared is a type I error. Nevertheless, clinicians may request that such a test be performed (cf. Laird (1983)].
2. The covariance matrix is of a special form, called a compound symmetric. This assumption may be relaxed.
3. The analysis leading to the RE above assumes that (4) is known. Clearly, this is not in general true; however, a full ANCOVA allows for the estimation of all the parameters.

4. A final complication can occur if the covariance matrices of the two groups are no longer identical, in which case ANCOVA is no longer appropriate. For such a situation Schafer (1981) suggests a technique originally proposed by Johnson and Neyman (1936) which seeks a so-called "region of equivalence." Essentially, the Johnson-Neyman technique establishes a range of values for x for which the treatments are not statistically different; outside this range the treatments produce statistically significant effects.

4.2 Baselines in the Two-Period Crossover

In the case of the two-period crossover, various models have been suggested for the incorporation of baseline measurements and for the subsequent analysis. In this section we consider three suggestions made by Willan and Pater (1986b), Varma and Chilton (1974), and Patel (1983) which are in increasing order of complexity.

Suppose that y_{ijk}, as in Section 2.1, denotes the posttreatment response of the jth patient in the ith sequence group in the kth period and that correspondingly x_{ijk} is the pretreatment response. Suppose further that y_{ijk} follows model I, and that x_{ijk} follows model I excluding the treatment effect, so that the cell means for the x_{ijk}'s are as shown in Table 5. Such a model was proposed by Willan and Pater (1986b), except that they introduced an additional random effect, which they characterize as a patient × period interaction, whose purpose is to model higher correlations between observations within the same period rather than between observations from different periods.

Define

$$\hat{\tau}_b = \frac{1}{4}(\bar{d}_{1\cdot 1} - \bar{d}_{1\cdot 2} - \bar{d}_{2\cdot 1} + \bar{d}_{2\cdot 2})$$

(where $d_{ijk} = y_{ijk} - x_{ijk}$), which has expectation τ and variance $m\sigma_\epsilon^2/4$. The null hypothesis of no treatment effect can then be tested using the

Table 5 Pretreatment Cell Means for Willan and Pater's Model

Sequence group	Period 1	Period 2
$A \to B$	$\mu + \pi$	$\mu - \pi + \gamma$
$B \to A$	$\mu + \pi$	$\mu - \pi - \gamma$

statistic

$$\text{FTB} = \frac{4(N-2)\hat{\tau}_b^2}{m\text{SSB}},$$

where SSB/$(N-2)$ is an estimate of σ_ϵ^2.

Varma and Chilton (1974) extend the Willan and Pater model by including, in addition to a carryover effect, an effect which they term the residual effect. This residual effect appears in the cell means for both pre- and posttreatment measurements in the second period, while the carryover effect appears only in the cells means of the posttreatment measurements. Under this model, inferences concerning treatment effect can only be made using data from both periods if the carryover effect is nonsignificant—in the same way as model I—and is essentially identical to the Willan and Pater analysis above. If the carryover effect is significant, the analysis reverts to Chassan's analysis of model IV.

Both of these approaches use the gain score method, and the discussion concerning ANCOVA in Section 4.1 is again relevant. Patel (1983) considers the ANCOVA approach to the analysis of Varma and Chilton's model, generalizing it by assuming arbitrary covariance matrices in the two sequence groups. He considers a number of different hypotheses of interest which may be tested using his model, for instance both carryover effect and period × treatment interaction are testable. Detailed considerations of Patel's approach are beyond the scope of this chapter; interested readers should consult Patel's original work.

That the use of baselines in the analysis of a two-period crossover design is not without danger is highlighted in a paper by Fleiss et al. (1985). These authors suppose that, given the length of a treatment period is one time unit and that the length of the washout period is w time units, the total length of time between the ends of the first and second treatment periods, $1+w$, is sufficiently long to ensure that there is no carryover effect, but that w itself is insufficiently long to eliminate the effect of the first-period treatment on the second period's baseline measurements. Explicitly, they assume that the y_{ijk}'s have model II cell means, while the x_{ijk}'s have the cell means shown in Table 6, where α is not necessarily a linear function of w.

Under this setup consider a gain-score analysis using $d_{ijk} = y_{ijk} - x_{ijk}$. Clearly, the d's have expected values

$$(\mu - \mu_0) + \pi + \tau, \qquad (\mu - \mu_1) - \pi - \tau - \alpha\tau$$

in sequence 1 and

$$(\mu - \mu_0) + \pi - \tau, \qquad (\mu - \mu_1) - \pi + \tau + \alpha\tau$$

Table 6 Pretreatment Cell Means for Fleiss et al.'s Model

Sequence group	Period 1	Period 2
$A \to B$	μ_0	$\mu_1 + \alpha\tau$
$B \to A$	μ_0	$\mu_1 - \alpha\tau$

in sequence 2, respectively, and the estimated carryover effect has expectation $-\alpha\tau$, which is opposite in sign to the treatment effect τ.

Fleiss et al. (1985) conclude that there are two serious consequences of the foregoing analysis. First, the use of baseline measurements may artificially induce an apparent carryover effect, which will cause the analysis of treatment effect to be carried out using period 1 data only, with a subsequent loss in efficiency. Second, it may have consequences for the conduct of future trials, in that clinicians may be wrongly dissuaded from using a crossover design in testing similar drugs in the same condition. They note that ANCOVA does not obviate the bias induced by using baseline measurements with an insufficiently long washout period.

5 EFFICIENCY, POWER, AND COST COMPARISONS

In the preceding sections a relatively straightforward presentation of the various analysis strategies for crossover and parallel studies, with and without baseline measurements, has been given, without explicitly comparing them. In this section the designs are compared with respect to RE, power, and cost.

5.1 Relative Efficiency

In Section 4.1 the RE of estimators was defined as the ratio of their respective variances, assuming that the relevant variance components were known. In this section we continue to use this definition and restrict attention to gain-score analyses in the case of baseline measurements. This approach has been chosen since we are only interested in order-of-magnitude qualitative comparisons. If more precise comparisons are required, account must be taken of the fact that the variance components need to be estimated.

Table 7 Estimators of the Treatment Effect and Their Variances

Type of design	Baseline	Estimator	Variance
Parallel	No	$(\bar{y}_{1\cdot} - \bar{y}_{2\cdot})/2$	$m\sigma^2/4$
	Yes	$(\bar{d}_{1\cdot} - \bar{d}_{2\cdot})/2$	$m\sigma^2(1-\rho)/2$
Crossover (No carryover)	No	$(\bar{y}_{1\cdot 1} - \bar{y}_{1\cdot 2} - \bar{y}_{2\cdot 1} + \bar{y}_{2\cdot 2})/4$	$m\sigma^2(1-\rho)/8$
	Yes	$(\bar{d}_{1\cdot 1} - \bar{d}_{1\cdot 2} - \bar{d}_{2\cdot 1} + \bar{d}_{2\cdot 2})/4$	$m\sigma^2(1-\rho)/8$
Crossover (carryover)	No	$(\bar{y}_{1\cdot 1} - \bar{y}_{2\cdot 1})/2$	$m\sigma^2/4$
	Yes	$(\bar{d}_{1\cdot 1} - \bar{d}_{2\cdot 1})/2$	$m\sigma^2(1-\rho)/2$

For each model, the unbiased estimator of the treatment effect τ and its associated variance are shown in Table 7, in which the variances have all been expressed in terms of σ^2 (the variance of an individual observation) and ρ (the correlation between two measurements on the same patient). Note that the crossover with baselines follows the models of Varma and Chilton. From Table 7 the REs of each pair of estimators may be calculated simply and are as shown above the diagonal in Table 8. A number of conclusions may be drawn from Table 8, among them the following:

Table 8 Relative Efficiences

Type of design		Parallel		Crossover (no carryover)		Crossover (carryover)	
	Baseline	No	Yes	No	Yes	No	Yes
Parallel	No	1	$\frac{1}{2(1-\rho)}$	$\frac{2}{1-\rho}$	$\frac{1}{1-\rho}$	1	$\frac{1}{2(1-\rho)}$
	Yes		1	4	2	$2(1-\rho)$	1
Crossover (no carryover)	No			1	$\frac{1}{2}$	$\frac{1-\rho}{2}$	$\frac{1}{4}$
	Yes				1	$1-\rho$	$\frac{1}{2}$
Crossover (carryover)	No					1	$\frac{1}{2(1-\rho)}$
	Yes						1

i. The use of baseline measurements in parallel studies is warranted only if the correlation between observations is greater than 0.5, since only in this case is the variance of the treatment effect estimate reduced.
ii. The use of baseline measurements in a crossover design in which there is no carryover effect reduces the efficiency by 50% [see also Hills and Armitage (1979, p.16)].
iii. The use of baseline measurements in a crossover design in which there is a carryover effect increases the efficiency if $\rho > 0$, and of course results in an unbiased estimate.
iv. Crossover designs in which there is no carryover effect are always more efficient than parallel designs, whether baseline measurements are used or not.

5.2 Power

Suppose that we wish to compare the various designs with respect to the required sample size for a given alternative and power. Assume that we wish to test the null hypothesis $\theta = 0$ using a statistic that has expectation θ and asymptotic variance ϕ^2/n and that a two-sided test is contemplated. Then a good approximation to the sample size, n, needed to achieve a power of $1 - \beta$ at level α against the alternative $\theta = \theta_0$ is

$$n = \frac{(z_{\alpha/2} + z_\beta)^2 \phi^2}{\theta_0^2},$$

where z_ξ is the upper ξ percentile of the standard normal distribution (Brown, 1980). For two statistics satisfying the assumptions above, having variances ϕ_1^2/n_1 and ϕ_2^2/n_2, respectively, the ratio of required sample sizes is clearly ϕ_1^2/ϕ_2^2. Thus Table 8 provides figures for the ratios of sample sizes, for given level and power, for those models that are considered in Table 7. Clearly, similar conclusions to those above also hold.

5.3 Costs

Brown (1980) compares the relative costs of the two-period crossover and parallel designs as follows. Suppose that C_0 is the cost of recruiting a patient (preliminary screening for eligibility etc.), and that C_1 is the cost of treatment and measurement in a given period (where we assume that the treatment cost is small relative to the measurement cost—this assumption can be relaxed but requires the introduction of a third cost). Then the total costs for parallel studies, with n_P patients in each group, are

$$2n_PC_0 + 4n_PC_1, \qquad 2n_PC_0 + 2n_PC_1,$$

with and without baseline measurements, respectively. The corresponding total costs for crossover designs, with n_C patients in each sequence, are

$$2n_C C_0 + 8n_C C_1, \qquad 2n_C C_0 + 4n_C C_1.$$

Suppose that the sample sizes are chosen so that the variances of the treatment effect estimates are equal; then a comparison of the relative costs may be made. From Table 7 we see that for the variances of the crossover design and parallel designs, without baselines, to be equal the sample sizes must satisfy the relationship

$$n_C = \frac{n_P(1-\rho)}{2},$$

and therefore their relative cost is

$$R_C = \frac{(1-\rho)(1+2C_1/C_0)}{1+C_1/C_0}.$$

This depends both on the correlation between individual observations on the same patient and on the relative costs of recruitment and treatment [see Brown (1980)]. Similar calculations can be made for other pairs of designs.

It is obviously difficult to make general statements about relative costs from the analysis above. Only in specific cases where there is some knowledge of the relative sizes of C_0 and C_1 can effective use be made of the results above.

6 DISCUSSION

Since 1978 there has been a great increase in research into the two-period crossover design for clinical trials. In large part this increase is due to the position taken by the U.S. Food and Drug Administration (FDA; cf. Section 1). In the main this research has been aimed at showing that the two-period crossover should not automatically be discarded at the planning stage, since it has something to offer to clinical research.

To evaluate this research it is worthwhile to summarize the findings of the BEMAC:

i. "The two-period crossover design is not the design of choice in clinical trials, where unequivocal evidence of treatment effect is required."
ii. "In most cases, the completely randomized (or randomized block) design with baseline measurements will be the design of choice."
iii. Experimental designs should be encouraged which yield unbiased estimates of treatment effects that are as model-free as possible.

iv. Persuasive evidence of the validity of any assumptions that are necessary to show unbiasedness of treatment estimates is required.
v. The two-period crossover should have sufficiently large patient numbers to detect and test an interaction of a given amount with a large power.

In looking at the more recent work we will not necessarily consider these five points in their given order.

Suppose that we wish to design a two-period crossover so that it has sufficient power to detect a substantial carryover effect, and that Grizzle's procedure, using a preliminary test, is contemplated. Brown (1980) assumes that if we were interested in a treatment effect τ, we would be interested in detecting a carryover effect of $\gamma = \tau/2$, which is the size of the bias (cf. Section 2.3). The variance of $\hat{\gamma}$ is $m(\sigma_\epsilon^2 + \sigma_\eta^2)/2$, and assuming equal numbers of patients in each sequence group, n_{CR}, the approximation in Section 5.2 may be used to show that at level α', a power of $1 - \beta'$ will be approximately achieved if

$$n_{CR} = \frac{(z_{\alpha'/2} + z_{\beta'})^2(\sigma_\epsilon^2 + 2\sigma_\eta^2)}{(\tau/2)^2}.$$

Brown further assumes that a test of power $1 - \beta$ at level α is required for the treatment effect, so that were a parallel design used, the required sample size, n_{PA}, in each group would be

$$n_{PA} = \frac{(z_{\alpha/2} + z_\beta)^2(\sigma_\epsilon^2 + \sigma_\eta^2)}{2\tau^2}.$$

The relative sample sizes of the two designs is therefore

$$\frac{n_{CR}}{n_{PA}} = \frac{8(z_{\alpha'/2} + z_{\beta'})^2(\sigma_\epsilon^2 + 2\sigma_\eta^2)}{(z_{\alpha/2} + z_\beta)^2(\sigma_\epsilon^2 + \sigma_\eta^2)},$$

which, as Brown shows, can be considerably larger than 1. For example, suppose that $\alpha = 5\%$, $\alpha' = 10\%$ (Grizzle's suggestion), $\beta = \beta' = 5\%$, $\sigma_\epsilon^2 = \sigma_\eta^2 (\rho = 0.5)$; then

$$\frac{n_{CR}}{n_{PA}} = \frac{8(3.2897)^2 \times 3}{(3.6048)^2 \times 2} = 10.$$

Brown concludes from his analysis that the crossover design is uneconomical for testing the assumption of no carryover effect.

This point of view is not accepted by all researchers; indeed, some argue against the necessity of there being absolutely no carryover effect. A group of British statisticians argue that it is only necessary that there be a small carryover in comparison to the treatment effect (Poloniecki and Daniel,

1981; Huitson et al., 1982; Barker et al., 1982; Poloniecki and Pearce, 1983). Poloniecki and Daniel (1981), for instance, argue that "the point about interaction is not that it should be absent in order to permit inferences about the treatment—since this is in the first place improbable, and in the second place impossible to establish—but that it should not be as great as the treatment effect, since this would mean that the drug is better than placebo in one period but not in the other."

Poloniecki and Pearce (1983) formalize this view, suggesting, in the notation of Section 2.5, that either

$$P[(\tau - \gamma > 0) \wedge (\tau > 0) \mid Y]$$

or

$$P[(\tau - \gamma < 0) \wedge (\tau < 0) \mid Y]$$

be calculated, depending on the sign of $\hat{\tau}$. Grieve (1985) shows that this is not a good idea since it is possible to have

$$P(\tau > 0 \mid Y) \approx 1 \qquad \text{and} \qquad P[(\tau - \gamma < 0) \wedge (\tau < 0) \mid Y] \approx 0,$$

the first probability indicating that conditional on any reasonable value of γ suggested by the data, the posterior probability of τ being positive is very high. Similar ideas are considered by Willan and Pater (1986a).

In considering the evidence required to show no carryover effect, BEMAC said: "It will require convincing support, from prior information or from the experimental data themselves ...." Racine et al. (1986) look at the possibility of incorporating prior information concerning γ, from, say, a pilot study, in the Bayesian analysis proposed by Grieve (1985). Racine et al. conclude that since a pilot study is in general far smaller than the main study, it would not provide sufficient information to remove bias from the treatment estimate. The alternative Bayesian approach, based on prior odds ratios and the Bayes factor, "has great potential for ... flexible sensitivity analysis displays." However, their experience suggests that "unequivocal evidence of no carryover effect will rarely be forthcoming and that the interpretation of such trial data ... must inevitably rest heavily on subjective assessment of the existence of such an effect." We return to these ideas when viewing the most recent standpoint of the FDA.

The BEMAC report strongly recommended the use of parallel designs with baseline measurements. As the analyses in Sections 4 and 5 have shown, this is not always advisable in terms of efficiency, and can introduce a bias which it is primarily supposed to eliminate (cf. Fleiss et al. (1985)]. Most of the work on baselines, an exception being Patel (1983), has assumed a mixed-model analysis, which constitutes an additional assumption that again has to be examined in each case (cf. item (iii) above).

Further work is also needed into the advisability of using the gain-score approach as opposed to ANCOVA.

Throughout this chapter we have considered only the simplest of crossover designs: the two-period, two-treatment crossover. Recently, there has been considerable interest in more complex designs, for instance, three-period two-treatment crossovers [see, e.g., Ebbutt (1984)]. Further work in this direction is reported by Kershner and Federer (1981), Laska et al. (1983), and Laska and Meisner (1985). Although such designs provide statistical improvements (optimality considerations) over the simple two-period design, it is not necessarily true that they provide practical alternatives since they may result in increased numbers of dropouts due to prolongation of the trial. Optimality results concerning crossovers with more than two treatments and periods are given by Hedayat and Afsarinejad (1975, 1978), for which the same concerns about high dropout rates are also valid.

Patel (1985) has considered the problem of dropouts in the two-period crossover, and shows that by utilizing information from patients who drop out at the end of the first treatment period, the powers of the tests for both carryover effects and treatment effects may be increased, at the cost of a more complicated analysis. The same problem, from a Bayesian perspective, is addressed in the reply to the discussion by Racine et al. (1986). Again the analysis is considerably more complicated, and numerical methods, for instance those of Naylor and Smith (1982), must be resorted to in order that the posterior distributions of interest may be calculated. An example of the application of these methods to missing data in the two-period crossover is given by Grieve (1987a).

In the introduction we noted that in certain circumstances the two-period crossover is inappropriate, and in Section 2.1 we noted that the carryover effect is sometimes termed the residual effect, or period×treatment interaction. These are essentially different sides of the same coin. In other words, what we have throughout this chapter termed carryover effect can have more than one cause. For instance, Hills and Armitage (1979) identify three possible causes of what we call carryover effect. First, the washout period may be inadequate, so the effect of the first-period treatment persists into the second period. Second, the first treatment may cause a change in the patients' physiological or psychological states. Third, the treatment effect may be proportional to patients' overall disease levels. In addition, there may be a difference between the sequence groups with respect to their average levels, but this is essentially a type I error. Unfortunately, these effects are indistinguishable from one another in the simple two-period crossover, and in the statistical model are completely confounded. Hecker (1986) investigates "carryover" and shows that there is no two-treatment, two-period design which can fully utilize data from both periods without assuming that one, or more, of the foregoing causes is nonexistent.

The review given in this chapter reflects the author's personal interests concerning the problem of crossover versus parallel designs. In my opinion there are no hard and fast rules as to the advisability, or not, of using a crossover design in any given circumstances, nor as to whether one should use baseline measurements. The most recent view from the FDA [see Dubey (1984)] suggests that the two-period crossover is not viewed as negatively as it was 10 years ago. Indeed, of the 22 clinical areas reviewed by Dubey, crossover designs are recommended in five, permitted in three, permitted by discouraged in eight, and not recommended in six. The saga of the crossover design for clinical trials is not yet over, and it is healthy that the debate over the applicability of these designs continues, and will continue in the future.

REFERENCES

Armitage, P., M. Hills (1982). The two-period crossover trial. *Statistician 31*, 119–131.

Barker, N., R. J. Hews, A. Huitson, and J. Poloniecki (1982). The two-period crossover trial. *Bull. Appl. Statist. 9*, 67–116.

Bock, R. D. (1975). *Multivariate Statistical Methods in Behavioral Research.* McGraw-Hill, New York.

Brogan, D. R., and M. H. Kutner (1980). Comparative analyses of pretest-postest research designs. *Amer. Statist. 34*, 229–232.

Brown, B. W. (1980). The crossover experiment for clinical trials. *Biometrics 36*, 69–79.

Chassan, J. B. (1970). A note on relative efficiency in clinical trials. *J. Clin. Pharmacol. 10*, 359–360.

Dubey, S. D. (1986). Current thoughts on crossover designs. *Clin. Res. Pract. Drug Regul. Aff. 4*, 127–142.

Ebbutt, A. F. (1984). Three-period crossover designs for two treatments. *Biometrics 40*, 219–224.

Farewell, V. T. (1985). Some remarks on the analysis of cross-over trials with a binary response. *Appl. Statist. 34*, 121–128.

Food and Drug Administration (1977). A report on the two-period crossover design and its applicability in trials of clinical effectiveness. Minutes of the Biometric and Epidemiology Methodology Advisory Committee (BEMAC) meeting.

Fidler, V. (1984). Change-over clinical trial with binary data: mixed model based comparison of test. *Biometrics 40*, 1063–1070.

Fleiss, J. L., S. Wallenstein, and R. Rosenfeld (1985). Adjusting for baseline measurements in the two-period crossover study: a cautionary note. *Controlled Clin. Trials 6*, 192–197.

Gart, J. J. (1969). An exact test for comparing matched proportions in crossover designs. *Biometrika 56*, 75–80.

Gart, J. J. (1975). The Poisson distribution. The theory and application of some conditional tests. In *Statistical Distributions in Scientific Work, Vol. 2* (G. P. Patil, S. Kotz, and J. K. Ord, eds.). D. Reidel, Dordrecht, The Netherlands.

Gomez-Marin, O., and R. B. McHugh (1984). Randomization modeling of the crossover experiment for clinical trials. *Biometrical J. 26*, 901–914.

Grieve, A. P. (1982). Letter to the editor. *Biometrics 38*, 517.

Grieve, A. P. (1985). A Bayesian analysis of the two-period crossover design for clinical trials. *Biometrics 42*, 979–990. Corrigenda *42*, 459 (1986).

Grieve, A. P. (1987a). Applications of Bayesian software: two examples. *Statistician 36*, 283–288.

Grieve, A. P. (1987b). A note on the analysis of the two-period crossover design when the period-treatment interaction is significant. *Biometrical J. 7*, 771–775.

Grizzle, J. E. (1965). The two-period change-over design and its use in clinical trials. *Biometrics 21*, 467–480. Corrigenda *30*, 727 (1974).

Hamilton, M. A., and G. K. Bissonnette (1975). Statistical inferences about injury and persistence of environmentally stressed bacteria. *J. Hyg. 74*, 149–155.

Hecker, H. (1986). Identification and interpretation of results from the two-period crossover designs. *EDV Med. Biol. 17*, 60–66.

Hedayat, A., and K. Afsarinejad (1975). Repeated measurements designs: I. In *A Survey of Statistical Design and Linear Models* (J. N. Srivastava, ed.). North-Holland, Amsterdam.

Hedayat, A., and K. Afsarinejad (1978). Repeated measurements designs: II. *Ann. Statist. 6*, 619–628.

Hews, R. J. (1981). Further note on the interpretation of results from the two-period cross-over trial. *Statist. Pharm. Indust. Newslett. 3*, No. 2.

Hills, M., and P. Armitage (1979). The two-period cross-over trial. *British J. Clin. Pharmacol. 8*, 7–20.

Huitson, A. (1980). A note on the interpretation of results from the two-period cross-over clinical trial. *Statist. Pharm. Indust. Newslett. 2*, No. 4.

Huitson, A., J. Poloniecki, R. J. Hews, and N. Barker (1982). A review of cross-over trials. *Statistician 31*, 71–80.

Johnson, P. O., and J. Neyman (1936). Tests of certain linear hypotheses and their application to some educational problems. *Statist. Res. Mem. 1*, 57–93.

Kenward, M. G., and B. Jones (1987). A log linear model for binary crossover data. *Appl. Statist. 36*, 192–204.

Kershner, R. P., and W. T. Federer (1981). Two-treatment crossover designs for estimating a variety of effects. *J. Amer. Statist. Assoc. 76*, 612–619.

Koch, G. G. (1972). The use of non-parametric methods in the statistical analysis of the two-period change-over design. *Biometrics 28*, 577–584.

Laird, N. (1983). Further comparative analyses of pretest-posttest research designs. *Amer. Statist. 37*, 329–330.

Larson, H. J., and T. A. Bancroft (1963). Biases in prediction by regression for incompletely specified models. *Biometrika 50*, 391–402.

Laska, E., and M. Meisner (1985). A variational approach to optimal two-treatment crossover designs: application to carryover effect models. *J. Amer. Statist. Assoc. 80*, 704–710.

Laska, E., M. Meisner, and H. B. Kushner (1983). Optimal crossover designs in the presence of carryover effects. *Biometrics 39*, 1087–1091.

Layard, M. W. J., and J. N. Arvesen (1978). Analysis of Poisson data in crossover trials. *Biometrics 34*, 421–428.

Lee, J. L. (1980a). A note on the interpretation of results of supplementation trials. *Amer. J. Nutr. 33*, 333–337.

Lee, J. L. (1980b). A note on the comparison of group means based on repeated measurements of the same subject. *J. Chronic Dis. 33*, 673–675.

Lord, F. M. (1967). A paradox in the interpretation of group comparisons. *Psychol. Bull. 68*, 304–305.

Nagelkerke, N. J. D., A. A. M. Hart, and J. Osting (1986). The two-period binary response crossover trial. *Biometrical J. 7*, 863–869.

Naylor, J. C., and A. F. M. Smith (1982). Applications of a method for the efficient computation of posterior distributions. *Appl. Statist. 31*, 214–225.

O'Neill, R. T. (1978). Subject-own-control designs in clinical drug trials: overview of the issues with emphasis on the two treatment problem. Presented at the Annual NCDEU Meeting, Key Biscayne, Fla.

Patel, H. I. (1983). Use of baseline measurements in the two-period crossover design. *Comm. Statist. A12*, 2693–2712.

Patel, H. I. (1985). Analysis of incomplete data in a two-period crossover design with reference to clinical trials. *Biometrika 72*, 411–418.

Patil, V. H. (1965). Approximation to the Behrens-Fisher distribution. *Biometrika 52*, 267–271.

Poloniecki, J. D., and D. Daniel (1981). Further analysis of Hills and Armitage enuresis data. *Statistician 30*, 225–229.

Poloniecki, J. D, and A. C. Pearce (1983). Letter to the editor. *Biometrics 39*, 798.

Prescott, R. J. (1981). The comparison of success rates in cross-over trials in the presence of an order effect. *Appl. Statist. 30*, 9–15.

Racine, A., A. P. Grieve, H. Flühler, and A. F. M. Smith (1986). Bayesian methods in practice: experiences in the pharmaceutical industry (with discussion). *Appl. Statist. 35*, 93–150.

Schafer, W. D. (1981). Letter to the editor. *Amer. Statist. 35*, 179.

Selwyn, M. R., A. P. Dempster, and N. R. Hall, (1981). A Bayesian approach to bioequivalence for the 2 × 2 changeover design. *Biometrics 37*, 11–21.

Varma, A. O., and N. W. Chilton (1974). Crossover designs involving two treatments. *J. Periodontal Res. 9, Suppl. 14*, 160–170.

Willan, A. R., and J. L. Pater (1986a). Carryover and the two-period crossover design. *Biometrics 42*, 593–599.

Willan, A. R., and J. L. Pater (1986b). Using baseline measurements in the two-period crossover clinical trial. *Controlled Clin. Trials 7*, 282–289.

Zimmermann, H., and V. Rahlfs (1978). Testing hypothesis in the two-period change-over trial with binary data. *Biometrical J. 20*, 133–141.

Zimmermann, H., and V. Rahlfs (1980). Model building and testing for the change-over design. *Biometrical J. 22*, 197–220.

9

Handling Dropouts and Related Issues

RICHARD G. CORNELL University of Michigan, Ann Arbor, Michigan

1 INTRODUCTION

A clinical trial carried out during an early phase of the development of a treatment regimen is often an explanatory trial, described by Sackett (1983) as dealing with a question such as "Can a certain drug reduce cancer size?" or "Under what conditions does the drug reduce cancer size?" This type of question is also asked in earlier laboratory experiments with respect to efficacy. In such an explanatory trial or experiment, if it were discovered that a switch to the wrong treatment had occurred for an experimental unit, or if problems developed which precluded observing the planned outcome, that experimental unit would weaken the final comparison of active treatment and control. No evidence is provided on whether or not a drug reduces cancer size if that drug is not given or the tumor not measured after administration of the drug. Thus great care should be taken in an explanatory trial to avoid changes in treatment, or patient dropouts, whatever the reason, even though this leads to limitations in the scope of the trial. The design and analysis of explanatory trials are discussed further in Section 2. See also the discussion of phase I trials in Chapter 1. General principles for the design and analysis of any clinical trial are also introduced in Section 2.

Most clinical trials are designed to answer a different question, a question such as "Does the use of a drug regimen in practice, for a regimen that features the drug under investigation as the primary treatment, lead to improvement in a patient's condition or prognosis?" Certainly, the last phases of the investigation of a clinical regimen would address a more general question of this type as indicated in the discussion of phase II and III trials in Chapter 1. A clinical trial that addresses this sort of question has been referred to as a management trial (Sackett, 1983) or a pragmatic trial (Armitage, 1983). Such a trial is very much like ordinary clinical practice. Information on a patient whose regimen involves a switch away from the primary drug is of interest here in addition to information on patients who stay on the treatment initially assigned to them. Was the primary drug avoided because of the complexity of the regimen? Was it taken initially but discontinued because of a lack of perceived efficacy or because of adverse effects? For patients who are lost to follow-up it is important, if possible, to find out why they dropped out. The reason may be treatment or response related. Thus, indicators of treatment changes, withdrawals, losses to follow-up, and protocol deviations are important, not just for a complete accounting, but also as outcome variables for the evaluation of treatment regimens. Various alternative patterns have to be anticipated and planned for in the design and analysis of a pragmatic clinical trial, not only because of the less restrictive nature of the question for which the trial seeks an answer, but also because of the greater scope and complexity of such a trial in comparison to an explanatory trial. Perspectives toward the analysis of pragmatic trials are presented in Section 3.1.

In some clinical trials withdrawals because of treatment efficacy or failure are not only anticipated but occur in substantial numbers among patients who follow the protocol. For instance, the purpose of treatment may be to reduce blood pressure. The protocol may call for entering patients with baseline diastolic blood pressures between 90 and 120. Dose adjustments based on blood pressure readings may be made during the first few weeks of the trial. Provision may also be made in the protocol to withdraw patients whose diastolic blood pressures rise above 120, and thus reflect treatment failure, whether on placebo or active drug, and to withdraw patients whose blood pressures fall below 90, which reflects treatment success. The analysis of a clinical trial of this type should be applied to data on early withdrawals, whether due to success or failure, as well as to data on patients who remain in the trial to the end. Approaches to trials with repeated measures and allowances for early withdrawal of failures or successes are discussed in Sections 3.7 and 3.8.

2 DESIGN CONSIDERATIONS

2.1 Basic Principles of Experimental Design

Two cornerstones of experimental design are basic to all clinical trials. One is comparison and the other is randomization. In many clinical trials only two treatments are compared, often an active drug and a control treatment. Whether the control treatment is a standard therapy or a placebo, or whether two or more treatments are included in a trial, the principle of comparison is compromised when departures from intended regimens occur. For instance, in an explanatory trial, a switch away from the treatment initially assigned may be made because of deterioration of a patient's condition or because of an adverse side effect. This switch may be in accord with the protocol. However, such a switch weakens the evidence on the effectiveness of the active drug, even if the patient is in the control group. This is of particular concern in an explanatory trial, which is usually focused on the effect of a single drug or treatment, not its effect as part of a broader treatment regimen in a pragmatic trial.

The concern with patients who depart from the intended treatment is not just because of a reduction in the number of patients who received only the treatment originally assigned. The primary analysis of a trial is a comparison of the treatment groups to which the patients were initially randomized. This is the only comparison for which a lack of bias is assured by the design of trial. Patients who switch would still be involved in the primary comparison, but with group membership identified by their initial assignments. Analyses by randomization groups are discussed in Sections 3.2 and 3.3.

Clearly, the difference in mean response between a treatment group that took the drug under study and a control group in which many of the patients switched from placebo to an active drug would be expected to be less than would have been observed if the control group had stayed on the placebo. Similarly, if many patients in the treatment group switched to a different active drug, an observed difference would not be attributed entirely to the drug assigned initially. This possible diminution of the treatment effect, based on a primary comparison of randomization groups, is important. For this reason, secondary analyses which are not limited to comparisons of randomization groups are important. These are discussed in Sections 3.4 and 3.6.

There is also concern for the bias that could be introduced by secondary comparisons of subgroups who remain on their initially assigned treatments, whether active drug or placebo. This bias could be considerable because those who switch are likely to be more severely ill, or less tractable, or less responsive to treatment, than those who remain on the same treatment throughout a trial.

Loss to follow-up may have a greater effect than just the loss of information to be entered into a comparison. It may introduce bias into a comparison based on the remaining data, since a loss to follow-up may be indirectly, not directly, related to a patient's treatment assignment. For instance, a patient may be lost from a clinical trial because of a move to a distant place to take advantage of a better employment opportunity for someone in the patient's family. This may seem completely unrelated to the treatment assignment in the clinical trial. Yet the patient may have been randomized to an ineffective treatment, perhaps a placebo, and may have not taken the termination of participation in the clinical trial into account in deciding on the move because of no change in health status. If the patient had been randomized to an active drug that was perceived to be beneficial, this might have been a prime consideration in the decision process of the family. If the patient desired continued care, the family might not have moved, or the patient might have delayed joining the rest of the family in order to complete the trial. On the other hand, the patient may have been randomized to a very effective treatment and moved happily, feeling cured.

Of course, a loss to follow-up may also be directly related to treatment and the resultant loss of information will surely bias treatment comparisons. Such losses can occur because of treatment failure or success, or because of adverse effects. Although such losses can be taken into account in the analysis, they are of particular concern in an explanatory trial which focuses on the potential of an active drug under ideal conditions.

The second cornerstone basic to the foundation of scientific inference in general, and clinical trials in particular, is randomization. One purpose of randomization is to avoid bias. Another is to form the basis for inference. If patients are assigned to treatments other than by randomization, the possibility of bias is introduced and the generalizability of the clinical trial through induction is impaired.

Randomization does not guarantee an equal distribution, or one not necessarily equal but representative of some population, over traits in a patient population within each treatment group. For instance, suppose that a given patient population is one-third female. A particular randomization of patients from that population to two treatment groups will not necessarily produce treatment groups with equal proportions of females, or if it did, with proportions of one-third as in the parent population. But randomization does avoid bias. Restricted randomization can be employed to control for a variable, through stratification, which is known to affect the outcome variable. An aspect of randomness is still important in the design of a clinical trail to avoid bias, not only with respect to variables which can be readily identified, measured, and controlled for in advance, but with respect to variables not measured and perhaps not yet known to be influential.

Randomization is also crucial for purposes of classical statistical inference. Quantitative inferences in the form of tests of hypotheses are based on the random assignment of patients to treatment groups. Thus valid induction as well as a lack of bias is possible with comparisons between treatment groups to which patients are initially randomized. This is the reason for the statement made earlier in this section that the primary comparison of patients is between randomization groups. This leads to an analysis based on the intent to treat, not necessarily on the actual treatment received. Secondary analyses by treatment regimen actually received, or by level of adherence, should also be carried out, but their interpretations should be guarded in view of the possible biases involved. If the conclusions drawn are to be generalized to a larger population of patients, as is usually the case, an assumption that the patients under study can be regarded as a random sample from the larger population is also crucial.

2.2 Implications for the Design of Explanatory Trials

The purpose of an explanatory trial is to attribute differences in the responses of treatment groups to a drug or other treatment alone. Thus to avoid bias and dilution of the evidence for a treatment effect, it is important to keep as many patients as possible in the trial and on the treatment initially assigned through a randomization procedure.

One way to avoid protocol deviations, withdrawals, and losses to follow-up is to restrict the patient population under study by imposing narrow entry criteria. This would be appropriate in a preliminary explanatory trial to see if a drug has the potential for use as a therapeutic agent. If would not be appropriate in a final pragmatic trial of the efficacy of a regimen in usual clinical practice.

Often patients are restricted in terms of the severity of their disease. Those most severely ill may be excluded because of comorbidity, and perhaps likelihood of death, which may make it unlikely that a drug would have adequate opportunity to show its effect in improved health. Perhaps those most severely ill have suffered from the disease longest and have been found refractory to treatment. Thus those most severely ill may be excluded to avoid withdrawal because of other illness, death, or ineffectual treatment.

Patients who are not very ill may also be excluded to avoid withdrawals because of treatment success, especially if a long period of observation is called for by the protocol. It is more likely that less ill patients will not be included because of a lack of potential for showing a demonstrable effect. This lack could be the result of either lower severity of disease or higher probability of misdiagnosis.

Patients may also be restricted to those who are thought likely to remain in the trial until its completion and to follow its protocol strictly. This is appropriate in a preliminary explanatory trial, but clearly would be expected to lead to an overestimate of treatment effectiveness in general practice. For further discussion of patient entry criteria, see Chapter 1.

Designers of explanatory trials may attempt to avoid problems with protocol deviations and dropouts in two other ways. The treatment regimen may be simplified relative to that which would be used in practice for a more diverse group of patients. This simplification could lead to better adherence to the prescribed regimen and less likelihood of noncompliance or withdrawal because of frustration with complicated procedures. On the other hand, lack of flexibility could lead to a higher probability of treatment failure and adverse reaction.

Second, the length of time for an explanatory trial may be limited to avoid problems with maintaining participation and compliance. A fairly short explanatory trial may be adequate to show that a drug or other treatment regimen can produce an efficacious effect. Afterward a larger, less restricted, pragmatic trial should be carried out to help assess its effectiveness in clinical practice under a broader range of conditions.

For instance, Bartlett et al. (1985) recently carried out an adaptive randomized controlled trial to determine if extracorporeal membrane oxygenation (ECMO) would enable newborns with severe respiratory distress to survive. This treatment involves surgically placing an infant on an artificial lung until its own lung matures. Clearly, this was a preliminary explanatory trial. It was not typical of explanatory clinical trials because it involved a novel adaptive treatment allocation procedure and limited comparison with the control treatment because of a lack of success with conventional intensive therapy in the past as well as during the trial. It was illustrative of the restrictions that may be placed on an explanatory trial. Patients were limited to those thought to have less than a probability of 0.2 of survival on conventional intensive therapy. They were also limited to newborns without other major complications and were relatively heavy considering that this affliction is most common in premature infants. This selection made a dramatic increase in survival rate possible and limited the risk in terms of an avoidable death due to ECMO. It also reduced the likelihood of a withdrawal after an initial assignment to ECMO, which would involve a continuation of conventional intensive care, since there was little likelihood of survival on conventional care.

In regular medical practice it would be desirable to use a lifesaving technique before an infant has such a tenuous grasp on life to avoid the effects of oxygen depravation. ECMO was found to be effective in terms of survival. A pragmatic trial is now under way with randomization to either ECMO or conventional therapy at an earlier stage of illness, and with ECMO as the backup treatment to conventional therapy in the event of deterioration in a newborn's condition. The treatment regimens are now more complex, and ECMO is involved in both regimens which will be compared in the primary analysis. Thus differences between randomization groups will not be attributable to ECMO alone. Since it is anticipated that most infants will survive, the main focus of this trial is on morbidity and cost.

2.3 Design Features for All Clinical Trials

Other measures that should be taken to avoid bias, because of a failure to maintain randomization groups and because of dropouts, are to make sure that information is provided on all patients randomized initially and to follow patients as intensely as possible, even if they withdraw from the study. The first can be accomplished by having patients entered into a patient log when they are first considered for the study. Background information should also be entered which can be useful in verifying patient eligibility decisions and in considering generalizations to other patient populations. This information can also be used to compare dropouts with those who remain in the trial to see if there is evidence that dropping out is related to variables such as disease severity, and hence to treatment efficacy.

For those who are eligible for the clinical trial and who give informed consent to participate, the initial randomization should be recorded, and ideally, sent to a central coordinating center. This avoids losing track of patients after randomization, which also introduces bias as well as resulting in a loss of information.

In addition to thorough data management practices throughout a trial, an effort should be made to follow up those who withdraw or drop out, perhaps through a final questionnaire or through a search of death certificates.

Another approach, which does not address the bias introduced by losses to follow-up, assures an adequate sample size for the subset of patients with attributes that enable them to complete a trial. With this approach the size of a trial is expanded with the anticipation that some patients will be lost to follow-up. Meinert (1986) suggests increasing the sample size by $1/(1-d)$, where d is the anticipated loss rate. He states that the choice of the value of d used should be based on relevant experience, and may range from zero in instances where follow-up is possible, say through death certificates even though a patient withdraws from the trial, to quite a high value when long periods of surveillance are required. Again, it should be stressed that increasing the sample size does not compensate for biases from losses.

Meinert also discusses increasing the sample size due to treatment noncompliance or other departures from protocol. The dilution of the treatment effect because of treatment switching has been discussed. An increased sample size would be required for an estimated treatment effect to be significant when protocol departures lead to less of an effect. Meinert illustrates the application of sample size formulas to a coronary drug project and a study of blood pressure change. For the first study he set $d = 0$ and for the second $d = 0.30$.

A patient log, intensive follow-up, and a sample size that allows for incomplete information are important in all clinical trials, perhaps more in pragmatic than in explanatory trials, because of the greater complexity and scope and longer time span of pragmatic trials. Many ways of dealing with problems of incomplete data in the analysis are also common to different types of trials. Discussion of approaches to analysis will be presented after a brief discussion of perspectives toward analysis for pragmatic trials.

3 APPROACHES TO STATISTICAL ANALYSIS

3.1 Perspectives Toward Analysis for Pragmatic Trials

It has already been indicated that a pragmatic clinical trial differs from an explanatory one in that the treatment protocol is more like that anticipated for use in regular medical practice, the patient population is more diverse, and the length of the trial and the period of follow-up is longer. One important aspect has not been mentioned. Namely, the outcome variable will usually be more complicated as well. Sometimes, instead, at an outcome at one point in time, there will be repeated measures. Also, because of the more complicated treatment regimens, there may be interest in more than one type of response. In addition, the longer time span may lead to greater emphasis on adverse reactions.

In a pragmatic trial there will also be a considerable amount of information on compliance, length of time in trial, and changes of status with respect to participation and availability for follow-up. Moreover, these variables should be viewed not just as variables to be recorded and reported as part of the monitoring and description of the trial, but should be thought of as informative outcome variables that reflect the acceptance of treatment as well as effectiveness. Not only should these variables be included as dependent variables in the comparisons of treatments, but care should be taken in interpreting analyses based on their use as stratification variables or covariates since they are likely to be correlated with the primary outcome variables of interest.

There is another change in perspective between an explanatory trial and a pragmatic one. In an explanatory trial with, say, a treatment involving an active drug and another involving placebo control, a comparison of treatment groups leads to an evaluation of the effect of the active drug. Even though that drug may be the primary component of a treatment regimen in a pragmatic trial, it is better to think of such a trial as a comparison of treatment strategies. These strategies usually have alternative treatments chosen for use in case of adverse reactions or deterioration in a patient's condition. In fact, the same active drug which is the primary component of one strategy may be the backup treatment in the another.

Another distinction between explanatory and pragmatic trials is that pragmatic trials are more likely to involve repeated measures on patients because of longer trial duration. So in a pragmatic trial it may be important to plan for the analysis of a vector of observations, instead of just a final outcome, or the difference between a final outcome and a baseline observation. Approaches that are unique to dependent variables that are vectors will be presented after discussion of approaches to analysis that are applicable to any type of dependent variable.

Methods of analysis for taking loss to follow-up into account are applicable to any clinical trial, yet it is helpful to keep the distinctive perspectives of a pragmatic trial in mind in the interpretation of statistical analyses.

3.2 Comparisons of Randomization Groups

The primary analysis in clinical trials should consist of comparisons between the treatment groups to which patients were randomized, regardless of the nature or course of their treatment. The dependent variables in these comparisons should be those determined in advance to reflect the clinical condition under study. Analyses should also be done on measures of participation and compliance, including dropout rates. Statistically significant differences in withdrawal rates or dropout rates should be interpreted as evidence of a differential effect of treatment strategies, just like a difference in measures of therapeutic response. Possible links between participation and treatment efficacy should be fully explored.

Despite the care with which different types of outcome variables are analyzed and the intensity with which relationships between them are investigated, the results of the analyses of dropout and withdrawal rates and of primary dependent variables may not be consistent with each other. For instance, one group may have a higher dropout rate than the other but better therapeutic results for those who continue to participate. The better therapeutic results may be because the dropouts were the most severely ill. To check on this, measures of severity could be compared between those who drop out and those who continue for each of the treatment groups. If, in fact, those who dropped out from the group with the better therapeutic results among continuing participants were not more severely ill, this might indicate that the treatment strategy for that group is more effective. Yet the question would still arise of whether or not there was another explanation that tied together the higher dropout rate and the apparent treatment efficacy. This would continue to shed doubt on whether or not it was the better treatment. If the high dropout rate were to continue to occur later in medical practice, the apparent efficacy of the treatment would be diminished by the failure of patients to adhere to its regimen. So an analysis that combines disparate aspects of treatment outcome, such as level of participation and therapeutic response, is needed.

3.3 Ranking

One way to achieve an overall evaluation is to convert all the information on outcome variables into a ranking of patients in terms of the desirability of their outcomes. For instance, suppose that one patient withdraws from a clinical trial early because of a lack of therapeutic response, while another continues until the trial is completed and shows improvement. Thus only an indication of a dropout and the reason for dropping out are available for one, but a final measurement of the clinical variable of main interest is available for the other. Although there is no common measurement scale, these outcomes could be ranked, first on the basis of the last time of observation and then on the basis of the clinical variable. Similarly, rankings that would be generally agreed upon could be assigned to deaths and to early withdrawals because of treatment success. Ties could be replaced by midranks, the average of ranks that would have been assigned had more information been available to assign unique ranks to patients with the same midrank.

The method of assigning ranks is attractive from another standpoint. Wilcoxon-type rank procedures are nearly as efficient as tests based on underlying normality assumptions, even when the assumption of normality holds exactly. So if the ranking obtained mirrors that which would have resulted without dropouts, little if anything would be lost through the use of a rank procedure.

3.4 Secondary Subgroup Analyses

Despite the fact that the primary analyses should involve the comparison of randomization groups and that withdrawal and dropout rates should be compared in addition to direct measures of disease severity or improvement, secondary analyses should also be done between subgroups and on variables that reflect only a direct treatment effect. The possibility of bias should be borne in mind in the interpretation of these analyses, and any treatment effect found to be significant for a subgroup of patients or for a particular circumstance in terms of the use of a treatment regimen should be subjected to additional scrutiny in another trial.

Of particular concern is narrowing consideration in secondary analyses to variables thought to be linked directly to treatment: for instance, limiting attention to death from a particular cause as opposed to all causes, limiting attention to a narrow time period and thus missing immediate or longer-term effects, or not taking adverse effects into account even though they may occur mainly in treatment groups that receive active drug therapy, perhaps at a high dose. This potential source of bias may seem to be outside the main concern of this chapter, the handling of treatment withdrawals and dropouts. However, the outcomes omitted often reflect adverse effects or death from other causes, which in turn lead to withdrawal, if not from the study, from the assigned treatment.

Problems that may arise in the interpretation of secondary analyses are illustrated by the reports on the Anturane Reinfarction Trial Research Group (1978, 1980). Anturane (sulfinpyrazone) and placebo were compared in this trial relative to the prevention of secondary attacks of myocardial infarction after at least one previous infarction. Correspondence in the *New England Journal of Medicine* and a paper by Temple and Pledger (1980) raise a number of issues about the exclusion of events and patients from study. Most relevant to our discussion is the grouping of the patients by whether or not they finished the prescribed course of treatment, as presented by Armitage (1983).

First, the perspective emphasized here of regarding the dropout rate as an outcome variable was taken. The number of patients who failed to complete their full course of treatment was compared among the 816 initially randomized to placebo as compared to the nearly equal number, 813, initially randomized to Anturane. The number of withdrawals from treatment were similar, 220 from the placebo group and 195 from the Anturane group. The reasons for withdrawal were also found to be similar. Data were given so that a comparison can be based on the total number of deaths in the randomization groups, namely, 89 for the placebo group and 74 for the Anturane group. The frequency of death is less for the Anturane group, but not by an amount that approaches statistical significance. In fact, the significance level $p = 0.22$ for a two-sided test using a standard normal deviate.

One complication that arose in this trial was that it was found that 33 patients who were randomized to placebo and 38 patients who were randomized to Anturane did not meet the eligibility criteria for the study. Again, these frequencies are similar for the two groups. It might seem that this would indicate that these patients could be omitted from further analysis, yet the possibility for bias exists, since it may be more likely that ineligibility with respect to some entry criterion may come to light under closer scrutiny as a result of a poor response to treatment. Four deaths in the placebo group and ten in the Anturane group were among patients found to be ineligible. Omission of ineligible patients would leave subgroups of eligible patients numbering 783 and 775 in the placebo and Anturane groups, with 85 and 64 deaths, respectively. The omission of more deaths, both in terms of frequency and proportion, in the Anturane group than in the placebo group has made the difference in the relative frequencies of death more pronounced, 0.026 instead of 0.018, although still not statistically significant ($p = 0.08$).

At the outset of this clinical trial it was decided to exclude events occurring within the first 7 days of treatment and more than 7 days after the end of treatment. This led to the exclusion of an additional 23 deaths from the placebo group and 20 from the Anturane group. This restriction imposed on the analysis led to a comparison between subgroups of the original randomization groups with 57 deaths omitted. The remaining numbers of deaths in the placebo and Anturane subgroups were 62 and 44 out of the 783 and 775 eligible subjects, respectively ($p = 0.08$).

Even though the deletions because of ineligibility or restriction of the time interval have seemed reasonable and of the same order of magnitude in each group, the effect on the analysis has been to make the estimated effect of Anturane more significant. Comparisons of subgroups are of interest, but great care should be taken in their interpretation, which at best can be suggestive of effects to be investigated further. The primary, more definitive, comparison is the one made between the original randomization groups, which led to a significance level of 0.22 for the Anturane example with death as the outcome variable.

3.5 Comparison of Baseline Variables

One basic comparison that should always be made in a clinical trial is the dropouts with the patients who complete a trial using baseline information collected at entry into the trial. If no significant differences are found with respect to variables that are possible precursors or predictors of the major outcome variables in the clinical trial, at least there is no evidence that the information from the trial is representative only of "completers."

If significant differences are found, the interpretation is more difficult and this casts doubts on the generalizability of the results. Should the results for completers be adjusted on the basis of baseline differences to be representative of the population mixture of completers and dropouts? Or should the difference in baseline values be explored to see if there is a selection bias toward completers in one of the treatment groups?

Suppose, for instance, that the completers and dropouts differ with respect to a baseline observation on a variable that is also measured at the end of the study for the patients who complete the study. Suppose that there are more dropouts in the placebo group. Suppose further that the baseline variable is proposed for use as a covariate to adjust for the unequal distribution among the active treatment and placebo groups. A covariance adjustment on the baseline variable would tend to adjust away any apparent treatment difference, when in fact it could be interpreted as indirect evidence of a treatment effect. Whether or not a patient drops out may be related to the baseline reading, or the reaction of the patient or the patient's physician to that reading. If the reading is abnormal, whether because of some underlying health condition or as a result of inherent random variation, the patient may be more apt to drop out under the suspicion, or knowledge in the absence of blinding, of an assignment to the placebo group. This tendency would make the active treatment group among completers worse off at baseline, and the baseline readings would become imperfect indicators of treatment assignment as opposed to predictors of outcome which are independent of treatment received.

This argument is speculative, but it illustrates the difficulty of interpretation when comparisons are made between subgroups other than the original randomization groups, in this case between completers and dropouts. It also illustrates the perspective that the dropout rate, and variables correlated with it, should be thought of as potential dependent variables for comparisons of treatment groups, not just as possible adjustment variables.

3.6 Analyses by Level of Adherence

When different treatments in an experiment consist of different doses of the same drug, including a dose of zero for the control group, it is desirable to analyze the data relative to a monotonic trend over increasing doses. In many clinical trials it is intended that all patients randomized to the active treatment group receive the same treatment regimen. However, if the active treatment is primarily a drug treatment, these patients actually receive different doses because of different levels of adherence to the treatment regimen or because of withdrawals from treatment, perhaps in accord with the protocol because of adverse effects. If it is possible to estimate the amount of drug received, it is possible to examine the data for evidence of a dose-response relationship.

Once again, care must be exercised. Different effects could have been observed because of different doses received, whatever the reason. On the other hand, different doses could have been taken as a response to different levels of effect with the original treatment regimen. If no dose effect is observed, this would support a conclusion of no treatment effect, provided that no difference in effect is observed in the primary comparison between the groups of patients randomized to active treatment and control. If a dose response is observed in the absence of differences among randomization groups, the dose response would be interpreted as only suggestive since evidence for it comes from a secondary analysis, which could also be interpreted as an indication of differential responses of patients to the treatment regimens.

Methods of carrying out analyses of dose-response curves are presented in Chapters 4 and 6. Analyses relative to levels of adherence are discussed in a report of the Committee for the Assessment of Biometric Aspects of Controlled Trials of Hypoglycemic Agents (Gilbert et al., 1975). One method presented in the latter report, referred to as the relative allocation method, consists of assigning a proportion of each patient's exposure and a proportion of each death to each of the several treatments involved based on relative times on the treatment regimens. The cardiovascular death rate for those who complied completely to the prescribed tolbutamide regimen was 21%, compared to 8% for patients randomized to tolbutamide who either did not adhere to the prescribed regimen completely or had a dose modification. Computation of this last rate utilized the relative allocation approach. The cardiovascular death rate for those who were randomized to placebo and adhered completely to the prescribed regimen was 6%. These last two rates are significantly less than the first one, and provide evidence of a dose-response relationship for tolbutamide. However, this analysis can only be considered to be suggestive of a relationship between exposure to tolbutamide and cardiovascular death.

Another method of analysis by level of adherence discussed by Gilbert et al. (1975) is the survival modeling method, presented initially by Cox (1972) and modified by Kalbfleisch and Prentice (1973) (see also Chapter 11). This method incorporates baseline covariates, institutional indicators, and extent of exposure to each treatment into a comparison of death rates for pairs of treatments, as well as comparisons with no treatment. The model assumes that the death rate bears the same proportional relationship to time in the study for all patients, with the proportionality constant determined by covariates and treatment exposures.

In particular, the model gives the logarithm of the probability of death for the ith patient, $\log \lambda_i(t)$, as

$$\log \lambda_i(t) = \log \lambda(t) + \sum_{j=1}^{p} \beta_j x_{ij}, \qquad i = 1, 2, \ldots, n,$$

where $\lambda(t)$ is a common underlying hazard rate modified by the linear combination of x_{ij} variables. The x_{ij}'s were chosen to represent seven demographic and health status variables, 12 institutions, and four treatments, so $p = 23$. For the ith patient, each x_{ij} which represented a treatment was set equal to the proportion of time the ith patient was on that treatment, so an individual patient could have nonzero entries for all four of these independent variables. Individual estimates of the β's for the four treatment terms provided estimates of the logarithms of the ratios of the death rates for the corresponding treatments relative to no treatment. Differences between these β estimates gave similar comparisons between the treatments in the protocol, including placebo. Similar results were obtained with this method and the relative allocation method for the UDGP data.

3.7 Repeated Measures

It has been emphasized that in clinical trials, particularly pragmatic trials which are likely to extend over a long interval, observations may be taken at many different times. The pattern of response over time may be of interest, not just the final observation. Missing observations will not be uncommon. Multivariate methods have been developed for such settings. Of concern here is each patient for whom all observations after a certain time are missing, either because of a withdrawal from treatment after experiencing success or failure, or because of a dropout for other reasons.

One approach to data of this type is to fit a model to the response patterns of each patient who remains in the study for a minimum period. Then statistics that summarize the profile for each patient could be analyzed in a comparison of patients by treatment group to which they were randomized. For instance, if a linear response pattern provides a reasonable fit to the data for each patient, a slope could be estimated for each patient. Then the slope would be the dependent variable in a comparison of treatment groups.

An analysis of summary statistics that describes trends over time allows information on withdrawals and dropouts to be used along with that on completers. Weights may be incorporated into the analysis which reflect different lengths of time of participation. However, this approach depends on the formulation of an appropriate model to represent time patterns, and assumes that no drastic changes in patterns would have resulted if every patient had continued to the end of the trial.

3.8 Endpoint Analysis

For an early withdrawal due to treatment success or failure, the time interval would be short and the observation at the time of withdrawal, which would reflect success or failure, would be at one of the extremes. Thus for early withdrawals the time and level of the last observation may reflect treatment efficacy. One approach to analysis uses only these data on time and level of last observation for all the subjects, completers as well as early withdrawals. Such an analysis is called an "endpoint" analysis.

For some trials, the long-term effectiveness of therapy may be the primary interest, but without regard to the time at which it is achieved. Moreover, the protocol may call for dosage adjustments during the early part of a trial, with increases in the dosage if no early response is observed, and decreases as a result of adverse reactions. This is common in clinical trials of psychoactive drugs, as discussed by Metzler and Schooley (1981). Since the dosage schedule would not be the same for all patients in such a trial, dose-response curves would not be of interest, but the level of response achieved would be. These trials often call for the withdrawal of patients for whom an upper bound is reached because of treatment failure, provided that a high score represents relatively severe disease. This is the case with several mood scales, such as the Hamilton Depression Scale, and with blood pressure as a measure of hypertension. Some protocols also call for the withdrawal of treatment successes who attain a low severity score because treatment is no longer needed.

In trials like these, data on early withdrawals and completers sometimes are analyzed together by confining the analysis to the last observation. However, when withdrawal is based on an extreme value of the dependent variable, which is used to indicate success or failure, a bias is introduced. The extreme level that triggers withdrawal might regress toward the mean if the patient remained in the trial. This regression effect is discussed in Chapter 1. A ranking of last observations, which takes the time of withdrawal into account for early withdrawals, but is not as sensitive to the magnitude of extreme observations as a parametric procedure, would be less subject to bias. Thus the full set of data may be analyzed together, using ranking procedures on "endpoint" data.

Gould (1980) proposed a ranking procedure for endpoint analysis that enables the last responses of treatment withdrawals, dropouts, and completers all to be ordered in the same scoring system. With Gould's approach, a score of L is assigned to early withdrawals, a score of U_1 to withdrawals due to intolerance and a score of U_2 to withdrawals due to lack of therapeutic effect. Completers receive scores equal to their final observations. For definiteness, assume that a low value indicates greater effectiveness than a high value. Any values may be assigned to L, U_1, and U_2 provided that $L <$ all final observations on completers $< U_1 \leq U_2$, since only the order of the scores is used in analysis with procedures based on ranks or ordered categories.

Pledger and Hall (1982) criticized the choice of a score for treatment intolerance near or equal to that for treatment failure. They reasoned that a potent drug might have the potential both for effective treatment and for adverse reaction. Gould's procedure would give withdrawals scores that would balance out with low and high rankings. This might cause the potential of the drug for effective treatment to be overlooked. In other words, they questioned Gould's scoring of withdrawals for treatment intolerance in the setting of an explanatory clinical trial.

In response, Gould (1982) took the perspective of a pragmatic trial. He reasoned that scoring treatment intolerance as a treatment failure or near failure makes sense because a drug that is not tolerated by a patient would not continue to be used by that patient, and could not prove to be effective for that patient in the long run. Any scoring system, including Gould's or a modification of it in the light of the comments of Pledger and Hall, is appropriate as long as it represents a preference ordering of treatment responses in a given setting.

Gould ranked all early withdrawals due to treatment failure equally. Alternatively, those occurring at the first time of observation could be given the highest ranks, either tied or ranked by the level of a dependent variable at the time of withdrawal. The next highest set of ranks could be assigned to those who withdraw due to failure at the second time, and so on. Then a set of lower ranks could be assigned to completers based on their endpoint levels. Still-lower sets of ranks could be assigned to withdrawals because of treatment success in reverse order by time of withdrawal. Unlike Gould's proposal, this procedure takes time of withdrawal into account.

Since the time of the last observation is given precedence over the level of that observation in the ranking, it presumably is less subject to bias due to the effect of regression toward the mean.

Another proposal for analysis provides for the last observation on completers to be projected forward to an estimated time of failure, relative to either a horizontal or decreasing line relating projected treatment responses to time. Then the time of withdrawal for early failures and the projected time of withdrawal for completers could be entered into a survival analysis. Patients who neither withdraw because of treatment failure nor exhibit a pattern indicative of failure in the future could be regarded as censored on the right. No allowance would be made for early withdrawals due to treatment success. Dropouts not known to be related to treatment response could be projected forward also. Since several survival analysis methods are extensions of common ranking methods, this is in the spirit of Gould's procedure but takes time of withdrawal into account for early withdrawals as does the alternative ranking procedure just described. However, this survival analysis proposal places completers on a projected failure time scale instead of representing their responses on an equally spaced rank scale.

4 SUMMARY

Approaches to statistical analysis have been discussed which incorporate information on withdrawals for reasons related to treatment and dropouts for other reasons into the overall evaluation of a clinical trial. It has been emphasized that the primary analysis and main conclusions of a trial should be based on a comparison of treatment groups, including control or placebo groups, as formed by the original randomization, even if the treatment of some subjects is subsequently modified. Subgroup comparisons or analyses by level of adherence can be suggestive of treatment effects and may strengthen conclusions if they are consistent with the results of the randomization group comparisons.

In order for group comparisons to lead to evidence on the direct effect of a drug in initial explanatory trials, withdrawals and dropouts should be minimized by strict entry criteria for patients, a relative short trial, and a simple treatment protocol. In longer pragmatic clinical trials, treatment strategies are compared, a more diverse sample of patients is sought in order to make generalizations to those encountered in practice, and withdrawals are viewed as informative responses about treatment regimens.

REFERENCES

Anturane Reinfarction Research Group (1978). Sulfinpyrazone in the prevention of cardiac death after myocardial infarction. *New England J. of Med. 298*, 289–295.

Anturane Reinfarction Research Group (1980). Sulfinpyrazone in the prevention of sudden death after myocardial infarction. *New England J. of Med. 302*, 250–256.

Armitage, P. (1983). Exclusions, losses to follow-up, and withdrawals in clinical trials. In *Clinical Trials: Issues and Approaches* (S. H. Shapiro and T. A. Louis, eds.), Marcel Dekker, New York.

Bartlett, R. H., D. W. Roloff, R. G. Cornell, A. F. Andrews, P. W. Dillon, and J. B. Zwischenberger (1985). Extracorporeal circulation in neonatal respiratory failure: a prospective randomized trial. *Pediatrics 76*, 479–487.

Cox, D. R. (1972). Regression models and life tables (with discussion). *J. Roy. Statist. Soc. B 34*, 187–220.

Gilbert, J. P., P. Meier, C. L. Rümke, R. Saracci, M. Zelen, and C. White, (1975). Report of the Committee for the Assessment of Biometric Aspects of Controlled Trials of Hypoglycemic Agents. *J. Amer. Med. Assoc. 231*, 583–608.

Gould, A. L. (1980). A new approach to the analysis of clinical drug trials with withdrawals. *Biometrics 36*, 721–727.

Gould, A. L. (1982). Letter to the editor on withdrawals from clinical trials. *Biometrics 38*, 277–278.

Kalbfleisch, J. D., and R. L. Prentice (1973). Marginal likelihoods based on Cox's regression and life model. *Biometrika 60*, 267–277.

Meinert, C. L. (1986). *Clinical Trials: Design, Conduct, and Analysis*. Oxford University Press, New York.

Metzler, C. M., and G. L. Schooley (1981). Design and analysis of clinical trials of psychoactive drugs. In *Statistics in the Pharmaceutical Industry* (C. R. Buncher and J.-Y. Tsay, eds.). Marcel Dekker, New York.

Pledger, G., and D. Hall (1982). Letter to the editor on withdrawals from clinical trials. *Biometrics 38*, 276–277.

Sackett, D. L. (1983). On some prerequisites for a successful trial. In *Clinical Trials: Issues and Approaches* (S. H. Shapiro and T. A. Louis, eds.), Marcel Dekker, New York.

Temple, R., and G. W. Pledger (1980). The FDA's critique of the Anturane Reinfarction Trial. *New England J. Med. 303*, 1488–1492.

10

Group Sequential Methods in Clinical Trials

PETER C. O'BRIEN Mayo Clinic, Rochester, Minnesota

1 INTRODUCTION AND HISTORICAL OVERVIEW

In this chapter we discuss the use of group sequential methods in evaluating drug efficacy. The therapy against which the new drug (*experimental therapy*) will be compared will be referred to as the *standard therapy*, with the recognition that in some instances standard therapy may consist of no intervention and be implemented using a placebo. Typically, the evaluation of a new drug in human subjects is performed in three phases. Phase I is a dose-seeking pilot study that evaluates pharmacokinetics and toxicity. When safe dose levels have been established, the drug is administered to a relatively small series of patients (phase II) to determine if there is sufficient preliminary evidence of efficacy (relative to historical data) to warrant further study. Ideally, in phase III, patients are randomly assigned to experimental or standard therapy in such a manner that neither the patient nor the physician is aware of the therapy used.

Discussion will focus primarily on group sequential methods in phase III trials, with only brief mention of phase II trials. Thus far, group sequential methods have not been found useful in phase I studies.

Patient recruitment into a phase III study usually is done over an extended period, so that data that measure response to treatment will accumulate during the course of the trial. Because of obvious ethical and cost considerations (measured in terms of money, time, or patient availability for future studies), it is desirable and often mandatory to monitor the data periodically as the trial progresses to determine if the evidence for or against drug efficacy is sufficient to warrant termination of the trial. There is also the analogous problem of monitoring for side effects. Armitage et al. (1969) demonstrated that if one repeatedly performs the conventional, single-sample test procedure during the course of the study, the overall probability of type I error will be increased over the nominal level used at each test. For example, five tests each performed at the $\alpha = 0.05$ level may result in an overall probability of 0.14 that an inactive drug would erroneously be judged efficacious.

The earliest procedures designed specifically for the sequential monitoring of the data while controlling the overall probability of type I error were *fully sequential*, with a statistical test performed after each observation. A prominent class of fully sequential procedures is defined by the *sequential probability ratio test* (SPRT). The test statistic, consisting of the ratio of the likelihoods under the null and alternative hypotheses (assuming both can be formulated as simple hypotheses), is compared to easily computed upper and lower boundaries. If either boundary is crossed, the study is terminated, accepting H_0 or H_a according to which boundary was violated.

Although fully sequential procedures occupy a prominent place in statistical theory, they have been used infrequently in practice. One impractical property of the SPRT is the absence of an upper boundary on the maximal number of observations that may be needed to complete the trial. Another is the impracticality of testing after each observation. These limitations have led to the advent of *group sequential methods*, with statistical analyses conducted only periodically during the study. For an early discussion of this approach, see Samuel-Cahn (1974a, 1974b).

One method for generating such group sequential procedures is to treat the sums of random variables accumulated between successive tests as the basic observation, then applying methods developed within the fully sequential context. Whitehead and Stratton (1983) give an extensive account of such procedures, including a discussion of triangular boundaries that impose an upper limit on the number of tests. Perhaps because of the somewhat greater complexity of the method, to date this approach has not been frequently used.

2 CLASSICAL GROUP SEQUENTIAL TEST PROCEDURES

2.1 Commonly Used Procedures

In describing the most commonly used group sequential procedures, we start by assuming an artificial, oversimplified setting. Specifically, suppose that groups of n subjects are to be recruited into each arm of the study, with a maximum of $2K$ groups (where n and K are prespecified numbers). The observation of the ith subject receiving the experimental treatment in group k, denoted by $X_{Eik}(i = 1, \ldots, n; k = 1, \ldots, K)$, is assumed to be observed immediately after administering the drug and to follow a normal distribution with mean μ_E and known variance σ^2. The notation for the standard therapy is similar. Extensions to more realistic settings are straightforward as described in Section 2.4.

For $k = 1, \ldots, K$ define T_k to be the usual single sample statistic for testing $H_0 : \mu_E = \mu_S$ against the alternative hypothesis $H_a : \mu_E \neq \mu_S$ after recruitment of $2k$ groups of subjects:

$$T_k = \frac{\sum_{l=1}^{k}(\bar{X}_{El} - \bar{X}_{Sl})\sqrt{n/2k}}{\sigma}.$$

We shall consider only the case of two-sided tests explicitly. The commonly used group sequential procedures are based on a boundary $\{(C_1, \alpha), \ldots, C(K, \alpha)\}$ and are defined as follows. Enter the first group of subjects and compute T_1. If $T_1 > C(1, \alpha)$, terminate the trial and reject H_0. Otherwise, recruit the second group of subjects. Continuing in this manner, compute T_k after the kth group is entered ($k = 1, 2, \ldots, K - 1$). If $T_k > C(k, \alpha)$, terminate the trial and reject H_0. Otherwise, recruit the $(k + 1)$st group. The trial ends upon completing the Kth test, with H_0 rejected if only if $T_K > C(K, \alpha)$. The boundary is chosen so that the overall probability of rejecting when H_0 is true is α.

Three of the most commonly used boundaries are listed below:

A. Constant boundary (Pocock, 1977):

$$C(k, \alpha) = C_P(K, \alpha), \qquad k = 1, \ldots, K$$

B. Monotone decreasing boundary (O'Brien and Fleming, 1979):

$$C(k, \alpha) = C_{O-F}(K, \alpha)\sqrt{K/k}$$

C. Ad hoc boundary (Haybittle, 1971; Peto et al., 1976):

$$C_k(k, \alpha) = \begin{cases} C_{H/P}, & k = 1, \ldots, K - 1 \\ Z_{1-\alpha/2}, & k = K. \end{cases}$$

where $Z_{1-\alpha/2}$ is the $(1 - \alpha/2)$ percentile of the standard normal distribution, and $C_{H/P}$ is a suitably large constant (e.g., $Z_{0.99}$).

The boundaries are provided for $K = 2$, 3, 4, and 5 in Table 1 and displayed graphically in Figure 1. The Pocock procedure offers the greatest opportunity for terminating at the outset. Conversely, however, when early termination does not occur (when all $2nK$ subjects are required), the Pocock procedure differs noticeably from the single-sample decision rule. The O'Brien–Fleming boundary is based on Monte Carlo simulations of 10,000 experiments. It attempts to mimic the manner in which a monitor-

Table 1 Group Sequential Stopping Bounds

	Pocock		O'Brien and Fleming		Haybittle and Peto	
k	Z	p	Z	p	Z	p
			$K = 2$			
1	2.178	0.0294	2.782	0.0054	2.576	0.0100
2	2.178	0.0294	1.967	0.0492	1.960	0.0500
			$K = 3$			
1	2.289	0.0221	3.438	0.0006	2.576	0.0100
2	2.289	0.0221	2.431	0.0151	2.576	0.0100
3	2.289	0.0221	1.985	0.0471	1.960	0.0100
			$K = 4$			
1	2.361	0.0182	4.084	5×10^{-5}	3.291	0.0010
2	2.361	0.0182	2.888	0.0039	3.291	0.0010
3	2.361	0.0182	2.358	0.0184	3.291	0.0010
4	2.361	0.0182	2.042	0.0412	1.960	0.0500
			$K = 5$			
1	2.413	0.0158	4.555	5×10^{-6}	3.291	0.0010
2	2.413	0.0158	3.221	0.0013	3.291	0.0010
3	2.413	0.0158	2.630	0.0085	3.291	0.0010
4	2.413	0.0158	2.277	0.0228	3.291	0.0010
5	2.413	0.0158	2.037	0.0417	1.960	0.0500

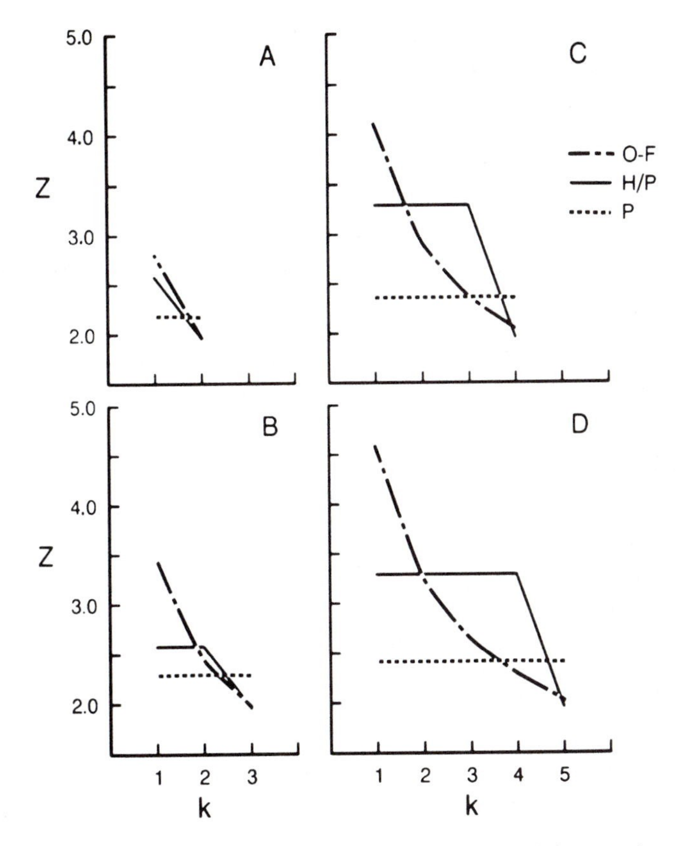

Figure 1 Companion of 3 group sequential stopping rules for designs allowing for 1, 2, 3, or 4 interim tests.

ing committee might approach early termination, requiring strongly convincing evidence of a difference to terminate the study initially, relaxing the stopping criteria during the course of the study, and adopting nearly a single-sample decision rule at the end (if the study is not terminated early). The possibilities for terminating at the first test with this procedure become remote for $K \geq 5$. In some applications, this may be viewed as an advantage. However, it may be unacceptable in others (see Section 4). Although the operating characteristics will be virtually unaffected if the decision rule is modified to stop after the first test when the corresponding single-sample p-value is less than 0.001, this type of ad hoc approach may be unappealing.

The Haybittle–Peto procedure represents something of a middle ground between the Pocock and the O'Brien–Fleming procedures. A disadvantage is the somewhat ad hoc choice for the interim testing levels. Another is the uncertainty regarding the overall probability of type I error, which in any case will exceed the specified level. Entries in the table were guided by the results presented by Fleming, Harrington, and O'Brien (1984).

Clearly, the number of group sequential rules that one could consider are unlimited. In fact, one could obtain boundaries based on Monte Carlo simulations designed specifically to meet the requirements of a given trial. The important consideration for any choice of boundary is that it be specified in a study protocol in advance of data collection. Some additional approaches to group sequential testing are described below.

2.2 Extensions of the Commonly Used Procedures

In an attempt to formalize the Haybittle–Peto approach, one may consider a procedure in which the null probability of terminating the trial at the kth test ($k = 1, \ldots, K-1$) is constant, $\alpha'/(K-1)$, say. For a given overall probability of type I error (α) and a specified probability of early termination (α'), one can determine the nominal significance levels (which will *not* be constant) for each group sequential test. This approach is discussed by Fleming, Harrington, and O'Brien (1984), who provide tables for the necessary nominal significance levels for values of K up to 10.

An advantage of this approach is that, under certain circumstances, the investigator is able to change the maximum number of tests (K) during the course of the study. The effect of such a change on the test procedure is to change the nominal significance level at the last test. This may be desirable, for example, if a monitoring committee is meeting at specified intervals (e.g, every 6 months) and the patient accrual rate is slower than expected, so that the maximal number of tests conducted will exceed the number anticipated initially.

In addition to achieving greater flexibility regarding the number of tests conducted, one might also wish to vary the time points at which the tests are conducted. For example, one may wish to review the data at regularly spaced time points in conjunction with periodic meetings of a monitoring committee, in which case the group sizes occurring between successive tests may be unequal. Although this situation represents a departure from the assumptions implicit in the group sequential procedures discussed thus far, it has been shown that the effect on size and power of the Pocock and the O'Brien–Fleming procedures is negligible (DeMets and Gail, 1985). A modification of these decision rules was developed by Lan and DeMets (1983) which allows the investigator to "spend" the overall error rate at various time points during the conduct of the study. The number of tests undertaken, and the timing of these tests, need not be specified in advance. Although they can depend on such factors as the study accrual rate, the number and timing of tests cannot depend on the data.

One objection to formal statistical stopping rules is that they tend to oversimplify the way in which the decision to terminate a trial actually is made. In practice many considerations will typically affect the decision whether or not to terminate early. To accommodate this concern, Jennison and Turnbull (1984) proposed exploiting the equivalence between hypothesis testing and confidence intervals. Specifically, one may formulate probability statements about the test statistics as a function of the unknown parameters,

$$\Pr[T_i \leq C(i,\alpha) \text{ for all } i = 1, \ldots, K \mid \mu_E - \mu_S] = \alpha,$$

and then invert it,

$$\Pr[T_i(\mu_E - \mu_S) \leq (C(i,\alpha); i = 1, \ldots, K] = \alpha,$$

to obtain a sequence of confidence intervals for $\mu_E - \mu_S$ having the property that all intervals will contain $\mu_E - \mu_S$ with probability $1 - \alpha$. Thus, at each review of the data, one may consider the values of $\mu_E - \mu_S$ which are consonant with the data and incorporate this information with other relevant considerations in deciding whether or not to terminate the trial.

2.3 Application to Clinical Trials

Thus far, consideration has been given to group sequential methods in the greatly oversimplified situation in which the endpoint was assumed to be (i) normally distributed, (ii) immediately observable, and (iii) univariate. In practice, of course, none of these assumptions are likely to be appropriate. Often the endpoint of interest is dichotomous (e.g, occurrence or nonoccurrence of tumor remission, dead/alive, success/failure). This is not a serious problem since, asymptotically, the sample proportions will be normally distributed. The appropriateness of the normal theory procedures is further indicated by small-sample simulations [see O'Brien and Fleming (1979) and Pocock (1977)], which indicate that the procedures provide accurate control over the size of the test even in small-scale studies.

A more formidable problem is the application of the methods to the study of chronic disease in which the endpoint is not immediately observable (e.g., long-term survivorship). In this situation, the natural extension of the classical group sequential tests would be to perform log-rank tests periodically, comparing the resulting relative deviate statistic to one of the group sequential boundaries described previously. Some theoretical justification for this approach is that the resulting sequence of test statistics can be described by a Brownian motion process with independent increments. The analogy with Brownian motion assumes that a constant number of deaths occur between successive tests. However, Monte Carlo simulations indicate that the size of the test is well controlled when this assumption is violated (DeMets and Gail, 1985).

The third assumption that must be considered is that the endpoint is univariate. In the conduct of a clinical trial, many aspects of drug safety and efficacy are of interest and it is undesirable to attempt to focus attention entirely on a single primary endpoint. The problem of multiple endpoints within the context of single-sample test procedures is not new [see Tukey (1960) and Meier (1975)]. For the conventional single-sample situation, an overall test for drug efficacy may be obtained by combining the individual normalized test statistics [see O'Brien (1984) and Pocock, Geller and Tsiatis (1987)]:

$$T = \frac{J'R^{-1}Z}{J'R^{-1}J},$$

where $J' = (1, \ldots, 1)$, R^{-1} is the estimated correlation matrix of individual measurements, and Z is the vector of normalized univariate test statistics. The distribution of T is closely approximated (even in small samples) by a t-distribution with $n - 2k$ df, where k is the number of endpoints. For endpoints that are not normally distributed, it may be possible to transform to normality or the observations could be replaced with their ranks. For censored data, log-rank scores may be substituted for the observation times.

For n sufficiently large, this approach could be extended to the group sequential setting in a straightforward manner. Specifically, at each test, one would compare T to the appropriate group sequential boundary. Initially (for small values of $n - 2k$) the distribution of T may be somewhat volatile, which in turn could cause an unacceptable increase in the probability of type I error for procedures that emphasize early stopping (e.g, Pocock's procedure). Conversely, the effect on procedures such as the O'Brien–Fleming procedure would be much less pronounced. This problem of multiple endpoints in group sequential studies is an area that warrants further study.

2.4 Point and Interval Estimation

Upon completing a group sequential test, it is desirable to obtain point and interval estimates of the drug effect on the various measurements studied. Just as a group sequential design will alter the operating characteristics of the usual test procedures, it also alters the properties of conventional single sample estimators. In general, studies that are terminated early will tend to overstate treatment differences (since, by definition, early termination occurs only when drug differences seem to be large). Conversely, group sequential studies that run their full course will tend to understate drug differences. Unfortunately, although the need for taking repeated testing into account in assigning significance levels is well recognized by statisticians, the importance of using corresponding, unbiased estimation procedures is often overlooked.

Consider first the problem of interval estimation. Procedures for phase II studies have been proposed by Jennison and Turnbull (1983) and Larson (1984). [Group sequential test procedures for phase II studies have been discussed by Fleming (1982).] An analogous procedure for phase III studies was proposed by Tsiatis et al. (1984). These procedures recognize that the relevant sample space at the conclusion of a group sequential study is two-dimensional, consisting of the number of tests undertaken ($k^* = 1, \ldots, K$) and the value of the test statistic at the last test (T^*). The approach is to transform to one dimension by ordering the sample space, first ordering on k^* and then ordering on T^*. Formally, one obtains $(k^*, T^*) \to Z(k^*, T^*)$, where $k_1 > k_2$ implies that $Z(k_1, T_1) < Z(k_2, T_2)$ and $k_1 = k_2 = k$, $T_1 > T_2$ implies that $Z(k, T_1) > (k, T_2)$. Conceptually, one inverts the probability statements about $Z(k^*, T^*)$ and the parameter of interest (θ) to obtain confidence intervals for θ. In practice, these procedures require special computing programs that are not available as part of standard statistical packages but which may be obtained from the respective authors.

One may also use these methods to obtain point estimates of parameters of interest. Specifically, obtaining 50% confidence limits will provide estimates that are "median unbiased." That is, the estimate will be greater than the true value with probability 0.5 and less than the true value with probability 0.5.

In addition to computational complexity, a limitation of these procedures is that the general method for ordering the sample space is ad hoc in nature and leads to confidence intervals that have intuitively undesirable properties. In particular, if a study terminates at the first test, the sequential adjusted confidence interval will be identically the same as the naive single-sample interval. This problem has been discussed by Chang and O'Brien (1986), who propose an alternative ordering based on maximum likelihood theory.

Perhaps owing to the newness or the computational complexity of the procedures described above, they seem to be rarely used in practice. A simple alternative approach is to incorporate interval estimation as part of the original study design using the repeated confidence interval approach described previously.

3 DECISION THEORETIC APPROACHES

Thus far, attention has been restricted to group sequential methods within the context of classical statistics. The focus has been on testing a null hypothesis of no treatment effect, with the operating characteristics of the test described by the probabilities of type I and type II errors. In practice, the information resulting from this type of analysis of a single clinical trial is informally combined with other sources of information to arrive at decisions regarding use or continued development of the new drug. Data analysis algorithms that aim at a more direct role in this decision making process are considered next.

3.1 Optimizing the Population Proportion Receiving Better Treatment

Assume that the number (N) of patients with the disease under study who might potentially receive the new treatment can be specified. In practice, a rough estimate of N will usually suffice. Some of these patients (n) will be entered into the trial, and n_E and n_S of these will receive the experimental and standard drugs, respectively. It is assumed that, upon conclusion of the trial, one drug will be selected and used for the remaining $N - n$ patients. Thus, one approach to the design of the trial and corresponding data analysis is to maximize the total number of subjects receiving the superior therapy. This expectation must of necessity take expectations over a priori distributions because it is unknown which drug is superior. Although the assumptions regarding the endpoints are often unrealistic, as is the assumption that the selected therapy will be used exclusively, these procedures may be considered as providing approximate guidelines for the design and analysis of the types of studies more typically encountered.

Canner (1970) proposed a fixed-sample-size procedure for the situation in which equal numbers of patients are assigned to each treatment in the experimental phase and the endpoint is dichotomous and immediately observable. A more general method not requiring the equal allocation of patients was developed by Berry and Pearson (1985). Group sequential analogs do not seem to be available at this time.

3.2 An Alternative Bayesian Procedure

One might argue (Anscombe, 1963; Berger and Berry, 1985) that when a physician chooses a therapy for his or her patients, the decision is based on a belief that the selected therapy is probably the most efficacious available—and that the probability statement inherent in this approach is the posterior

Bayes probability based on prior beliefs and available data. In this context, the primary goal of a clinical trial is to obtain sufficient evidence to ascertain if the experimental therapy is better than the standard therapy with a suitably high posterior probability.

To illustrate, consider the following example (Berger and Berry, 1985). Suppose that a randomized double-blind experiment is performed to compare the efficacy of an experimental drug with that of standard therapy. Specifically, it will be assumed that randomization occurs within pairs of patients, and after 24 hours, which therapy was associated with greater improvement in disease status is determined. In this admittedly simplistic setting, the results in the initial 18 patients are listed in Table 2. The first step in the proposed analysis is to specify a suitable prior probability (p) that H_0 is true (E not better than S). In this example, $p = 1/2$.

Table 2 Results in 18 Pairs of Patients

Pair number	Preference	Preference for E minus preference for S	Unconditional error probability	Final probability that treatment E is better
1	E	1	—	0.750
2	S	0	—	0.500
3	E	1	—	0.687
4	E	2	—	0.812
5	E	3	—	0.891
6	S	2	—	0.773
7	E	3	—	0.855
8	E	4	—	0.910
9	E	5	—	0.945
10	E	6	—	0.967
11	E	7	—	0.981
12	E	8	—	0.989
13	E	9	—	0.994
14	S	8	—	0.982
15	E	9	—	0.989
16	E	10	—	0.994
17	E	11	—	0.996
18	E	12	0.05	0.998

Source: Berger and Berry (1985).

Computation of a posterior probability also requires specifications regarding the probability (θ) that in a given pair E will be observed to be superior to S. We will assume that θ is uniformly distributed over the interval (0,1). For this model and the data at hand, the posterior probability that H_0 is true is given in Table 2. In monitoring the accumulating data, one could have used a group sequential approach. For example, evaluating the data after every 5 pairs, it would have become apparent at the second analysis (after 10 pairs) that the posterior probability that treatment E was superior was 0.967; the odds that E is better is $0.967/0.033 = 29.3$. It is important to note that for this type of analysis, the motivation for using a group sequential rather than fully sequential approach is entirely based on convenience. There is no penalty for repeated looks at the data and, in fact, the analysis completely ignores the number of times the data have been analyzed and the preceding (or future) considerations regarding termination of the trial.

3.3 Decision Theoretic Procedures for Drug Development Programs

Thus far we have assumed that the purpose of the trial and corresponding data analysis was to evaluate safety or efficacy with a view toward obtaining the definitive answer to these questions. We now turn attention to the situation where a pharmaceutical company is in the process of developing an experimental drug and wishes to perform internal evaluations to determine if continuing developmental efforts are justified. This phase of the investigation is therefore assumed to be separate from, and well in advance of, publications in the medical literature and presentations to the FDA for permission to market the drug. The method described below [and discussed in greater detail by Berry and Ho (1988)] is designed to allow early termination of the development program if interim results are sufficiently negative. The simplistic setting of Section 2 (and corresponding notation) is used in which response to therapy is observed immediately and normally distributed with known variance. Now, however, one asks at each interim analysis: Are the results sufficiently negative to terminate the development effort? Letting $\zeta = \mu_E - \mu_S$, assume that $\zeta \sim N(\Delta, \sigma_0^2)$. The possible decisions at any point in the trial are

d_1. terminate development
d_2. do not terminate

The future loss associated with d_i is $L_i(\zeta)$, $i = 1, 2$. The consequences of attempting to market the drug are assumed to be reasonably approximated by

$$L_2(f) = \begin{cases} -C\zeta & \text{if } \zeta \geq 0 \\ L & \text{if } \zeta < 0, \end{cases}$$

where C and L are specified positive constants. The decision procedure takes the following form: Before initiating the trial, compute a quantity denoted by $R(v_0, 0)$ and undertake the trial only if $R(v_0, 0) < 0$. The study proceeds by admitting the first group of patients and concluding d_1 if $R(v_1, 1) = 0$ and d_2 otherwise. Continuing in this manner, the trial is completed and marketing of the drug pursued if and only if $R(v_k, k) < 0$, $k = 1, \ldots, K$. For any specified values of $\{C, L, \sigma^2, \sigma_0^2, \Delta, n, \text{ and } K\}$ the

Table 3 Stopping Boundaries for Various Values of K, n, Δ, and σ_0^2 with $C = 5000$, $L = 2000$, and $\sigma^2 = 2$[a]

K	n	σ_0^2	Δ	b_1	d_1	b_2	d_2	b_3	d_3
2	30	1	−1	−0.072		0.125			
					0.067		0.034		
			0	−0.139		0.091			
					0.067		0.033		
			1	−0.206		0.058			
		2	−1	−0.127		0.097			
					0.016		0.008		
			0	−0.143		0.089			
					0.017		0.008		
			1	−0.160		0.081			
2	60	1	−1	0.022		0.101			
					0.034		0.017		
			0	−0.012		0.085			
					0.033		0.017		
			1	−0.045		0.068			
3	20	1	−1	−0.478		−0.026		0.125	
					0.100		0.050		0.034
			0	−0.578		−0.076		0.091	
					0.100		0.050		0.033
			1	−0.678		−0.126		0.058	

Source: Berry and Ho (1988).
[a]The d_m are differences as Δ varies.

critical values of $\{R_k(v_k, k), k = 1, \ldots, K\}$ must be calculated by numerical interpretation. The relevant calculations are described by Berry and Ho (1988), who consider explicitly the case in which $K = 2$, $C = 5000$, $L = 2000$, $\sigma^2 = 2$, $n = 30$, $\sigma_0^2 = 1$, $\Delta = -1$, and the sampling cost is 1 unit per patient. For this situation, the optimal rule will result in completion of the study and marketing of the drug if and only if the difference in sample means exceeds -0.072 at the first test and exceeds 0.125 at the second test. Stopping boundaries for various alternative choices of K, n, Δ, and σ_0^2 with $C = 5000$, $L = 2000$, and $\sigma^2 = 2$ are listed in Table 3.

4 CONTROVERSIES

The advent of group sequential methods that are designed to meet the specific needs of investigators concerned with the monitoring of accumulating data in clinical trials is relatively recent. As the availability of such methods rapidly multiplies, there is a need to consider carefully what the needs really are. Disagreement on this point leads to different views on the appropriateness and relative usefulness of the methods that have been considered herein. In this part, some of the major controversies will be reviewed, with the discussion necessarily consisting mostly of generalities. Although this type of discussion may be illuminating and somewhat typical of the type of discussion found in much of the statistical literature on this subject, in practice the answers will depend on the specific needs of individual clinical trials and may vary greatly depending on the circumstances of each study. Although I have attempted to present both sides of the issues, my opinions are freely expressed and should be recognized as such.

4.1 Is It Desirable to Terminate a Study Early?

Many advocates of group sequential methods seem to take as a given that the obvious answer to this question is an unqualified yes. There are strong motivations for monitoring accumulating data. The ethical need to terminate a study when the welfare of the patient is at stake and the superiority of one therapy over another has been clearly demonstrated is unquestioned. The opportunity to terminate early may also result in cost savings which, in some instances, may be substantial. Furthermore, an early answer to the scientific question at issue may facilitate the initiation of additional studies, either as a result of the completed study indicating new areas of investigation or freeing up patients to participate.

However, from a scientific standpoint, there are often powerful incentives for continuing a trial. Because the ultimate goal of the science is patient care, these incentives also translate into ethical arguments.

1. One of the disadvantages of early termination is that it may preclude obtaining satisfactory answers to secondary (but nonetheless important) questions pertaining to drug safety and efficacy. Typically, there are many such questions. However, as alluded to previously, a limitation of the group sequential method is that, of necessity, the goals of the study must be oversimplified, often resulting in the formal consideration of only a single endpoint.
2. A related and equally important concern is the need for subgroup analyses, because the drug efficacy and toxicity will often vary among different types of patients.
3. The use of group sequential monitoring rules necessitates a corresponding estimation strategy that will provide unbiased estimates of drug efficacy. In addition to greatly complicating the analysis, the need for such methods increases the difficulties of communicating study results to nonstatisticians.
4. The criterion that may be appropriate for addressing the immediate ethical question (which therapy should I select for my next patient?) may be less satisfactory for obtaining a definitive answer to the scientific questions. Although $p < 0.05$ or $p < 0.10$ may suffice for the former, $p < 0.01$ may be desirable for the latter.
5. When the endpoint of primary interest is survival, the long-term effect of therapy may not become apparent until the latter part of the trial and may differ substantially from the early effects. For example, some forms of therapy (surgery or chemotherapy) may be sufficiently hazardous that early (e.g., 1-year) mortality might actually be increased, with a benefit becoming apparent only much later (e.g., 5- to 10-year mortality). The converse, an early transient benefit with no subsequent difference in survival, is also a possibility.
6. The interpretation of "sequentially adjusted" p-values is often difficult to communicate to medical investigators. In fact, there is often disagreement among statisticians on this point [see Dupont (1983) and related discussion]. For example, interpretation of the results of a group sequential trial may be controversial if the trial did not terminate early and did not achieve statistical significance using a group sequential boundary, but the single-sample p-value is less than 0.05.
7. Finally, many investigators are reluctant to have their studies terminated early for reasons unrelated to either the ethical or the scientific issues that motivated the study, owing to the considerable effort re-

quired to launch a well-designed clinical trial and the practical need of providing stable financing both for themselves and for their supporting staff. Uncertainty regarding continuity of funding for *individual studies* raised by the possibility of early termination may jeopardize the long-term prospects for research *programs*. The answer to this question will vary from one study to the next.

Is it desirable to terminate a study early? Rather than attempt a simple, universally acceptable answer, I would recommend incorporating group sequential testing into the study design and choosing a boundary that appropriately reflects the perceived desirability of early termination.

4.2 What Is the Usefulness of Formal Stopping Rules in Studies Subject to Early Termination?

It is assumed for the present purposes that the decision has been made to review the accumulating data periodically during the course of a trial and that such review will be a consideration in deciding whether or not to terminate the trial. The question here is: Should the decision-making process regarding termination incorporate a formal algorithm, based entirely on a probability statement? One point of view is that the decision-making process should incorporate such an algorithm and, furthermore, the decision as to whether or not to terminate should depend entirely on the outcome of the corresponding statistical test. That is, one continues the study *if and only if* the agreed-upon group sequential test boundary has not been crossed. The rationale for this approach is that such discipline is required to make valid statements regarding the probability of type I error.

At the other extreme, one might argue that a decision to terminate a study early will depend on so many factors, many of which are difficult to quantify or even anticipate, that the decision should be recognized as inherently subjective. Thus any attempt to prespecify a decision-making algorithm is doomed to failure. Some of the factors that must be considered are the need to consider multiple endpoints, the feasibility of continuing the trial (e.g., the availability of patients, funding, or enthusiasm among the investigators), information obtained concurrently from similar studies, and availability of new alternative therapies.

As alluded to previously, some statisticians question the appropriateness and interpretability of "sequential p-values." Others go so far as to question the appropriateness of considering the probability of type I error at all in the context of clinical trials. Anscombe (1963) argues that because the purpose of a clinical trial is to identify the most effective therapy, the therapy that is observed to be most effective should be selected. Berger and Berry (1985) raise the fundamental issue regarding the appropriateness of classical versus Bayesian statistical methods. They argue that, a priori, there are two basic principles guiding the analysis of data from a clinical trial:

PRINCIPLE 1 For any experiment and assumed statistical model, data that might have been observed but were not should have no effect on conclusions drawn.

PRINCIPLE 2 Thoughts or intentions of the experimenter that were concerned solely with the reasons for stopping or continuing experimentation, and that had no physical effect on the data reported (i.e., precisely the same data would have resulted in any case), should not affect the conclusions drawn.

Not unexpectedly, the authors conclude that Bayesian methods are preferable to classical statistical methods generally and in the clinical trial setting in particular.

In practice, stopping rules based on classical statistical concepts are increasingly being incorporated into the design of clinical trials. One possible explanation for the evident lack of enthusiasm for Bayesian methods is that the decision-making processes involved in evaluating the results of a clinical trial are complex and to some extent not even quantifiable. Although it may be true that "medical researchers ... act like Bayesians" (Berry, 1985), they typically do so with the aid of classical statistics. For the reasons alluded to above, they may do it better than Bayesians who rely entirely on mathematical algorithms.

It seems that, in practice, study designs that incorporate the opportunity for early termination often prespecify group sequential stopping bounds but with the understanding that they will provide guidelines helpful to the decision-making process. From this perspective, it seems that the practice of inverting group sequential tests to obtain repeated confidence intervals may be useful.

4.3 Formulation of One-Sided and Two-Sided Tests

The decision as to whether tests of hypotheses should be one-or two-sided has been debated well before the advent of group sequential methods. My view is that the purpose of data analysis is to answer the questions which motivated the study, as stated in the specific aims of the study protocol. Questions which were originally formulated as one-sided should be translated statistically into the corresponding one-sided hypotheses and tested using the corresponding one-sided tests. For example, a study which is conducted to answer the one-sided question "Is experimental therapy superior to placebo?" would appropriately use a one-sided test. Other (exploratory) analyses in which unanticipated or secondary questions or findings are evaluated may appropriately be evaluated using two-sided tests.

The problem of choosing a one-or two-sided test is more problematic in the group sequential setting, in which the purposes of testing may be different at different time points. For example, during the course of interim monitoring, ethical issues are usually paramount and the decision to terminate will be made if a convincing difference occurs in either direction. Thus interim testing may be two-sided. At the end of the study, however, assuming that early termination did not occur, emphasis shifts to the scientific question that initially motivated the study, and that question may be one-sided. This situation can be further complicated by the fact that the need to terminate early may not be symmetric: one may require convincing evidence of a treatment effect to terminate with a conclusion of efficacy, while requiring less convincing evidence of little or no treatment benefit. As indicated previously, resolution of this controversy, as well as those that preceded it, will depend on the circumstances and perceived needs surrounding an individual study. Typically, serious controversy will be avoided in practice if resolution of these issues is dealt with at the outset in the study protocol.

REFERENCES

Anscombe, F. J. (1963). Sequential medical trials. *J. Amer. Statist. Assoc. 58*, 365–383.

Armitage, P. (1975). *Sequential Medical Trials*, 2nd ed. Blackwell Scientific, Oxford.

Armitage, P., C. K. McPherson, and B. C. Rowe (1969). Repeated significance tests on accumulating data. *J. Roy Statist. Soc. A 132*, 235–244.

Berger, J. O., and D. A. Berry (1985). Analyzing data: the great conditioning debate, unpublished manuscript.

Berger, J. O., and D. A. Berry (1988). Statistical analysis and the illusion of objectivity. *American Scientist 76*, 159–165.

Berry, D. A. (1983). Interim analyses in clinical trials: classical vs. ad hoc vs. Bayesian approaches, *Tech. Rep. 418*. University of Minnesota, Minneapolis.

Berry, D. A. (1985). Interim analyses in clinical trials: classical vs. Bayesian approaches. *Statist. Med. 4*, 521–526.

Berry, D. A. (1987). Interim analysis in clinical trials: the role of the likelihood principle. *Amer. Statist. 41*, 117–122.

Berry, D. A., and C. Ho (1988). One-sided sequential stopping boundaries for clinical trials: A decision-theoretic approach. Unpublished manuscript.

Berry, D. A., and L. M. Pearson (1985). Optimal designs for clinical trials with dichotomous responses. *Statist. Med. 4*, 497–508.

Brown, B. W., Jr. (1983). Comments on the Dupont manuscript. *Controlled Clin. Trials 4*, 11–12.

Canner, P. L. (1970). Selecting one of two treatments when the responses are dichotomous. *J. Amer. Statist. Assoc. 65*, 293–306.

Canner, P. L. (1984). Monitoring long-term clinical trials for beneficial and adverse treatment effects. *Comm. Statist. 13* (19), 2369–2394.

Chang, M. N., and P. C. O'Brien (1986). Confidence intervals following group sequential tests. *Controlled Clin. Trials 7*, 18–26.

DeGroot, M. H. (1970). *Optimal Statistical Decisions*. McGraw-Hill, New York.

DeMets, D. L. (1984). Stopping guidelines vs. stopping rules: a practitioner's point of view. *Comm. Statist. 13* (19), 2395–2418.

DeMets, D. L., and M. H. Gail (1985). Use of log rank tests and group sequential methods at fixed calendar times. *Biometrics 41*, 1039–1044.

DeMets, D. L., and K. K. G. Lan (1984). An overview of sequential methods and their application in clinical trials. *Comm. Statist. 13* (19), 2315–2338.

DeMets, D. L., and J. H. Ware (1980). Group sequential methods in clinical trials with a one-sided hypothesis. *Biometrika 67*, 651–660.

DeMets, D. L., and J. H. Ware (1982). Asymmetric group sequential boundaries for monitoring clinical trials. *Biometrika 69*, 661–663.

Dupont, W. D. (1983). Sequential stopping rules and sequentially adjusted P-values: does one require the other? *Controlled Clin. Trials 4*, 3–10.

Fairbanks, K., and R. Madsen (1982). P-values for tests using a repeated significance test design. *Biometrika 69*, 69–74.

Fleming, T. R. (1982). One sample multiple testing procedure for phase II clinical trials. *Biometrics 38*, 143–151.

Fleming, T. R., D. P. Harrington and P. C. O'Brien (1984). Designs for group sequential tests. *Controlled Clin. Trials 5*, 348–361.

Freedman, L. S., D. Lowe, and P. Macaskill (1984). Stopping rules for clinical trials incorporating clinical opinion. *Biometrics 40*, 575–586.

Gail, M., D. L. DeMets, and E. V. Slud (1982). Simulation studies on increments of the two-sample logrank score tests for survival time data with application to group sequential boundaries. In *Survival Analysis*, IMS Monograph Series, 287–301.

Haybittle, J. L. (1971). Repeated assessment of results in clinical trials of cancer treatment. *British J. Radiol. 44*, 793–797.

Jennison, C., and B. W. Turnbull (1983). Confidence intervals for a binomial parameter following a multistage test with application to MIL-STD 105D and medical trials. *Technometrics 25*, 49–58.

Jennison, C., and B. W. Turnbull (1984). Repeated confidence intervals for group sequential clinical trials. *Controlled Clin. Trials 5*, 33–45.

Jones, D. R., and J. Whitehead (1979). Sequential forms of the log rank and modified Wilcoxon tests for censored data. *Biometrika 66*, 105–113.

Lai, T. L. (1984). Incorporating scientific, ethical and economic considerations into the design of clinical trials in the pharmaceutical industry: a sequential approach. *Comm. Statist. 13* (19), 2355–2368.

Lan, K. K. G., and D. L. DeMets (1983). Discrete sequential boundaries for clinical trials. *Biometrika 70*, 659–663.

Lan, K. K. G., D. L. DeMets, and M. Halperin (1984). More flexible sequential and non-sequential designs in long-term clinical trials. *Comm. Statist. 13* (19), 2339–2353.

Larson, S. O. (1984). APL programs for outcome probabilities and confidence limits in sequential binomial trials. *Controlled Clin. Trials 5*, 245–249.

Lindgren, B. W. (1976). *Statistical Theory*, 3rd ed. Macmillan, New York.

Meier, P. (1975). Statistics and medical experimentation. *Biometrics 31*, 511–529.

O'Brien, P. C. (1984). Procedures for comparing samples with multiple endpoints. *Biometrics 40*, 1079–1087.

O'Brien, P. C., and T. R. Fleming (1979). A multiple testing procedure for clinical trials. *Biometrics 35*, 549–556.

Paulson, E. (1962). A sequential procedure for comparing several experimental categories with a standard or control. *Ann. Math. Statist. 33*, 438–443.

Paulson, E. (1964). A sequential procedure for selecting the population with the largest mean from k normal populations. *Ann. Math. Statist. 35*, 174–180.

Peto, R., M. C. Pike, P. Armitage, et al. (1976). Design and analysis of randomized clinical trials requiring prolonged observation of each patient: I. Introduction and design. *British J. Cancer 34*, 585–612.

Pocock, S. J. (1977). Group sequential methods in the design and analysis of clinical trials. *Biometrika 64*, 191–199.

Pocock, S. J. (1982). Interim analyses for randomized clinical trials: the group sequential approach. *Biometrics 38*, 153–162.

Pocock, S. J., N. L. Geller, and A. A. Tsiatis (1987). The analysis of multiple endpoints in clinical trials, *Biometrics 43*, 487–498.

Raiffa, H., and R. Schlaifer (1961). *Applied Statistical Decision Theory.* Harvard University, Cambridge, Mass.

Samuel-Cahn, E. (1974a). Repeated significance test II, for hypotheses about the normal distribution. *Comm. Statist. 3*, 711–733.

Samuel-Cahn, E. (1974b). Two kinds of repeated significance tests, and their application for the uniform distribution. *Comm. Statist. 3*, 419–431.

Siegmund, D. (1977). Repeated significance tests for a normal mean. *Biometrika 64*, 177–189.

Siegmund, D. (1978). Estimation following sequential tests. *Biometrika 65*, 341–349.

Siegmund, D. (1980). Sequential $\chi 2$ and F tests and the related confidence intervals. *Biometrika 67*, 389–402.

Slud, E. V., and L. J. Wei (1982). Two-sample repeated significance tests based on the modified Wilcoxon statistics. *J. Amer. Statist. Assoc. 77*, 862–868.

Tsiatis, A. A. (1982). Repeated significance testing for a general class of score statistics used in censored survival analysis. In *Survival Analysis*, IMS Monograph Series, 257–268.

Tsiatis, A. A., G. L. Rosner, and C. R. Mehta (1984). Exact confidence intervals following a group sequential test. *Biometrics 40*, 797–803.

Tukey, J. W. (1960). Where do we go from here? *J. Amer. Statist. Assoc. 55*, 80–93.

Wald, A. (1947). *Sequential Analysis*. Wiley, New York.

Wald, A., and J. Wolfowitz (1948). Optimum character of the sequential probability ratio test. *Ann. Math. Statist. 19*, 326–339.

Wetherill, G. B. (1975). *Sequential Methods in Statistics*, 2nd ed. Wiley, New York.

Whitehead, J. (1983). *The Design and Analysis of Sequential Clinical Trials*. Ellis Horwood, Chichester, West Sussex, England.

Whitehead, J., and D. R. Jones (1979). The analysis of sequential clinical trials. *Biometrika 66*, 443–452.

Whitehead, J., and I. Stratton (1983). Group sequential clinical trials with triangular continuation regions. *Biometrics*.

11

Survival Analysis

JOHN D. KALBFLEISCH University of Waterloo, Waterloo, Ontario, Canada

JAMES O. STREET Boehringer Ingelheim Pharmaceuticals, Inc., Ridgefield, Connecticut

1 INTRODUCTION

In this chapter we summarize a number of methods that have proved useful for the analysis of failure-time data. These methods are important in many pharmaceutical applications where the primary endpoint is the time until an event occurs. For example, the methods are relevant in clinical trials where the primary endpoint is the patient's survival time, the duration of remission, or the time to some other event in the patient's life history. These methods are also useful in many laboratory trials. Peto et al. (1976, 1977) provide a comprehensive discussion of scientific issues related to clinical trials with prolonged observation of patients.

Our main emphasis in this chapter is on semiparametric methods which arise in the analysis of the proportional hazards or relative risk model proposed by Cox (1972). The extensive literature on fully parametric models receives little of our attention here, due to space limitations. We consider primarily applications in which the purpose of experimentation is to compare two or more treatments, or to evaluate the effect of covariates on the risk of an event occurring over time. For these applications, the methodology based on the proportional hazards model has high efficiency compared with its parametric competitors and provides a great deal of flexibility in modeling. We present some of the theoretical underpinnings of the methodology, and discuss and illustrate simple methods of data summary and presentation that are closely allied with the formal analyses and that help communicate the principal results to nonstatisticians.

To set the stage for illustrating some of the methods, we give an example of a clinical trial on 64 patients with severe aplastic anemia. Prior to the trial, all the patients were treated with high-dose cyclophosphamide followed by an infusion of marrow from an HLA-identical family member. Half were then assigned to each of two treatment groups: cyclosporine and methotrexate (CSP + MTX), and methotrexate alone (MTX). One endpoint of interest was the time from assignment until life-threatening stage (≥ 2) of acute graft versus host disease (AGVHD).

These data, which were provided to us by V. Farewell with the permission of R. Storb of the Fred Hutchinson Cancer Research Center in Seattle, are shown in Table 1. The times are given in days until AGVHD of stage ≥ 2, death, or last contact. Also included are two covariates: the patient's age in years and an indicator of whether or not a laminar airflow (LAF) isolation room was used. Storb et al. (1986) report on the subset of 46 patients who were randomly assigned to treatment, with stratification by age group and LAF. For purposes of illustrating the various methods of analysis, we shall treat the data as though all 64 patients had been randomly assigned. However, to assure the absence of bias in any inferences, only the randomized patients should be considered.

In this trial, only 20 of the 64 patients actually reached the endpoint (severe AGVHD or death); the remaining 44 patients were "right censored," meaning they had not reached the endpoint at last contact. The presence of right censoring is a common feature of survival studies, and is one of the key reasons that special methods have been developed for survival analysis.

2 GENERAL BACKGROUND

2.1 Failure-Time Distributions

Let $T > 0$ be a random variable representing the time until the occurrence of some event, which we shall call a failure. It is crucial that T be measured with reference to some well defined and biologically meaningful origin, and that failure itself be unambiguously defined. The distribution of T can be specified by the survivor function

$$S(t) = P(T > t), \qquad 0 < t < \infty.$$

Table 1 Time in Days to Severe (Stage ≥ 2) Acute Graft Versus Host Disease (AGVHD), Death, or Last Contact for Patients Treated with Cyclosporine and Methotrexate (CSP + MTX) or with Methotrexate Only (MTX)[a].

Time	LAF[b]	Age	Time	LAF	Age	Time	LAF	Age
			CSP + MTX					
3[c]	0	40	98[c]	1	10	449[c]	1	37
8	1	21	155[c]	0	27	490[c]	1	35
10	1	18	189[c]	1	9	528[c]	1	32
12[c]	0	42	199[c]	1	19	547[c]	1	32
16	0	23	247[c]	1	14	691[c]	1	38
17	0	21	324[c]	0	23	767[c]	0	18
22	1	13	356[c]	1	13	1111[c]	0	20
64[c]	0	29	378[c]	1	34	1173[c]	0	12
65[c]	1	15	408[c]	1	27	1213[c]	0	12
77[c]	1	34	411[c]	1	5	1357[c]	0	29
82[c]	1	14	420[c]	1	23			
			MTX					
9	1	35	31	1	17	316[c]	1	15
11	1	27	35	1	21	393[c]	1	27
12	0	22	35	1	25	395[c]	0	2
20	1	21	46	1	35	428[c]	0	3
20	1	30	49	0	19	469[c]	1	14
22	0	7	104[c]	1	21	602[c]	1	18
25	1	36	106[c]	1	19	681[c]	0	23
25	1	38	156[c]	1	15	690[c]	1	9
25[c]	0	20	218[c]	1	26	1112[c]	1	11
28	0	25	230[c]	0	11	1180[c]	0	11
28	0	28	231[c]	1	14			

[a]Age is age in years at the time of transplant. Also recorded is laminar airflow isolation (LAF).
[b]0, no; 1, yes.
[c]Censored.

Note that $S(t) = 1 - F(t)$, where $F(t)$ is the cumulative distribution function of T. The function $S(t)$ is nonincreasing with $S(0) = 1$ and $S(\infty) = 0$.

When T is continuous, its probability density function is

$$f(t) = -\frac{d}{dt}S(t) = \frac{\lim_{\Delta t \to 0} P\{T \in (t, t + \Delta t]\}}{\Delta t}, \qquad 0 < t,$$

and its hazard function is

$$\lambda(t) = \frac{\lim_{\Delta t \to 0} P\{T \in (t, t + \Delta t] \mid T > t\}}{\Delta t}, \qquad 0 < t;$$

this is the rate of failure at time t among individuals who survive to time t. It can be seen that

$$\lambda(t) = \frac{f(t)}{S(t)} = -\frac{d}{dt}\log S(t).$$

Integrating, and using $S(0) = 1$, we obtain

$$S(t) = \exp[-\Lambda(t)], \tag{1}$$

where $\Lambda(t) = \int_0^t \lambda(s)ds$ is termed the cumulative hazard function. Thus the hazard function $\lambda(t)$ determines the distribution of T.

When T is discrete with probability mass points at $y_1, y_2, \ldots$, where $0 < y_1 < y_2 < \cdots$, similar results are available. Here the hazard function is defined by

$$\lambda_j = P(T = y_j \mid T \geq y_j), \qquad j = 1, 2, \ldots.$$

Survival to time $t > 0$ requires survival through all points $y_j < t$. It follows that

$$S(t) = P(T > t) = \prod_{j|y_j \leq t} (1 - \lambda_j). \tag{2}$$

The probability function is similarly obtained as

$$f_j = P(T = y_j) = \lambda_j \prod_{j|y_j < t} (1 - \lambda_j) = \lambda_j S(y_j^-), \tag{3}$$

where $S(a^-) = \lim_{t \uparrow a} S(t)$. That is, to fail at y_j, the individual must survive at time points $y_1, \ldots, y_{j-1}$ [with probability $S(y_j^-)$] and then fail at y_j (with probability λ_j).

Both the CDF (or the survivor function) and the probability density function are commonly used in statistical modeling. The hazard function is of particular value in survival analysis. As (2) and (3) make evident, the discrete hazard function invites an interpretation whereby an individual on trial is viewed as undergoing a sequence of Bernoulli trials with varying probabilities of failure λ_j until the first failure occurs (see Figure 1). This

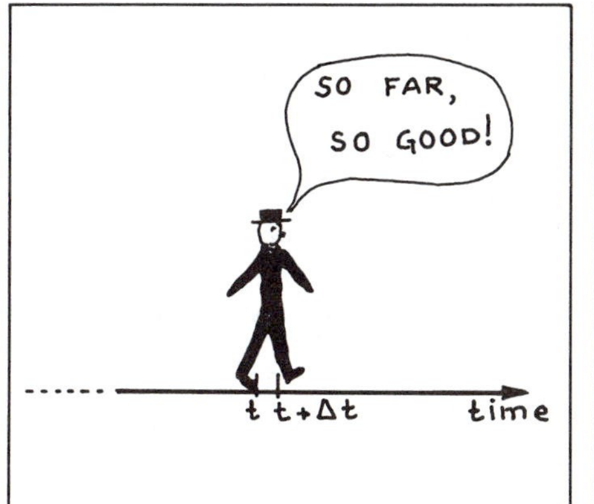

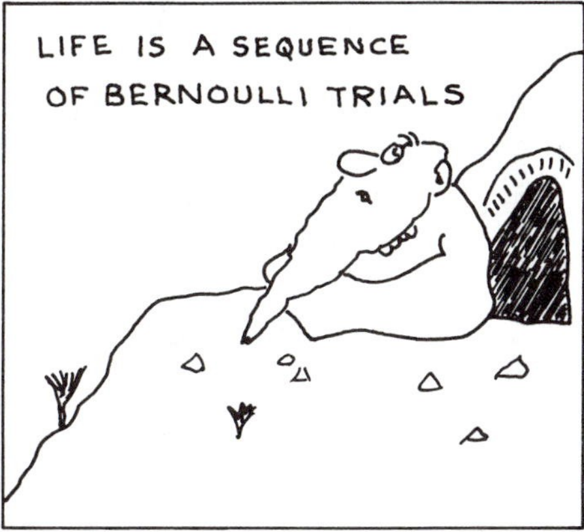

Figure 1 Sequential interpretation of a failure-time mechanism.

sequential interpretation has been the basis of many recent developments in survival analysis, and focuses attention on the hazard function as the primary modeling tool.

The interpretation as a sequence of Bernoulli trials, which is clear in the discrete case, also holds in the continuous case. The relationship (1) between the survivor function and the hazard function has a "product integral" representation in which the continuous survivor function can be expressed as the limit of instantaneous survival probabilities [see, e.g., Kalbfleisch and Prentice (1980, pp. 8, 9)].

The hazard function has several other advantages as a modeling tool. For instance, the general form of the hazard may provide insight into the nature of the failure mechanism. By specifying the failure rate for individuals at a given time t, a monotone-increasing hazard function indicates deterioration with age, whereas a monotone-decreasing hazard indicates improvement with age. In the case of human mortality, the hazard function is initially high, decreases rapidly to a relatively low level, then remains constant until, at about age 35, it starts to increase exponentially, giving the familiar "bathtub" shape of Figure 2.

The sequential nature of the hazard function is also suited to modeling risk factors whose effects vary with time. For example, the event of interest may be the healing of an ulcer, and the use of tobacco over time may be thought to affect the rate of healing. In this case, the hazard allows us to consider a model in which the rate of healing at time t depends on the recent use of tobacco. Thus, as discussed in Section 4, we might modulate the hazard function using time-varying covariates.

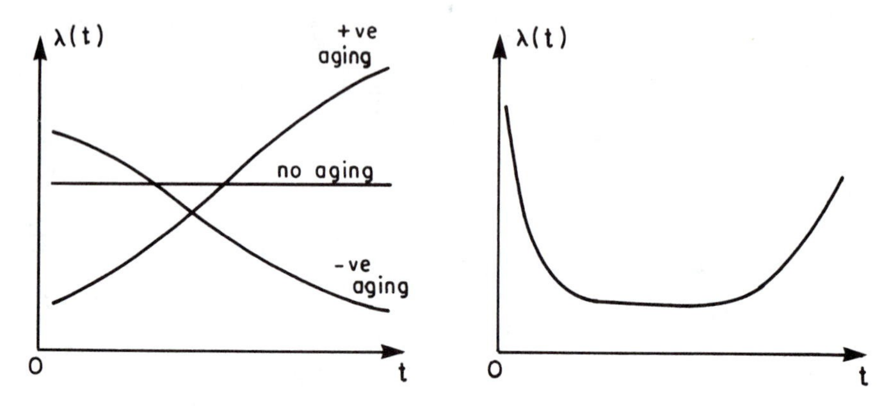

Figure 2 Some general shapes of hazard functions showing deterioration with age, improvement with age, and the "bathtub."

Many parametric models have been used in survival analysis. Lawless (1982) gives a thorough summary of many of the standard models used. As noted in the introduction, we will not review parametric models in this chapter except to mention two that we utilize in later sections. We describe these next.

The exponential distribution with constant hazard $\lambda(t) = \theta > 0$ is the baseline continuous survival model. Its PDF and survivor functions are

$$f(t) = \theta e^{-\theta t}, \qquad S(t) = e^{-\theta t} \tag{4}$$

for $t > 0$. The memoryless property of this distribution is described by the constant failure rate θ that applies at all times the individual is on test.

One generalization of the exponential distribution that is particularly useful in informal data analysis is the piecewise exponential distribution. This has hazard function

$$\lambda(t) = \theta_j, \qquad t \in (a_{j-1}, a_j], \qquad j = 1, \ldots, k, \tag{5}$$

where $a_0 = 0 < a_1 < \cdots < a_k = \infty$ are prespecified constants. This provides a flexible model which, for moderate k, describes with reasonable accuracy a variety of shapes for the hazard (see Figure 3). As can be shown by direct calculation using (1), the survivor function is

$$S(t) = \exp[-\theta_i(t - a_{i-1})] \prod_{j=1}^{i-1} \exp[-\theta_j(a_j - a_{j-1})] \tag{6}$$

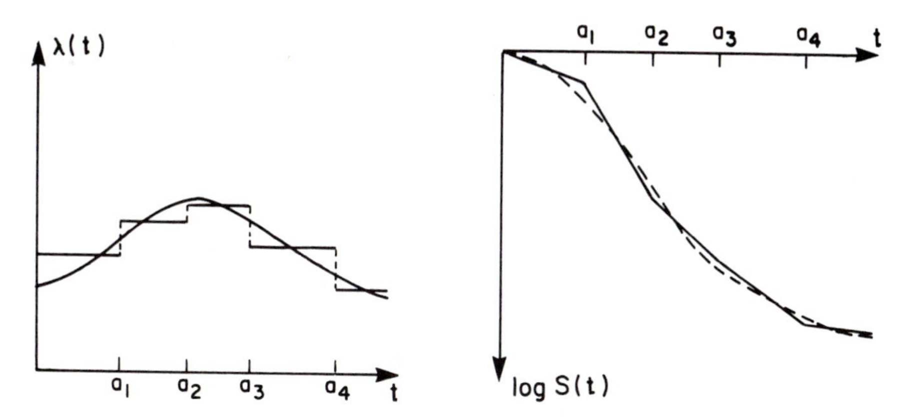

Figure 3 Piecewise exponential approximations to a smooth hazard function and the related approximation to the survivor function.

for $t \in (a_{i-1}, a_i]$, $i = 1, \ldots, k$, and the density in this interval is $f(t) = \theta_i S(t)$.

2.2 Independent Right Censoring

As noted earlier, most survival studies include some individuals who do not fail during their observation period; the data on these individuals are said to be right censored. Often, right censoring occurs because some of the individuals under observation have not failed at the end of the study when the statistical analysis is done. In other cases, individuals may move outside the study area or be unable to participate due to an accident. In some clinical trials, an individual may withdraw from study due, for example, to dissatisfaction with the treatment. As is intuitively apparent, some of these censoring mechanisms have the potential to introduce bias into the estimation of survival probabilities, or into treatment comparisons.

A censoring mechanism is called independent right censoring if the failure rates that apply to the individuals on trial at each time $t > 0$ are unaffected by the censoring. Suppose that the failure rate at time t that applies in the absence of censoring for each member of a homogeneous group is $\lambda(t; \mathbf{x})$, where $\mathbf{x}$ is a vector of covariates containing information such as treatment assignment or measures of physical and medical condition at time 0. Suppose now that, within this group, individuals are to be right censored according to some specific mechanism. Consider the subset of individuals who are at risk of failure (not failed and uncensored) at some time $t > 0$. The censoring scheme is independent if, for an individual selected at random from this subset, the failure rate is $\lambda(t; \mathbf{x})$. Thus we require that at each time t,

$$\lim_{\Delta t \to 0} \frac{P\{T \in (t, t + \Delta t] \mid \mathbf{x},\ T \geq t\}}{\Delta t} = \lim_{\Delta t \to 0} \frac{P\{T \in (t, t + \Delta t] \mid \mathbf{x},\ T \geq t,\ \text{uncensored at } t\}}{\Delta t}. \tag{7}$$

Independent censoring includes many censoring schemes that commonly arise, such as independent random censoring and type II censoring. In the former scheme, each individual in the group $\mathbf{x}$ has a random censoring time C which, conditionally on $\mathbf{x}$, is distributed independently of the failure time T; we observe $\min(T, C)$. In the latter scheme, all individuals are placed on trial at time 0 and followed until the kth failure occurs, when all surviving individuals are censored. In general, a censoring scheme is independent if the probability of censoring at time t depends only on the covariates $\mathbf{x}$, the observed pattern of failures and censoring up to time t in the trial, or on random processes that are independent of the failure times in the trial. Mechanisms in which individuals are censored because they appear to be at unusually high (or low) risk of failure are not independent. For these mechanisms, (7) is violated and the methods discussed in this chapter are inappropriate.

Dependent censoring makes all ordinary methods for the analysis of survival data inadmissible. It is, therefore, very important to follow all randomized patients as completely as possible. If there is censoring that is thought to be dependent, there is no straightforward method of analysis. A very conservative approach would assume that a censored individual in the treatment group is a failure while one in the control group survives to the end of the study period. However, this is generally too conservative. In some trials, a strongly predictive variable, such as a measure of general physical condition, may be observed repeatedly over time. If the censoring is dependent, it may be possible to base the analysis on the predictive factor as an endpoint. Generally, if there is evidence that some individuals have been subject to dependent censoring, one needs to explore different assumptions about the censored individuals to see whether the inferences remain stable.

Suppose now that the time to failure T has PDF $f(t; \theta)$, hazard function $\lambda(t; \theta)$, and survivor function $S(t; \theta)$, where θ is an unknown parameter or vector of parameters. The exponential (4) or piecewise exponential (5) models provide examples. Suppose that n individuals are on trial and that these individuals are subject to independent right censoring so that (7) holds. The likelihood function of θ can then be shown to be

$$L(\theta) = \prod_{i=1}^{n} f(t_i;\theta)^{\delta_i} S(t_i;\theta)^{1-\delta_i}, \tag{8}$$

where $t_1, \ldots, t_n$ are the observed times to either failure or censoring, and δ_i is 1 if t_i is a failure or 0 if t_i is a censoring. Thus, for independent censoring, the contribution to likelihood (8) of a failure at t_i is the density function $f(t_i;\theta)$, while a censoring at t_i contributes only the information that the time of failure exceeds the time of censoring, $S(t_i;\theta) = P(T_i > t_i)$.

EXAMPLE 1 Let $(t_1, \delta_1), \ldots, (t_n, \delta_n)$ be an independently censored sample from the exponential distribution with PDF $\theta e^{-\theta t}$ and survivor function $e^{-\theta t}$. The likelihood function (4) in this case reduces to

$$L(\theta) = \theta^r \exp(-U\theta), \tag{9}$$

where $r = \sum_1^n \delta_i$ is the number of failures and $U = \sum_1^n t_i$ is the total exposure time, that is, the sum of all observed times whether censorings or failures. The score function is obtained as the logarithmic derivative of (9):

$$s(\theta) = \frac{r}{\theta} - U,$$

and the maximum likelihood estimate of θ is $\hat{\theta} = r/U$. Under some specific type II censoring schemes, the exact distribution of $\hat{\theta}$ can be obtained. But for most censoring schemes this distribution is intractable, as is the joint distribution of the sufficient statistics r and U. Consequently, inferences in both parametric and semiparametric models are based primarily on asymptotic results.

EXAMPLE 2 If (t_i, δ_i), $i = 1, \ldots, n$, is an independently censored sample from the piecewise exponential (5), the calculations are very similar. After some algebra (or, more efficiently, by interpreting the survival experience sequentially across successive intervals), we obtain the likelihood function

$$L(\theta_1, \ldots, \theta_k) = \prod_{j=1}^{k} \theta_j^{r_j} \exp(-U_j \theta_j), \tag{10}$$

where r_j is the number of individuals observed to fail in the jth interval, $I_j = (a_{j-1}, a_j]$, and U_j is the total exposure in the jth interval. Thus

$$U_j = n_j(a_j - a_{j-1}) + \sum_{i|t_i \in I_j} (t_i - a_{j-1}),$$

where n_j is the number of individuals surviving and under observation at a_j, $j = 1, \ldots, k$. The maximum likelihood estimate is

$$\hat{\theta}_j = \frac{r_j}{U_j}, \qquad j = 1, \ldots, k. \tag{11}$$

This is illustrated in Section 3 on the data from the aplastic anemia trial.

3 SOME SIMPLE AND FLEXIBLE METHODS

In this section we introduce some simple, yet very effective methods for the analysis of survival data. These methods are useful for preliminary investigation of the data and also provide flexible tools for presenting the results of more formal statistical analyses. Empirical distributions play an important role in statistics by providing information about distributional shape and useful summaries about the sample of interest. The generalizations of the empirical distribution that allow independent right censoring in the data are of fundamental importance in the analysis of survival data. In Section 3.1 we discuss these methods, including the important Kaplan–Meier (1958) technique, and methods based on the piecewise exponential distribution. In Section 3.2 we discuss some comparative techniques which allow tests of the differences between two or more samples as defined, for instance, by treatment groups.

Throughout this section, we treat the derivations somewhat informally and stress the intuitive basis of the procedures in terms of the sequential interpretation of the time until failure.

3.1 Estimation of the Survivor Function

Again, we consider a sample (t_i, δ_i), $i = 1, \ldots, n$, of independently right censored data from some distribution with unknown survivor function $S(t)$. Our purpose is to construct a nonparametric estimate of $S(t)$. If there were no censoring in the sample, the empirical survivor function

$$\hat{S}(t) = \frac{\#\{t_i > t\}}{n}$$

would be the estimate. The generalization of this to censored data is the Kaplan–Meier estimate.

Let $t_{(1)} < \cdots < t_{(k)}$ be the distinct failure times and let d_i be the number of failures at time $t_{(i)}$. We adopt a convention whereby individuals censored at $t_{(i)}$ are taken to be censored at $t_{(i)} + \delta$, where $\delta > 0$ is small. Let m_i be the number of items censored in the interval $[t_{(i)}, t_{(i+1)})$, where

$t_{(0)} = 0$ and $t_{(k+1)} = \infty$, and let n_i be the number of items at risk at $t_{(i)}^-$ (just prior to time $t_{(i)}$) so that $n_i = \sum_i^k (d_j + m_j)$. As in the uncensored case, we seek an estimate with mass concentrated at the observed failure times, that is, a discrete survivor function with hazard contributions $\hat{\lambda}_1, \ldots, \hat{\lambda}_k$ at the observed failure times $t_{(1)}, \ldots, t_{(k)}$. Recalling the sequential interpretation of the failure mechanism, we have, at time $t_{(i)}$, n_i independent Bernoulli trials with d_i failures. The hazard component can be estimated by

$$\hat{\lambda}_i = \frac{d_i}{n_i}, \qquad i = 1, \ldots, k.$$

At any time t where individuals are exposed but no failures are observed, the hazard contribution is estimated to be zero. Thus we are led to the Kaplan–Meier estimator

$$\hat{S}(t) = \prod_{i|t_{(i)} \le t} \left(1 - \frac{d_i}{n_i}\right); \tag{12}$$

this is defined for all t if $m_k = 0$ (the largest observation is a failure at $t_{(k)}$) or for t less than the largest observation time if $m_k > 0$. The resulting estimate is a step function with discontinuities at the observed failure times. It is a discrete failure time distribution in which the hazard component at $t_{(i)}$ is chosen to match exactly the proportion of individuals at risk at $t_{(i)}^-$ who fail at $t_{(i)}$.

A frequently used alternative estimator of $S(t)$ is the Nelson–Aalen estimator, which is a first-order approximation to the Kaplan–Meier estimator (12). The Nelson–Aalen estimator is given by

$$\log \hat{S}_{\mathrm{NA}}(t) = \sum_{i|t_{(i)} \le t} \frac{d_i}{n_i} \tag{13}$$

and arises naturally as an estimator of the cumulative hazard function

$$\Lambda(t) = \int_0^t \lambda(u) du.$$

In the continuous case, $\Lambda(T) = -\log S(t)$ from (1). Since, however, the estimators are discrete, this relationship between the estimated cumulative hazard and the estimated survivor function does not hold exactly. In the discrete case, the relationship between the survivor function and the hazard function is given by (2).

In large samples, the distribution of $\hat{S}(t)$ of $\hat{S}_{\mathrm{NA}}(t)$ is approximately normal with mean $S(t)$ and variance estimated by Greenwood's formula:

$$\widehat{\mathrm{var}}(\hat{S}(t)) = \hat{S}^2(t) \sum_{i|t_{(i)} \leq t} \frac{d_i}{n_i(n_i - d_i)}. \tag{14}$$

In fact, the distribution of $\log[-\log \hat{S}(t)]$ is, for moderate sample sizes, more nearly normal than that of $\hat{S}(t)$. The asymptotic variance of $\log[-\log \hat{S}(t)]$ can be estimated by

$$\widehat{\mathrm{var}}(\log[-\log \hat{S}(t)]) = \sum_{i|t_{(i)} \leq t} \frac{d_i}{n_i(n_i - d_i)} \Big/ [\log \hat{S}(t)]^2. \tag{15}$$

The Kaplan–Meier or Nelson–Aalen estimators can be used to provide information on distributional form. For example, if the distribution of the failure time variable T is exponential, then $\log S(t) = -\lambda t$, and a plot of $\log \hat{S}(t)$ versus t should approximate a straight line through the origin with slope equal to the negative of the failure rate.

In many instances, the piecewise exponential model (5) provides an attractive continuous alternative to the Kaplan–Meier estimator. For this, we choose interval endpoints $a_0 = 0 < a_1 < a_2 < \cdots < a_k = \infty$ and, from the data, estimate the hazard rate θ_j for the jth interval using (11). The corresponding survivor function estimate is

$$\hat{S}_{\mathrm{PE}}(t) = \exp\left[-\sum_{j=0}^{i-1} \hat{\theta}_j(a_j - a_{j-1}) - \hat{\theta}_i(t - a_{i-1})\right] \tag{16}$$

for $t \in (a_i, a_{i+1}]$, which follows from (6). On a logarithmic scale, this estimate is a connected series of straight lines, the slope of the line in the ith interval being $-\hat{\theta}_i$. As with any statistical procedure that requires grouping into intervals, there is arbitrariness in the choice of k and $a_1, \ldots, a_{k-1}$. The primary use of survivor function estimation is descriptive, however, and not inferential. If the a_i's are chosen independently of the data and based, perhaps, on experience in previous trials, this approach yields reasonably descriptive plots.

EXAMPLE 3 Table 2 outlines the calculation of the Kaplan–Meier estimate for the clinical trial data in Table 1 for each of the two treatment groups; the estimates are displayed in Figure 4. There appear to be essentially no differences during the first 22 days of follow-up, after which time the CSP + MTX group does markedly better, with no additional failures observed. An alternative display using the piecewise exponential estimate is given in Figure 5. The intervals (0,10], (10,20], (20,30], (30,40], (40,50], and $(50, \infty]$ were chosen for convenience, and the plot on the log scale

Table 2 Calculation of the Kaplan–Meier Estimates

CSP + MTX					MTX				
$t_{(i)}$	d_i	n_i	$1-\hat{\lambda}_i$	$\hat{S}(t_{(i)})$	t_i	d_i	n_i	$1-\hat{\lambda}_i$	$\hat{S}(t_{(i)})$
8	1	31	30/31	0.968	9	1	32	31/32	0.969
10	1	30	29/30	0.935	11	1	31	30/31	0.938
16	1	28	27/28	0.902	12	1	30	29/30	0.906
17	1	27	26/27	0.868	20	2	29	27/29	0.844
22	1	26	25/26	0.835	22	1	27	26/27	0.813
					25	2	26	24/26	0.750
					28	2	23	21/23	0.685
					31	1	21	20/21	0.652
					35	2	20	18/20	0.586
					46	1	18	17/18	0.554
					49	1	17	16/17	0.522

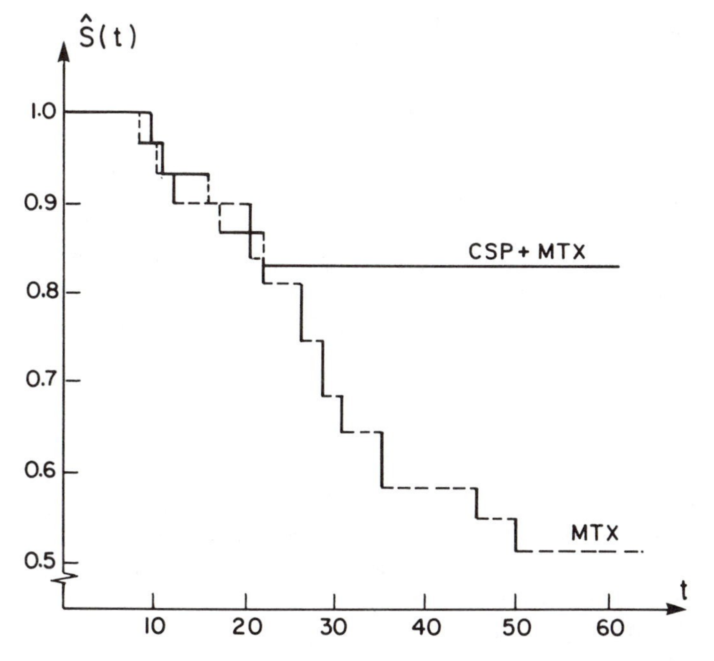

Figure 4 Kaplan–Meier estimates for the data of Table 1.

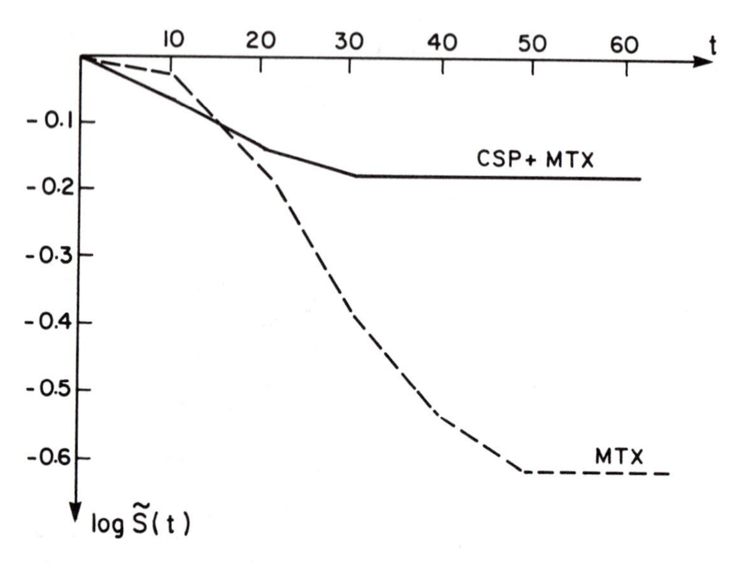

Figure 5 Piecewise exponential estimates of the log survivor functions for the data of Table 1.

gives a connected sequence of straight lines with slopes $-0.0064 = -2/312$ $-0.0072 = 2/275$, -0.0040, 0.0, 0.0, and 0.0 for CSP + MTX and -0.0031, -0.0136, -0.0206, -0.0157, -0.0114, and 0.0 for MTX. This plot is simpler to view and conveys essentially the same information as does Figure 4.

Had it been identified in advance that patient status at, say, time 60 days after transplant was of primary interest, the Kaplan–Meier estimates together with the Greenwood estimates of variance would provide a suitable method for comparing the treatments. For CSP + MTX, we find $\hat{S}_1(60) = 0.835$, and for MTX, $\hat{S}_2(60) = 0.522$, with estimated variances from (14) of $\hat{G}_1 = 0.00454$ and $\hat{G}_2 = 0.00802$, respectively. Thus a test of no treatment difference with respect to the survival probabilities at $t = 60$ is based on the statistic

$$\frac{\hat{S}_1(60) - \hat{S}_2(60)}{\sqrt{\hat{G}_1 + \hat{G}_2}} = -2.79,$$

which, when compared with the $N(0,1)$ table, offers strong evidence against the null hypothesis. In fact, the normal approximations are somewhat suspect; the approximation in the CSP + MTX group is similar to the normal approximation of a binomial distribution with $n = 31$ and $p = 0.83$. A better approximation would be based on the asymptotic distribution of $\log\left\{-\log(\hat{S}(t))\right\}$ and the variance estimate (15) as discussed above. This yields the analogous test statistic

$$\frac{-1.713 + 0.431}{\sqrt{0.2002 + 0.0697}} = -2.47,$$

which suggests somewhat weaker evidence against the null hypothesis than does the test based directly on the Kaplan–Meier estimate, although both tests provide substantial evidence against the null hypothesis of no difference at $t = 60$.

In fact, 60 days was not prespecified as a time point of particular interest. Here, as usual, we wish to evaluate treatment differences across the entire time scale—not at a single time point only. The tests developed in the next section provide alternative procedures that compare the failure rates over the whole course of the study.

3.2 Censored Data Rank Tests

In this section we develop some simple and very useful inferential techniques for the two- and k-sample problems. As we shall see in Section 4, these methods relate closely to the proportional hazards or relative risk model and are of particular value in communicating the results of analyses based on that model to nonstatisticians.

Consider first a two-sample problem. Suppose that the distinct failure times in the combined sample are $t_{(1)} \ldots, t_{(k)}$ and that at $t_{(i)}$ there are d_{1i} failures in sample 1 and d_{0i} in sample 0. Suppose further that, just prior to $t_{(i)}$, there are n_{1i} items at risk in sample 1 and n_{0i} in sample 0. The log-rank, or Mantel–Haenszel (1959) [see also Chapter 13 and Mantel (1966)] procedure involves the construction of a 2×2 table at each observed failure time. Thus at $t_{(i)}$ we have

	Failures	Survivals	At risk
Sample 0	d_{0i}	$n_{0i} - d_{0i}$	n_{0i}
Sample 1	d_{1i}	$n_{1i} - d_{1i}$	n_{1i}
Total	d_i	$n_i - d_i$	n_i

Under the hypothesis of no difference between the two populations, and conditional upon n_{0i}, n_{1i} and d_i, the distribution of d_{1i} is hypergeometric. Its conditional expected value and variance are given by

$$e_{1i} = \frac{n_{1i} d_i}{n_i}$$

and

$$v_{1i} = \frac{n_{0i} n_{1i} d_i (n_i - d_i)}{n_i^2 (n_i - 1)}.$$

The log-rank or Mantel–Haenszel test is obtained by summing $d_{1i} - e_{1i}$ across all k tables to obtain

$$O_1 - E_1 = \sum_{i=1}^{k} (d_{1i} - e_{1i}),$$

where O_1 is the observed failure count in sample 1 and E_1 is an "expected" failure count (actually a sum of conditional expectations). Under the hypothesis of no difference between the two populations, it can be shown that the variance of $O_1 - E_1$ can be estimated by $V_1 = \sum v_{1i}$, and that the statistic

$$T_{\text{MH}} = \frac{O_1 - E_1}{\sqrt{V_1}} \tag{17}$$

is approximately $N(0, 1)$ in moderately large samples.

An alternative statistic,

$$\sum_{0}^{1} \frac{(O_j - E_j)^2}{E_j}, \tag{18}$$

is approximately $\chi^2_{(1)}$ under the null hypothesis and is sometimes used. In fact, (18) can be shown to be less than or equal to T^2_{MH} and so gives a conservative test. Although this statistic is slightly easier to compute by hand, (17) is not difficult and should be used in preference to (18).

If $r + 1$ samples are under comparison, a natural generalization of the procedure above involves an $(r + 1) \times 2$ contingency table at each failure time with corresponding expected frequencies $e_{01}, e_{1i}, \ldots, e_{ri}$ for the $r + 1$ samples. The log-rank statistic is then of the form

$$(\mathbf{O} - \mathbf{E})' \mathbf{V}^{-1} (\mathbf{O} - \mathbf{E}). \tag{19}$$

Here $\mathbf{O}' = (O_1, \ldots, O_r)$ where $O_j = \sum_{i=1}^{k} d_{ji}$ is the vector of observed frequencies, $\mathbf{E}' = (E_1, \ldots, E_r)$, where $E_j = \sum_{i-1}^{k} e_{ji}$ is the vector of "expected" frequencies, and $\mathbf{V} = \sum_{i=1}^{k} \mathbf{V}_i$, where $\mathbf{V}_i$ is the covariance matrix from the multivariate hypergeometric distribution obtained in the ith table by conditioning on $d_i, n_{0i}, \ldots, n_{ki}$. Specifically,

$$e_{ji} = \frac{n_{ji} d_i}{n_i}$$

and

$$(V_i)_{jj} = n_{ji}(n_i - n_{ji})d_i(n_i - d_i)n_i^{-2}(n_i - 1)^{-1},$$
$$(V_i)_{jk} = -n_{ji}n_{ki}d_i(n_i - d_i)n_i^{-2}(n_i - 1)^{-1}.$$

Under the null hypothesis of no treatment differences, (19) has an approximate $\chi^2_{(r)}$ distribution. Again, a conservative test is obtained from the statistic

$$\frac{\sum_{j=0}^{r}(O_j - E_j)^2}{E_j},$$

although the result (19) is preferable and simple to compute.

EXAMPLE 3 (CONTINUED) The two treatment groups in Table 1 can be compared using the log-rank procedure. Table 3 describes the relevant calculations, and we obtain

$$\frac{O_1 - E_1}{\sqrt{V_1}} = -2.34$$

which, when compared to the $N(0,1)$ distribution, indicates that the data are significant at the 2% level under the hypothesis of no treatment difference.

Flexibility is increased by considering an extension in which the population under study is divided into strata. Suppose, for example, that there are s strata defined by some auxiliary variable and that interest centers on the comparison of $r + 1$ treatment groups. In this case, let $\mathbf{O}^{(l)}$ be the vector of observed frequencies in the lth stratum, $\mathbf{E}^{(l)}$ the corresponding vector of "expected" frequencies, and $\mathbf{V}^{(l)}$ the covariance matrix. The stratified log-rank statistic is

$$\sum_{l=1}^{s}(\mathbf{O}^{(l)} - \mathbf{E}^{(l)})' \left(\sum_{l=1}^{s}\mathbf{V}^{(l)}\right)^{-1} \sum_{l=1}^{s}(\mathbf{O}^{(l)} - \mathbf{E}^{(l)}), \tag{20}$$

which in reasonably large samples has an approximate chi-squared distribution on r degrees of freedom under the usual hypothesis of no treatment differences.

The log-rank test is an example of what is often termed a censored data rank test. This test is fully efficient against alternatives in which the hazard rates between samples are proportional across time. The reasons for its efficiency in this case will become apparent in the next section. A versatile class of censored data rank tests can be constructed by introducing a weight w_i into the comparison between observed and expected frequencies

Table 3 Calculation of the log-Rank Statistic

$t_{(i)}$	d_{1i}	$e_{1i} = n_{1i}d_i/n_i$	$d_{1i} - e_{1i}$	v_{1i}	w_i[a]
8	1	31 × 1/63	0.508	0.250	1.00
9	0	30 × 1/62	−0.438	0.250	0.984
10	1	30 × 1/61	0.508	0.250	0.969
11	0	29 × 1/60	−0.484	0.250	0.953
12	0	29 × 1/59	−0.491	0.250	0.938
16	1	28 × 1/57	0.508	0.250	0.922
17	1	27 × 1/56	0.518	0.250	0.906
20	0	26 × 2/55	−0.945	0.490	0.890
22	1	26 × 2/53	0.019	0.490	0.858
25	0	25 × 2/51	−0.980	0.490	0.827
28	0	25 × 2/48	−1.041	0.489	0.795
31	0	25 × 1/46	−0.543	0.248	0.762
35	0	25 × 2/45	−1.111	0.482	0.746
46	0	25 × 1/43	−0.581	0.243	0.713
49	0	25 × 1/42	−0.595	0.241	0.697
			$O_1 - E_1 = -5.196$	$v_i = 4.922$	

[a]Weights for the Prentice (1978) generalization of the Wilcoxon test.

at the ith failure time $t_{(i)}$. Considering the two-sample case for simplicity, the test statistic then becomes

$$T_w = \left[\sum w_i(d_{1i} - e_{1i})\right]^2 \left(\sum w_i^2 v_{1i}\right)^{-1}. \tag{21}$$

Under the null hypothesis, the distribution of T_w is again approximately $\chi^2_{(1)}$ and, if $w_i = 1$ for all i, the log-rank test is obtained. If $w_i = \tilde{S}(t^-_{(i)})$, where $\tilde{S}$ is an estimate of the survivor function based on the pooled data,

$$\tilde{S}(t) = \prod_{j|t_j \le t} \left(1 - \frac{d_j}{n_j + 1}\right),$$

then T_w is the Prentice (1978) generalization of the Wilcoxon test.

The weights w_i can be prespecified to emphasize an expected pattern of treatment effect. For example, if it were thought that the treatment would tend to decrease the hazard for early times, but that after some period this effect would diminish and the hazards converge, it would be natural to pick monotone-decreasing weights such as $w_i = \tilde{S}(t_{(i)})$. By weighting the earlier comparisons more heavily, this choice would avoid a loss in power due to the decreasing hazard ratio.

A further generalization allows the weights w_i to be arbitrary functions of time as well. Thus, at time $t_{(i)}$, the weights $w_i(t_{(i)})$ are applied. Such tests are efficient against alternatives in which the relative risk is time dependent and will be discussed further in Section 4.3 Examples of the use of the stratified log-rank test are discussed in Section 4.2 A complete and very elegant treatment of censored data rank tests and their asymptotic properties is given by Andersen et al. (1982).

EXAMPLE 3 (CONTINUED) The Prentice generalization of the Wilcoxon test can be applied to the data in Table 1 using the weights given in the final column of Table 3. We find in this case that $\sum w_i(d_{1i} - e_{1i}) = -3.996$ and $\sum w_i^2 v_i = 3.636$, so that the corresponding standard normal test statistic is $T_w = -3.996/\sqrt{3.636} = -2.10$, which suggests somewhat weaker evidence than did the log-rank test (a significance level of about 4% versus 2%). This happens because the Prentice weights place more emphasis on the early times, and as Figure 5 illustrates, the treatment differences are apparently greater for the later times. Weights which increased with i would give nominal significance levels of less than 2%, but weights must not be chosen after the data have been examined. If, however, from previous studies we had expected to see little difference until some initial period had passed, we might have chosen weights such as $w_i^* = w_i^{-1}$ (the inverse of the Prentice weights) for our primary analysis. These weights give a $N(0,1)$ statistic of $T_{w*} = -2.57$, compared with -2.34 for the log-rank and -2.10 for the Prentice weights.

4 COMPARATIVE STUDIES AND REGRESSION MODELS

In many applications it is important to have regression models for failure time. The covariates in these models may reflect treatment assignments, baseline characteristics, or even measurements of variables taken repeatedly across time (time-varying covariates). In this section we consider regression models for the hazard function and develop a number of techniques that are suitable for the estimation of regression effects or comparison of treatment groups. The emphasis will be on the semiparametric regression models of the type proposed by Cox (1972).

4.1 Relative Risk Regression Models

Suppose that a vector of covariates $\mathbf{x}' = (x_1, \ldots, x_r)$ is observed on an individual prior to the study, and let $\lambda(t; \mathbf{x})$ be the hazard function for this individual. It is usually convenient to define the origin of measurement of the covariates $\mathbf{x}$ so that $\mathbf{x} = \mathbf{0}$ represents some baseline condition (e.g., control group); in any case, let $\lambda_0(t) = \lambda(t; \mathbf{0})$ represent the baseline hazard that applies when $\mathbf{x} = \mathbf{0}$. The relative risk function is

$$\mathrm{RR}(t; \mathbf{x}) = \frac{\lambda(t; \mathbf{x})}{\lambda_0(t)},$$

which measures the multiplicative effect on the hazard of the covariate $\mathbf{x}$ at time t. Alternatively, we write

$$\lambda(t; \mathbf{x}) = \lambda_0(t)\, \mathrm{RR}(t; \mathbf{x}).$$

The semiparametric modeling strategy that we examine in this section leaves $\lambda_0(t)$ arbitrary, but specifies particular parametric models for $\mathrm{RR}(t; \mathbf{x})$. If $\mathrm{RR}(t; \mathbf{x})$ does not depend on t, we say that the model is a proportional hazards model. More generally, when the relative risk varies with time, the model is referred to as a relative risk model.

It should be noted that full parametric modeling can be achieved by introducing a parametric model for $\lambda_0(t)$. For example, if $\lambda_0(t) = \theta$ is taken to be constant in t, exponential regression models are obtained. These can be combined with various forms of the relative risk function. A full discussion of parametric regression models of both the relative risk and log-linear forms can be found in Lawless (1982) or Kalbfleisch and Prentice (1980). In most cases, full parametric modeling gives relatively small efficiency gains in the estimation of the regression parameters. The semiparametric procedures that we shall outline have good properties and do not depend for their validity on a particular parametric form of the baseline hazard.

In the simplest case, with arbitrary $\lambda_0(t)$, $\mathrm{RR}(t; \mathbf{x})$ does not depend on t. If $\mathbf{z}' = (z_1, \ldots, z_k)$ is a vector of derived covariates comprising elements of $\mathbf{x}$, powers or other functions of these elements, and possibly cross-product terms, it is often assumed that

$$\mathrm{RR}(t; \mathbf{x}) = r(\mathbf{z}'\boldsymbol{\beta}), \tag{22}$$

where $\boldsymbol{\beta}' = (\beta_1, \ldots, \beta_k)$ is a vector of regression parameters. Various forms for the relative risk $r(w)$ have been suggested, including $r(w) = 1 + w$, $r(w) = (1 + w)^{-1}$, and $r(w) = \exp(w)$. The choice of relative risk will depend to some extent on the application. One choice, $r(w) = \exp(w)$, is particularly convenient from a mathematical point of view, and is often an adequate description for suitably chosen $\mathbf{z}$. In this case

$$\lambda(t;\mathbf{x}) = \lambda_0(t)\exp(\mathbf{z}'\boldsymbol{\beta}), \tag{23}$$

a log-linear model for the failure rate $\lambda(t;\mathbf{x})$. It should be noted, however, that the general methodology used here would apply equally to other choices of $r(w)$.

More generally, the relative risk may be a function of time. The derived covariate vector $\mathbf{z}(t)' = (z_1(t),\ldots,z_k(t))$ comprises elements of $\mathbf{x}$, powers of these elements, cross-product terms, and possibly products of these with functions of time. Here again, we might take

$$\mathrm{RR}(t;\mathbf{x}) = r(\mathbf{z}(t)'\boldsymbol{\beta})$$

and for $r(w) = \exp(w)$, obtain

$$\lambda(t;\mathbf{x}) = \lambda_0(t)\exp[\mathbf{z}(t)'\boldsymbol{\beta}]. \tag{24}$$

We conclude this section with an example of relative risk modeling.

EXAMPLE 4 Consider a trial in which individuals are randomly assigned to one of two treatment groups so that $x_1 = 0$ or 1 is a treatment indicator. In addition, suppose that x_2 is measured on each patient and is thought to be predictive of failure, as for example when x_2 measures the baseline severity of disease. For a constant relative risk model, we might take $z_1 = x_1$, $z_2 = x_2$ and specify

$$\lambda(t;\mathbf{x}) = \lambda_0(t)\exp(\mathbf{z}'\boldsymbol{\beta}). \tag{25}$$

Here, β_1 measures the treatment effect, with negative values of β_1 indicating a decreased failure rate for treatment 1. Under this model, inferences about β_1 are adjusted for the effect of z_2, assuming that this effect is accurately described as linear on the log failure rate. The model can be extended to test the adequacy of (25) against specific alternatives. In some applications, for example, one may wish to add $z_3 = x_2^2$ to allow for a possible quadratic dependence on the covariate x_2; in this extended model, a test of $\beta_3 = 0$ would provide a test for linearity. In other cases, one might wish to include $z_4 = x_1x_2$ in the model to allow for a possible interaction between the treatment and the covariate.

Models that allow time-dependent relative risks can also be considered. Thus we might take $z_1(t) = x_1$, $z_2(t) = x_1t$, $z_3(t) = x_2$ and consider

$$\lambda(t;\mathbf{x}) = \lambda_0(t)\exp(x_1\beta_1 + x_1t\beta_2 + x_2\beta_3). \tag{26}$$

The coefficient β_2 measures the interaction between x_1 and time, where a positive value of β_2, for example, corresponds to a relative risk function that is increasing with time. If a time-dependent effect is expected, model (26) may be an adequate description. One important use of (26) is to check the assumption of constant relative risk; thus a test of $\beta_2 = 0$ provides a check for the constant relative risk model (25) against the alternative (26).

4.2 Proportional Hazards; Constant Relative Risk

As in Section 4.1, let $\mathbf{x}_1$ be a vector of covariates observed on the ith individual, and suppose that the hazard function is

$$\lambda(t;\mathbf{x}) = \lambda_0(t) r(\mathbf{z}'\boldsymbol{\beta}), \tag{27}$$

where $\mathbf{z}$ is a vector of derived covariates. We consider estimation first of the regression parameters $\boldsymbol{\beta}$, and then of the baseline hazard function $\lambda_0(t)$.

Let $t_{(1)} < t_{(2)} < \cdots < t_{(k)}$ be the observed failure times of individuals $(1), \ldots, (k)$, respectively, and suppose for the moment that no ties are present in the data. Suppose further that the censoring mechanism is independent, and let $R(t)$ be the set of labels of all individuals at risk just prior to t. At time $t_{(i)}$ we find that

$$\begin{aligned} P\{&\text{item } (i) \text{ fails} \mid \text{failure at } t_{(i)}, R(t_{(i)})\} \\ &= \frac{P\{(i) \text{ fails in } (t_{(i)}, t_{(i)} + dt_{(i)}) \mid R(t_{(i)})\}}{P\{\text{failure in } (t_{(i)}, t_{(i)} + dt_{(i)}) \mid R(t_{(i)})\}} \\ &= \frac{\lambda(t_{(i)}; \mathbf{x}_{(i)}) dt_{(i)}}{\sum_{l \in R(t_{(i)})} \lambda(t_{(i)}; \mathbf{z}_l) dt_{(i)}} = \frac{r(\mathbf{z}'_{(i)}\boldsymbol{\beta})}{\sum_{l \in R(t_{(i)})} r(\mathbf{z}'_l\boldsymbol{\beta})} \end{aligned} \tag{28}$$

under relative risk model (27). The "likelihood function" is obtained as a product over the failure times $t_{(i)}$ of the conditional probabilities (28). Thus

$$L(\boldsymbol{\beta}) = \prod_{i=1}^{k} \frac{r(\mathbf{z}'_i\boldsymbol{\beta})}{\sum_{l \in R(t_{(i)})} r(\mathbf{z}'_{(i)}\boldsymbol{\beta})}. \tag{29}$$

This likelihood has been constructed as though the experiments at each failure time were independent of each other. In fact, they are not independent since the items at risk at time $t_{(i)}$ will depend on the outcome of the experiment at $t_{(i-1)}$. It can be shown, however, that the contributions to the score function from the separate terms in (29) are uncorrelated and have expectation zero. As a consequence, the usual asymptotic properties for likelihood inference might be expected to apply to (29); Andersen and Gill (1982) use martingale central limit theorems to establish this result. Cox (1975) examines the general argument leading to (29) and terms the result a partial likelihood, since it is composed of selected conditional components of the full likelihood. The full likelihood will involve the nuisance function $\lambda_0(t)$, whereas (29) involves only the parameter $\boldsymbol{\beta}$. Only the time points at which failures occur contribute to the partial likelihood; no information about $\boldsymbol{\beta}$ can be obtained from intervals in which no failures occur when $\lambda_0(t)$ is completely unspecified since $\lambda_0(t) = 0$ on these intervals would account completely for these data. If external information on $\lambda_0(t)$ is available in the form of a parametric model, these intervals would contribute to the likelihood, and we might be able to improve on (29).

In what follows we restrict attention to the exponential relative risk model $r(w) = e^w$, for which the partial likelihood is

$$L(\boldsymbol{\beta}) = \prod_{1}^{k} \frac{\exp(\mathbf{z}'_{(i)}\boldsymbol{\beta})}{\sum_{l \in R(t_{(i)})} \exp(\mathbf{z}'_l \boldsymbol{\beta})}. \tag{30}$$

However, the methods can be applied to other forms of relative risk, and another form [e.g., $r(w) = 1 + w$] may be more appropriate in a given application.

The argument leading to (29) is essentially the same as that used to derive the log-rank test in Section 3.2. Suppose that $r = p = 1$ and $z = x = 0$ or 1 is a sample indicator. In this case, the proportional hazards model gives hazards $\lambda_0(t)$ in sample 0 and $\lambda_0(t)\exp(\beta)$ in sample 1. The partial likelihood (30) reduces to

$$L(\beta) = \prod_{l}^{k} \frac{\exp(z_{(i)}\beta)}{n_{0i} + n_{1i}\exp(\beta)}$$

where n_{0i} and n_{1i} are the numbers of items at risk at $t^-_{(i)}$ in samples 0 and 1, respectively. At time $t_{(i)}$, consider the 2×2 table, which, in the absence of ties, is one of the following two forms:

	Fail	Survive
Sample 0	1	$n_{0i} - 1$
Sample 1	0	n_{1i}

	Fail	Survive
Sample 0	0	n_{0i}
Sample 1	1	$n_{1i} - 1$

depending on whether $z_{(i)} = 0$ or $z_{(i)} = 1$. Given the risk set $R(t_{(i)})$ (or equivalently, the row totals n_{0i} and n_{1i}) and the fact that one item fails at time $t_{(i)}$ (or equivalently, the column total), the probability that item (i) fails is

$$\frac{\lambda_0(t_{(i)})dt_{(i)}}{n_{0i}\lambda_0(t_{(i)})dt_{(i)} + n_{1i}\lambda_0(t_{(i)})\exp(\beta)dt_{(i)}} = \frac{1}{n_{0i} + n_{1i}\exp(\beta)}$$

if $z_{(i)} = 0$ and $\exp(\beta)/[n_{0i} + n_{1i}\exp(\beta)]$ if $z_{(i)} = 1$. The product over i generates the partial likelihood (30) specialized to this case.

This close parallel between the derivation of the partial likelihood and the log-rank test is reflected in the fact that the log-rank test arises as a score test based on (30). Continuing the scalar case, the score function arising from (30) is

$$S(\beta) = \frac{\partial}{\partial\beta}\log L(\beta) = \sum_{1}^{k}\left[z_{(i)} - \sum_{l\in R(t_{(i)})}\frac{z_l\exp(z_l\beta)}{\sum_{l\in R(t_{(i)})}\exp(z_l\beta)}\right]$$

and, at $\beta = 0$, we obtain

$$S(0) = \sum_{i=1}^{k}\left(z_{(i)} - \frac{n_{1i}}{n_i}\right) = O_1 - E_1,$$

where O_1 is the observed number of failures in sample 1 (with $z = 1$) and E_1 is the "expected" number of failures. This is exactly the log-rank statistic of the preceding section. Its variance can be estimated by $I(0)$, where $I(\beta) = -\partial^2\log L(\beta)/\partial\beta^2$ is the observed information; this is the variance estimate V_1 in (17). The log-rank test provides a simple way of summarizing an analysis based on the proportional hazards model, and is, as was noted in the preceding section, particularly efficient against constant relative risk alternatives.

Heretofore, we have assumed that there are no tied failure times in the data. In fact, even when a continuous model is appropriate, there are often a few ties due to the discreteness of the measurements taken. If the ties are not too numerous, a satisfactory generalization of (30) is

$$L(\boldsymbol{\beta}) = \prod_{i=1}^{k}\frac{\exp(\mathbf{s}_i'\boldsymbol{\beta})}{[\sum_{l\in R(t_{(i)})}\exp(\mathbf{z}_l'\boldsymbol{\beta})]^{d_i}}, \tag{31}$$

where d_i is the number of individuals that fail at $t_{(i)}$ and $\mathbf{s}_i$ is the sum of their covariate values. If each $d_i = 1$, (31) reduces to (30). Expression (31) is utilized in most statistical packages currently available, although other approximations are somewhat preferable. With numerous ties, a discrete model may be more appropriate; discrete models are discussed in Section 5.

The partial likelihood (31) can be used to estimate $\boldsymbol{\beta}$ by applying standard asymptotic results for maximum likelihood estimation. For example, the score vector $\mathbf{S}(\boldsymbol{\beta})$ has jth component

$$S_j(\boldsymbol{\beta}) = \frac{\partial\log L}{\partial\beta_j} = \sum_{i=1}^{k}\mathbf{s}_{ji} - \frac{\sum_{l\in R(t_{(i)})}z_{jl}\exp(\mathbf{z}_l'\boldsymbol{\beta})}{\sum_{l\in R(t_{(i)})}\exp(\mathbf{z}_l'\boldsymbol{\beta})}.$$

It can be used to test the global null hypothesis $\boldsymbol{\beta} = \mathbf{0}$ by comparing

$$\mathbf{S}(\mathbf{0})'I(\mathbf{0})^{-1}\mathbf{S}(\mathbf{0}) \tag{32}$$

with $\chi^2_{(p)}$, where $I(\boldsymbol{\beta})$ is the observed information matrix

$$I(\boldsymbol{\beta}) = \left(-\frac{\partial^2 \log L(\boldsymbol{\beta})}{\partial\beta_j \partial\beta_k}\right)_{p\times p},$$

for which simple formulas are available. The maximum likelihood estimate $\hat{\boldsymbol{\beta}}$ is obtained as the unique solution to the system of simultaneous equations

$$S_j(\boldsymbol{\beta}) = 0, \qquad j = 1, \ldots, p,$$

and the covariance matrix of $\boldsymbol{\beta}$ can be estimated by $I(\hat{\boldsymbol{\beta}})^{-1}$. Thus, in large samples

$$\hat{\boldsymbol{\beta}} \approx N_p(\boldsymbol{\beta}, I(\hat{\boldsymbol{\beta}})^{-1}). \tag{33}$$

Inference about particular elements of $\boldsymbol{\beta}$, say β_1, can be made by using marginal distribution derived from (33),

$$\hat{\beta}_1 \approx N(\beta_1, I^{11}(\hat{\boldsymbol{\beta}})),$$

where $I^{11}(\boldsymbol{\beta})$ is the (1,1) element of $I(\boldsymbol{\beta})^{-1}$. The likelihood ratio test of $\boldsymbol{\beta} = \boldsymbol{\beta}_0$ is obtained by comparing the statistic

$$-2r(\boldsymbol{\beta}_0) = -2[\log L(\boldsymbol{\beta}_0) - \log L(\hat{\boldsymbol{\beta}})] \tag{34}$$

with the $\chi^2_{(p)}$ distribution. In like manner, a test of $\beta_1 = \beta_1^0$ can be based on the comparison of the generalized likelihood ratio statistic

$$-2r_M(\beta_1^0) = -2\log\frac{\max_{\beta_2,\ldots,\beta_p} L(\beta_1^0, \beta_2, \ldots, \beta_p)}{L(\hat{\boldsymbol{\beta}})} \tag{35}$$

with the $\chi^2_{(1)}$ distribution. Approximate confidence intervals for the parameters can be obtained from (33) or from the likelihood ratio statistic. Thus, for example, an approximate 95% confidence interval for β_1 based on (35) is

$$\{\beta_1 : -2r_M(\beta_1) \leq 3.84\},$$

where 3.84 is the upper 5% point of the $\chi^2_{(1)}$ distribution.

It is always difficult to give guidelines as to when a normal or chi-squared approximation is adequate. Nevertheless, experience indicates that in most applications, approximation (33) and the approximate distributions of (34) and (35) have proved satisfactory. As a rough guideline, the number of deaths should be considerably greater than the number p of parameters to be estimated. Extreme elements of $\mathbf{z}$ can greatly influence the estimates, and the presence of such elements suggests caution in applying the asymptotic results. A rather informal check for the appropriateness of approximation (33) is to compare the intervals obtained from it with those obtained from the likelihood ratio statistic. The latter generally provides a better approximation for moderate sample sizes, but the asymptotic distribution of $\hat{\boldsymbol{\beta}}$ is the simplest asymptotic result to use in practice.

Once $\boldsymbol{\beta}$ has been estimated, we can estimate the baseline hazard function $\lambda_0(t)$ or the baseline survivor function $S_0(t) = \exp[-\int \lambda_0(u)du]$ by developing estimates analogous to the Kaplan–Meier estimate (13) or to the Nelson–Aalen estimate (14). In this discussion, however, we extend the methods based on the piecewise exponential model for $\lambda_0(t)$. Therefore, we suppose that $\lambda_0(t) = \theta_j$ for $t \in (a_{j-1}, a_j] = I_j$, where $0 = a_0 < a_1 < \cdots < a_k = \infty$. If $\boldsymbol{\beta}$ is taken as given, the likelihood function for $\theta_1, \ldots, \theta_k$ is

$$L(\theta_1, \ldots, \theta_k) = \prod_{j=1}^{k} \theta_j^{r_j} \exp[-U_j(\boldsymbol{\beta})\theta_j], \tag{36}$$

where r_j is the number of failures in the jth interval and $U_j(\boldsymbol{\beta})$ is the "adjusted exposure" in this interval:

$$U_j(\boldsymbol{\beta}) = \sum_{i|t_i \in I_j} (t_i - a_{j-1})e^{\mathbf{z}_i'\boldsymbol{\beta}} + \sum_{i \in R(a_j)} (a_j - a_{j-1})e^{\mathbf{z}_i'\boldsymbol{\beta}}.$$

Taking $\boldsymbol{\beta} = \hat{\boldsymbol{\beta}}$ and maximizing (36), we obtain the estimated exponential rates as

$$\hat{\theta}_j = \frac{r_j}{U_j(\hat{\boldsymbol{\beta}})}, \qquad j = 1, \ldots, k,$$

and the estimated survivor function

$$\tilde{S}_0(t) = \exp\left[-\sum_{j=0}^{i-1} \hat{\theta}_j(a_j - a_{j-1}) - \hat{\theta}_i(t - a_{i-1})\right] \tag{37}$$

for $t \in [a_{i-1}, a_i)$. The estimate of the survivor function $S(t; \mathbf{z})$ corresponding to covariate level $\mathbf{z}$ is

$$\tilde{S}(t; \mathbf{z}) = \tilde{S}_0(t)^{\exp(\mathbf{z}'\hat{\boldsymbol{\beta}})}. \tag{38}$$

EXAMPLE 3 (CONTINUED) The proportional hazards model can be fitted to the data of Table 1. Consider first a model that includes treatment only, coded 0 for CSP + MTX and 1 for MTX. Newton's algorithm converges quickly from an initial value of $\beta = 0$ to give $\hat{\beta} = 1.143$ with an estimated standard error of $I(\hat{\beta})^{-1/2} = 0.517$. Thus a test of the null hypothesis is provided by the statistic $\hat{\beta}\sqrt{I(\hat{\beta})} = 2.21$, which gives an approximate significance level of 0.027. At $\beta = 0$, the log partial likelihood (31) has value -79.124; at $\hat{\beta}$, the maximized log likelihood has value -76.293. Therefore, $-2r(0) = -2[\log L(0) - \log L(\hat{\beta})] = 5.661$, which yields a significance level of 0.017. These results can be compared with the log-rank analysis of Section 3.2, which gave a significance level of 0.028. All these procedures are in reasonable agreement, and all suggest the presence of a treatment effect.

The estimated size of the effect is measured by $\hat{\beta} = 1.143$, or a relative risk of $\exp(\hat{\beta}) = 3.136$. This indicates that failures in the MTX group occur at about three times the rate of failures in the CSP + MTX group. An approximate 95% confidence interval for β is $\hat{\beta} \pm 1.96 I(\hat{\beta})^{-1/2} = (0.13, 2.16)$ corresponding to the interval (1.14, 8.67) for the relative risk e^{β}. The study is small and the confidence intervals are correspondingly large. Figure 6 gives a plot of the log relative likelihood $r(\beta) = \log[L(\beta)/L(\hat{\beta})]$ for these data. The 95% confidence interval arising from the likelihood ratio statistic in (34) is $\{\beta : r(\beta) > -1.92\} = (0.19, 2.24)$ or (1.21, 9.39) for the relative risk e^{β}, in good agreement with the intervals based on $\hat{\beta}$. The approximating normal log likelihood, $-(\hat{\beta} - \beta)^2 I(\hat{\beta})/2$, is also plotted in Figure 6, and the approximation is seen to be quite good.

Table 4 presents the results of fitting a number of models. Model 1 gives the baseline likelihood assuming no dependence of the failure rate on any covariates; model 2 presumes a dependence on treatment only and was just discussed. In model 3, age was considered as a continuous covariate, resulting in a substantially better fit and increasing the estimated size of the treatment effect. The regression coefficient of 0.057 suggests that the rate of AGVHD increases with age, a 10-year increase in age resulting in a relative risk of $\exp(0.57) = 1.77$. With a continuous covariate such as age, it is often a good idea to code the variable into a few levels since this limits the leverage of outlying values. Model 4 incorporates age as a factor on three levels, ≤ 15, 15 to 25, ≥ 26, and indicates that the two oldest groups did significantly worse than the youngest group but differed little from one another. Models 5 and 6 include LAF and LAF interacting with treatment. There is no evidence of any dependence of failure rates on LAF nor of an interaction effect. Had there been indication of an interaction, the effect could have been further assessed by analyzing age and treatment within each level of LAF.

As noted earlier, the log-rank analysis of Section 3 provides a simpler way to describe the results of model 2. Similarly, the treatment effect of

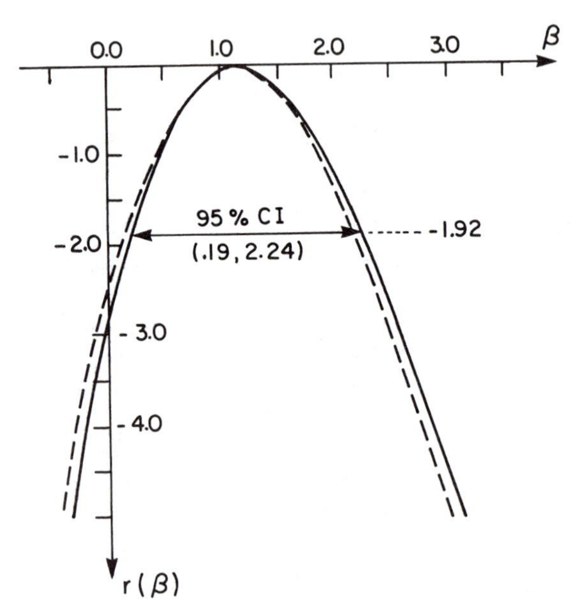

Figure 6 Log relative likelihood of β, $r(\beta = \log[L(\beta)/L(\hat{\beta})]$, arising from the proportional hazards model and the data of Table 1. The dashed curve is the likelihood arising from the normal approximation to the distribution of $\hat{\beta}$.

model 4 can be described by means of the stratified log-rank test (20), with age group as the stratification variable. This provides the same simple O versus E comparison of treatment groups while adjusting for possible age effects, and is closely related to the stratified proportional hazards model discussed in the next section. Table 5 presents the results of the stratified log-rank test, which yields a test statistic of 5.760, giving a significance level of 0.016 when compared with $\chi^2(1)$. As can be seen by looking at the components of the log-rank, the apparent treatment differences are concentrated among patients of age ≥ 26. This can also be seen by fitting separate proportional hazards models within the age groups.

Applying (37) to model 4 in Table 4, we can estimate the baseline hazard functions in the two treatment groups corresponding to age group ≤ 15. As before, we select the intervals $(0, 10]$, $(10, 20]$, $(20, 30]$, $(30, 40]$, $(40, 50]$, $(50, \infty]$, and present the estimated survivor functions in Figure 7. This adjusts the comparison for age; unfortunately, the plots are constrained by the proportional hazards model and may give an inaccurate impression of

Table 4 Proportional Hazards Models Fitted to the Data of Table 1.[a]

Model	Treatment	Age	Age group: 16–25	Age group: ≥ 26	LAF	LAF × Treatment	Log likelihood
1	—	—	—	—	—	—	−79.124
2	1.143/0.517 (0.027)	—	—	—	—	—	−76.143
3	1.388/0.554 (0.009)	0.057/0.025 (0.025)	—	—	—	—	−73.709
4	1.165/0.537 (0.030)	—	1.907/0.771 (0.013)	1.678/0.810 (0.038)	—	—	−71.577
5	1.181/0.544 (0.030)	—	1.904/0.771 (0.014)	1.700/0.818 (0.038)	−0.097/0.488 (0.843)	—	−71.557
6	1.248	—	1.911/0.794 (0.014)	1.706/0.820 (0.038)	−0.017	−0.109/1.07 (0.919)	−71.552

[a]The numerator is the estimated regression coefficient, the denominator is the estimated standard error, and the number in parentheses is the significance level.

Table 5 Stratified log-Rank Test for Data of Table 1 with Age Group Defining Strata[a]

Age group	$O_1^{(l)} - E_1^{(l)}$	$V_1^{(l)}$	$\left\{O_1^{(l)} - E_1^{(l)}\right\} / \sqrt{V_1^{(l)}}$
≤ 15 ($l = 1$)	$1 - 0.950$	0.005	0.07
16–25 ($l = 2$)	$4 - 4.327$	2.557	−0.20
≥ 26 ($l = 3$)	$0 - 4.596$	1.515	−3.73
	−4.875	4.119	

[a]The notation is that of (20).

consistent treatment differences over time. If no covariate like age is included, the Kaplan–Meier comparison of Figure 6 is preferable as a graphical method of presenting treatment comparisons. To adjust the treatment comparison for age effects without imposing a proportional hazards constraint, we can use the stratified analysis discussed in the next section; this yields the better graphical presentation in Figure 8.

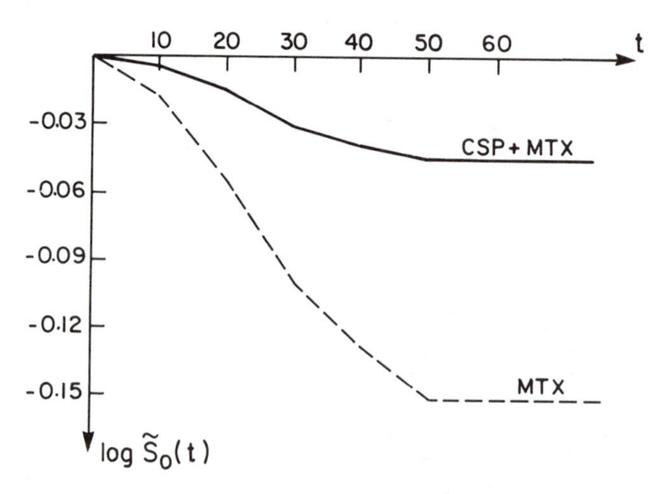

Figure 7 Comparison of survival experience for the two treatment groups adjusted for age to age ≤ 15. Treatment is included as a regression variable in the model and the comparison is constrained by the model, giving an erroneous impression of consistent differences in the rates across time. Figure 8 gives an alternative and preferable comparison.

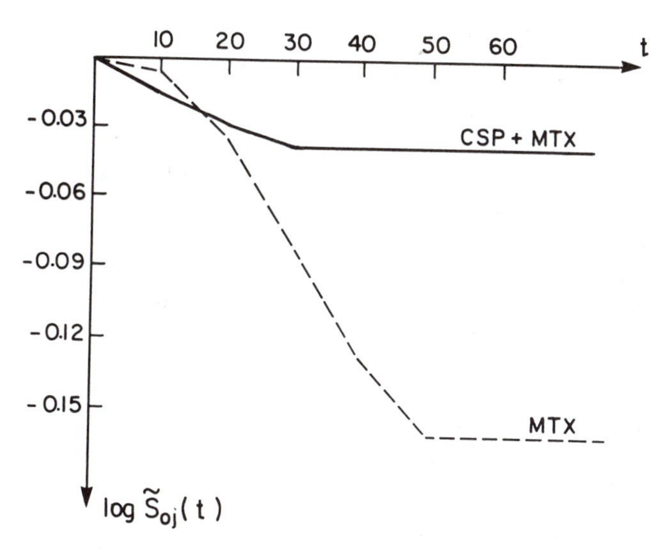

Figure 8 Comparison of survival experience for the two treatment groups adjusted for age to age ≤ 15 years. Treatment defines the strata here, and the comparison is not constrained by the proportional hazards assumption.

4.3 Extensions of the Relative Risk Model

An important extension of the relative risk model (31) allows the baseline hazard rates to vary between strata. Suppose that the s levels of some factor are taken to define the strata; this might be done, for example, if there were a factor for which the proportional hazards assumption was quite inadequate, the hazard rates for different levels not being proportional across time. We might then postulate a model of the form

$$\lambda_j(t; \mathbf{x}) = \lambda_{0j}(t) \exp(\mathbf{z}'\boldsymbol{\beta}) \tag{39}$$

for the hazard in the jth stratum, $j = 1, \ldots, s$. It is assumed in (39) that the baseline hazards are unknown and unrelated, whereas the effect of the covariate $\mathbf{z}$ (the relative risk function) is the same across all strata.

The analysis of (39) proceeds in the same way as for the simpler unstratified model. A partial likelihood $L_j(\boldsymbol{\beta})$ can be obtained for the data on individuals in the jth stratum. The overall likelihood is then

$$L(\boldsymbol{\beta}) = \prod_{j=1}^{s} L_j(\boldsymbol{\beta}) \tag{40}$$

and likelihood inference proceeds as before. The stratified log-rank test (20) arises as the score test (32) of $\beta = 0$ based on (40) when the covariate z is an indicator variable and β is a scalar. Estimation of the baseline survivor function in the jth stratum, $S_{oj}(t) = \exp[-\int_0^t \lambda_{oj}(u)du]$, proceeds by using (37) with only the data from the jth stratum contributing. Figure 8 presents the estimates when treatment defines the strata and age is incorporated in the model.

The assumption that the covariate effect is the same in each stratum can also be tested and relaxed if necessary. It is possible, for example, to allow some components of $\boldsymbol{\beta}$ to be stratum dependent without complicating the analysis.

Finally, no new analytical complications are introduced by allowing the covariates to vary with time, although interpretation and computation become more difficult. Consider the (unstratified) model

$$\lambda(t; \mathbf{X}(t)) = \lambda_0(t) \exp(\mathbf{z}(t)'\boldsymbol{\beta}), \tag{41}$$

where $\mathbf{X}(t) = \{\mathbf{x}(s) : 0 < s < t\}$, $\mathbf{x}(t)$ is a vector of basic (possibly time-varying) covariates, and $\mathbf{z}(t)$ is a vector of derived covariates, which might include functions of $\mathbf{X}(t)$ or cross products between functions of $\mathbf{X}(t)$ and time. The arguments leading to the partial likelihood go through unchanged to yield

$$L(\boldsymbol{\beta}) = \prod_{i=1}^{k} \frac{\exp[\mathbf{s}_i(t_{(i)})'\boldsymbol{\beta}]}{\left\{\sum_{l \in R(t_{(i)})} \exp[\mathbf{z}_l(t_{(i)})'\boldsymbol{\beta}]\right\}^{d_i}}. \tag{42}$$

Of software currently available, the package offered by BMDP (Dixon, 1985, p. 576 ff.) offers the most flexibility in allowing time-varying covariates and stratification.

One important use of time-varying relative risk models is to incorporate interactions between fixed covariates and time. For example, in a two-sample problem with $x = 0$ or 1, we might define $z_i(t) = x$ and $z_2(t) = xg(t)$, where $g(t)$ might be t, or $\log t$, or some other function of time that describes the departures from constant relative risk of interest. In this case

$$\lambda(t; x) = \lambda_0(t) \exp[x\beta_1 + xg(t)\beta_2]. \tag{43}$$

The regression parameter β_2 measures the interaction of x with $g(t)$ and provides a test of the proportional hazards assumption.

The same model can be useful for modeling nonproportional effects. For example, if there were a priori reason to suppose that the treatment effect would be large initially, but minimal later, (43) with $g(t) = t$ or $\log t$ would describe a relative risk function of this type. Simultaneous estimation and testing of β_1 and β_2 can be accomplished using likelihood (42). Both β_1

and β_2 are required to characterize the nature of the treatment effect, which can be summarized graphically by plotting the estimated relative risks over time.

EXAMPLE 3 (CONTINUED) Figure 7 (or Figure 5) suggest that in the aplastic anemia trial, the effect of treatment is not well described by the proportional hazards model: the relative risk of severe AGVHD or death appears to increase with time on study when MTX is compared with CSP+ MTX. To investigate this further, we fit a model that incorporates age (on three levels), treatment, and the interaction of treatment with $g(t) = t$. The maximized log likelihood with no interaction term (see model 4 of Table 4) is -71.577; this increases to -68.194 when the interaction term is included. Thus the likelihood ratio statistic is 6.766, giving an approximate significance level of less than 0.01. Similar results are found with models that incorporate other monotone functions of time [e.g., $g(t) = \log t$].

The likelihood ratio test provides a better test for interaction with time than does a test based on the maximum likelihood estimate, since the likelihood function is positively skewed with respect to this coefficient. In this case, the MLE of the regression coefficient of the treatment by time interaction is 0.1608 with an estimated standard error of 0.0813, giving an approximate significance level of 0.05. An approximate 95% confidence interval based on the likelihood ratio statistic is (0.032, 0.362), compared with (0.002, 0.320) based on the MLE.

It is reasonable to conclude that there is strong evidence of a net benefit from adding CSP to MTX. There is evidence suggesting that the size of this effect increases with time since treatment, so that the addition of CSP delays or avoids late occurrences of AGVHD. There is, as well, some indication that the treatment effect is concentrated among the older patients (≥ 26), as in Table 5. This is an unexpected and not easily explained feature of the data. A confirmatory study is needed to examine further this possible interaction between treatment and age.

In some instances, the covariates $\mathbf{x}(t)$ in (41) may be measures of some covariate that is changing over time. In a leukemia trial, for example, repeated white blood cell counts may be taken on patients over time; in a study of asthma, measurements of environmental pollution levels may be relevant predictors of attacks. When the covariates $\mathbf{x}(t)$ include repeated measures on an individual in a comparative clinical trial, care is required in the interpretation. If, for example, the covariate used is responsive (i.e., its levels are affected by the treatment), including that covariate in the model may mask an important treatment effect or create a spurious effect.

This can provide useful information when exploring possible mechanisms of action of the treatment.

One particular time-dependent model arises sufficiently often to deserve special mention. Suppose that individuals on study may or may not experience an intermediate event prior to failure, and that particular interest centers on the difference in failure rates when the event has or has not occurred. The event histories can be described with reference to Figure 9. The intermediate event may represent, for instance, transplant in a transplantation study in which, at time 0, individuals enter the program and wait for an available donor organ. Alternatively, the intermediate event may be reinfarction in a trial on patients with previous myocardial infarctions. In both cases, death would be the relevant terminal event.

One approach to modeling that has proved to be particularly useful is to define a time-varying covariate $x_1(t)$ which takes the value 0 if the intermediate event has not occurred by time t, and the value 1 thereafter. If $\mathbf{x}_2$ represents the other covariates, we can consider modeling the hazard of the terminal event:

$$\lambda(t;\mathbf{X}(t)) = \lambda_0(t)\exp[\beta_1 x_1(t) + \mathbf{x}_2'\boldsymbol{\beta}_2],$$

where β_1 measures the effect of the intermediate event on the rate at which the terminal event occurs. This model can be extended to allow for interaction between $x_1(t)$ and components of $\mathbf{x}_2$ to check whether the effects of the intermediate event vary across the levels of prognostic or treatment variables. For additional discussion of models of this type, see Kalbfleisch and Prentice (1980, Chap. 5 and references therein) and Cox and Oakes (1984 and references therein).

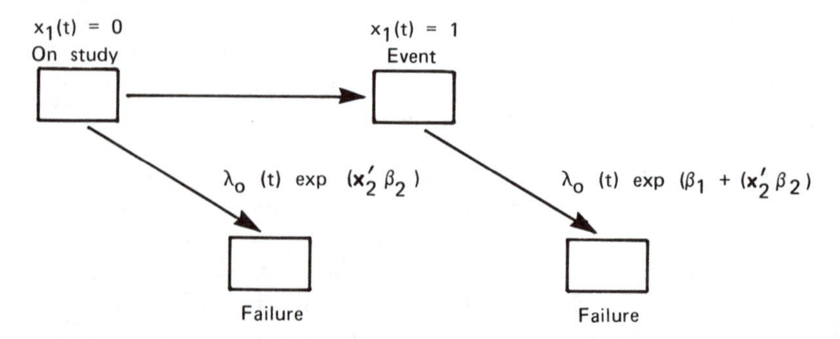

Figure 9 Simple model involving an intermediate event and a terminal failure. The dependence of failure rate on the presence or absence of the event can be assessed using time-dependent covariates.

5 DISCRETE SURVIVAL MODELS

In some applications, the time to the event of interest is a discrete random variable either inherently (as, for example, when "time" is measured by the number of treatment episodes until a cure is obtained) or because continuous failure times have been grouped in the observational process (as, for example, when times to observed ulcer healing are grouped at biweekly endoscopies). The same modeling principles as in the continuous case can then be applied to the discrete hazard function.

5.1 Discrete Regression Models

As before, let $\mathbf{x}$ be a vector of r basic covariates, $\mathbf{z}$ a vector of p derived covariates, and suppose that failures can occur (or be observed) at times $y_1, y_2, \ldots,$ where $0 < y_1 < y_2 \cdots$. Let

$$\lambda_j(\mathbf{x}) = P(T = y_j \mid T \geq y_j, \mathbf{x}), \qquad j = 1, 2, \ldots$$

be the discrete hazard applying at time y_j to an individual with covariate vector $\mathbf{x}$. We shall consider regression models which, as in the continuous case, relate $\lambda_j(\mathbf{x})$ to $\lambda_j(\mathbf{0})$. For the most part, we restrict attention to the logistic model proposed by Cox (1972), which specifies that

$$\log \frac{\lambda_j(\mathbf{x})}{1 - \lambda_j(\mathbf{x})} = \log \frac{\lambda_j(\mathbf{0})}{1 - \lambda_j(\mathbf{0})} + \mathbf{z}'\boldsymbol{\beta}, \tag{44}$$

where $\boldsymbol{\beta}$ is a vector of p regression parameters. Note that (44) can be written as

$$\frac{\lambda_j(\mathbf{x})}{1 - \lambda_j(\mathbf{x})} = \frac{\lambda_j(\mathbf{0})}{1 - \lambda_j(\mathbf{0})} \exp(\mathbf{z}'\boldsymbol{\beta}), \tag{45}$$

from which it can be seen that the covariates act multiplicatively on the baseline conditional odds of failure at y_j. This application of the logistic model to the sequential evolution of a survival study has the same basic motivation as its applications to binary data [see, e.g., Cox (1970, Chap. 2)].

As we shall see in Section 5.2, the logistic model (45) is particularly convenient since we can form a partial likelihood that can be used for estimation as in the continuous-time models. In fact, the choice of $\exp(\mathbf{z}'\boldsymbol{\beta})$ as the constant odds ratio (analogous to the relative risk) can be altered to $r(\mathbf{z}'\boldsymbol{\beta})$, and the analyses can proceed with little change. Finally, the model can be extended to allow time-varying covariates just as in the continuous case. We shall not deal with these extensions here.

There are many other discrete models that could be considered. In fact, we can write quite generally

$$\text{link}(\lambda_j(\mathbf{x})) = \text{link}(\lambda_j(\mathbf{0})) + \mathbf{z}'\boldsymbol{\beta},$$

where "link" is a continuous mapping of (0,1) onto $(-\infty, \infty)$. Any choice of link gives a corresponding discrete model. For example, the logit link,

$$\text{link}(q) = \log \frac{q}{1-q}$$

gives the logistic model (45), whereas the complementary log log link

$$\text{link}(q) = \log[-\log(1-q)]$$

gives the model

$$\lambda_j(\mathbf{x}) = 1 - [1 - \lambda_j(\mathbf{0})]^{\exp(\mathbf{z}'\boldsymbol{\beta})}, \tag{46}$$

which was proposed by Kalbfleisch and Prentice (1973) and studied by Prentice and Gloeckler (1978). The discrete model (46) bears a particularly close relationship to the continuous proportional hazards model; it is obtained when the continuous model is discretized by grouping along the time axis.

There seems to be little difference in $\boldsymbol{\beta}$ estimation when different links are selected. The logistic model (45) gives rise to a partial likelihood which allows estimation of $\boldsymbol{\beta}$ in the presence of the nuisance parameters $\lambda_j(\mathbf{0})$, but other choices of link will require joint estimation of $\lambda_j(\mathbf{0})$ and $\boldsymbol{\beta}$. This joint estimation is more complicated; more important, it can be subject to substantial bias in the estimation of $\boldsymbol{\beta}$, particularly in a stratified analysis with relatively few observations in each stratum. Further, these biases tend to exaggerate treatment effects. For these reasons we think that the model (45), together with the analysis presented in the next section, is sufficiently flexible to be the method of choice.

5.2 Estimation from the Discrete Model

Suppose that data, possibly with independent right censoring, are available from the model (45). As noted above, one might consider joint maximum likelihood estimation of $\boldsymbol{\beta}$ and $\lambda_j(\mathbf{0})$, $j = 1, 2, \ldots$. With the logistic model, this can be accomplished in a straightforward manner using standard software for binary logistic models. The data are organized as if they arose from a sequence of experiments with binary outcomes for all individuals at risk at each failure time y_j; therefore, we have a categorical variable for time, as well as the covariate vector $\mathbf{z}$. This approach is satisfactory in most applications, but can lead to biased estimation of $\boldsymbol{\beta}$ in highly stratified analyses, as noted above.

The construction of a partial likelihood based on the discrete model (45) follows closely the development in the continuous case (see Section 4.2). Let D_j be the set of labels of the d_j items observed to fail at time y_j, and let R_j be the risk set just prior to y_j. Given R_j and the fact that d_j items fail at y_j, the probability that they are the items in D_j is, after some algebra,

$$P(D_j \mid R_j, d_j \text{ items fail at } y_j)$$

$$= \frac{P(D_j \mid R_j)}{P(d_j \text{ items fail at } y_j \mid R_j)}$$

$$= \frac{\prod_{l \in D_j} \lambda_j(\mathbf{x}_l)/[1 - \lambda_j(\mathbf{x}_l)]}{\sum_{V \in C(R_j, d_j)} \prod_{l \in V} \lambda_j(\mathbf{x}_l)/[1 - \lambda_j(\mathbf{x}_l)]}, \tag{47}$$

where $C(R_j, d_j)$ denotes the set of all subsets of R_j of size d_j. This calculation is essentially the same as that leading to the Fisher exact test in the 2×2 contingency table. Under the logistic model (44), the common factor $\lambda_j(\mathbf{0})/[1 - \lambda_j(\mathbf{0})]$ cancels in (47), and a product over j gives the partial likelihood

$$L(\boldsymbol{\beta}) = \prod_j \frac{\exp(\mathbf{s}_j' \boldsymbol{\beta})}{\sum_{V \in C(R_j, d_j)} \exp(\mathbf{s}_V' \boldsymbol{\beta})}, \tag{48}$$

where $\mathbf{s}_j = \sum_{l \in D_j} \mathbf{z}_l$ and $\mathbf{s}_V = \sum_{l \in V} \mathbf{z}_l$.

The argument leading to (48) is again sequential and exploits the conditional binomial structure at the ith failure time. It is closely related to the Mantel–Haenszel or log-rank test of Section 3.2: if $\mathbf{z}$ is a vector of group indicators for the $r+1$ sample problem, the log-rank test for this problem arises as the score test based on (48). Recall that (30) also yields the log-rank test when no ties are present in the data. Indeed, the likelihood (48) reduces to (30) if there are no ties, and offers a method of incorporating ties that is superior to (31).

Direct calculation of (48) or its derivatives is apparently very complicated due to the sum in the denominator over $\binom{n_j}{d_j}$ terms where n_j is the number of individuals at risk just prior to y_j. In fact, efficient algorithms are available as first outlined by Howard (1972) and later developed by Storer, Wacholder, and Breslow (Storer et al., 1983). The algorithms are not currently implemented in standard software packages; however, they are used in the package EGRET soon to be marketed by SERC.

5.3 An Application to Discrete Failure-Time Data

As a final example, we consider the data reported in Table 6, which were drawn from a randomized, double-blind, multiclinic trial to evaluate a drug

Table 6 Randomized Multicenter Clinical Trial with Endoscopies at 2, 4, and 6 Weeks (Coded as 1, 2, 3)

Placebo			Treatment			Placebo			Treatment		
Tob.[a]	Diam.[b]	Time	Tob.[a]	Diam.[b]	Time	Tob.[a]	Diam.[b]	Time	Tob.[a]	Diam.[b]	Time
Clinic 1						Clinic 5					
0	5	2	0	5	1	0	10	1[c]	0	5	3
0	10	1[c]	0	4	1	0	4	2[c]	1	4	3[d]
1	5	2	0	7	1[c]	1	4	3	1	4	3
0	6	2	1	10	3	1	10	3[d]	0	12	3[d]
1	5	3	1	7	1	0	12	1[c]	0	10	1[c]
0	8	3[d]				0	10	3[d]	0	10	1[c]
0	8	2				0	5	3	0	8	3
						0	3	2	0	4	2
						0	4	2	1	5	2
Clinic 2						Clinic 6					
1	5	3[d]	1	7	3[d]	0	3	1[c]	1	2	1[c]
0	9	1[c]	1	8	2	1	20	2[c]	0	10	3[d]
0	7	3	1	8	2	1	10	3	1	12	2
0	11	3[d]	1	5	1	1	4	2	1	10	2
1	12	1[c]	1	7	1	1	10	3[d]	0	7	2
1	5	3[d]	1	6	2	1	5	3[d]	0	4	2
1	7	1[c]	1	5	2	0	20	3[d]	1	8	3[d]
0	8	2	0	8	2	1	8	3	0	3	1
1	3	1	1	5	1	0	3	3	0	10	2
1	6	3[d]	0	5	2	1	18	3[d]	0	10	3[d]
1	6	1				0	10	1			
1	7	2									

Clinic 3					
1	10	3[d]	0	8	1
1	7	3[d]	0	8	3[d]
0	7	1	0	5	1
0	7	1	0	6	3[d]
0	5	2	0	5	2
0	7	3	0	8	2
0	5	1	0	5	2
0	5	1	0	10	2
0	5	3[d]	0	4	1
0	7	1	0	10	3[d]

Clinic 4					
0	15	3	0	10	1
0	8	1	0	10	1
0	4	2	0	5	3[d]
0	20	3[d]	1	10	1
0	10	3[d]	0	4	1
0	8	2	1	6	1
0	7	2	0	8	3[d]
1	10	3	0	8	3[d]

Clinic 7					
0	5	2	0	2	2
1	3	3[d]	0	8	3
1	10	2	0	5	3
1	10	3[d]	1	3	1
0	6	1[c]	1	2	1
0	8	3[d]	1	5	2
			0	15	2
			1	6	2
			1	5	1
			1	5	1

[a] For tobacco, 0, no; 1, yes.
[b] Diameter is measured in mm.
[c] Withdrawal—treated as a failure through 6 weeks.
[d] Independently censored.

for the treatment of active duodenal ulcers. These data were selected and rearranged from a much larger set; the analyses are presented here solely to illustrate the statistical methodology.

Table 6 gives the times to observed healing (or censoring) for 125 patients with baseline ulcer craters between 3 and 20 mm in longest dimension, as determined by endoscopic examination at time zero. The patients were randomized within clinics to treatment or control, and were endoscoped again after 2, 4, and 6 weeks of treatment or until complete reepithelialization. Thirteen patients withdrew prior to 6 weeks of study due to adverse events or severe ulcer symptoms; their ulcers are assumed to be unhealed through 6 weeks. Patients who reached 6 weeks of study with unhealed ulcers are viewed as independently censored. In addition to clinic and time, Table 6 includes two baseline variables: ulcer diameter (mm) and an indicator as to whether or not the patient used tobacco.

As discussed earlier, one approach to estimation and testing utilizes a standard package for binary logistic regression. Time is then included as a factored variable on three levels and clinic as a factored variable on seven levels. Table 7 presents the results of an analysis with the additional regression variables of treatment, diameter, and tobacco use. The log odds ratio for treatment is estimated as 0.764 with standard error 0.288, giving a significance level of 0.008. Also, there are substantial differences between

Table 7 Maximum Likelihood Estimation Based on a Binary Logistic Regression Model for the Data in Table 6

	Estimate	Standard error	Significance level
Grand mean	−0.1973	0.605	—
Treatment	0.764	0.288	0.008
Time:			
2 weeks	1.010	0.326	0.002
4 weeks	0.737	0.389	0.058
Clinic:			
2	−0.319	0.552	0.564
3	−0.029	0.558	0.958
4	0.231	0.594	0.698
5	−1.07	0.573	0.062
6	−0.744	0.565	0.188
7	−0.346	0.585	0.554
Diameter	−0.178	0.053	< 0.001
Tobacco	0.033	0.317	0.916

Table 8 Maximum Partial Likelihood Estimates for the Data in Table 6 with Clinics Defining Strata

	Estimate	Standard error	Significance level
Treatment	0.687	0.285	0.016
Diameter	−0.176	0.053	< 0.001
Tobacco	0.072	0.319	0.821

clinics, ulcer diameter is an important predictor, and there is no indication of any dependence of cure rate on tobacco use. The odds ratio of ulcer healing and its associated 95% confidence interval, (1.22, 3.78), indicates that there is a substantial benefit of treatment with respect to healing rates.

Since many parameters are fitted, there is potential here for bias in the estimate of the treatment effect. A preferable approach would allow the clinics to define the strata, and fit a discrete proportional model (45) with different baseline hazards $\lambda_{lj}(0)$ for each of the clinics $l = 1, \ldots, 7$. The partial likelihood for the regression parameters β associated with treatment, diameter, and tobacco use is then composed of seven components, each of the form (48). Table 8 presents the results of this analysis. The estimated log odds ratio corresponding to treatment is 0.687 with standard error 0.285 and significance level 0.016. Although there is still strong evidence of a treatment effect, it is clear that maximum likelihood based on the binary logistic model tends to overstate this effect. Ulcer diameter is again seen to be an important predictor, and tobacco usage does not appear to be related to healing rates.

The inclusion of diameter in the model substantially reduces the apparent treatment effect. This arises since patients in the treatment group had a smaller mean ulcer diameter at the outset, despite the randomization. There is also some suggestion of an interaction between treatment and tobacco use ($p = 0.048$), in which treatment appears more effective among smokers than among nonsmokers. Clinics could also be incorporated as factored variables in the discrete proportional hazards analysis. This gives essentially the same results as the stratified analysis in Table 8 and again avoids the bias in the maximum likelihood estimate.

6 DISCUSSION

We have sketched some of the methods in current use for the analysis of survival data. More complete treatments can be found in various books [e.g., Kalbfleisch and Prentice (1980), Lawless (1982), and Cox and Oakes (1984)]. Due to space limitations, we have kept references to a minimum; these books have extensive bibliographies. We have not discussed parametric models, although in some applications, these are important and appropriate. In general, the methods based on the proportional hazards model and the related log-rank tests have wide applicability and offer flexible approaches to modeling, data analysis, and inference.

There are important generalizations of the ideas and techniques presented here to problems in competing risks. In such problems, individuals under study are subject to several different modes of failure, and one wishes to evaluate treatment and covariate effects on only one or two of the failure modes, or to evaluate possible dependencies between them. The interested reader is referred to Prentice et al. (1978). More generally, the response of interest may involve the timing of occurrences of several different lifetime events. For example, in a cancer trial, one may wish to examine the effect of treatment on time to remission as well as on the period from remission to death. In investigations of asthma, the sequence and timing of asthma attacks on an individual may be the response of interest. The methods described here can be extended to address these sorts of questions as well. The work of Prentice, Williams, and Peterson (Prentice et al., 1982) provides a good introduction to the area.

Acknowledgments. We would like to thank R. Storb for his permission to use the data in Table 1 and to acknowledge his research funding from NHLBI grant HL36444. This work was supported in part by a grant from the Natural Sciences and Engineering Research Council of Canada. We also wish to thank Boehringer Ingleheim Pharmaceuticals, Inc., for making the data in Table 4 available to us.

REFERENCES

Andersen, P. K., O. Borgan, R. D. Gill, and N. Keiding (1982). Linear nonparametric tests for comparison of counting processes with applications to censored survival data. *Internat. Statist. Rev. 50*, 219–258.

Andersen, P. K., and R. D. Gill (1982). Cox's regression model for counting processes: a large sample study. *Ann. Statist. 10*, 1100–1120.

Cox, D. R. (1970). *Analysis of Binary Data.* Chapman & Hall, London.

Cox, D. R. (1972). Regression models and life tables (with discussion). *J. Roy. Statist. Soc. B 34*, 187–220.

Cox, D. R. (1975). Partial likelihood. *Biometrika 62*, 269–276.

Cox, D. R., and D. Oakes (1984). *Analysis of Survival Data.* Chapman & Hall, London.

Dixon, W. J., ed. (1985). *BMDP Statistical Software Manual.* University of California Press, Berkeley.

Howard, S. (1972). Discussion of paper by D. R. Cox. *J. Roy Statist. Soc. B 34*, 210–211.

Kalbfleisch, J. D., and R. L. Prentice (1973). Marginal likelihoods based on Cox's regression and life model. *Biometrika 60*, 267–278.

Kalbfleisch, J. D., and R. L. Prentice (1980). *The Statistical Analysis of Failure Time Data.* Wiley, New York.

Kaplan, E. L., and P. Meier (1958). Nonparametric estimation from incomplete observations. *J. Amer. Statist. Assoc. 53*, 457–481.

Lawless, J. F. (1982). *Statistical Models and Methods for Lifetime Data*, Wiley, New York.

Mantel, N. (1966). Evaluation of survival data and two new rank order statistics arising in its consideration. *Cancer Chemother. Rep. 50*, 163–170.

Mantel, N. and W. Haenszel (1959) Statistical aspects of the analysis of data from retrospective studies of disease. *J. Nat. Cancer Inst. 22*, 719–748.

Peto, R., M. C. Pike, P. Armitage, N. E. Breslow, D. R. Cox, S. V. Howard, N. Mantel, K. McPherson, J. Peto, and P. G. Smith (1976). Design and analysis of randomized clinical trials requiring prolonged observation of each patient: I. Introduction and design. *British J. Cancer 34*, 585–612.

Peto, R., M. C. Pike, P. Armitage, N. E. Breslow, D. R. Cox, S. V. Howard, N. Mantel, K. McPherson, J. Peto, and P. G. Smith (1977). Design and analysis of randomized clinical trials requiring prolonged observation of each patient: II. Analysis and examples. *British J. Cancer 35*, 1–39.

Prentice, R. L. (1978). Linear rank tests with right censored data. *Biometrika 65*, 167–179.

Prentice, R. L., and L. A. Gloeckler (1978). Regression analysis of grouped survival data with applications to breast cancer. *Biometrics 34*, 57–67.

Prentice, R. L., J. D. Kalbfleisch, A. V. Peterson, N. Flournoy, V. T. Farewell, and N. E. Breslow (1978). The analysis of failure times in the presence of competing risks. *Biometrics 34*, 541–554.

Prentice, R. L., B. J. Williams, and A. V. Peterson (1981). On the regression analysis of multivariate failure time data. *Biometrika 68*, 373–380.

Storb, R., H. J. Deeg, V. Farewell, K. Doney, F. Appelbaum, P. Beatty, W. Bensinger, C. D. Buckner, R. Clift, J. Hansen, R. Hill, G. Longton, L. Lum, P. Martin, R. McGuffin, J. Sanders, J. Singer, P. Stewart, K.

Sullivan, R. Witherspoon, and E. D. Thomas (1986). Marrow transplantation for severe aplastic anemia: methotrexate alone compared with a combination of methotrexate and cyclosporine for prevention of acute graft-versus-host disease. *Blood 68*, 119–125.

Storer, B. E., S. Wacholder, and N. E. Breslow (1983). Maximum likelihood fitting of general risk models to stratified data. *J. Roy. Statist. Soc. C 32*, 172–181.

12

Robust Data Analysis

ROBERT V. HOGG The University of Iowa, Iowa City, Iowa

STEPHEN J. RUBERG and LIANNG YUH Merrell Dow Research Institute, Cincinnati, Ohio

1 INTRODUCTION

The method of least squares and its generalizations have served statisticians well for many years. Most of the statistical computer packages are based on these theories, and thus will be used for many years to come and rightfully so. Statisticians should question, however, whether the assumptions underlying these theories are met in each application. Statisticians are doing this more often now with various procedures that involve examination of the residuals from the fitted model—whether the model is a one-sample estimation problem or a multiple linear regression problem. For example, if the residuals are skewed to the right, transformations like the square root and the logarithm can make the underlying distribution more symmetric and, in particular, more normal.

The use of transformations has been a popular approach to applied problems in the past, and extensions to general power transformations have received much attention. Of course, the power transformation is not a panacea because incorrect selection of the power could cause difficulties, and other methods have been developed. Two popular areas of development have been M-estimation and nonparametric or rank procedures. These methods are frequently referred to as robust methods because they have good statistical properties for many different underlying probability structures, although they may not be optimal for any one situation.

In this chapter we deal with such robust procedures. In Section 2 robust estimation through weighted least squares will be approached because most statisticians are familiar with that technique. Using the one-sample location problem as a starting point, we will develop M-estimation procedures involving regression applications. Hypothesis testing is presented in Section 3 using the Wilcoxon test for the two-sample location problem as the foundation for development. Extensions to more general linear rank statistics and methods for broader alternative hypotheses will also be discussed. In each section, examples from actual data analysis problems in the pharmaceutical industry will be used to demonstrate the application and utility of the robust procedures. We conclude in Section 4 with practical suggestions for robust data analysis.

2 M-ESTIMATION

Let $X_1, X_2, \ldots, X_n$ be a random sample from a continuous distribution with cumulative distribution function (CDF) $F(x-\theta)$, where F is symmetric about zero. There are three major classes of robust point estimators for θ: the L-estimate, which is a linear combination of the sample order statistics; the R-estimate, which is a nonparametric method resulting from ranking; and the M-estimate, which was proposed by Huber (1964). In this section we concentrate on the M-estimates and their applications.

2.1 One-Sample Case

The M-estimate for a one-sample parameter is defined as follows. With a nonnegative function, ρ, choose the value of θ that minimizes

$$\sum_{i=1}^{n} \rho(X_i - \theta),$$

where $X_1, X_2, \ldots, X_n$ are random observations from the symmetric distribution $F(x-\theta)$ and $\rho(x)$ is usually monotone increasing in $|x|$. In particular, if $\rho(x) = x^2$, the solution is the least squares estimate (the sample mean). The M-estimate is actually a maximum likelihood estimator for the location parameter θ when the underlying density function $f(x)$

exists and $\rho(x) = -ln[f(x)]$; this is the reason the modifier M is used. The asymptotic behavior of these M-estimators and some of their properties are considered in detail by Huber (1981).

To provide an estimator for θ, a robust estimate for the scale, say σ, of the underlying distribution is needed when this scale is unknown. Many statisticians use $s = \text{median}[|X_i - M|/0.6745]$, where M is the sample median and the median $|X_i - M|$ is usually taken over the nonzero deviations, or perhaps $s = (75\text{th percentile} - 25\text{th percentile})/[2(0.6745)]$. The constant 0.6745 in these estimates is used so that each is a consistent estimate of σ when the sample arises from a normal distribution. Thus $\hat{\theta}$ is then the solution of

$$\sum_{i=1}^{n} \psi\left(\frac{X_i - \theta}{s}\right) = 0, \tag{1}$$

where $\psi = \rho'$. Equations of this form may be difficult to solve for certain functions (like the Cauchy case), and iterative numerical methods are required. There are three iteration schemes that can be used to solve equation (1). The first is Newton's method and the second is applying the H-method; details of these schemes can be found in Hogg (1979). The third scheme is to take the kth iteration to be

$$T_k = \frac{\sum_{i=1}^{n} w_{i,k-1} X_i}{\sum_{i=1}^{n} w_{i,k-1}},$$

where the weight function is defined by

$$\begin{aligned} w_{i,k-1} &= 1, \qquad \text{when} \qquad X_i - T_{k-1} = 0, \\ &= \frac{\psi[(X_i - T_{k-1})/s]}{(X_i - T_{k-1})/s}, \qquad \text{when } X_i - T_{k-1} \neq 0, \end{aligned}$$

for $i = 1, 2, \ldots, n$, where T_0 is some reasonable robust starting value, like the sample median. Note that the weight function is defined by $w(z) = \psi(z)/z$.

Let us follow through this development with a simple illustration, finally computing a robust estimate when $n = 5$. Suppose we believe that the random sample $X_1, X_2, \ldots, X_n$ arises from a Student's t distribution with r degrees of freedom with location parameter θ and scale parameter σ (which is not necessarily the standard deviation). That is, the underlying density is

$$f(x; \theta, \sigma) = \frac{c}{[1 + \left(\frac{x-\theta}{\sigma}\right)^2 / r]^{(r+1)/2}}, \qquad -\infty < x < \infty,$$

where the constant c is a function of σ. Let us not worry about the estimation of σ at present. The logarithm of the likelihood function, $L(\theta)$, is

$$\ln L(\theta) = \text{constant} - \frac{r+1}{2}\sum_{i=1}^{n} \ln\left[1 + \left(\frac{x_i - \theta}{\sigma}\right)^2 \Big/ r\right].$$

Equating the derivative of this expression, with respect to θ, to zero, we obtain

$$\frac{r+1}{r\sigma}\sum_{i=1}^{n} \frac{\frac{x_i-\theta}{\sigma}}{1+(\frac{x_i-\theta}{\sigma})^2/r} = 0$$

or, equivalently,

$$\sum_{i=1}^{n} \frac{1}{1+(\frac{x_i-\theta}{\sigma})^2/r}(x_i - \theta) = 0.$$

Inserting the preliminary estimates of θ and σ, namely,

$$T_0 = M = \text{median}, \qquad s = \frac{\text{median } |x_i - M|}{0.6745},$$

into the first factor, we obtain

$$\sum_{i=1}^{n} w_{i,0}(x_i - T_1) = 0,$$

where

$$w_{i,0} = \frac{1}{1+(\frac{x_i-T_0}{s})^2/r}, \qquad i = 1, 2, \ldots, n.$$

That is, the one-step estimate is

$$T_1 = \frac{\sum_{i=1}^{n} w_{i,0}x_i}{\sum_{i=1}^{n} w_{i,0}}.$$

Often, this is used without further computation, but it is easy to iterate any number of times if you like. For illustration, T_1 and s (either the original s or one constructed using T_1 as the preliminary estimate of θ) are used as the preliminary estimates to obtain the two-step estimate T_2, and so on.

For an explicit computation, suppose we believe that our distribution has somewhat heavier tails than those of the normal and we choose a Student's t with $r = 6$ d.f. Here r can be thought of as a "tuning constant," and its selection depends upon experience or the actual data (Hogg et al., 1987). However, many applied statisticians would agree with the selection of r

about equal to 6 for many data sets. Say that $n = 5$ and the ordered observations are

$$x_{(1)} = 72, \qquad x_{(2)} = 95, \qquad x_{(3)} = 101, \qquad x_{(4)} = 104, \qquad x_{(5)} = 113.$$

Thus

$$T_0 = M = 101 \qquad \text{and } s = \frac{\text{med}\{29, 6, 3, 12\}}{0.6745} = \frac{9}{0.6745} = 13.34.$$

The respective weights of the five points are

$$w_{1,0} = \frac{1}{1 + \left(\frac{72-101}{13.34}\right)^2/6} = 0.56,$$
$$w_{2,0} = \frac{1}{1 + \left(\frac{95-101}{13.34}\right)^2/6} = 0.97,$$
$$w_{3,0} = \frac{1}{1 + \left(\frac{101-101}{13.34}\right)^2/6} = 1.00,$$
$$w_{4,0} = \frac{1}{1 + \left(\frac{104-101}{13.34}\right)^2/6} = 0.99,$$
$$w_{5,0} = \frac{1}{1 + \left(\frac{113-101}{13.34}\right)^2/6} = 0.88.$$

Notice how the outlying observation, 72, is downweighted substantially, while the weights of the other observations are fairly close to 1. This yields the one-step estimate of

$$T_1 = \frac{\sum_{i=1}^{5} w_{i,0} x_{(i)}}{\sum_{i=1}^{5} w_{i,0}} = \frac{436}{4.40} = 99.$$

Of course, this process can be repeated any number of times, although we have often been satisfied with one-step estimates.

Some standard weight functions, along with the corresponding ψ-functions, are given in Table 1. It is noted that some of the standard weight functions, such as Tukey's biweight, do not even have corresponding density functions, but they still provide excellent estimation procedures. The graphs of these functions are given in Figure 1. Note that the ψ-functions for all but the normal case are bounded. Moreover, those of Student and Tukey redescend to zero as $|x|$ becomes large. Satisfactory values of the tuning constants for the last three weight functions in Table 1 are $K = 1.25$, $r = 6$, and $b = 4.82$, respectively. With these values, the efficiencies of the robust estimators are fairly large (above 90% compared to the least squares

Table 1 Standard ψ and Weight Functions

Distribution	ψ	Weight function
Normal	x	1
Double exponential	$\begin{cases} -1, & x < 0 \\ 1, & x > 0 \end{cases}$	$1/\lvert x\rvert, \quad x \neq 0$
Huber (K) ($K = 1.25$)	$\begin{cases} x, & \lvert x\rvert \leq K \\ K\,\text{sign}(x), & \lvert x\rvert > K \end{cases}$	$\begin{cases} 1, & \lvert x\rvert \leq K \\ k/\lvert x\rvert, & \lvert x\rvert > K \end{cases}$
Student $T(r)$ ($r = 6$)	$\dfrac{2x}{1 + x^2/r}$	$\dfrac{1}{1 + x^2/r}$
Tukey (b) ($b = 4.82$)	$\begin{cases} x(1 - x^2/b^2)^2, & \lvert x\rvert \leq b \\ 0, & \lvert x\rvert > b \end{cases}$	$\begin{cases} (1 - x^2/b^2)^2, & \lvert x\rvert \leq b \\ 0, & \lvert x\rvert > b \end{cases}$

method) if the underlying distribution is normal, but these estimators give excellent protection against outliers if the distributions have long and thick tails, say like a Student t-distribution with $r = 1$, 2, or 3. Of course, we believe in adaptive robust estimation and would decrease the values of these tuning constants if we really thought, through some preliminary investigation of the data, that the underlying distribution had extremely long and thick tails. On the other hand, if the data indicate a light-tailed distribution, larger values of these tuning constants would be used.

EXAMPLE 1 We studied the behavior of several M-estimators using the distribution of the blood chemistry serum glutoxyacetic transaminase (SGOT) measurements. The measurements were taken from 203 male patients following treatment with an investigational drug. The data were collected to estimate the location of the underlying distribution. Statistical programs such as BMDP7D and BMDP2D (Dixon, 1983) compute several M-estimators. We used PROC NLIN and PROC UNIVARIATE in SAS (Yuh and Sullivan, 1988) for the numerical computation. Robust estimators, which included the median, Huber's ψ, and Tukey's biweight, were compared to the sample mean. The results of this comparison are presented in Table 2. Robust estimators provide a markedly different estimate than the sample mean. Since the underlying distribution of SGOT is asymmetric as demonstrated by Hill and Dixon (1984), these robust estimators are preferred as measures of location (Table 3).

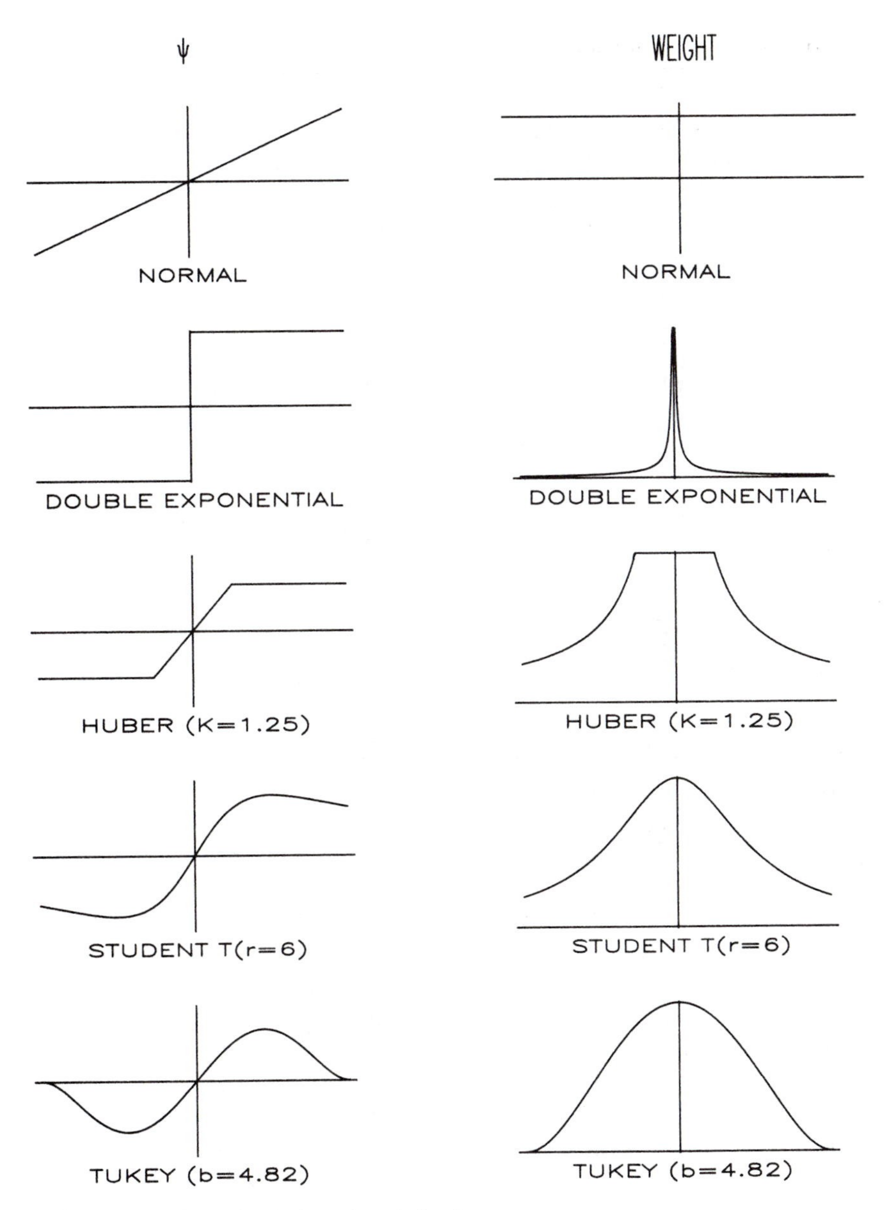

Figure 1 Standard ψ and weight functions.

Table 2 Raw Data for Example 1

Patient	SGOT (units/liter)	Patient	SGOT (units/liter)	Patient	SGOT (units/liter)
1	12	35	30	69	36
2	20	36	18	70	34
3	19	37	45	71	20
4	33	38	137	72	25
5	45	39	32	73	27
6	40	40	37	74	16
7	61	41	20	75	230
8	46	42	104	76	28
9	33	43	29	77	34
10	37	44	60	78	56
11	32	45	15	79	40
12	23	46	53	80	23
13	38	47	28	81	20
14	28	48	19	82	22
15	31	49	37	83	35
16	30	50	33	84	21
17	36	51	14	85	39
18	24	52	14	86	25
19	39	53	21	87	47
20	32	54	29	88	22
21	38	55	22	89	16
22	20	56	14	90	55
23	38	57	3500	91	44
24	30	58	27	92	49
25	58	59	29	93	68
26	32	60	21	94	17
27	16	61	29	95	39
28	30	62	19	96	38
29	20	63	52	97	22
30	29	64	8	98	14
31	12	65	47	99	14
32	42	66	34	100	10
33	38	67	28	101	26
34	24	68	28	102	16

Table 2 (*continued*)

Patient	SGOT (units/liter)	Patient	SGOT (units/liter)	Patient	SGOT (units/liter)
103	14	137	17	171	20
104	8	138	7	172	24
105	20	139	17	173	157
106	24	140	36	174	39
107	14	141	17	175	1
108	89	142	10	176	34
109	105	143	33	177	26
110	11	144	26	178	45
111	23	145	15	179	55
112	23	146	25	180	47
113	22	147	24	181	256
114	12	148	68	182	375
115	27	149	60	183	69
116	39	150	50	184	48
117	10	151	72	185	53
118	86	152	56	186	47
119	17	153	31	187	150
120	18	154	70	188	19
121	21	155	50	189	26
122	73	156	42	190	37
123	15	157	24	191	34
124	34	158	39	192	31
125	870	159	32	193	89
126	26	160	29	194	46
127	16	161	31	195	25
128	22	162	30	196	31
129	13	163	15	197	17
130	37	164	56	198	30
131	23	165	35	199	32
132	37	166	30	200	30
133	29	167	12	201	49
134	25	168	9	202	21
135	25	169	30	203	31
136	16	170	35		

Table 3 Robust Estimators for One-Sample Location Problem

Estimator	$\hat{\theta}$
Sample mean	58.71
Sample median	30.00
Huber ($K = 1.25$)	30.46
Tukey ($b = 4.82$)	29.21

2.2 Regression

The M-estimate can easily be extended to the regression problem. Suppose that we have the linear model

$$\mathbf{Y} = \mathbf{X}\boldsymbol{\beta} + \boldsymbol{\epsilon},$$

where $\mathbf{Y}$ is an $n \times 1$ random vector, $\mathbf{X}$ is an $n \times k$ full-rank design matrix, $\boldsymbol{\beta}$ is a $k \times 1$ vector of unknown parameters, and $\boldsymbol{\epsilon}$ is a $n \times 1$ random vector with elements like a random sample from a distribution (usually symmetric about zero, but not necessarily normal) with δ as a measure of the scale. We wish to minimize with an appropriate ρ-function,

$$\sum_{i=1}^{n} \rho\left(\frac{Y_i - \mathbf{X}_i\boldsymbol{\beta}}{\delta}\right),$$

where Y_i is the ith element of $\mathbf{Y}$ and $\mathbf{X}_i$ is the ith row of $\mathbf{X}$. If $\rho' = \psi$, then equating the first partial derivatives of the summation with respect to the elements of $\boldsymbol{\beta}$ equal to zero, we obtain

$$\sum_{i=1}^{n} X_{ij}\psi\left(\frac{Y_i - \mathbf{X}_i\boldsymbol{\beta}}{\delta}\right) = 0, \qquad j = 1, 2, \ldots, k, \tag{2}$$

where X_{ij} is the element in the ith row and jth column of $\mathbf{X}$.

Obviously, if (2) has a closed-form solution in $\boldsymbol{\beta}$, no iterations are required. This is the case with $\psi(x) = x$, for which the solution is the least squares estimate. For ψ-functions that do not yield closed-form solutions, X_i's of a univariate sample are replaced by the residuals from some initial estimates; namely $\mathbf{R} = \mathbf{Y} - \mathbf{X}\hat{\boldsymbol{\beta}}_0$, where $\hat{\boldsymbol{\beta}}_0$ is a good robust starting value. To obtain a robust estimate of δ and these starting values, Kroenker and Bassett (1978) have developed "regression quantiles" (L_p), which generalize the notion of the $(100p)$th quantile of the sample for the regression case. For simple linear regression, their estimate is defined to be any $\boldsymbol{\beta}$ that minimizes

$$p \sum_{R_1} |Y_i - \mathbf{X}_i \boldsymbol{\beta}| + (1-p) \sum_{R_2} |Y_i - \mathbf{X}_i \boldsymbol{\beta}|,$$

where

$$R_1 = [i : Y_i \geq \mathbf{X}_i \boldsymbol{\beta}], \qquad R_2 = [i : Y_i < \mathbf{X}_i \boldsymbol{\beta}],$$

and $0 < p < 1$. The least absolute value (LAV) is the value of $\boldsymbol{\beta}$ that minimizes

$$\sum_{i=1}^{n} |Y_i - \mathbf{X}_i \boldsymbol{\beta}|$$

and is a special case of L_p with $p = 1/2$. The LAV estimate is frequently used as the robust starting value. If this $\hat{\boldsymbol{\beta}}_0$ is used, then take

$$\hat{\delta} = \frac{\text{median } |Y_i - \mathbf{X}_i \hat{\boldsymbol{\beta}}_0|}{0.6745},$$

where the median is that of the nonzero deviations $|Y_i - \mathbf{X}_i \hat{\boldsymbol{\beta}}_0|$. Other robust starting estimates include those of Brown and Mood (1951), which are easy to use, and those of Dutter (1977), which give estimates for $\boldsymbol{\beta}$ and δ simultaneously.

After obtaining good robust estimates of $\boldsymbol{\beta}$ and scale by using the LAV, Dutter's algorithm, or another scheme, we could treat outliers more severely by using these robust estimates as starting values, say $\hat{\boldsymbol{\beta}}_0$ and $\hat{\delta}$, with a redescending ψ such as Student's $T(r)$ or Tukey's biweight. In those cases, a weighted least squares procedure is a good algorithm. In this method we replace the k equations

$$\sum_{i=1}^{n} X_{ij} \psi \left(\frac{Y_i - \mathbf{X}_i \boldsymbol{\beta}}{\delta} \right) = 0, \qquad j = 1, 2, \ldots, k,$$

or, equivalently when $Y_i - \mathbf{X}_i \boldsymbol{\beta} \neq 0$,

$$\sum_{i=1}^{n} X_{ij} \frac{\psi[(Y_i - \mathbf{X}_i \boldsymbol{\beta})/\delta]}{(Y_i - \mathbf{X}_i \boldsymbol{\beta})/\delta} (Y_i - \mathbf{X}_i \boldsymbol{\beta}) = 0,$$

with the approximations

$$\sum_{i=1}^{n} X_{ij} w_{i,0} (Y_i - \mathbf{X}_i \boldsymbol{\beta}) = 0, \qquad j = 1, 2, \ldots, k,$$

where

$$w_{i,0} = \frac{\psi[(Y_i - \mathbf{X}_i\hat{\boldsymbol{\beta}}_0)/\hat{\delta}]}{Y_i - \mathbf{X}_i\hat{\boldsymbol{\beta}}_0/\hat{\delta}}, \qquad Y_i \neq \mathbf{X}_i\hat{\boldsymbol{\beta}}_0,$$

and $w_{i,0} = 1$ when $Y_i = \mathbf{X}_i\hat{\boldsymbol{\beta}}_0$. In matrix notation, in which $\mathbf{W}_0$ is the $n \times n$ diagonal matrix with $w_{1,0}, w_{2,0}, \ldots, w_{n,0}$ on the principal diagonal, the one-step estimator is

$$\hat{\boldsymbol{\beta}}_1 = (\mathbf{X}'\mathbf{W}_0\mathbf{X})^{-1}\mathbf{X}'\mathbf{W}_0\mathbf{Y}.$$

The iteration requires that on each step, we recompute the weights and thus the inverse $(\mathbf{X}'\mathbf{W}_k\mathbf{X})^{-1}$ for the $(k+1)$th iteration. With good estimates $\hat{\boldsymbol{\beta}}_0$ and $\hat{\delta}$ only a few iterations are usually needed to obtain good redescending estimates.

What should be used for the error structure of the robust estimators $\hat{\boldsymbol{\beta}}$ associated with the final iteration? It is true that under certain reasonable conditions (one is a known scale $\delta = \sigma$), $\hat{\boldsymbol{\beta}}$ has an approximate normal distribution with mean $\boldsymbol{\beta}$ and variance-covariance matrix

$$\frac{\sigma^2 E[\psi^2(Z/\sigma)](\mathbf{X}'\mathbf{X})^{-1}}{E[\psi'(Z/\sigma)]^2},$$

where Z represents an element of the random vector $\boldsymbol{\epsilon}$ (Huber, 1973). An approximation of this variance-covariance matrix is

$$\frac{(n\hat{\delta}^2)\left\{(1/n)\sum_{i=1}^{n}\psi^2[(Y_i - \mathbf{X}_i\hat{\boldsymbol{\beta}})/\hat{\delta}]\right\}(\mathbf{X}'\mathbf{X})^{-1}}{(n-p)\left\{(1/n)\sum_{i=1}^{n}\psi'[(Y_i - \mathbf{X}_i\hat{\boldsymbol{\beta}})/\hat{\delta}]\right\}^2}.$$

Of course, a weighted least squares program usually provides another estimate of this variance-covariance matrix. Two other suggestions are given by Welsch (1975), but there is no general agreement on which of these variance approximations is best. Nevertheless, whichever one we choose, we do have some idea about the error structure of $\hat{\boldsymbol{\beta}}$, and we can thus make some approximate statistical inferences about $\boldsymbol{\beta}$ by using the usual normal theory.

EXAMPLE 2 An example involving the dose-response of a positive inotropic agent, which is used in the treatment of congestive heart failure, is used to demonstrate these robust procedures. Twenty-four dogs were randomly assigned to four dose groups (six for each dose level). One objective is to estimate the effective dose level that produces a 10% increase (ED_{10}) in mean blood pressure, defined as (1/3) systolic blood pressure + (2/3) diastolic blood pressure (cf. Chapter 4). The response variable is the percent of mean blood pressure change from the baseline measurement, and the independent variable is the logarithm (base 10) of the dose. The raw data are presented in Table 4.

Using PROC NLIN in SAS (Yuh and Sullivan, 1988), the weights associated with each observation are computed and given in the same table. Note that the last observation at the high dose level received a much smaller weight than other observations. The estimates of the slope based on Tukey's biweight and Huber's ψ are 5.54 and 6.60, respectively, while the least squares procedure produces a much larger estimate of the slope (see Table 5). The order of the slopes, namely LAV $<$ Tukey ($b = 4.82$) $<$

Table 4 Dog Data and Weights from Robust Estimators

Dose level (mg/kg IV)	Mean blood pressure (% change)	Weight (Huber's ψ)	Weight (Tukey's ψ)
0.3	−2.11	1.000	0.875
0.3	1.90	1.000	0.991
0.3	4.00	1.000	0.998
0.3	5.56	1.000	0.980
0.3	6.41	1.000	0.962
0.3	10.00	0.798	0.823
1	1.05	1.000	0.886
1	2.11	1.000	0.927
1	3.77	1.000	0.973
1	6.72	1.000	0.999
1	8.33	1.000	0.982
1	8.49	1.000	0.980
3	2.11	0.755	0.811
3	4.44	1.000	0.916
3	7.14	1.000	0.986
3	11.38	1.000	0.975
3	11.50	1.000	0.972
3	14.89	1.000	0.855
10	5.31	0.731	0.827
10	8.51	1.000	0.953
10	11.63	1.000	1.000
10	19.66	0.845	0.757
10	19.67	0.843	0.756
10	32.61	0.287	0.007

Table 5 Intercept, Slope, and ED Estimates for Dog Data

Estimator	$\hat{\beta}_0$	$\hat{\beta}_1$	$\widehat{\mathrm{ED}}_{10}$
Least squares	6.69	7.79	2.66
LAV	6.72	4.91	4.66
Huber ($K = 1.25$)	6.41	6.60	3.51
Tukey ($b = 4.82$)	6.30	5.54	4.66

Huber ($K = 1.25$) < LS, indicates that Tukey's biweight and Huber's ψ functions do, in fact, "down-weight" the extreme observation. The least squares line is influenced by this extreme point, and its slope is much steeper than those of the robust procedures (Figure 2).

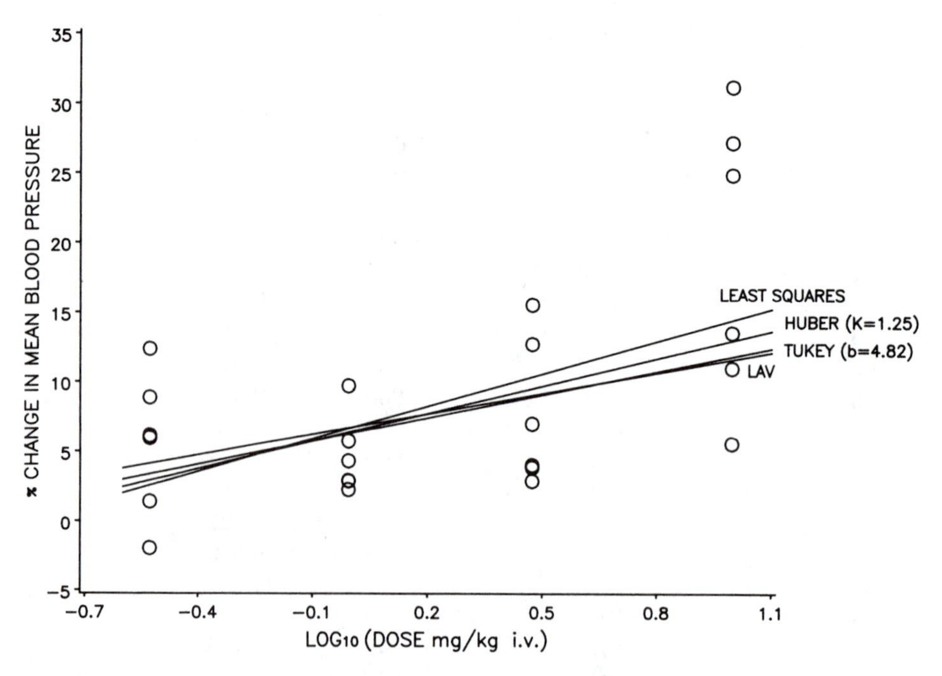

Figure 2 Fitted regression lines for dog data.

2.3 Extensions of Robust Estimation

We close this section with a remark about nonlinear models. Let $\mathbf{Y} = \mathbf{h}(\boldsymbol{\beta}) + \boldsymbol{\epsilon}$, where $\mathbf{h}(\cdot)$ is a nonlinear function of $\boldsymbol{\beta}$, and $h_i(\boldsymbol{\beta})$ is $\mathbf{h}(\boldsymbol{\beta})$, which is associated with Y_i. We wish to minimize

$$\sum_{i=1}^{n} \rho \left\{ \frac{Y_i - h_i(\boldsymbol{\beta})}{\hat{\delta}} \right\},$$

where an estimate $\hat{\delta}$ of the scale can be found by using a preliminary estimate $\hat{\boldsymbol{\beta}}_0$. Equating the first partial derivatives to zero, we have

$$\sum_{i=1}^{n} \frac{\partial h_i(\boldsymbol{\beta})}{\partial \beta_j} \psi \left\{ \frac{Y_i - h_i(\boldsymbol{\beta})}{\hat{\delta}} \right\} = 0, \qquad j = 1, 2, \ldots, k.$$

With the preliminary estimate $\hat{\boldsymbol{\beta}}_0$ and a weighted nonlinear least squares algorithm available in packages such as BMDP and SAS, it is easy to solve

$$\sum_{i=1}^{n} \frac{\partial h_i(\boldsymbol{\beta})}{\partial \beta_j} w_{i,0}[Y_i - h_i(\boldsymbol{\beta})] = 0 \qquad j = 1, 2, \ldots, k,$$

where

$$w_{i0} = \frac{\psi[(Y_i - h_i(\hat{\boldsymbol{\beta}}_0))/\hat{\delta}]}{[Y_i - h_i(\hat{\boldsymbol{\beta}}_0)]/\hat{\delta}}, \qquad Y_i \neq h_i(\hat{\boldsymbol{\beta}}_0)$$

and $w_{i0} = 1$ when $Y_i = h_i(\hat{\boldsymbol{\beta}}_0)$, $i = 1, 2, \ldots, n$.

Other applications include analysis of variance (ANOVA), time series, splines, multivariate analysis, and discrimination. For example, Lenth (1977) has produced some robust splines that give excellent fits to data points for which the usual (least squares) splines fail. Also, Randles et al. (1978) have found robust estimates of mean vectors and variance-covariance matrices that are used in discrimination problems. Robust ANOVA procedures are discussed by Schrader and McKean (1977).

3 HYPOTHESIS TESTING

There are many situations where the comparison of treatment effects is of primary interest. Although many different designs are used in the pharmaceutical industry, the focus of this section will be on the two-sample problem. This is one of the most fundamental problems in statistics. In the pharmaceutical industry this type of experiment arises frequently because the comparison of a standard treatment and a test treatment or an active compound versus a placebo is of interest (cf. Chapter 7). Extensions to ANOVA problems will be mentioned later in this section.

For now, the focus is on the two-sample location problem. Specifically, let $X_1, \ldots, X_m$ and $Y_1, \ldots, Y_n$ be independent random samples from continuous distributions with CDF $F(x)$ and $F(x - \Delta)$, respectively, with $-\infty < \Delta < \infty$. Thus the distributions are identical in every respect except for the possible shift in location, Δ. Typically, the null hypothesis of interest is H_0: $\Delta = 0$, in which case $X_1, \ldots, X_m$ and $Y_1, \ldots, Y_n$ represent a single random sample of size $N = m + n$ with cumulative distribution function $F(x)$.

The performance of any test statistic for detecting a shift in location is dependent on the underlying distribution from which the data arise. If the data are normally distributed, it is well known that the t-test is the best test for detecting the shift. Because of the misgivings that many statisticians have about using only normal theory results, nonparametric distribution-free methods have gained importance as helpful tools for data analysis when the underlying distribution is unknown. In the case of the two-sample location problem, many nonparametric procedures exist and are known to be more efficient than the t-test for underlying distributions other than normal.

3.1 The Wilcoxon Test

The Wilcoxon test is probably the most widely used nonparametric test for detecting shifts in location. If R_i is the rank of X_i and R_{m+i} is the rank of Y_i in the combined sample of the $N = m + n$ observations $X_1, \ldots, X_m$, $Y_1, \ldots, Y_n$, the test statistic proposed by Wilcoxon (1945) is simply

$$W = \sum_{i=1}^{n} R_{m+i}.$$

That is, the test statistic is merely the sum of the ranks of the Y-sample observations.

Under H_0: $\Delta = 0$, the rank vector, $\mathbf{R}$, of the combined sample is uniformly distributed over the set of all permutations of the integers 1, 2, ..., N. That is, each of the $N!$ arrangements of these integers occurs with equal probability. Thus the exact null distribution of the Wilcoxon statistic can be derived by enumerating all $\binom{N}{n}$ possible combinations of the ranks and tabulating the relative frequency of each rank sum.

Most nonparametric texts contain a table of the null distribution of the Wilcoxon rank-sum statistic for a variety of sample sizes. Clearly, as N gets large, examining all permutations of the ranks is extremely tedious. In those situations, a large-sample approximation can be used. The distribution of the standardized W converges to the standard normal distribution. It can be shown that the mean and variance of W are

$$E(W) = \frac{n(N+1)}{2}$$

and

$$\mathrm{var}(W) = \frac{mn(N+1)}{12},$$

and thus critical values for the test based on

$$Z = \frac{W - E(W)}{\sqrt{\mathrm{var}(W)}}$$

can be taken from the standard normal distribution. Using the large-sample normal test for sample sizes as small as $m = n = 8$ provides a reasonable approximation to upper tail probabilities of the exact null distribution, especially for p-values of 0.05 or less.

When there are two or more observations that have the same value (ties), the values can be assigned average ranks. For example, if the two smallest observations are the same, each would receive a rank of $(1+2)/2 = 1.5$. When using the normal approximation, the variance should be corrected by the formula

$$\mathrm{var}(W) = \frac{mn}{12}\left[(N+1) - \frac{\sum_{i=1}^{k} t_i(t_i^2 - 1)}{N(N-1)}\right],$$

where k is the number of tied groups (every untied observation is considered a tied group of size 1) and t_i is the size of the ith tied group. Note that this variance formula reduces to the previous variance formula when there are no ties ($t_i = 1$ for all i).

3.2 Linear Rank Statistics

The Wilcoxon test is a special case of the class of statistics called linear rank statistics. By creating functions of the ranks, known as scores, linear rank statistics provide a useful distribution-free approach to testing hypotheses. We begin with some definitions.

Let $a(1), \ldots, a(N)$ and $c(1), \ldots, c(N)$ be two sets of N constants such that the numbers within each set are not all the same. Then

$$S = \sum_{i=1}^{N} c(i)a(R_i)$$

is a linear rank statistic. The constants $a(1), \ldots, a(N)$ are the scores, and $c(1), \ldots, c(N)$ are termed the regression constants. For the two-sample problem, the regression constants are chosen to be

$$c(i) = \begin{cases} 0 & i = 1, \ldots, m \\ 1 & i = m+1, \ldots, N. \end{cases}$$

In the sequel, these regression constants will always be used so that the linear rank statistic simplifies to

$$S = \sum_{i=1}^{n} a(R_{m+i}),$$

where again R_{m+i} is the rank of Y_i in the combined sample. Clearly, if $a(i) = i (i = 1, 2, \ldots, N)$, the linear rank statistic defined above is the Wilcoxon statistic. Consequently, the scores $a(i) = i$ are called Wilcoxon scores.

There are many functions of the ranks that one might consider in creating a linear rank statistic, and the choice of scores for testing the hypothesis H_0: $\Delta = 0$ has been investigated in detail (Hajek and Sidak, 1967). If $F(x)$ is a CDF of a continuous distribution,

$$f(x) = \frac{dF(x)}{dx}$$

and

$$f'(x) = \frac{d^2F(x)}{dx^2}$$

exists at all but at most a countable number of x-values, then, with F^{-1} being the inverse of F, it is known that

$$\phi(u, f) = \frac{-f'(F^{-1}(u))}{f(F^{-1}(u))}$$

is the optimal score function for the two-sample location problem. Suppose now that the support of F is the whole real line and $f'(x)$ exists at all but a countable number of x-values. Then, under certain regularity conditions, the locally most powerful rank test for detecting a shift in the distribution F uses the optimum expected value scores given by

$$a(i) = E[\phi(U_{(i)}, f)], \qquad i = 1, 2, \ldots, N,$$

where $U_{(i)}$ is the ith-order statistic of a random sample of size N from a uniform (0,1) distribution. If F is the logistic distribution, the optimal score function is equivalent to $\phi(u, f) = u$, which corresponds to the Wilcoxon scores. Although this test is locally most powerful, $\phi(u, f)$ cannot be evaluated unless the underlying distribution is assumed to be known. While methods have been developed for efficiently estimating $\phi(u, f)$ asymptotically, they are beyond the scope of this presentation. Rather, several popular scores will be presented and their utility discussed.

Let the scores for a two-sample linear rank statistic be

$$a(i) = \begin{cases} 1, & i > (N+1)/2 \\ 0, & i \leq (N+1)/2. \end{cases}$$

The resulting linear rank statistic is equivalent to the number of Y_i's that are greater than the median of the combined sample. These scores are called the median scores and the resulting linear rank statistic is called the median test (Mood, 1950). This is a very simple test statistic (denoted M) with a hypergeometric null distribution

$$P(M = k) = \frac{\binom{n}{k}\binom{m}{[N/2]-k}}{\binom{N}{[N/2]}},$$

where $[x]$ is the greatest integer less than or equal to x. This test is the locally most powerful rank test when the underlying distribution is the double-exponential distribution, which is a symmetric, heavy-tailed, peaked distribution.

The scores

$$a(i) = \Phi^{-1}\left(\frac{i}{N+1}\right), \qquad i = 1, 2, \ldots, N,$$

where $\Phi^{-1}(\cdot)$ is the inverse of the CDF $\Phi(\cdot)$ for the standard normal distribution, were developed by van der Waerden (1952, 1953a, 1953b). These scores (VW) are asymptotically equivalent to the normal scores (NS) proposed by Fisher and Yates (1938):

$$a(i) = E[\Phi^{-1}(U_{(i)})], \qquad i = 1, 2, \ldots, N$$

where $U_{(i)}$ is the ith-order statistic for a sample of size N from a uniform (0,1) distribution. The VW test and the NS test are asymptotically efficient for detecting shifts in location for the normal distribution, making them asymptotically equivalent to the t-test. Furthermore, the asymptotic relative efficiency of the NS test to the t-test (T) is greater than or equal to 1 for any underlying distribution.

The Savage test (SV) is based on the scores

$$a(i) = \sum_{j=N+1-i}^{N} \frac{1}{j}, \qquad i = 1, 2, \ldots, N,$$

which can also be defined as

$$a(i) = E[F^{-1}(U_{(i)})],$$

where $F(\cdot)$ is the CDF for the exponential distribution and $U_{(i)}$ is defined as before. This test is actually the desirable rank test for detecting changes of scale when the data arise from an exponential distribution with lower bound limit of zero, but a change in scale in the exponential case also means a change in location.

Under H_0: $\Delta = 0$, the mean and variance of a linear rank statistic are

$$E(S) = n\bar{a}$$

and

$$\text{var}(S) = \frac{mn}{N(N-1)} \sum_{i=1}^{N} [a(i) - \bar{a}]^2,$$

where $\bar{a} = \sum a(i)/N$. Furthermore, under some weak regularity conditions governing the scores, the standardized linear rank statistic

$$Z = \frac{S - E(S)}{\sqrt{\text{var}(S)}}$$

has a limiting standard normal distribution as m and n simultaneously tend to infinity. Thus significance testing using a properly standardized linear rank statistic can be approximated by comparing Z with the standard normal critical values. The following example will illustrate the aforementioned test statistics.

EXAMPLE 3 An experimental antiarrhythmic compound was tested using a guinea pig model. Following setup and stabilization of the preparation, the coronary artery was ligated and the number of premature ventricular contractions (PVCs) were counted over the next hour. For the treatment group, the experimental compound was administered just prior to ligation. The data for the $m = 48$ control and $n = 16$ treated preparations are given in Table 6. It is clear from the histogram (Figure 3A) that the data are highly skewed to the right. Furthermore, the usual transformations for skewed data (log and square root) do not appear to yield symmetrical distributions (Figure 3B and C). Note that the log transformation requires the addition of a constant in order to accommodate the zero response. While log(PVC+1) was chosen for this particular histogram, the additive constant is arbitrary and may be selected to minimize the skewness of the observed data. For example, log(PVC + 100) produces a more symmetric set of data. However, the estimation of this additive constant complicates the hypothesis testing and may increase the potential for bias. This is also a problem with power transformations when the response may take on negative values (e.g., change in blood pressure). Although other

Table 6 Premature Ventricular Contraction Data with Associated Scores

Control group ($n = 48$)

PVC	W	VW	NS	SV
27	3	−1.68	−1.75	0.05
36	5	−1.43	−1.46	0.08
54	6	−1.33	−1.36	0.10
56	7	−1.24	−1.27	0.11
60	8	−1.16	−1.18	0.13
66	9	−1.09	−1.11	0.15
74	11	−0.96	−0.97	0.19
88	12	−0.90	−0.91	0.21
90	13	−0.84	−0.85	0.23
91	14	−0.79	−0.80	0.24
114	15	−0.74	−0.75	0.26
122	17	−0.64	−0.65	0.31
154	21	−0.46	−0.47	0.39
164	23	−0.38	−0.38	0.44
187	24	−0.33	−0.34	0.47
208	25	−0.29	−0.30	0.49
228	26	−0.25	−0.26	0.52
234	27	−0.21	−0.22	0.54
255	29	−0.14	−0.14	0.60
272	30	−0.10	−0.10	0.63
320	32	−0.02	−0.02	0.69
323	33	0.02	0.02	0.72
327	34	0.06	0.06	0.75
344	35	0.10	0.10	0.78
355	36	0.14	0.14	0.82
394	38	0.21	0.22	0.89
401	39	0.25	0.26	0.93
458	41	0.33	0.34	1.01
478	42	0.38	0.38	1.05
502	43	0.42	0.42	1.10
547	45	0.50	0.51	1.20
551	46	0.55	0.55	1.25
559	47	0.59	0.60	1.30
655	48	0.64	0.65	1.36
658	49	0.69	0.70	1.43
674	50	0.74	0.75	1.49
839	51	0.79	0.80	1.56
858	52	0.84	0.85	1.64
907	53	0.90	0.91	1.72
934	54	0.96	0.97	1.81
941	55	1.02	1.04	1.91
949	56	1.09	1.11	2.03
1100	58	1.24	1.27	2.29
1125	59	1.33	1.36	2.46
1208	61	1.54	1.59	2.91
1439	62	1.68	1.75	3.24
1591	63	1.87	1.96	3.74
1796	64	2.16	2.34	4.74

Treatment group ($n = 16$)

PVC	W	VW	NS	SV
0	1	−2.16	−2.34	0.02
1	2	−1.87	−1.96	0.03
31	4	−1.54	−1.60	0.06
67	10	−1.02	−1.04	0.16
120	16	−0.69	−0.70	0.29
137	18	−0.59	−0.60	0.33
139	19	−0.55	−0.55	0.35
140	20	−0.50	−0.51	0.37
155	22	−0.42	−0.42	0.42
241	28	−0.17	−0.18	0.57
284	31	−0.06	−0.06	0.66
388	37	0.17	0.18	0.85
443	40	0.29	0.30	0.97
515	44	0.46	0.47	1.15
1072	57	1.16	1.18	2.15
1165	60	1.43	1.46	2.66
$\sum a(i)$	409	−6.06	−6.37	11.04
$\sum[a(i) - \bar{a}]^2$	21,840	57.08	61.36	59.26
Z	−1.72	−1.84	−1.86	−1.48

The median scores are not given on this table; they are zero for ranks of 32 or less and are 1 for ranks of 33 or more. Thus $\sum a_M(i) = 5$, $\sum[a_M(i) - \bar{a}_M]^2 = 16$, and $Z_M = -1.72$.

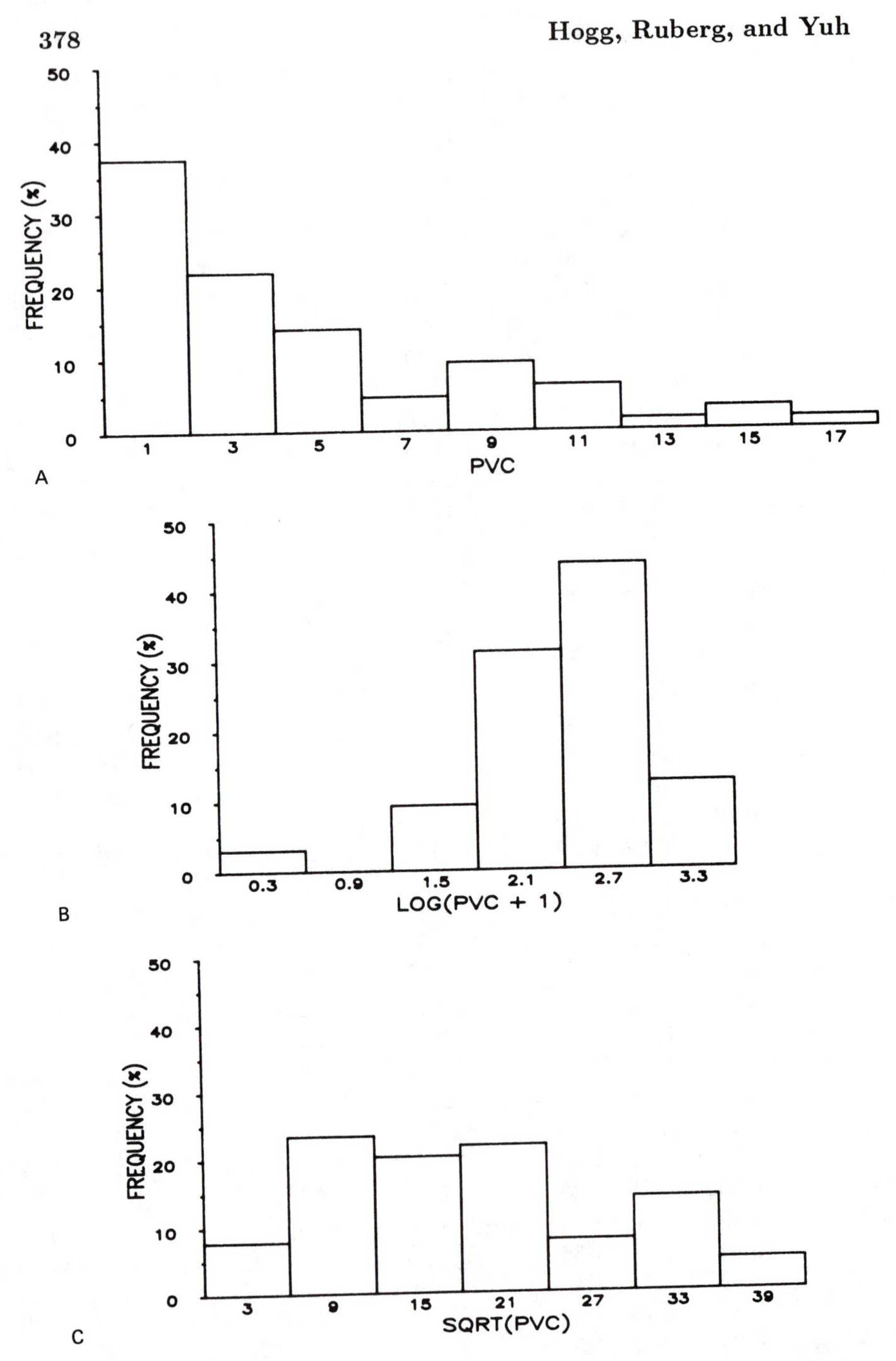

Figure 3 (A) Raw PVC data (in hundreds); (B) log-transformed PVC data; (C) square root-transformed PVC data.

transformations could be tried, a rank test may be most appropriate for these data, especially the Savage test, since the data appear approximately exponentially distributed.

The ranks from the joint sample and the various scores are also presented in Table 6. The sum of the scores and the corrected sums of squares for the scores are also presented in that table. The various standardized test statistics and associated two-tailed p-values from the large-sample approximations were computed to be

$$\begin{aligned}
T &= -1.56 \qquad (p = 0.122),\\
W &= -1.72 \qquad (p = 0.086),\\
M &= -1.72 \qquad (p = 0.086),\\
VW &= -1.84 \qquad (p = 0.066),\\
NS &= -1.86 \qquad (p = 0.063),\\
SV &= -1.48 \qquad (p = 0.139).
\end{aligned}$$

The various linear rank test statistics are quite similar for this example, with the exception of the SV test.

There are many other score functions that can be used to test for shifts in location depending on the knowledge of the underlying distribution of the data [see, e.g., Randles and Wolfe (1979)]. The asymptotic relative efficiency of several of these test statistics compared to the Wilcoxon test has been investigated for a broad class of unimodal distributions which may be encountered in practice (Ruberg, 1986a).

3.3 Tests for Broad Alternatives

The discussion in Sections 3.1 and 3.2 focused on testing for a shift in location of the underlying distribution. There may be some instances, however, when the nature of the treatment effect is not clear, and a broader alternative hypothesis is of interest. Suppose that the test of interest is

$$H_0\colon F = G \quad \text{versus} \quad H_a\colon F \neq G,$$

where F and G are the CDFs for the two populations. Thus any difference in location, scale, or shape of the underlying distribution is of interest.

Let $Z_1 < Z_2 < \cdots < Z_N$ be the order statistics of a random sample of size N. The sample cumulative distribution function, denoted $F_N(x)$, is simply defined as

$$F_N(x) = \frac{\text{number of } Z\text{'s} \leq x}{N}.$$

Thus $F_N(x)$ is a step function with step sizes $1/N$ occurring at each Z_i. It seems natural that a suitable test statistic for detecting differences in the CDFs of two populations should involve a function of the two sample CDFs.

The Kolmogorov–Smirnov (KS) statistic (Smirnov, 1939) is defined as the maximum vertical distance between the sample CDFs of the two populations, or

$$D_{m,n} = \max_x |G_n(x) - F_m(x)|.$$

If this distance is sufficiently large, the null hypothesis H_0: $F = G$ is rejected. Computationally, one only need consider the differences between F_m and G_n for the $N = m + n$ points at which either one of the sample distribution functions has a jump. Since the vertical distance $|G_n(x) - F_m(x)|$ depends only on the ranks of the observations, the test has the same distribution-free property under H_0, as do the rank tests described previously. Tables for exact critical values for $D_{m,n}$ are given in Lehmann (1975) for $m = n = 1$ to 30, while selected critical values for $m \neq n$ are given in Hollander and Wolfe (1973). For large sample sizes, the statistic $D_{m,n}$ does not tend toward a normal distribution. For a discussion of the large-sample approximation and the handling tied observations, see Lehmann (1975).

It may be argued that looking at the single point for which the distance between the two-sample CDFs is a maximum does not make efficient use of all the data. For example, $|G_n(x) - F_m(x)|$ may be substantial over most of the range of X, suggesting that F and G are different, but not quite large enough at any particular x for KS to reject H_0. The Cramér–von Mises (CVM) test for the two-sample problem (Rosenblatt, 1952) is useful in just such a situation and is defined as

$$C = \frac{mn}{(m+n)^2} \sum_{i=1}^{N} [G_n(Z_{(i)}) - F_m(Z_{(i)})]^2.$$

Again, if C is too large, H_0: $F = G$ is rejected. Anderson (1962) shows that the CVM test can be expressed as a function of the ranks. By examining all possible arrangements of the ranks, tables of exact critical values for small samples are given in Anderson (1962) and Burr (1963). Based on the fact that

$$E(C) = \frac{N+1}{6N}$$

and

$$\text{var}(C) = \left(\frac{1}{45}\right)\left(\frac{N+1}{N^2}\right)\left(\frac{4mnN - 3(m^2+n^2) - 2mn}{4mn}\right),$$

we can use the standardized test statistic

$$T = \frac{C - E(C)}{\sqrt{\text{var}(C)}}.$$

Selected critical values for the asymptotic null distribution of T, which is not a normal distribution, are also given in the references cited above, while the limiting distribution is described further in Anderson and Darling (1952).

Finally, the empirical quantile-quantile (EQQ) plot can be viewed as a graphical comparison of the sample CDFs for the two populations. Briefly, if $m = n$, the order statistics from each sample are paired—$(X_{(1)}, Y_{(1)})$, $(X_{(2)}, Y_{(2)})$, ..., $(X_{(n)}, Y_{(n)})$—and plotted. If $m \neq n$, the smaller sample is used as the reference sample, and the comparable percentiles (quantiles) from the larger sample must be found and paired with the reference sample. Under H_0: $F = G$, these points should fall randomly about the line $Y = X$. If $F \neq G$, there are essentially three possibilities:

1. The points fall randomly about a straight line with slope equal to 1, but translated up or down from the line $Y = X$, indicating a difference in locations.
2. The points fall randomly about a straight line with a slope not equal to 1, indicating differences in scale.
3. The points fall randomly about a curved line, indicating differences in shape.

EXAMPLE 4 The following data set will illustrate the preceding tests. Two antihypertensive medications were employed in a double-blind study to compare their effects on blood pressure. The change in blood pressure, posttreatment value minus the pretreatment value, was calculated for each patient and is presented in Table 7. Because the sample sizes are equal, $m = n = 59$, the calculations are made simpler by multiplying $F_m(x)$ and $G_n(x)$ by 59. The values in the table are grouped since there were a large number of tied observations in the data set. The sample CDFs are plotted in Figure 4.

The KS statistic is $10/59 = 0.169$. Using the large-sample approximation and the tables from Lehmann (1975), the observed probability value is about $p = 0.365$, which implies that there is little evidence to reject H_0: $F = G$. However, this asymptotic approximation is conservative in the presence of ties, making the actual p-value for the test less than 0.365. Because there were a large number of ties in the data, it is not known how much the asymptotic distribution and resulting p-value are affected.

The CVM test is standardized and compared to its asymptotic distribution, given in Table 3 of Burr (1963). The associated p-value is approx-

Table 7 Grouped Values for Change in Blood Pressure with Sample CDFs ($m = n = 59$)

BP change	Number of tied values (g)	Treatment A $mF_m(x)$	Treatment B $nG_n(x)$	Difference $m[F_m - G_n]$	$g \cdot$ Difference^2
−40	2	2	0	2	8
−29	1	3	0	3	9
−28	2	4	1	3	18
−26	2	6	1	5	50
−24	6	10	3	7	294
−22	2	12	3	9	162
−20	1	13	3	10	100
−18	6	15	7	8	384
−16	4	16	10	6	144
−15	2	17	11	6	72
−14	5	20	13	7	245
−13	2	21	14	7	98
−12	6	24	17	7	294
−10	9	28	22	6	324
−9	1	29	22	7	49
−8	13	36	28	8	832
−6	4	36	32	4	64
−5	1	37	32	5	25
−4	12	42	39	3	108
−3	1	42	40	2	4
−2	8	44	46	−2	32
0	12	52	50	2	48
2	4	53	53	0	0
4	5	57	54	3	45
8	2	57	56	1	2
9	2	58	57	1	2
12	1	59	57	2	4
24	1	59	58	1	1
46	1	59	59	0	0
Sum	118				3418

KS test: $D_{m,n} = 10/59;\ \sqrt{\dfrac{mn}{m+n}}D_{m,n} = 0.921 \quad (p \leq 0.365)$

CVM test: $C = [(59)(59)/118^2][3418/59^2] = 0.245$

$T = (0.245 - 0.168)/0.022 = 0.52 \quad (p \approx 0.035)$

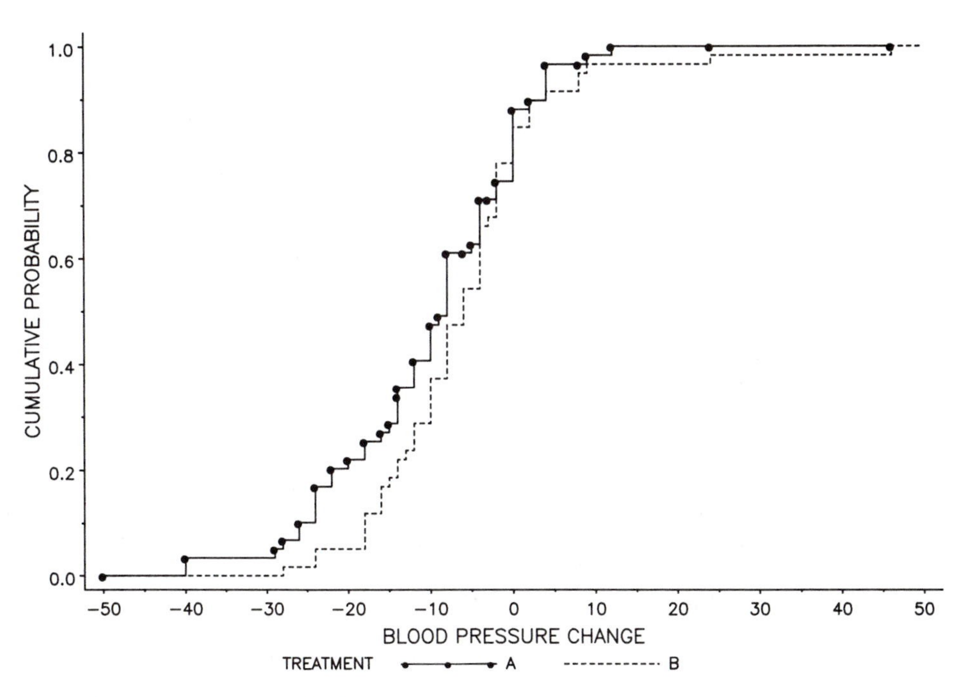

Figure 4 Sample CDFs for change in blood pressure.

imately 0.035, suggesting that $F \neq G$. It appears that the CVM test is more sensitive than the KS test for detecting a difference between the two distributions, although this is not completely clear since the exact p-value of the KS test is unknown. In viewing the EQQ plot for these data (Figure 5), one can quickly recognize that the two sample CDFs have different shapes even though their sample means ($\bar{x}_A = -10.2$, $\bar{x}_B = -5.9$) and standard deviations ($s_A = 11.3$, $s_B = 11.2$) are quite similar.

Some people may naively do a two-sample t-test to compare these two treatment groups. Although the t-statistic is 2.08 ($p = 0.04$), the conclusion that the two underlying distributions differ in location may be misleading. Treatment A appears to be skewed left with two extreme observations pulling the mean down, and treatment B appears to be skewed right with two large observations pulling the mean up. Thus any apparent shift in location is probably a result of the difference in skewness, and the interpretation of the pharmacologic activity of the two compounds could be quite different.

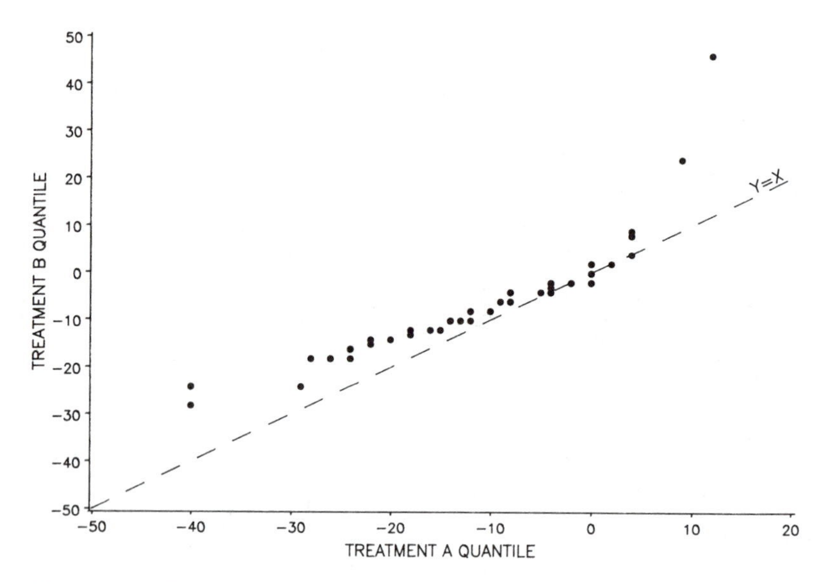

Figure 5 EQQ plot for change in blood pressure.

3.4 Extensions to Other ANOVA Settings

Many of the test statistics discussed in this section have been extended to the one-way ANOVA setting where the comparison of k treatment locations is of interest. The general form of a rank test based on the scores $a(R_j)$ is given by Hajek and Sidak (1967) as

$$Q = \frac{N-1}{\sum_{i=1}^{N}[a(i)-\bar{a}]^2}\left(\sum_{j=1}^{k}\frac{1}{n_j}S_j^2 - N\bar{a}^2\right),$$

where S_j is the sum of the scores in the jth group, n_j is the sample size for the jth group, and $N = \sum n_j$. The scores presented in this section are the ones most commonly used for this k-sample setting; furthermore, Q has a χ^2 distribution with $k-1$ degrees of freedom for these scores as min $\{n_j\}$ tends to infinity. Other extensions of the KS test are also discussed in Hajek and Sidak (1967).

The Wilcoxon scores (ranks) have also been used in more complicated ANOVA problems, multiple comparisons, regression, and correlation. Hollander and Wolfe (1973) and Hettmansperger (1984) have provided good texts that cover in detail many of the topics presented in this section as well as applications of rank tests to the areas mentioned above.

4 CONCLUSION

The appropriate statistical analysis of any data depends on the underlying distribution from which the data arise. A variety of robust methods have been discussed in this chapter, and each has its merits. In practice, the statistician is faced with a choice of $\psi(x)$ or $a(R_j)$. It seems logical to suggest that this choice be made adaptively; that is, the selection of the estimation or testing procedure occurs after observing the data (Hogg, 1974; Hogg and Lenth, 1984; Yuh and Hogg, 1988). For example, the tuning constants for the function $\psi(x)$ or the form of the scores $a(R_j)$ could be selected based on what the observed sample tells us about the underlying distribution. After all, if the various M-estimators or rank tests are good, wouldn't adaptive ones be better (particularly because the former are included in the latter)? Moreover, it seems as if statisticians would find adaptation very appealing since we do it all the time. For example, choosing a nonparametric procedure versus a parametric procedure or analyzing the raw data versus the log transformed data are adaptive approaches, although we do not always formalize them as such.

Some attempts have been made to formalize adaptive procedures, especially in the area of robust or nonparametric statistical methods. Of course, asymptotically, we can select the best $\psi(x)$ or $a(R_j)$, but in practice we are working with finite sample sizes. Hence we must find some reasonable procedures for practical applications. In the hypothesis testing framework, methods have been developed which make the selection of a rank test independent of the rank test itself, thereby maintaining the nominal significance level of the test. For the most part, these methods use the order statistics from the entire sample to compute measures of skewness and tail length, which are in turn used for selecting an appropriate rank test (Hogg et al., 1975; Ruberg, 1986b). In the setting of estimation, adaptive robust methods have been developed (Moberg et al., 1978; Yuh and Hogg, 1988), but they, too, may suffer from bias similar to what may occur in choosing the power for a power transformation.

In any case, good statisticians have always been on guard for outliers or bad data points, discarding them or investigating them further as is appropriate. In complicated data sets, however, spotting some of these extreme points is most difficult. A formal robust procedure can definitely help us in this regard. Hence it is recommended that in our statistical investigations we do the following:

1. Perform the usual least squares analyses.
2. Also use a robust procedure.

3. If conclusions from methods 1 and 2 are in essential agreement, report the agreement and the usual statistical summaries associated with method 1.
4. If the conclusions from methods 1 and 2 do not agree very well, take another hard look at the data. For example, when using M-estimation, look at those points with low weights or large residuals from the robust fit (the weights and residuals of the points should always be displayed on the last iteration). Then the usual questions can be asked about these points: "Has someone made a simple recording error?" or "Is this outlier trying to tell us something significant about our experiment?"

If a robust element is added to our present methods, we will detect many simple, and some not so simple, errors, or discover interesting relationships in the data. Our hope is that statistical investigations routinely include a robust aspect. Certainly, researchers in robust methods will continue to develop new and better procedures to propose to the statistical community.

Acknowledgment. We would like to thank Laura P. Ragouzis for her assistance with the graphics.

REFERENCES

Anderson, T. W. (1962). On the distribution of the two-sample Cramér–von Mises criterion. *Ann. Math. Statist. 33*, 1148–1159.

Anderson, T. W., and D. A. Darling (1952). Asymptotic theory of certain "goodness of fit" criteria based on stochastic processes. *Ann. Math. Statist. 23*, 193–212.

Brown, G. W., and A. M. Mood (1951). On median tests for linear hypotheses. In *Proceedings of the Second Berkeley Symposium on Mathematical Statistics and Probability* (J. Neyman, ed.). University of California Press, Berkeley, pp. 159–166.

Burr, B. J. (1963). Distribution of the two-sample Cramér–von Mises criterion for small equal samples. *Ann. Math. Statist. 34*, 95–101.

Dixon, W. J., ed. (1983). *BMDP Statistical Software.* University of California Press, Los Angeles.

Dutter, R. (1977). Numerical solution of robust regression problems: computational aspects, a comparison. *J. Statist. Comput. Simulation 5*, 207–238.

Fisher, R. A., and F. Yates (1938). *Statistical Tables for Biological Agriculture, and Medical Research.* Oliver & Boyd, Edinburgh. (1st ed., 1938; 5th ed., 1957.)

Hajek, J., and Z. Sidak (1967). *Theory of Rank Tests.* Academic Press, New York.

Hettmansperger, T. P. (1984). *Statistical Inference Based on Ranks.* Wiley, New York.

Hill, M. A., and W. J. Dixon (1984). Robustness in real life: a study of clinical laboratory data. *Biometrics 38*, 377–396.

Hogg, R. V. (1974). Adaptive robust procedures: a partial review and some suggestions for future application and theory. *J. Amer. Statist. Assoc. 69*, 909–923.

Hogg, R. V. (1979). Introduction to robust estimation. In *Robustness in Statistics*, (R. L. Launer, ed.). Academic Press, New York, pp. 1–17.

Hogg, R. V., and R. V. Lenth (1984). A review of some adaptive statistical techniques. *Comm. Statist. A13*, 1551–1579.

Hogg, R. V., D. M. Fisher, R. H. Randles (1975). A two-sample adaptive distribution-free test. *J. Amer. Statist. Assoc. 70*, 655–661.

Hogg, R. V., G. K. Bril, S. M. Han, and L. Yuh (1988). An argument for adaptive robust estimation. In *Probability and Statistics, Essays in Honor of F. A. Graybill*, (J. N. Srivastava, ed.). North-Holland, New York, pp. 135–148.

Hollander, M., and D. A. Wolfe (1973). *Nonparametric Statistical Methods.* Wiley, New York.

Huber, P. J. (1964). Robust estimation of a location parameter. *Ann. Math. Statist. 35*, 73–101.

Huber, P. J. (1973). Robust regression: asymptotics, conjectures and monte carlo. *Ann. Statist. 1*, 799–821.

Huber, P. J. (1981). *Robust Statistics.* Wiley, New York.

Kroenker, R., and G. Bassett (1978). Regression quantiles. *Econometrica 46*, 33–50.

Lehmann, E. L. (1975). *Nonparametrics: Statistical Methods Based on Ranks.* Holden-Day, San Francisco.

Lenth, R. V. (1977). Robust splines. *Comm. Statist. A6*, 847–854.

Moberg, T. F., J. S. Ramberg, and R. H. Randles (1978). An adaptive M-estimator and its application to a selection problem. *Technometrics 20*, 255–263.

Mood, A. M. (1950). *Introduction to the Theory of Statistics.* McGraw-Hill, New York.

Randles, R. H., and D. A. Wolfe (1979). *Introduction to the Theory of Nonparametric Statistics.* Wiley, New York.

Randles, R. H., J. D. Brofitt, J. S. Ramberg, and R. V. Hogg (1978). Generalized linear and quadratic descriminant functions using robust estimates. *J. Amer. Statist. Assoc. 73*, 564–568.

Rosenblatt, M. (1952). Limit theorems associated with variants of the von Mises statistic. *Ann. Math. Statist. 23*, 617–623.

Ruberg, S. J. (1986a). Efficiencies of some two-sample location tests for a broad class of distributions. *Comm. Statist. A15*, 2991–3004.

Ruberg, S. J. (1986b). A continuously adaptive nonparametric two-sample test. *Comm. Statist. A15*, 2899–2920.

Schrader, R. M., and J. W. McKean (1977). Robust analysis of variance. *Comm. Statist. A6*, 879–894.

Smirnov, N. V. (1939). On the estimation of the discrepancy between empirical curves of distribution for two independent samples. *Bull. Univ. Moscow 2*, 3–14.

van der Waerden, B. L. (1952). Order tests for the two-sample problem and their power. *Indag. Math 14*, 453–458. Correction *15* 80, (1953).

van der Waerden, B. L. (1953a). Order tests for the two-sample problem: II. *Indag. Math. 15*, 303–310.

van der Waerden, B. L. (1953b). Order tests for the two-sample problem: III. *Indag. Math. 15*, 311–316.

Welsch, R. E. (1975). Confidence regions for robust regression, Working paper 3. National Bureau of Economic Research, Cambridge, Mass.

Wilcoxon, F. (1945). Individual comparisons by ranking methods. *Biometrics 1*, 80–83.

Yuh, L., and R. V. Hogg (1988). On adaptive M-regression. *Biometrics 44*, 433–445.

Yuh, L., and W. A. Sullivan (1988). Robust estimation using SAS software. *SAS User's Group International Conference Proceedings: SUGI 13*, 805–810.

13

Categorical Data Analysis

GARY G. KOCH and GREGORY J. CARR University of North Carolina, Chapel Hill, North Carolina

INGRID A. AMARA Quintiles, Inc., Chapel Hill, North Carolina

MAURA E. STOKES SAS Institute, Inc., Cary, North Carolina

THOMAS J. URYNIAK Fisons Corporation, Bedford, Massachusetts

1 INTRODUCTION

Many studies in the pharmaceutical sciences are concerned with the relationships between categorical response variables which describe favorable or unfavorable outcome and one or more explanatory variables. The explanatory variables include experimental factors such as treatment in clinical trials and background characteristics such as age, sex, and baseline status of subjects; additional factors that often need to be taken into account are "center" in multicenter studies and "visit" in multivisit studies. Since the explanatory variables which are considered can have either a categorical (e.g., sex) or continuous (e.g., age) nature, the distinguishing feature of situations which require categorical data analyses is that the response variables are categorical.

The statistical questions of interest for categorical data analysis are addressed in this chapter through a specific example from a multicenter, multivisit clinical trial for patients with a respiratory disorder. The data for this example are displayed as case records in Table 1. There are two centers

Table 1 Data from a Multicenter, Multivisit Clinical Trial to Compare Two Treatments for Patients with a Respiratory Disorder[a]

Center	Patient	Drug	Sex	Age	Base	Visit 1	Visit 2	Visit 3	Visit 4
1	53	A	F	32	1	2	2	4	2
	18	A	F	47	2	2	3	4	4
	54	A	M	11	4	4	4	4	2
	12	A	M	14	2	3	3	3	2
	51	A	M	15	0	2	3	3	3
	20	A	M	20	3	3	2	3	1
	16	A	M	22	1	2	2	2	3
	50	A	M	22	2	1	3	4	4
	03	A	M	23	3	3	4	4	3
	32	A	M	23	2	3	4	4	4
	56	A	M	25	2	3	3	2	3
	35	A	M	26	1	2	2	3	2
	26	A	M	26	2	2	2	2	2
	21	A	M	26	2	4	1	4	2
	08	A	M	28	1	2	2	1	2
	30	A	M	28	0	0	1	2	1
	33	A	M	30	3	3	4	4	2
	11	A	M	30	3	4	4	4	3
	42	A	M	31	1	2	3	1	1
	09	A	M	31	3	3	4	4	4
	37	A	M	31	0	2	3	2	1
	23	A	M	32	3	4	4	3	3
	06	A	M	34	1	1	2	1	1
	22	A	M	46	4	3	4	3	4
	24	A	M	48	2	3	2	0	2
	38	A	M	50	2	2	2	2	2
	48	A	M	57	3	3	4	3	4
	05	P	F	13	4	4	4	4	4
	19	P	F	31	2	1	0	2	2
	25	P	F	35	1	0	0	0	0
	28	P	F	36	2	3	3	2	2
	36	P	F	45	2	2	2	2	1
	43	P	M	13	3	4	4	4	4
	41	P	M	14	2	2	1	2	3
	34	P	M	15	2	2	3	3	2
	29	P	M	19	2	3	3	0	0
	15	P	M	20	4	4	4	4	4
	13	P	M	23	3	3	1	1	1

Table 1 (*Continued*)

Center	Patient	Drug	Sex	Age	Base	Visit 1	Visit 2	Visit 3	Visit 4
	27	P	M	23	4	4	2	4	4
	55	P	M	24	3	4	4	4	3
	17	P	M	25	1	1	2	2	2
	45	P	M	26	2	4	2	4	3
	40	P	M	26	1	2	1	2	2
	44	P	M	27	1	2	2	1	2
	49	P	M	27	3	3	4	3	3
	39	P	M	28	2	1	1	1	1
	02	P	M	28	2	0	0	0	0
	14	P	M	30	1	0	0	0	0
	31	P	M	37	1	0	0	0	0
	10	P	M	37	3	2	3	3	2
	07	P	M	43	2	3	2	4	4
	52	P	M	43	1	1	1	3	2
	04	P	M	44	3	4	3	4	2
	01	P	M	46	2	2	2	2	2
	46	P	M	49	2	2	2	2	2
	47	P	M	63	2	2	2	2	2
2	30	A	F	37	1	3	4	4	4
	52	A	F	39	2	3	4	4	4
	23	A	F	60	4	4	3	3	4
	54	A	F	63	4	4	4	4	4
	12	A	M	13	4	4	4	4	4
	10	A	M	14	1	4	4	4	4
	27	A	M	19	3	3	2	3	3
	47	A	M	20	2	4	4	4	3
	16	A	M	20	2	1	1	0	0
	29	A	M	21	3	3	4	4	4
	20	A	M	24	4	4	4	4	4
	25	A	M	25	3	4	3	3	1
	15	A	M	25	3	4	4	3	3
	02	A	M	25	2	2	4	4	4
	09	A	M	26	2	3	4	4	4
	49	A	M	28	2	3	2	2	1
	55	A	M	31	4	4	4	4	4
	43	A	M	34	2	4	4	2	4
	26	A	M	35	4	4	4	4	4
	14	A	M	37	4	3	2	2	4
	36	A	M	41	3	4	4	3	4

Table 1 (*Continued*)

Center	Patient	Drug	Sex	Age	Base	Visit 1	Visit 2	Visit 3	Visit 4
	51	A	M	43	3	3	4	4	2
	37	A	M	52	1	2	1	2	2
	19	A	M	55	4	4	4	4	4
	32	A	M	55	2	2	3	3	1
	03	A	M	58	4	4	4	4	4
	53	A	M	68	2	3	3	3	4
	28	P	F	31	3	4	4	4	4
	05	P	F	32	3	2	2	3	4
	21	P	F	36	3	3	2	1	3
	50	P	F	38	1	2	0	0	0
	01	P	F	39	1	2	1	1	2
	48	P	F	39	3	2	3	0	0
	07	P	F	44	3	4	4	4	4
	38	P	F	47	2	3	3	2	3
	08	P	F	48	2	2	1	0	0
	11	P	F	48	2	2	2	2	2
	04	P	F	51	3	4	2	4	4
	17	P	F	58	1	4	2	2	0
	39	P	M	11	3	4	4	4	4
	40	P	M	14	2	1	2	3	2
	24	P	M	15	3	2	2	3	3
	41	P	M	15	4	3	3	3	4
	33	P	M	19	4	2	2	3	3
	34	P	M	20	3	2	4	4	4
	13	P	M	20	1	4	4	4	4
	45	P	M	33	3	3	3	2	3
	22	P	M	36	2	4	3	3	4
	18	P	M	38	4	3	0	0	0
	35	P	M	42	3	2	2	2	2
	44	P	M	43	2	1	0	0	0
	06	P	M	45	3	4	2	1	2
	46	P	M	48	4	4	0	0	0
	31	P	M	52	2	3	4	3	4
	42	P	M	66	3	3	3	4	4

[a]0, terrible; 1, poor; 2, fair; 3, good; 4, excellent.

(center 1, center 2) within which patients were randomly assigned to two treatments (active, placebo) in successive blocks of 6. The status of each patient was classified relative to a set of five ordinal categories (0 = terrible, 1 = poor, 2 = fair, 3 = good, 4 = excellent) at baseline and at each of four visits (visit 1, visit 2, visit 3, visit 4) during the time period over which the treatments were administered. Data for the age and sex of all patients were obtained at the time of entry to the study.

The categorical response variables for the example are the classifications of the status of patients at the four visits. These response variables have an ordinal measurement scale which expresses an ordering of possible outcomes from most unfavorable (i.e., terrible), to most favorable (i.e., excellent). The simplification of the observed classifications to the dichotomous measurement scale of (terrible, poor, or fair) versus (good or excellent) provides another set of response variables of interest. Dichotomous classifications and ordinal classifications are the most prominent types of categorical response variables in the pharmaceutical sciences, so this chapter focuses primary attention on methods for their analysis. Other measurement scales for categorical data and references for their discussion are as follows:

i. Discrete counts: for example, number of infected quarters of the udder of dairy cows receiving treatment for mastitis (Koch et al., 1978) or number of hours with little or no pain for women receiving treatment for obstetrical-related pain (Koch et al., 1985a); methods for this type of data are similar to those for ordinal classifications.
ii. Grouped survival data: for example, time interval between periodic evaluations for healing of duodenal ulcer (Koch and Edwards, 1987) or time interval between periodic evaluations for death or recurrence of duodenal ulcer (Koch et al., 1986); methods for this type of data are analogous to those for dichotomous data; they include the Mantel–Haenszel statistic (Mantel and Haenszel, 1959) as extended by Mantel (1966) to a life-table format, Poisson regression for piecewise exponential models (Holford, 1980), and extensions of logistic models (Chapter 11).
iii. Nominal classifications: for example, type or site of pain or infection with there being no ordering for three or more outcomes; one strategy for this type of data is the application of methods for dichotomous classifications to the presence or absence of each outcome separately or to specified combinations of outcomes; extensions of the Mantel–Haenszel statistic (Landis et al., 1978; Koch et al., 1985a) and log-linear models (Bishop et al., 1975; Fienberg, 1980; Imrey et al., 1981, 1982) are useful for the joint analysis of all outcomes.

The explanatory variables for the example further illustrate the different types of measurement scales for data from studies in the pharmaceutical sciences. Center, sex, and treatment are dichotomous classifications; baseline status is an ordinal classification; visit is a nominal classification (since the ordering of visits in time may not be relevant to their relationship with the response variables); and age has a continuous distribution. Thus categorical data analyses for the response variables from the example need to include consideration of both categorical and continuous explanatory variables.

The subsequent sections of this chapter address the statistical questions of interest for the data in Table 1. Section 2 is concerned with comparisons between treatment groups for the background variables of age, sex, and baseline status. Such analysis is of interest because any background variable that does not have equivalent distributions for the two treatments might partly explain the observed differences between treatments for response variables if it is also strongly associated with the response variables. For this reason, potentially important associations between background variables and response variables are evaluated to identify those background variables for which the framework for treatment comparisons for response variables requires statistical adjustment; these are background variables that are both strongly associated with response variables and have different distributions for the two treatments. Two methods for adjustment of treatment comparisons for such background variables are stratification and covariance analysis. Adjustment by one of these methods is necessary for observed differences between treatment groups to be interpretable as due to treatment (as opposed to a random lack of equivalence of the treatment groups for a background variable with strong association with the response variables). Stratification and covariance analysis are useful for other purposes besides adjustment for differences between treatment groups for background variables. One of these is a capability for more powerful statistical tests through the relatively smaller variances which are provided for the estimates of treatment differences. Another is that their scope enables questions concerning homogeneity of treatment differences across subgroups based on background variables to be addressed through tests of treatment $\times$ background variable interaction. More specific aspects of stratification and covariance analysis are discussed subsequently through the roles they serve for the analysis of the data in Table 1.

Univariate methods for the analysis of the response variables at each visit separately are presented in Section 3. Attention is initially given to nonparametric statistical tests for comparisons between treatments under minimal assumptions. These include Fisher's exact test for (2×2) contingency tables and rank tests (with adjustments for ties) for ordinal data within each center separately, and the Mantel–Haenszel test and its extensions for the combined centers. An alternative analysis strategy that is more useful for descriptive purposes is based on statistical models for the relationship between response variables and explanatory variables for treatment, center, and background variables. Methods include logistic regression for dichotomous data, the proportional odds model for ordinal data, and weighted least squares for mean scores or other relevant functions of response distributions. Their range of application enables the evaluation of the similarity of treatment differences across centers through tests of treatment × center interaction and across subgroups based on background variables through tests of treatment × background variable interaction. Also, background variables without equivalent distributions for treatments need to be included in the statistical model for covariance adjustment purposes. A noteworthy limitation of model-based methods is their requirement of assumptions about how data from a clinical study are representative of a general population.

In Section 4, multivariate methods for the analysis of the response variables at all four visits jointly are discussed. They include both nonparametric statistical tests of comparisons between treatments under minimal assumptions, and statistical models which account for variation of response across visits as well as treatment and center. An important feature of the statistical models is that they enable the evaluation of the similarity of treatment differences across visits through tests of treatment × visit interaction.

The roles of the alternative methods in Sections 3 and 4 are summarized in Section 5. Relative strengths and limitations are also discussed there. Throughout Sections 2 to 5, concepts, analysis procedures, results, and interpretation are emphasized. The reader is assumed to have general familiarity with statistical issues for studies in the pharmaceutical sciences and basic methods for the statistical analysis of categorical data and contingency tables. Some background references for these topics are: Everitt (1977), Fienberg (1980), Fleiss (1981, 1986), Friedman et al. (1981), Koch and Sollecito (1984), Shapiro and Louis (1983), and Tygstrup et al. (1982). Also, the scope of this chapter does not include a substantial discussion for the statistical theory and technical structure of available methods for the analysis of categorical data; some references for these topics are: Agresti (1984), Bishop et al. (1975), Cox (1970), Forthofer and Lehnen (1981), Freeman (1987), Imrey et al. (1981, 1982), Koch et al. (1985a), and McCullagh and Nelder (1983). All computations to illustrate the application of the methods in this chapter were performed with the SAS System (1985); the types of statements that were used are described in the appendix to this chapter.

2 EVALUATION OF BACKGROUND VARIABLES

The case record data in Table 1 are from $n = 111$ patients of whom $n_1 = 56$ participated at center 1 and $n_2 = 55$ participated at center 2. The numbers of patients n_{hi} who received active (A) and placebo (P) treatment were $n_{1A} = 27$ and $n_{1P} = 29$ at center 1 and $n_{2A} = 27$ and $n_{2P} = 28$ at center 2 (where $h = 1, 2$ indexes center and $i = A, P$ indexes treatment). The total numbers of patients $n_{+i} = (n_{1i} + n_{2i})$ for the two treatment groups were $n_{+A} = 54$ for active and $n_{+P} = 57$ for placebo.

Three background variables that characterized patients prior to treatment in the clinical trial were age, sex, and baseline status. For most clinical trials, patients are selected for study by convenience mechanisms related to their need or eligibility for treatment at a particular time as opposed to a probabilistic sampling process. Similarly, centers are selected according to judgmental criteria for their qualifications and willingness to conduct the study. These considerations imply that the patients in a clinical trial might not represent a general target population in a formal statistical way. Thus distributions of background variables such as age, sex, and baseline status in the study population (which the patients in a clinical trial constitute) might be different from those in the target population (to which conclusions concerning treatments are to be generalized). For example, the study population for a clinical trial might have relatively more patients who are younger, male, or have more favorable baseline status than the target population.

One way to evaluate treatments in a clinical trial relative to the issue about how a study population represents a target population is for the statistical analysis to have the following two parts:

I. Usage of nonparametric statistical tests to compare treatment groups with respect to background variables and response variables in the study population under minimal assumptions that involve only study design considerations

II. Usage of statistical models to describe the relationships between response variables and treatment, center, and background variables for the target population under the (not provable) assumption that the conditional distributions of response variables given treatment, center, and background variables for patients in the study reasonably represent those in the target population

The objective for part I is the determination of the existence of a treatment difference for the study population; whereas the objective for part II is the evaluation of the extent to which a treatment difference is generalizable throughout a target population. Since the nonparametric methods for part I are based only on study design considerations, the conclusions from them are often called design-based inferences (for the study population). In a similar spirit, the conclusions from analysis in part II are often called model-based inferences (for the target population). Both parts I and II serve important roles. The primary advantage of part I is its applicability without assumptions external to the study design; but this is counterbalanced by the limitation of its scope of inference to the study population. In contrast, part II has the advantage of providing conclusions about the target population, but its applicability has the limitation of requiring potentially debatable assumptions that express how patients in the study population are conceptually representative of their counterparts in the target population. Also, any need for assumptions about model structure would be another concern. Since the advantages and limitations of parts I and II are in some sense complementary, the combined usage of both is recommended in this chapter. Other references that discuss this strategy are Koch et al. (1980b, 1982), Koch and Gillings (1983), Koch and Sollecito (1984), and Koch and Edwards (1987). The remainder of this section is concerned with aspects of the application of nonparametric statistical tests to address the comparisons in part I for the background variables and related questions concerning the association between background variables and response variables. Both parts I and II are discussed for the response variables in Sections 3 and 4.

2.1 Comparisons Between Treatment Groups Within Centers

For the specific example in this chapter, the patients at each center were separately assigned to the two treatments through random partitions of successive blocks of six patients (i.e., within each block, three patients received active treatment and three patients received placebo). These blocks are ignored henceforth on the basis of the assumption that the order of entry of patients to the study was sufficiently random for them to have no association with either background variables or response variables. The randomization process in the study design and the ignorability of blocks jointly imply that the patients in each treatment group at each center are a simple random sample of the finite subpopulation of all patients in the study at the corresponding center (if blocks needed to be taken into account, each treatment group would be a stratified simple random sample and the methods in Section 2.2 would apply).

The statistical properties of sums or means of observations from simple random samples [as discussed in Cochran (1977)] then enables the construction of nonparametric statistical tests for comparisons between treatment groups. To be specific, let x_{hik} denote the value of a background variable for the kth patient with the ith treatment at the hth center. Since treatment has no effect on background variables (as a consequence of their determination prior to treatment), the subpopulation mean μ_h and variance v_h for all patients at each of the centers are known constants, that is,

$$\mu_h = \frac{\sum_{i=A}^{P} \sum_{k=1}^{n_{hi}} x_{hik}}{n_h}, \qquad v_h = \frac{\sum_{i=A}^{P} \sum_{k=1}^{n_{hi}} (x_{hik} - \mu_h)^2}{n_h}. \tag{1}$$

The status of each treatment group as a simple random sample from the finite subpopulation at the corresponding center implies that the expected values and covariance structure for their observed means $\bar{x}_{hi} = \{\sum_{k=1}^{n_{hi}} x_{hik}/n_{hi}\}$ are

$$E\{\bar{x}_{hi}\} = \mu_h, \qquad \text{var}\{\bar{x}_{hi}\} = \frac{(n_h - n_{hi})v_h}{n_{hi}(n_h - 1)},$$

$$\text{cov}\{\bar{x}_{hA}, \bar{x}_{hP}\} = \frac{-v_h}{n_h - 1}. \tag{2}$$

When the sample sizes for the two treatment groups are sufficiently large (e.g., the $n_{hi} \geq 15$), the mean score statistic relative to either treatment $i = A,\ P$,

$$Q_{S,h} = \frac{(\bar{x}_{hi} - \mu_h)^2}{\text{var}\{\bar{x}_{hi}\}} = \frac{n_h - 1}{n_h}(\bar{x}_{hA} - \bar{x}_{hP})^2 \Big/ \left(\frac{1}{n_{hA}} + \frac{1}{n_{hP}}\right) v_h, \tag{3}$$

approximately has the chi-square distribution with one degree of freedom (i.e., $d.f. = 1$). Thus the p-value from this chi-square approximation for outcomes $\geq Q_{S,h}$ enables evaluation of the extent to which randomization has provided the treatment groups with similar distributions for the background variable. In this regard, small p-values (e.g., $p \leq 0.05$) correspond to large values of $Q_{S,h}$ and hence identify background variables with noteworthy differences between treatment groups due to chance (since treatment should have no effect on background variables). The determination of p-values for situations with small samples requires consideration of the exact distribution of the $\bar{x}_{hi}$ across all possible randomizations of patients to treatments at each center.

The mean score statistic $Q_{S,h}$ in (3) has forms that encompass well-known methods for particular types of background variables. Dichotomous variables such as sex are handled with indicator variables such as $x_{hik} = 1$ if male or $x_{hik} = 0$ if female. It then follows that $\bar{x}_{hi}$ is the proportion of males with the ith treatment at the hth center and $n_{hi}\bar{x}_{hi} = n_{hiM}$ is the number of males with the ith treatment at the hth center. Similarly, μ_h is the proportion of males at the hth center and $n_h\mu_h = n_{h+M}$ is the number of males at the hth center. Also, $v_h = (n_{h+F}n_{h+M})/n_h^2$, where n_{h+F} is the number of females at the hth center. It then follows that

$$Q_{S,h} = \left(n_{hiM} - \frac{n_{hi}n_{h+M}}{n_h}\right)^2 \Big/ \left[\frac{n_{hA}n_{hP}n_{h+M}n_{h+F}}{n_h^2(n_h-1)}\right]$$
$$= \frac{n_h - 1}{n_h}\sum_i\sum_j \frac{(n_{hij} - m_{hij})^2}{m_{hij}} = \frac{(n_h-1)Q_{P,h}}{n_h}; \quad (4)$$

here $i = A$, P and $j = F$, M index treatment and sex; n_{hij} and $m_{hij} = (n_{hi}n_{h+j}/n_h)$ denote the observed and expected numbers of patients with the jth sex in the ith treatment group under randomization at the hth center; and $Q_{P,h}$ denotes the well-known Pearson chi-square statistic for the (2×2) contingency table of frequencies n_{hij} from the cross-classification of treatment and sex for each center. For the data in Table 1, the (2×2) contingency tables for treatment $\times$ sex are:

Center 1	Female	Male	Center 2	Female	Male
Active (A)	2	25	Active (A)	4	23
Placebo (P)	5	24	Placebo (P)	12	16

(5)

Their corresponding mean score statistics are $Q_{S,1} = 1.21$ with $p = 0.271$ and $Q_{S,2} = 5.15$ with $p = 0.023$. However, for (2×2) contingency tables, the determination of exact p-values through Fisher's exact test is straightforward and usually desirable unless sample sizes are clearly large enough for a chi-square approximation (e.g., all $m_{hij} \geq 10$).

The p-values for Fisher's exact test is determined by identification of all possible (2×2) contingency tables with the same row and column sums as the observed table, computation of the probability of occurrence of each with respect to the randomization-induced hypergeometric distribution, and the summation of those probabilities that are less than or equal to the probability of the observed table. One-sided p-values for a specified alternative are obtained by summation of all probabilities for tables in the corresponding direction for differences $(\bar{x}_{hA} - \bar{x}_{hP})$ between treatments at least as large as that for the observed table. The two-sided p-values from Fisher's exact test for sex are $p_1 = 0.42$ at center 1 and $p_2 = 0.037$ at center 2. These results suggest the presence of an imbalance in the sex distributions for the treatment groups at center 2 with a substantially larger percentage of males being randomly assigned to A (85.2%) than to P (57.1%). Also, at center 1, somewhat more males were assigned to A (92.6%) than to P (82.8%).

The percentages of males for A and P at each center and the two-sided p-values from Fisher's exact test are displayed in Table 2. These

Table 2 Descriptive Statistics and p-Values from Treatment Comparisons for Background Variables[a]

Background variable	Treatment	Statistic	Center 1	Center 2	Combined centers[b]
Number of patients	Active (A)	n	27	27	54
	Placebo (P)	n	29	28	57
	Total	n	56	55	111
Age	Active (A)	Mean	29.93	35.85	32.89
		SE	2.16	3.07	1.88
	Placebo (P)	Mean	30.69	36.71	33.65
		SE	2.25	2.70	1.75
	A vs. P	p-value	0.93	0.69	0.73
Sex	Active (A)	% male	92.6	85.2	88.9
		SE	5.1	7.0	4.3
	Placebo (P)	% male	82.8	57.1	70.2
		SE	7.1	9.5	5.9
	A vs. P	p-value	0.42	0.037[c]	0.013[c]
Baseline status	Active (A)	Mean	1.96	2.78	2.37
		SE	0.22	0.20	0.15
	Placebo (P)	Mean	2.17	2.61	2.39
		SE	0.17	0.17	0.12
	A vs. P	p-value	0.57	0.55	0.98
Dichotomous baseline status	Active (A)	% $\geq$ good	33.3	55.6	44.4
		SE	9.2	9.7	6.7
	Placebo (P)	% $\geq$ good	31.0	60.7	45.6
		SE	8.7	9.4	6.4
	A vs. P	p-value	1.00	0.79	0.88

[a]The p-values for age and baseline status are based on the Wilcoxon rank sum statistic via (3) for centers 1 and 2 separately and on the extended Mantel–Haenszel statistic (12) relative to within-center standardized ranks (or the van Elteren statistic) for the combined centers; midranks were used to account for ties via (16). The p-values for sex and dichotomous baseline status are based on Fisher's exact test for centers 1 and 2 separately [as described relative to (5)] and the Mantel–Haenszel statistic (13) for the combined centers. Computations were performed with the FREQ Procedure in the SAS System (1985).
[b]Means for the combined centers are based on the pooled data for the two centers; their standard errors are adjusted for center via (21). The p-values for the combined centers are adjusted for centers by the stratification for the extended Mantel–Haenszel statistic (12).
[c]Treatment comparisons with $p \leq 0.05$.

types of results are also given there for the dichotomous classification of baseline status as (good or excellent) or not. For both sex and dichotomous baseline status, standard errors (SE) are shown in Table 2 for the reported percentages. They were obtained via

$$(\mathrm{SE})_{hi} = 100 \left[\frac{p_{hij}(1 - p_{hij})}{n_{hi} - 1} \right]^{1/2} \tag{6}$$

where $p_{hij} = (n_{hij}/n_{hi})$ denotes the proportion of patients with the jth category of the background variable for the ith treatment group at the hth center; the multiplication by 100 accounts for percentages being $100p_{hij}$. The purpose of the SE's is to describe the variability of the reported percentages relative to the general setting of simple random sampling from corresponding infinite populations, so their computation from (6) presumes this framework (by involving no finite population correction and being based only on the data for the ith treatment at the hth center).

For age and baseline status, the means $\bar{x}_{hi}$ and their standard errors

$$(\mathrm{SE})_{hi} = \left[\frac{\sum_{k=1}^{n_{hi}} (x_{hik} - \bar{x}_{hi})^2}{n_{hi}(n_{hi} - 1)} \right]^{1/2} \tag{7}$$

are given in Table 2 for each treatment group at each center; the SE's in (7) apply to infinite populations for the same reasons stated for (6). Although the actual values of age and baseline status can be used in the mean score statistic $Q_{S,h}$ for the comparison of the two treatment groups at each center, their transformation to ranks for this purpose is often preferable. An advantage of ranks for an ordinal variable such as baseline status (for which midranks are used to account for ties) is that they basically express the relative ordering of the observed categories as opposed to an explicit scaling such as 0, 1, 2, 3, 4, which might be debatable (the issue of using 0, 1, 2, 3, 4 for means and standard errors is discussed further in Section 3.1). For continuous variables such as age with distributions that may be nonsymmetric and may have a wide range, use of ranks can enhance the applicability of chi-square approximations to $Q_{S,h}$ for the available sample sizes. Also, when the $\{x_{hik}\}$ are ranks, the sum $n_{hi}\bar{x}_{hi}$ of observed values for the ith treatment is the Wilcoxon rank sum statistic, so analysis for small samples can be undertaken with exact p-values. An algorithm due to Mehta et al. (1984) can be used to obtain such exact p-values for ordinal variables with a small number of categories and possibly many ties; for continuous variables with only a few ties, tables like those in Owen (1962) for the Wilcoxon rank sum statistic (or its Mann–Whitney counterpart) are applicable.

In Table 2, the p-values for the comparison of the two treatment groups with respect to age and baseline status are based on the Wilcoxon rank-sum statistic. They were obtained through the approximate chi-square distribution of the mean score statistics $Q_{S,h}$ for which the $\{x_{hik}\}$ were the ranks of the kth patient relative to all patients at the hth center. This method is considered to be suitably supported by the available sample size (i.e., all $n_{hi} \geq 25$).

The statistical comparisons in Table 2 for the separate centers generally confirm that randomization has provided similar distributions of background variables for the two treatment groups. Only the p-value for sex at center 2 suggests a noteworthy imbalance by its ≤ 0.05 status; the other seven p-values for within center comparisons had ≥ 0.25 status and hence were clearly compatible with what might be expected from randomization.

2.2 Comparisons Between Treatment Groups for the Combined Centers

The patients from the combined centers constitute a stratified population (with centers as the strata), and the patients in the two treatment groups are stratified simple random samples of this population (since the random assignment of patients to treatments was undertaken separately at the two centers). Thus the question of whether the distribution of background variables for the two treatment groups is similar is equivalent to the question of whether the distribution of background variables for each treatment group is similar to what would be expected from the structure of its corresponding stratified simple random sample. The latter question can be addressed for the ith treatment group by comparing the across-center sum

$$x_{+i+} = \sum_{h=1}^{2} \sum_{k=1}^{n_{hi}} x_{hik} = \sum_{h=1}^{2} n_{hi} \bar{x}_{hi} \tag{8}$$

of its observations to their expected value

$$E\{x_{+i+}\} = \sum_{h=1}^{2} n_{hi} \mu_{h}. \tag{9}$$

The stratified structure of the randomization of patients to treatments implies that the means $\bar{x}_{hi}$ from different centers are independent of one another; so

$$\operatorname{cov}\{\bar{x}_{1i}, \bar{x}_{2i}\} = 0 \qquad \text{for } i = A, P. \tag{10}$$

Also, for (10), it is implicitly assumed that the x_{hik} are obtained either without any measurement error or with mutually independent measurement errors (which are ignorable by restriction of attention to the data as given). From (2) and (10), the variance of x_{+i+} is

$$\operatorname{var}(x_{+i+}) = \frac{\sum_{h=1}^{2} n_{hi}(n_h - n_{hi})v_h}{n_h - 1}. \tag{11}$$

Thus an approximate test statistic for the comparison of the two treatment groups for the combined centers is

$$\begin{aligned} Q_{EMH} &= \frac{(x_{+i+} - E\{x_{+i+}\})^2}{\operatorname{var}\{x_{+i+}\}} \\ &= \frac{[\sum_{h=1}^{q}(n_{hA}n_{hP}/n_h)(\bar{x}_{hA} - \bar{x}_{hP})]^2}{\sum_{h=1}^{q}(n_{hA}n_{hP}/n_h)^2\tilde{v}_h}, \end{aligned} \tag{12}$$

where $q = 2$ is the number of centers (or strata), $\tilde{v}_h = \operatorname{var}\{\bar{x}_{hA} - \bar{x}_{hP}\}$ and x_{+i+} can refer to either $i = A$ or $i = P$. This criterion is often called the extended Mantel–Haenszel statistic. It approximately has the chi-square distribution with d.f. = 1 when the two treatment groups have sufficiently large sample sizes $\{n_{+i}\}$ for the combined centers ($e.g., n_{+i} \geq 20$). Small p-values (e.g., $p \leq 0.05$) relative to this chi-square approximation indicate background variables for which atypically large differences between the two treatment groups for the combined centers resulted from randomization. For situations with small samples, the determination of p-values for Q_{EMH} needs to be based on the exact distribution of x_{+i+} across all possible randomizations of patients to treatments at the two centers. Regardless of whether sample sizes are large or small, the p-values for Q_{EMH} are adjusted for centers in the sense of being based on the within-center differences of the means $(\bar{x}_{hA} - \bar{x}_{hP})$ for the two treatments.

The definition of Q_{EMH} in (12) for dichotomous background variables with possible categories $j = 1, 2$ provides the usual Mantel–Haenszel (Mantel and Haenszel, 1959) statistic,

$$\begin{aligned} Q_{MH} &= \frac{[\sum_{h=1}^{q}(n_{hA}n_{hP}/n_h)(p_{hA1} - p_{hP1})]^2}{\sum_{h=1}^{q}[n_{hA}n_{hP}n_{h+1}n_{h+2}/n_h^2(n_h - 1)]} \\ &= \frac{[\sum_{h=1}^{q}(n_{hA1} - m_{hA1})]^2}{\sum_{h=1}^{q}[n_{hA}n_{hP}n_{h+1}n_{h+2}/n_h^2(n_h - 1)]}, \end{aligned} \tag{13}$$

where $q = 2$, $n_{h+j} = (n_{hAj} + n_{hPj})$ and $m_{hij} = (n_{hi}n_{h+j}/n_h)$. In (13), Q_{MH} is specified relative to the p_{hi1}, but the same result would be obtained relative to the p_{hi2}; also, Q_{MH} would remain the same if the $(n_{hA1} -$

m_{hA1}) were replaced by the $(n_{hij} - m_{hij})$ for some other i, j. Through its definition in terms of frequencies $\{n_{hij}\}$, Q_{MH} is a method for the combined analysis of a set of (2×2) contingency tables like those shown in (5) for treatment × sex at each center. A criterion due to Mantel and Fleiss (1980) is available for confirming the appropriateness of the chi-square approximation to the distribution of Q_{MH} for this data structure. It is that the difference between the across-center sum of expected values $\{\sum_{h=1}^{2} m_{hij}\}$ for any i, j and both the minimum possible value and the maximum possible value for the corresponding sums of the observed values exceed 5. For the situations where the Mantel and Fleiss (1980) criterion is not satisfied, the methods reviewed in Gart (1971) can be used to determine an exact p-value for Q_{MH}. Algorithms for the computation of such exact p-values or other types of exact results for sets of (2×2) contingency tables are discussed in Thomas (1975) and Mehta et al. (1985).

The extended Mantel–Haenszel statistic in (12) was proposed by Mantel (1963) for the comparison of two groups with respect to an ordinal variable in a way that adjusts for a set of strata. Although (12) expressed how Q_{EMH} is obtained from the case record data $\{x_{hik}\}$ for patients, a common framework for its usage is a set of $(2 \times r)$ contingency tables for group × ordinal variable. In this setting, computation of Q_{EMH} would also be based on (12), but with the modifications that the

$$\bar{x}_{hi} = \frac{\sum_{j=1}^{r} a_{hj} n_{hij}}{n_{hi}} \tag{14}$$

become means with respect to scores $\{a_{hj}\}$ at the hth center for the numbers of patients $\{n_{hij}\}$ with the jth category of the observed variable in the ith treatment group at the hth center and

$$\begin{aligned} \tilde{v}_h &= \frac{n_h}{n_h - 1}\left(\frac{1}{n_{hA}} + \frac{1}{n_{hP}}\right) v_h \\ &= \left(\frac{1}{n_{hA}} + \frac{1}{n_{hP}}\right) \frac{\sum_{j=1}^{r}(a_{hj} - \mu_h)^2 n_{h+j}}{n_h - 1} \end{aligned} \tag{15}$$

where $n_{h+j} = n_{hAj} + n_{hPj}$ and $\mu_h = \sum_{j=1}^{r} a_{hj} n_{h+j} / n_h$. As discussed in Section 2.1 for the within-center mean score statistic $Q_{S,h}$ in (3), analyses based on ranks have important advantages. A nonparametric rank procedure with a locally most powerful property was proposed by van Elteren (1960) and is discussed by Lehmann (1975). It has essentially the same structure as Q_{EMH} relative to scores that are called within-center, standardized midranks here [and modified ridits in the documentation for the FREQ Procedure in the SAS System (1985)]. The definition of these scores with respect to a set of ordinal categories is

$$a_{hj} = \begin{cases} 0 & \text{for all } j \text{ such that } \sum_{j'=1}^{j} n_{h+j'} = 0 \\ \dfrac{\sum_{j'=1}^{j} n_{h+j'} - (1/2)n_{h+j} + 1/2}{n_h + 1} & \text{for all } j \text{ such that } \sum_{j'=1}^{j} n_{h+j'} \geq 0. \end{cases} \tag{16}$$

It also applies to variables with continuous distributions through the special case where all $n_{h+j} = 1$. Thus the extended Mantel–Haenszel statistic for within-center, standardized midranks is the categorical data counterpart to the van Elteren statistic.

Consistent tendencies for one treatment group to have larger means than the other treatment group across the strata (centers) are the types of imbalance which the Mantel–Haenszel statistic most effectively detects for the distribution of a background variable. This aspect of its performance is a consequence of the differences $(\bar{x}_{hA} - \bar{x}_{hP})$ reinforcing one another in the numerator of Q_{EMH} when they predominantly have the same sign (i.e., nearly all are positive or nearly all are negative). Accordingly, Q_{EMH} is often said to provide a test of average partial association [see Landis et al. (1978)]. Aside from the previous considerations about the optimal setting for its performance, Q_{EMH} is a valid test statistic for the comparison of treatment groups for a combined set of strata regardless of the pattern of differences across them. Thus use of Q_{EMH} has the important advantage of being unconditionally specifiable in the protocol for a study (i.e., at a time prior to data collection or data analysis).

When the directions of the differences between treatments for a background variable conflict to the extent that positive ones offset negative ones, a potential limitation of Q_{EMH} is an inability to detect the extent to which their absolute magnitudes for the respective strata might collectively suggest an atypical distribution from randomization. Two more effective methods for evaluating this pattern for the means $\bar{x}_{hi}$ are the total association, mean score statistic

$$Q_{S,T} = \sum_{h=1}^{q} Q_{S,h}, \tag{17}$$

where $q = 2$, and the pseudohomogeneity statistic

$$Q_{S,PH} = Q_{S,T} - Q_{EMH}. \tag{18}$$

When the sample sizes within each center are sufficiently large (e.g., all $n_{hi} \geq 15$) for the $Q_{S,h}$ to have approximate chi-square distributions with d.f. = 1, then $Q_{S,T}$ and $Q_{S,PH}$ approximately have the chi-square distributions with d.f. = $q = 2$ and d.f. = $(q-1) = 1$, respectively. This sample size requirement is more stringent than that for Q_{EMH} relative to the sample sizes $\{n_{+i}\}$ for the combined strata, so Q_{EMH} has the advantage that its chi-square approximation is applicable in a broader range of situations than those for $Q_{S,T}$ or $Q_{S,PH}$; these include the case of matched pairs where there is $n_{hi} = 1$ observation per treatment and for which Q_{EMH} is analogous to the paired t-test for continuous data and the sign test (or McNemar's test) for dichotomous data.

Another reason why Q_{EMH} is used more extensively than $Q_{S,T}$ or $Q_{S,PH}$ is that the consistent patterns of imbalance which it is better able to detect are typically of greater interest than the more general patterns which it may be less able to detect. Regardless of their somewhat different capabilities, there is merit in evaluating the results for Q_{EMH}, $Q_{S,T}$, and $Q_{S,PH}$ together when within-center sample sizes are sufficiently large for such analysis. For these situations, $Q_{S,T}$ is directed at general patterns of treatment differences which may or may not have consistent direction; Q_{EMH} is directed at the specific pattern of differences with consistent direction; and $Q_{S,PH}$ is directed at patterns of differences which are not encompassed by Q_{EMH} in the sense of its definition in (18). However, $Q_{S,PH}$ needs to be interpreted cautiously because it is not a test of homogeneity of treatment differences across the strata (or centers), although it can often shed light on whether such homogeneity seems to apply. Appropriate methods for evaluating homogeneity of treatment differences are described in Section 3 through tests of treatment × center interaction in statistical models. Other discussion of the roles of Q_{EMH}, and $Q_{S,PH}$ is given in Koch et al. (1985a).

Statistical results pertaining to comparisons between treatment groups for the combined centers are summarized for the background variables in the last column of Table 2. For sex, application of the Mantel–Haenszel statistic in (13) to the set of (2×2) contingency tables shown in (5) yielded $Q_{MH} = 6.15$; so $p = 0.013$ relative to the chi-square distribution with d.f. = 1. A chi-square approximation was considered reasonable here because the Mantel and Fleiss (1980) criterion was satisfied. More specifically, the minimum and maximum possible values for $(n_{1AF} + n_{2AF})$ are 0 and 23, and both are different from $(m_{1AF} + m_{2AF}) = 11.23$ by at least 5. If consideration is given to the exact distribution for (5) through the algorithm of Thomas (1975), one-sided $p = 0.011$ is obtained. Both this result and that from the chi-square approximation agree in indicating that an atypically larger percentage of males were randomly assigned to active treatment than to placebo for the combined centers.

When the one-sided exact p-value requires a close approximation (and is not available in its own right), some references, such as Breslow and Day (1980) and Fleiss (1981), recommend usage of a continuity correction; that is, (13) is modified to

$$Q_{MH,C} = \frac{[|\sum_{h=1}^{q}(n_{hA1} - m_{hA1})| - 0.5]^2}{\sum_{h=1}^{q}[n_{hA}n_{hP}n_{h+1}n_{h+2}/n_h^2(n_h - 1)]}, \tag{19}$$

and the one-sided p-value from its chi-square approximation with d.f. = 1 is determined.

The total association statistic in (17) for the comparison of the sex distributions for the two treatments is $Q_{S,T} = 6.36$ with d.f. = 2; so the pseudohomogeneity statistic in (18) is $Q_{S,PH} = (6.36 - 6.15) = 0.21$ with d.f. = 1. Since $Q_{S,PH}$ is a relatively small component of $Q_{S,T}$, these results indicate that the imbalance in sex distributions for the two treatments is due primarily to a consistent pattern of treatment differences (i.e., a larger percentage of males for A than for P for both centers). Chi-square approximations are not used here to determine p-values for $Q_{S,T}$ and $Q_{S,PH}$ because the sample sizes at center 1 are not considered large enough for this purpose (e.g., $m_{1iF} \leq 5$ for $i = A, P$).

The distribution of baseline status for the two treatment groups at the two centers is described by the following set of (2×5) contingency tables:

Center 1	Terrible (0)	Poor (1)	Fair (2)	Good (3)	Excellent (4)
Active (A)	3	6	9	7	2
Placebo (P)	0	7	13	6	3

(20)

Center 2	Terrible (0)	Poor (1)	Fair (2)	Good (3)	Excellent (4)
Active (A)	0	3	9	6	9
Placebo (P)	0	4	7	13	4

Since baseline status is an ordinal variable, its comparison for the two treatments is based on the extended Mantel–Haenszel statistic in (12) for the within-center, standardized midrank scores in (16). This method corresponds to the van Elteren statistic. For center 1 the standardized midrank scores are $a_{1j} = (2/57), (10/57), (27.5/57), (45/57), (54/57)$; and for center 2, they are $a_{2j} = (0), (4/56), (15.5/56), (33/56), (49/56)$. The result of this analysis was $Q_{EMH} = 0.001$, for which $p = 0.98$. It clearly confirms the fact that randomization has provided similar distributions of baseline status for the two treatment groups at the two centers. Such similarity was also evident for dichotomous baseline status on the basis of $Q_{MH} = 0.023$

with $p = 0.88$, and for age on the basis of $Q_{EMH} = 0.122$ with $p = 0.73$. Thus, among the four background variables for which statistical comparisons between treatments were evaluated for the combined centers, only sex exhibited a noteworthy imbalance. Although such a finding is not a substantial departure from what might be expected from randomization (relative to the framework of four statistical tests), it does merit some concern by identifying the possibility that any treatment difference for the response variables might be due partly to differences in the sex distributions for the two treatment groups. Analyses to address this issue are undertaken in Sections 2.3, 3.2, and 3.3.

A description is given in Table 2 for the distributions of background variables for all patients in each treatment group through the means $\bar{x}_{+i+}$ for the pooled data from the two centers and their corresponding standard errors $(\text{S.E.})_{+i}$ relative to stratified sampling from an infinite population. These results were obtained via

$$\bar{x}_{+i+} = \frac{\sum_{h=1}^{2} n_{hi}\bar{x}_{hi}}{n_{+i}}, \qquad (\text{SE})_{+i} = \left[\frac{\sum_{h=1}^{2} n_{hi}^2 (\text{SE})_{hi}^2}{n_{+i}^2}\right]^{1/2}, \tag{21}$$

where the $(\text{SE})_{hi}$ are defined by (6) for dichotomous variables and by (7) for variables with reasonably meaningful scores for ordinal categories or measured numerical values on a continuum. The $\bar{x}_{+i+}$ are the quantities at which Q_{EMH} in (12) is directed; but the $(\text{SE})_{+i}$ are not based on (11), but rather are stratified counterparts to (6) and (7) in the sense of being based on the data for the ith treatment within each of the respective centers and not involving any finite population corrections.

2.3 Association Between Background Variables and Response Variables

An atypically large difference in the sex distributions for the two treatment groups was identified through the analyses in Sections 2.1 and 2.2. As discussed in Section 1, comparisons between treatments for response variables would need to be adjusted for sex if important associations between sex and the response variables existed in the study population (to avoid potential bias from the imbalance in sex distributions favoring one of the treatments). Since sex is a dichotomous variable, one way to evaluate its effects under minimal assumptions is through nonparametric statistical tests like the mean score statistic in (3) for the separate centers and the extended Mantel–Haenszel statistic in (12) for the combined centers. For such analysis, sex defines the groups, and comparisons are directed at distributions of the response variables at each of the four visits. However, sex is a known characteristic of patients at the time of entry to a study rather than a randomly allocated condition, so the application of (3) and (12) to it requires somewhat different justification than that which applies to treatment comparisons. One strategy here is to argue that no association between sex and a response variable is hypothetically equivalent to sex categories being perceivable as randomly assigned labels for response distributions. In other words, randomization is invoked by hypothesis; and this provides the framework for sex comparisons with the same statistical properties as that discussed for treatment comparisons in Sections 2.1 and 2.2. Thus under the hypothesis of no association between response variables and groups based on sex (or those based on any other background variable), the counterparts to the mean score statistic in (3) for the separate centers and the extended Mantel–Haenszel statistic in (12) for the combined centers approximately have chi-square distributions when sample sizes are sufficiently large; also, exact methods are applicable for small-sample situations. The occurrence of small p-values for these methods is interpreted as contradicting the hypothesis of no association which provided the basis for their determination, thereby indicating the presence of an association. Additional discussion of this analysis strategy is given in Landis, et al. (1978) and Koch et al. (1980b).

Approximate p-values from the analyses of the association between sex and the response variables at visits 1 to 4 are shown in the upper part of Table 3. For the separate centers, these results are obtained from the Wilcoxon rank sum statistic through its specification in (3) as a mean score statistic; and for the combined centers, they are from the extended Mantel–Haenszel statistic in (12) for within-center, standardized midranks (i.e., the van Elteren statistic). The ≥ 0.10 status of all p-values in Table 3 for sex comparisons suggests that there is little or no association between sex and response variables. On this basis, the imbalance in sex distributions for the two treatments is interpreted as ignorable in the sense of only inducing negligible bias on treatment comparisons for response variables. Thus analyses of treatment effects are not considered to need any adjustment for sex. Nevertheless, the role of sex is evaluated further in Section 3.4 and found to have a possible interaction with treatment at visits 3 and 4; for this reason, the discussion there does include analyses that are adjusted for sex.

Since baseline status reflects the condition of patients prior to treatment, its association with response variables is of natural interest. A relevant consideration for the analysis of such association is that both baseline status and the response variables have ordinal measurement scales. A method that effectively accounts for this data structure within each center sepa-

Table 3 p-Values for Association of Sex and Baseline Status with Response Variables at Visits 1, 2, 3, and 4[a]

Background variable	Response variable	Degrees of freedom	Center 1	Center 2	Combined centers
Sex	Visit 1	1	0.36	0.61	0.34
	Visit 2	1	0.47	0.24	0.17
	Visit 3	1	0.87	0.30	0.47
	Visit 4	1	0.77	0.59	0.54
Baseline status	Visit 1	1	< 0.001[b]	0.012[c]	< 0.001[b]
	Visit 2	1	< 0.001[b]	0.29	< 0.001[b]
	Visit 3	1	< 0.001[b]	0.15	< 0.001[b]
	Visit 4	1	< 0.001[b]	0.059	< 0.001[b]

[a]The p-values for sex are based on the Wilcoxon rank sum statistic via (3) for centers 1 and 2 separately and on the extended Mantel–Haenszel statistic (12) relative to within-center standardized ranks (or the van Elteren statistic) for the combined centers; midranks were used to account for ties via (16). The p-values for baseline status are based on the Spearman rank correlation statistic (25) for centers 1 and 2 separately and on its Mantel–Haenszel extension (26) with standardized ranks for the combined centers. Computations were performed with the FREQ Procedure in the SAS System (1985).
[b]Relationships with $p \leq 0.01$.
[c]Relationships with $p \leq 0.05$.

rately is the Spearman rank correlation statistic (with midranks applied to ties). The relevant quantities for the expression of this criterion for categorical data are frequencies $\{n_{hh'j}\}$ for the frequency of the h'th category of baseline status and the jth category for a response variable at the hth center, standardized midranks $\{c_{hh'}\}$ as scores for baseline status, and standardized midranks $\{a_{hj}\}$ as scores for the response variable. Then let

$$f_h = \frac{\sum_{h'=0}^{4} \sum_{j=0}^{4} c_{hh'} a_{hj} n_{hh'j}}{n_h}. \tag{22}$$

Relative to the perspective that the hypothesis H_0 of no association between baseline status and a response variable for each center is equivalent to each being randomly distributed relative to the other, it follows that

$$E\{f_h \mid H_0\} = \frac{\sum_{h'=0}^{4} \sum_{j=0}^{4} c_{hh'} a_{hj} n_{hh'+} n_{h+j}}{n_h^2}$$

$$= \frac{\sum_{h'=0}^{4} c_{hh'} n_{hh'+}}{n_h} \frac{\sum_{j=0}^{4} a_{hj} n_{h+j}}{n_h} \tag{23}$$

$$= \mu_{hc} \mu_{ha},$$

$$\text{var}\{f_h \mid H_0\} = \frac{\sum_{h'=0}^{4} (c_{hh'} - \mu_{hc})^2 n_{hh'+}}{n_h} \frac{\sum_{j=0}^{4} (a_{hj} - \mu_{ha})^2 n_{h+j}}{n_h(n_h - 1)}$$

$$= \frac{v_{hc} v_{ha}}{n_h(n_h - 1)}, \tag{24}$$

where $n_{hh'+} = \sum_{j=0}^{4} n_{hh'j}$ and $n_{h+j} = \sum_{h'=0}^{4} n_{hh'j}$. The test statistic that emerges from this framework is

$$Q_{CS,h} = \frac{(f_h - E\{f_h \mid H_0\})^2}{\text{var}\{f_h \mid H_0\}}$$

$$= \frac{(n_h - 1)[\sum_{h'=0}^{4} \sum_{j=0}^{4} (c_{hh'} - \mu_{hc})(a_{hj} - \mu_{ha}) n_{hh'j}]^2}{n_h^2 v_{hc} v_{ha}}$$

$$= (n_h - 1) r_{ca,h}^2, \tag{25}$$

where $r_{ca,h}$ denotes the correlation coefficient between the baseline status scores and the response variable scores for the hth center. When standardized midranks are used for baseline status and the response variable, $r_{ca,h}$ becomes the Spearman rank correlation coefficient. Since $Q_{CS,h}$ approximately has the chi-square distribution with d.f. = 1 when the sample size for the corresponding center is large (e.g., $n_h \geq 30$), it is often called a correlation chi-square statistic.

A synthesis of the principles underlying the $\{Q_{CS,h}\}$ in (25) and the extended Mantel–Haenszel statistic in (12) provides the basis for a test statistic suggested by Mantel (1963) for the association between two ordinal variables for a combined set of strata (e.g., centers). It is given by

$$Q_{CSMH} = \frac{[\sum_{h=1}^{q} n_h (f_h - E\{f_h \mid H_0\})]^2}{\sum_{h=1}^{q} n_h^2 \text{var}\{f_h \mid H_0\}}$$

$$= \frac{[\sum_{h=1}^{q} n_h (v_{hc} v_{ha})^{1/2} r_{ca,h}]^2}{\sum_{h=1}^{q} [n_h^2 v_{hc} v_{ha} / (n_h - 1)]}, \tag{26}$$

where $q = 2$ is the number of strata. Sufficiently large sample size for the combined strata (e.g., $\sum_{h=1}^{q} n_h \geq 40$) supports usage of an approximate chi-square distribution with d.f. = 1 for Q_{CSMH}.

The lower part of Table 3 displays approximate p-values for statistical tests of the association between baseline status and the response variables at visits 1 to 4. The results for the separate centers are based on the Spearman rank correlation chi-square statistic in (25), and those for the combined centers are based on its extended Mantel–Haenszel counterpart in (26) for within-center, standardized midranks. For the combined centers, all p-values have ≤ 0.01 status, so the hypothesis of no association between baseline status and response variables is clearly contradicted. This conclusion applies equally strongly to center 1, but it has somewhat weaker support in center 2. Further evaluation of differences between centers for the relationship of response variables to baseline status requires methods analogous to the pseudohomogeneity statistic in (18) or usage of appropriate statistical models along the lines described in Section 3. Aside from this issue, the strong relationship between baseline status and the response variables for the combined centers suggests that treatment comparisons for response variables would be more effective (in the sense of involving relatively smaller variances) if they were adjusted for baseline status.

Other nonparametric strategies are available for the analysis of the association between background variables and response variables. Comparisons among more than two groups can be based on the Kruskal–Wallis statistic (Kruskal and Wallis, 1953) for the separate centers and its extended Mantel–Haenszel counterpart for the combined centers. Also, scores other than within-center, standardized midranks can be used, and strata can be based on treatment × center or other cross-classifications. For further discussion of extended Mantel–Haenszel statistics and related nonparametric methods based on randomization principles, see Landis et al. (1978, 1979), Koch and Bhapkar (1982), Koch et al. (1980b, 1982, 1985a), and Koch and Edwards (1987).

2.4 Computations

The p-values in Tables 2 and 3 were obtained with the FREQ Procedure in the SAS System (1985). The MEANS Procedure was used to determine descriptive statistics for the separate centers, and algorithms in the IML Procedure were used to determine descriptive statistics for the combined centers. Additional documentation for computations is given in the footnotes of Tables 2 and 3 and in the appendix.

3 UNIVARIATE METHODS FOR RESPONSE VARIABLES

As discussed at the beginning of Section 2, the analysis of a categorical response variable in a clinical trial often requires the use of more than one method in order to address the questions of statistical interest. These questions include:

a. Is there a difference between treatments for a response variable under minimal assumptions and no (or only necessary) adjustment for background variables?
b. Is there a difference between treatments for a response variable after adjustments for appropriate background variables and under minimal assumptions?
c. Is any difference between treatments for a response variable homogeneous across centers?
d. Is any difference between treatments for a response variable homogeneous across background variables?

The rationale for question a is that randomization usually is successful in providing the treatment groups with equivalent distributions of background variables. Moreover, the imbalances that may occasionally occur are often ignorable because the corresponding background variables have little or no association with the response variables (e.g., sex for the data in Table 1) or have offsetting associations (i.e., one may favor active treatment while another may favor placebo). Thus, for most situations, no adjustment for any background variable is necessary to avoid bias in treatment comparisons from imbalances, and any that is applied may have the potential limitation of seeming judgmental and thereby debatable unless its role was well justified (e.g., by inclusion in the protocol for a study or by the argument that substantial bias from no adjustment will be misleading, etc.). In Section 3.1, analysis of the direct comparisons in question a is undertaken with minimal assumptions for each response variable by the same nonparametric statistical tests that were discussed in Section 2. These methods and certain refinements are also applicable to the adjusted comparisons between treatments in question b. The objective of the latter analyses, which are discussed in Section 3.2, is the confirmation that conclusions are as well supported when adjustments for relevant background variables are applied as when they are not. For the data in Table 1, adjustment for sex is evaluated because of the imbalance in its distribution in the two treatment groups; and adjustment for baseline is evaluated because of the strong association between baseline and the response variable.

Statistical models are used to address questions c and d. For these analyses, the patients in the study are assumed to represent a general target population along the lines indicated in part II at the beginning of Section 2. The homogeneity of treatment effects across centers in question c is evaluated in Section 3.3 by determining whether a model with components for treatment and center needs to be expended to include the treatment × center interaction. Such analysis is applied to the dichotomous response variables of (good or excellent) or not through maximum likelihood procedures for fitting logistic regression models. For the scaling of the ordinal classification of response with successive integers, it is applied through weighted least squares procedures for fitting linear models. The evaluation of the homogeneity of treatment differences across background variables is undertaken in Section 3.4 with similar strategies. Attention is given there to whether relatively comprehensive models with components for treatment, center, and background variables also need to include treatment × background variable interactions. Logistic regression is used for such analysis of the dichotomous response variable of (good or excellent) or not, and its extension to the proportional odds model [as discussed in McCullagh (1980) and Harrell (1986)] is used for the ordinal expression of each response variable.

3.1 Direct Comparisons Between Treatments Under Minimal Assumptions

The primary conceptual difference between response variables and background variables is that the response variables for a patient may be substantially influenced by the treatment that is received. However, under the hypothesis H_0 of equivalence of treatment effects for each patient (i.e., the responses of each patient to the assigned treatment are identical to what would occur for the other treatment), the statistical framework provided by the randomization process in the study design is essentially the same for both response variables and background variables. In other words, the observed values of a response variable for all patients under H_0 constitute a finite population (which would hypothetically remain the same relative to all possible randomizations), and those for the two treatment groups are corresponding stratified simple random samples. Thus the nonparametric statistical tests described in Sections 2.1 and 2.2 for comparisons between treatment groups for background variables are also appropriate for such analyses of response variables. However, the role they serve for response variables involves somewhat different considerations. One is that maintenance of study design integrity is presumed; the basis for this includes double blinding and other mechanisms for avoiding bias in treatment comparisons from possible associations between response variables and inconsistencies in study management or measurement procedures. Another is that a small p-value ≤ 0.05 is interpreted as a contradiction to the equivalence of treatment groups for the distribution of a response variable. Both together enable the contradiction to apply to the hypothesis H_0 of equivalence of treatment effects, and thereby support the evaluation of p-values ≤ 0.05 as indicative of a significant difference in treatment effects.

Results for the comparison of the two treatment groups are given in Table 4 for the dichotomous response variables of (good or excellent) or not at visits 1 to 4. For each center $\times$ treatment $\times$ visit, the percentages of patients with good or excellent response are reported with their corresponding standard errors. These descriptive statistics were obtained from the frequencies $\{n_{ghij}\}$ of the jth response category at the gth visit for patients in the ith treatment group at the hth center via

$$
\begin{aligned}
(\%)_{ghi} &= 100 p_{ghi} = 100 \left(\frac{\sum_{j=3}^{4} n_{ghij}}{n_{hi}} \right), \\
(\mathrm{SE})_{ghi} &= 100 \left[\frac{p_{ghi}(1 - p_{ghi})}{n_{hi} - 1} \right]^{1/2}
\end{aligned}
\tag{27}
$$

As was the case with (6) for dichotomous background variables, the standard errors in (27) apply to random samples for infinite populations. Within each center, the p-values for each visit are based on Fisher's exact test. Those at visits 1 to 3 for center 2 are ≤ 0.05, and thus indicate that the percentages of good or excellent response for A in these settings are significantly larger than those for P. A directional tendency for good or excellent response to be more prevalent for A than for P also is apparent for each of the other center $\times$ visit combinations. The comparisons of the treatment groups for the combined centers are based on the Mantel–Haenszel statistic (13). The approximate p-values from this method are significant ($p \leq 0.05$) at visits 1 to 3 and nearly so at visit 4 ($p = 0.063$). These results provide the principal basis for the conclusion that the percentages of good or excellent response are significantly greater for A than P since they are based on all patients in the study population. They also do this more effectively than their within-center counterparts because of the consistency of the pattern of treatment differences across centers. A descriptive statistic for the treatment difference at which the Mantel–Haenszel statistic is directed for the gth visit response is

$$
d_g = 100 \left[\frac{\sum_{h=1}^{2} w_h (p_{ghA} - p_{ghP})}{\sum_{h=1}^{2} w_h} \right] = 100(p_{g*A} - p_{g*p}), \tag{28}
$$

Table 4 Descriptive Statistics and p-Values from Treatment Comparisons for Percentages of Patients with Good or Excellent Response at Visits 1, 2, 3, and 4

Response variable	Treatment	Statistic[a]	Center 1	Center 2	Combined centers[b]
Visit 1	Active (A)	% ≥ good	51.9	85.2	68.4
		SE	9.8	7.0	6.0
	Placebo (P)	% ≥ good	41.4	57.1	49.2
		SE	9.3	9.5	6.7
	A vs. P	Difference	10.5	28.0	19.2
		SE	13.5	11.8	9.0
		p-value	0.59	0.037[c]	0.036[c]
Visit 2	Active (A)	% ≥ good	59.3	81.5	70.3
		SE	9.6	7.6	6.2
	Placebo (P)	% ≥ good	34.5	42.9	38.6
		SE	9.0	9.5	6.5
	A vs. P	Difference	24.8	38.6	31.6
		SE	13.2	12.2	9.0
		p-value	0.11	0.005[d]	0.001[d]
Visit 3	Active (A)	% ≥ good	63.0	81.5	72.1
		SE	9.5	7.6	6.1
	Placebo (P)	% ≥ good	41.4	50.0	45.7
		SE	9.3	9.6	6.7
	A vs. P	Difference	21.6	31.5	26.5
		SE	13.3	12.3	9.0
		p-value	0.12	0.023[c]	0.005[d]
Visit 4	Active (A)	% ≥ good	44.4	77.8	61.0
		SE	9.7	8.2	6.4
	Placebo (P)	% ≥ good	31.0	57.1	44.0
		SE	8.7	9.5	6.5
	A vs. P	Difference	13.4	20.6	17.0
		SE	13.1	12.5	9.1
		p-value	0.41	0.15	0.063

[a] The p-values are based on Fisher's exact tests [as described relative to (5)] for centers 1 and 2 separately and on the Mantel–Haenszel statistic (13) for the combined centers. Computations were performed with the FREQ Procedure in the SAS System (1985).

[b] Descriptive statistics for the combined centers are based on weighted averages (28)–(30) for which the weights reflect adjustment for centers through their relative contributions to the Mantel–Haenszel statistic; that is, the weight for the hth center is $w_h/(w_1 + w_2)$ with $w_h = n_{h1}n_{h2}/(n_{h1} + n_{h2})$, where the n_{hi} denote the numbers of patients in the ith treatment group at the hth center.

[c] Treatment comparisons with $p \leq 0.05$.

[d] Treatment comparisons with $p \leq 0.01$.

where $w_h = n_{h1}n_{h2}/(n_{h1} + n_{h2})$; its standard error relative to stratified random sampling from an infinite population is

$$\mathrm{SE}(d_g) = 100 \left(\frac{\left\{ \sum_{h=1}^{2} w_h^2 [(\mathrm{SE})_{ghA}^2 + (\mathrm{SE})_{ghP}^2] \right\}^{1/2}}{\sum_{h=1}^{2} w_h} \right); \tag{29}$$

corresponding statistics that describe each treatment group's percentage of good or excellent response for the combined centers are

$$(\%)_{g*i} = 100(p_{g*i}), \qquad (\mathrm{SE})_{g*i} = \frac{[\sum_{h=1}^{2} w_h^2 (\mathrm{SE})_{ghi}^2]^{1/2}}{\sum_{h=1}^{2} w_h}, \tag{30}$$

where the p_{g*i} are defined in (28). The $(\%)_{g*i}$, the d_g, and their standard errors are given in Table 4. The range for the percentage of good or excellent response over the four visits is about 40 to 50% for P and about 60 to 70% for A. The difference between A and P has a range of about 20 to 30% and a standard error of about 10%.

The analysis of treatment comparisons for the ordinal expression of the response variables at visits 1 to 4 is similar to that which was described for baseline status in Sections 2.1 and 2.2. Means with respect to the integer scores 0, 1, 2, 3, 4 for the ordinal categories of terrible, poor, fair, good, and excellent, respectively, and their standard errors are used to describe the response distribution for each center × treatment × visit. These statistics were obtained from the frequencies $\{n_{ghij}\}$ in contingency tables such as (20) via

$$\bar{y}_{ghi} = \frac{\sum_{j=0}^{4} j n_{ghij}}{n_{hi}}, \qquad (\mathrm{SE})_{ghi} = \left[\frac{\sum_{j=0}^{4} (j - \bar{y}_{ghi})^2 n_{ghij}}{n_{hi}(n_{hi} - 1)} \right]^{1/2}. \tag{31}$$

Alternatively, if y_{ghik} denotes the response at the gth visit for the kth patient in the ith treatment group at the hth center, they could have been computed directly via

$$\bar{y}_{ghi} = \frac{\sum_{k=1}^{n_{hi}} y_{ghik}}{n_{hi}}, \qquad (\mathrm{SE})_{ghi} = \left[\frac{\sum_{k=1}^{n_{hi}} (y_{ghik} - \bar{y}_{ghi})^2}{n_{hi}(n_{hi} - 1)} \right]^{1/2}. \tag{32}$$

In accordance with (6), (7), and (27), the standard errors in (31) and (32) apply to random samples from infinite populations in order to describe the observed experience of the patients for this general setting.

A potential concern for the interpretation of the means and standard errors in (31) or (32) is that the integer scores on which they are based are not necessarily clinically meaningful values. One way to address this issue is to rewrite $\bar{y}_{ghi}$ in (31) as

$$\bar{y}_{ghi} = \frac{\sum_{j=0}^{4} j n_{ghij}}{n_{hi}} = \frac{\sum_{j=1}^{4} \sum_{j'=1}^{j} n_{ghij}}{n_{hi}}$$

$$= \frac{\sum_{j'=1}^{4} \sum_{j=j'}^{4} n_{ghij}}{n_{hi}} = \frac{\sum_{j'=1}^{4} N_{ghij'}}{n_{hi}} = \sum_{j'=1}^{4} P_{ghij'}, \tag{33}$$

where the $P_{ghij'}$ are the proportions of patients in the ith treatment group at the hth center with response at the gth visit at least as favorable as the j'th category. In view of (33), the difference between the treatment groups for the gth visit and hth center is

$$d_{gh} = (\bar{y}_{ghA} - \bar{y}_{ghP}) = \sum_{j=1}^{4} (P_{ghAj} - P_{ghPj}). \tag{34}$$

Through (34), the $\{d_{gh}\}$ have a meaningful interpretation as measures of the consistency with which the differences $\{(P_{ghAj} - P_{ghPj})\}$ across $j = 1$, 2, 3, 4, favor active treatment (or placebo). This rationale for the use of integer scores in the determination of the d_{gh} is considered to provide reasonable support for their usage in the means $\bar{y}_{ghi}$. As a consequence of (31) and (34), the standard errors for the d_{gh} are given by

$$(\text{SE})_{gh*} = [(\text{SE})_{ghA}^2 + (\text{SE})_{ghP}^2]^{1/2}. \tag{35}$$

For each center, the means $\bar{y}_{ghi}$, the differences d_{gh}, and their standard errors are given in Table 5 for the responses at each visit. Approximate p-values are also given there for the comparison between treatments through two specifications of the mean score statistic in (3). One of these is based on the integer scores 0, 1, 2, 3, 4 for the ordinal categories and hence has the advantage of being directed at the treatment difference that is described by the d_{gh}. The other is based on standardized midranks and hence is equivalent to the Wilcoxon rank-sum statistic; it has the advantage of only making use of the ordering of response categories rather than involving an explicit scaling. As often occurs in practice, the results from these methods support essentially the same conclusions. In Table 5, both methods indicate significantly ($p \leq 0.05$) more favorable response for A than P for all visits at center 2 and visit 2 at center 1; for the other visits at center 1, the positive values of the d_{gh} indicate directional tendencies in favor of active treatment.

For the combined centers, the statistical comparisons between the treatments for the ordinal response variables are assessed with the extended Mantel–Haenszel statistic in (12). Results were obtained for both inte-

Table 5 Descriptive Statistics and *p*-Values from Treatment Comparisons for Ordinal Response at Visits 1, 2, 3, and 4

Response variable	Treatment	Statistic[a]	Center 1	Center 2	Combined centers[b]
Visit 1	Active (A)	Mean	2.52	3.33	2.92
		SE	0.19	0.16	0.12
	Placebo (P)	Mean	2.24	2.82	2.53
		SE	0.25	0.19	0.16
	A vs. P	Difference	0.28	0.51	0.39
		SE	0.31	0.25	0.20
		p-value(int)	0.38	0.043[c]	0.053
		p-value(sr)	0.45	0.045[c]	0.052
Visit 2	Active (A)	Mean	2.85	3.41	3.13
		SE	0.19	0.19	0.13
	Placebo (P)	Mean	2.00	2.29	2.14
		SE	0.25	0.25	0.17
	A vs. P	Difference	0.85	1.12	0.99
		SE	0.31	0.31	0.22
		p-value(int)	0.011[c]	0.001[d]	$<$ 0.001[d]
		p-value(sr)	0.016[c]	0.001[d]	$<$ 0.001[d]
Visit 3	Active (A)	Mean	2.81	3.30	3.05
		SE	0.23	0.19	0.15
	Placebo (P)	Mean	2.24	2.21	2.23
		SE	0.27	0.28	0.19
	A vs. P	Difference	0.57	1.08	0.83
		SE	0.35	0.34	0.24
		p-value(int)	0.11	0.004[d]	0.001[d]
		p-value(sr)	0.13	0.005[d]	0.002[d]
Visit 4	Active (A)	Mean	2.48	3.26	2.87
		SE	0.20	0.24	0.16
	Placebo (P)	Mean	2.03	2.46	2.25
		SE	0.24	0.31	0.19
	A vs. P	Difference	0.45	0.79	0.62
		SE	0.31	0.39	0.25
		p-value(int)	0.16	0.047[c]	0.015[c]
		p-value(sr)	0.22	0.037[c]	0.020[c]

[a]The *p*-values are based on randomization chi-square statistics (3) to compare mean scores for treatments within centers 1 and 2 separately and on

ger scores and within-center, standardized midrank scores; use of the latter corresponds to the van Elteren statistic. Approximate p-values from these analyses are given in the last column of Table 5. For visits 2 to 4, they are significant ($p \leq 0.05$); and for visit 1, they are nearly significant ($p = 0.053, 0.052$). The extent to which the responses for active treatment are more favorable than those for placebo are described in a spirit similar to (28)–(29) with weighted linear combinations of the d_{gh} and their corresponding standard errors. These statistics have the form

$$d_g = \frac{\sum_{h=1}^{2} w_h(\bar{y}_{ghA} - \bar{y}_{ghP})}{\sum_{h=1}^{2} w_h},$$

$$\mathrm{SE}(d_g) = \frac{\left\{\sum_{h=1}^{2} w_h^2[(\mathrm{SE})_{ghA}^2 + (\mathrm{SE})_{ghP}^2]\right\}^{1/2}}{\sum_{h=1}^{2} w_h}, \tag{36}$$

where $w_h = n_{h1}n_{h2}/(n_{h1} + n_{h2})$ and the $\bar{y}_{ghi}$ and the $(\mathrm{SE})_{ghi}$ are given in (32). The counterparts to (36) for describing each treatment group's response distributions for the combined centers are

$$\bar{y}_{g*i} = \frac{\sum_{h=1}^{2} w_h \bar{y}_{ghi}}{\sum_{h=1}^{2} w_h}, \qquad (\mathrm{SE})_{g*i} = \frac{[\sum_{h=1}^{2} w_h^2 (\mathrm{SE})_{ghi}^2]^{1/2}}{\sum_{h=1}^{2} w_h}. \tag{37}$$

The $\bar{y}_{g*i}$, the d_g, and their standard errors are given in Table 5. The difference between the two treatments over the four visits is indicated there to have a range of about 0.4 to 1.0 and a standard error of about 0.2.

The results in Table 4 and Table 5 have the attractive feature of being based on methods with minimal assumptions for which justification usually is reasonably supported by study design considerations. These assumptions were randomization, ignorability of blocks in the randomization, and maintenance of study design integrity. Of particular importance, no

---

the extended Mantel–Haenszel statistic (12) for such analysis of the combined centers. Results for both integer scores (int) and within center, standardized ranks (sr) via (16) are presented; the latter correspond to the Wilcoxon rank sum statistic for the separate centers and the van Elteren statistic for the combined centers. Computations were performed with the FREQ Procedure in the SAS System (1985).

[b]Descriptive statistics for the combined centers are based on weighted averages (36)–(37) for which the weights reflect adjustment for centers through their relative contributions to the extended Mantel–Haenszel statistic; that is, the weight for the hth center is $w_h/(w_1 + w_2)$ with $w_h = n_{h1}n_{h2}/(n_{h1} + n_{h2})$, where the n_{hi} denote the numbers of patients in the ith treatment group at the hth center.

[c]Treatment comparisons with $p \leq 0.05$.

[d]Treatment comparisons with $p \leq 0.01$.

assumption about specific structure for the distribution of response variables within the two centers nor the homogeneity of treatment differences across centers is required. Thus the conclusions from Table 4 and Table 5 are design-based inferences. Another important advantage of the methods used to obtain the descriptive statistics and p-values for the treatment comparisons in Tables 4 and 5 is that they are a priori specifiable in the protocol of a study. In this role, the extended Mantel–Haenszel statistic is a valid method for the analysis of all patients in a way that is particularly effective for detecting treatment differences with consistent direction across centers. As indicated in Section 2.2, it is not useful when treatment differences predominantly have conflicting direction, but the detection of such patterns of contradictory results is rarely an objective of a clinical trial. When necessary, these situations can be addressed with either methods like the total association statistic in (17) or separate tests for each center. Most clinical trials, however, are undertaken to detect a consistent pattern of treatment differences, and their analysis for this purpose is well served by the extended Mantel–Haenszel statistic. Since its usage is a priori specifiable, involves only minimal assumptions, and encompasses all patients, the extended Mantel–Haenszel statistic is often the most appropriate method for the inferential analysis of categorical data from multicenter clinical trials.

3.2 Adjusted Comparisons Between Treatments Under Minimal Assumptions

In Section 2, an imbalance in the sex distributions for the treatment groups was identified. This imbalance merits attention since it might partially account for any treatment differences for the response variables. The extent of such a confounding influence is determined by the strength of the association between sex and the response variable. Since analyses reported in Section 2.3 indicate little or no association between sex and the response variables, the imbalance in the sex distributions for the treatment groups was interpreted as ignorable. Thus direct comparisons between treatments in Section 3.1 are considered to provide appropriate conclusions for the response variables.

Alternatively, if there had been substantial association between sex and the response variables, treatment comparisons for response variables would need to be adjusted for sex to avoid any bias from the imbalance in its distribution. Such analyses are undertaken here to confirm that they yield the same conclusions as the direct comparisons in Section 3.1. A way of implementing adjustment for a categorical background variable like sex for a nonparametric statistical test is through its use for the post-stratification of patients (i.e., sex is "held constant" in subgroups of the center × sex × treatment cross-classification). Then treatment comparisons for response variables are combined across center × sex strata through the extended Mantel–Haenszel statistic. Results from such analysis (which involves minimal assumptions) are given in Table 6 for both the dichotomous and ordinal expressions of the response variables at visits 1 to 4; also, those for the ordinal response variables are based on within center × sex standardized midranks. The conclusions from Table 6 agree very well with those in Tables 4 and 5 from direct comparisons between treatments for the combined centers. For the ordinal response variables, the stratification adjusted p-values in Table 6 indicate that the differences between treatments are significant ($p \leq 0.05$) at visits 2 to 4 and nearly significant ($p = 0.066$) at visit 1. Those for the dichotomous response variable are significant ($p \leq 0.05$) at visits 2 and 3 and nearly significant at visits 1 and 4 ($p = 0.063, 0.081$).

Analysis of baseline status in Section 2 supported the following two conclusions: the two treatment groups had equivalent distributions of baseline status (see Table 2); and baseline status had strong relationships with the response variables (see Table 3). As a consequence of the former, no adjustment for baseline status is necessary for the avoidance of bias in treatment comparisons for response variables. However, the latter suggests that adjustment can strengthen statistical tests for treatment comparisons; this

Table 6 p-Values for Association of Treatment with Response Variables at Visits 1, 2, 3, and 4 under Stratification Adjustment for Center and Sex

Response variable	Degrees of freedom	Good or excellent response[a]		Ordinal response[b]	
		Q_{MH}	p-value	Q_{EMH}	p-value
Visit 1	1	3.46	0.063	3.37	0.066
Visit 2	1	10.07	0.002[c]	15.22	< 0.001[c]
Visit 3	1	6.45	0.011[d]	7.76	0.005[c]
Visit 4	1	3.04	0.081	4.57	0.032[d]

[a]The p-values for (good or excellent response) are based on the Mantel–Haenszel statistic (13) with adjustment for center × sex strata.
[b]The p-values for the ordinal response are based on the extended Mantel–Haenszel statistic (12) relative to within center, standardized ranks via (16) and adjustment for center × sex strata (i.e., the van Elteren statistic).
[c]Treatment comparisons with $p \leq 0.01$.
[d]Treatment comparisons with $p \leq 0.05$.

occurs through a reduction in the relative variability of the applicable distributions for estimates of treatment differences.

Poststratification could be used to adjust for baseline status along the lines discussed previously in this section for sex. This strategy has two limitations: it does not account for the ordinality of baseline status, and the center × baseline status cross-classification produces 10 strata within many of which the numbers of patients may be too small to contribute effectively to the detection of a treatment difference. In this regard, any stratum for which all patients correspond to one treatment or one response category merits particular concern because of the zero values for their components in the numerator and denominator of the extended Mantel–Haenszel statistic; that is, they provide no information, and this essentially implies the exclusion of such patients from the analysis. The issue here is that when results are not effectively based on all patients, their ability to support conclusions may become debatable.

The previously stated limitations of poststratification provide the rationale for the consideration of another method for adjustment. It involves the synthesis of nonparametric covariance analysis principles [described in Quade (1967) for ranks] with the randomization framework of the extended Mantel–Haenszel test. For each center separately, covariance analysis is applied by the construction of the residuals from the ordinary least squares prediction of a response variable as a linear function of baseline status. These residuals for the response variable at the gth visit are given by

$$z_{ghik} = (y_{ghik} - \bar{y}_{gh*}) - \lambda_{gh}(x_{hik} - \mu_h); \tag{38}$$

here $\bar{y}_{gh*} = \sum_{i=A}^{P} \sum_{k=1}^{n_{hi}} y_{ghik}/n_h$ and $\mu_h = \sum_{i=A}^{P} \sum_{k=1}^{n_{hi}} x_{hik}/n_h$ denote the means for the response levels y_{ghik} and baseline levels x_{hik} for all patients in the finite study population at the hth center; and

$$\lambda_{gh} = \frac{\sum_{i=A}^{P} \sum_{k=1}^{n_{hi}} (y_{ghik} - \bar{y}_{gh*})(x_{hik} - \mu_h)}{\sum_{i=A}^{P} \sum_{k=1}^{n_{hi}} (x_{hik} - \mu_h)^2} \tag{39}$$

denotes the least squares slope for the linear prediction of the response at the gth visit by baseline status for the finite population of patients at the hth center. Under the hypothesis H_0 of equivalence of treatment effects for each patient (as discussed in Section 3.1), $\bar{y}_{gh*}$, μ_h, and λ_{gh} are constants that apply to all possible randomizations. Thus the observed values of the residuals z_{ghik} for all patients constitute a finite population under H_0, and those for the two treatment groups within each center are simple random samples. These considerations provide the basis for the usage of the mean score statistic in (3) for the comparison of the two treatment groups with respect to the distribution of the response residuals z_{ghik}. This statistic has the form

$$Q_{z,gh} = \frac{(\bar{z}_{ghA} - \bar{z}_{ghP})^2}{\text{var}\left\{(\bar{z}_{ghA} - \bar{z}_{ghP}) \mid H_0\right\}}$$
$$= \frac{[(n_h - 1)/n_h][(\bar{y}_{ghA} - \bar{y}_{ghP}) - \lambda_{gh}(\bar{x}_{hA} - \bar{x}_{hP})]^2}{(1/n_{hA} + 1/n_{hP})(1 - r^2_{xg,h})v_{g,h}}, \tag{40}$$

where $v_{g,h} = \sum_{i=A}^{P} \sum_{k=1}^{n_{hi}} (y_{ghik} - \bar{y}_{gh*})^2/n_h$ and $r^2_{xg,h} = \lambda^2_{gh} v_h / v_{g,h}$, with v_k given by (1). The test statistic $Q_{z,gh}$ in (40) approximately has the chi-square distribution with d.f. = 1 when the sample sizes for the two treatment groups are sufficiently large (e.g., the $n_{hi} \geq 15$). For the situation where the y_{ghik} and the x_{hik} are ranks, it is equivalent to the rank analysis of covariance statistic discussed in Quade (1967). Another noteworthy feature of $Q_{z,gh}$ is that its addition to the mean score statistic $Q_{x,h}$ from (3) for baseline status yields the bivariate mean score statistic $Q_{xg,h}$ for the comparison of the two treatment groups with respect to the response variable at the gth visit and baseline status simultaneously; that is,

$$Q_{xg,h} = Q_{x,h} + Q_{z,gh} = \mathbf{f}'\mathbf{V}_f^{-1}\mathbf{f},$$

where

$$\mathbf{f} = \begin{bmatrix} (\bar{y}_{ghA} - \bar{y}_{ghP}) \\ (\bar{x}_{hA} - \bar{x}_{hP}) \end{bmatrix}, \qquad \mathbf{V_f} = \mathbf{var}(\mathbf{f} \mid H_0). \tag{41}$$

Under H_0, $Q_{xg,h}$ approximately has the chi-square distribution with d.f. = 2 for large-sample situations. The partition (41) is of interest because it enables $Q_{z,gh}$ to be interpreted as applying to the comparison of adjusted means of the response variables for the prediction setting where the treatment groups have the same mean for baseline status [see Koch et al. (1982) for further explanation].

The counterpart to the $Q_{z,gh}$ for the combined centers is formulated by applying the principles underlying the extended Mantel–Haenszel statistic in (12) to the z_{ghik}. It is given by

$$Q_{z,g} = \frac{[\sum_{h=1}^{q}(n_{hA}n_{hP}/n_h)(\bar{z}_{ghA} - \bar{z}_{ghP})]^2}{\sum_{h=1}^{q}[n_{hA}n_{hP}/(n_h - 1)](1 - r^2_{xg,h})v_{g,h}}, \tag{42}$$

where $q = 2$ is the number of strata (e.g., centers). An approximate chi-square distribution with d.f. = 1 applies to $Q_{z,g}$ under H_0 when the two treatment groups have sufficiently large sample sizes n_{+i} for the combined centers (e.g., $n_{+i} \geq 20$). As summarized in this discussion, $Q_{z,g}$ is based on randomization, accounts for centers through stratification, and provides covariance adjustment for baseline status through the residuals z_{ghik}; so its usage is describable as stratified randomization covariance analysis. Another important feature of this nonparametric method is its applicability under the same minimal assumptions as the extended Mantel–Haenszel statistic (see Section 3.1). In this regard, no assumption about the relationship between the y_{ghik} and the x_{hik} is required even though the definition of the z_{ghik} involves a linear structure.

Results from randomization covariance analysis with baseline adjustment of treatment comparisons are shown in Table 7 for the ordinal re-

Table 7 p-Values from Randomization Covariance Analysis Relative to Baseline Status for Ordinal Response at Visits 1, 2, 3, and 4

Response variable	Statistic[a]	Center 1	Center 2	Combined centers	Combined for center × sex
Visit 1	Q_Z ($d.f. = 1$)	3.03	3.67	6.64	6.65
	p-value	0.082	0.055	0.010[c]	0.010[c]
Visit 2	Q_Z ($d.f. = 1$)	11.63	11.17	22.59	20.95
	p-value	0.001[c]	0.001[c]	< 0.001[c]	< 0.001[c]
Visit 3	Q_Z ($d.f. = 1$)	4.69	7.68	12.33	10.50
	p-value	0.030[b]	0.006[c]	< 0.001[c]	0.001[c]
Visit 4	Q_Z ($d.f. = 1$)	2.99	4.00	6.97	6.19
	p-value	0.084	0.046[b]	0.008[c]	0.013[b]
All visits	Q_Z ($d.f. = 4$)	12.34	11.74	23.41	21.58
	p-value	0.015[b]	0.019[b]	< 0.001[c]	< 0.001[c]
Average over 4 visits	Q_Z ($d.f. = 1$)	8.76	8.97	17.47	16.09
	p-value	0.003[c]	0.003[c]	< 0.001[c]	< 0.001[c]

[a]The p-values for each center are based on randomization chi-square statistics (40) to compare mean scores for treatment with covariance adjustment for baseline status. For both response variables and baseline status, within center, standardized midranks are used as framework for analysis. Stratification adjustment in a spirit similar to that for the Mantel–Haenszel statistic is used via (42) to determine the p-values for treatment comparisons for the combined centers and the combined (center × sex) strata with covariance adjustment for baseline status. Computations were performed with the procedures documented in Amara and Koch (1980).
[b]Treatment comparisons with $p \leq 0.05$.
[c]Treatment comparisons with $p \leq 0.01$.

sponse variables at each visit. The approximate p-values for each center are based on the mean score statistics $Q_{z,gh}$ in (40) for within center, standardized midranks of both the response variable and baseline status; i.e., they correspond to rank analysis of covariance. For center 1, these p-values are significant ($p \leq 0.05$) at visits 2 and 3 and nearly significant at visits 1 and 4 ($p = 0.082, 0.084$); and for center 2, they are significant at visits 2 to 4 and nearly significant at visit 1 ($p = 0.055$). These patterns of results agree well with their counterparts in Table 5 from direct comparisons between treatments, although those for center 1 are slightly stronger and those for center 2 are slightly weaker; the reason for these minor variations is the association of more favorable baseline status with more favorable response status, so adjustment offsets the somewhat less favorable baseline status of active treatment in center 1 and its somewhat more favorable status in center 2. Adjusted treatment comparisons for the combined centers are evaluated with the stratified randomization covariance statistic $Q_{z,g}$ in (42); this method was also applied with stratification adjustment for both center and sex. The approximate p-values from these analyses indicated significant ($p \leq 0.05$) differences between treatments at all visits. Thus they supported somewhat stronger conclusions than their counterparts in Table 5 from direct comparisons between treatments and in Table 6 from stratification-adjusted comparisons with respect to sex.

More general versions of randomization covariance statistics such as the $Q_{z,gh}$ and the $Q_{z,g}$ are available. They encompass comparisons among more than two groups, stratification adjustment for cross-classifications of center with one or more background variables, covariance adjustment for more than one background variable, and usage of scores other than ranks. Also, as described in Section 4.1, multivariate analyses of more than one response variable can be undertaken. For some background variables, such as sex, either stratification adjustment or covariance adjustment could be applied, so the choice between them requires attention. The basic consideration here is that stratification provides a more explicit adjustment by "holding the background variable constant" at the individual patient level, whereas covariance analysis involves adjustment for which equivalence of means of background variables is induced for groups of patients. The usefulness of each method is greater when adjustment is for background variables which are strongly associated with response variables. Further discussion of nonparametric methods for covariance analysis is given in Quade (1967, 1982), Puri and Sen (1971), Amara and Koch (1980), Huitema (1980), and Koch et al. (1982).

3.3 Evaluation of Treatment × Center Interaction

At the beginning of Section 2 the conduct of the statistical analysis of a clinical trial in two parts was identified as an effective strategy for having the evaluation of treatments account for how the study population was selected and how it conceptually represents some target population. Part I is concerned with the existence of a treatment difference for the study population under minimal assumptions. It was addressed with the nonparametric methods in Sections 2, 3.1, and 3.2. The results of these analyses indicated the existence of a significant difference between treatments for the patients in the study population (by the contradiction of the hypothesis of no difference with p-values ≤ 0.05). This significant difference was due to the tendency for patients with active treatment to have more favorable responses than placebo patients.

After the determination of the existence of a difference between treatments for a study population in part I of the statistical analysis of a clinical trial, the objective for part II is the evaluation of whether this difference is homogeneous across study factors such as center or subgroups based on background variables such as age, sex, and baseline status. When homogeneity applies, a treatment difference is interpretable as being independent of study factors and background variables; in this sense, it is generalizable throughout some large target population that the patients conceptually represent (i.e., it applies to younger persons, older persons, females, males, etc.). An important consideration here is that generalizability is an issue for the target population, so its evaluation requires assumptions about how patients in the study population represent those in the target population. Since the target population can be viewed as containing patients like those in the study population, a reasonable (but not provable) assumption is that representation is provided by a process equivalent to stratified simple random sampling where the strata are based on the cross-classification of center × treatment (i.e., representation is assumed for the conditional distributions of response variables given center and treatment). Through this assumption, statistical models are formulated in this section for the relationship of response variables to treatment and center. Then, homogeneity of treatment effects across centers is evaluated by the determination of whether such statistical models need to be expanded to include the treatment × center interaction. In Section 3.4 attention is given to homogeneity of treatment effects across subgroups based on background variables through statistical models which include components for treatment, center, and background variables. For these analyses, the assumed sampling process for the representation of the target population has its stratification structure based on the cross-classification of center, treatment, and the background variables.

On the basis of the assumption that the patients within each center × treatment group represent a target population in a sense equivalent to stratified simple random sampling, the frequencies n_{ghij} for the distribution of the response variable at the gth visit have the product multinomial distribution

$$\Pr(\{n_{ghij}\}) = \prod_{h=1}^{2} \prod_{i=A}^{P} n_{hi}! \frac{\prod_{j=0}^{4} \pi_{ghij}^{n_{ghij}}}{n_{ghij}!}; \tag{43}$$

here the π_{ghij} denote the probabilities with which a randomly selected patient from the stratum corresponding to the hth center and ith treatment is observed to have the jth response category at the gth visit. From the structure in (43), it follows that the frequencies $N_{ghi*} = n_{ghi3} + n_{ghi4}$ for good or excellent response have the product binomial distribution

$$\Pr(\{N_{ghi*}\}) = \frac{\prod_{h=1}^{2} \prod_{i=A}^{p} n_{hi}! \theta_{ghi}^{N_{ghi*}} (1-\theta_{ghi})^{(n_{hi}-N_{ghi*})}}{N_{ghi*}!(n_{hi}-N_{ghi*})!}, \tag{44}$$

for which $\theta_{ghi} = \pi_{ghi3} + \pi_{ghi4}$; that is, the θ_{ghi} denote the probabilities of good or excellent response at the gth visit for a randomly selected patient from the stratum corresponding to the hth center and ith treatment.

A useful analysis of the relationship between a dichotomous response variable and a set of explanatory variables (e.g., center, treatment) is provided by logistic regression. It is based on the fitting of a logistic model to the probabilities of favorable (i.e., good or excellent) response. For the θ_{ghi} in (44), this model has the specification

$$\theta_{ghi} = \left[1 + \exp\left(-\xi_g - \sum_{G=1}^{u} \beta_{gG} x_{Ghi}\right)\right]^{-1}, \tag{45}$$

where the x_{Ghi} are the values of u explanatory variables for the respective center × treatment strata, the $\{\beta_{gG}\}$ are corresponding regression parameters, and ξ_g is an intercept parameter. The parameters ξ_g and $\{\beta_{gG}\}$ can have any value in $(-\infty, \infty)$ since values of $(\xi_g + \sum_{G=1}^{u} \beta_{gG} x_{Ghi})$ in $(-\infty, \infty)$ correspond to values of the θ_{ghi} in (0,1). Additional insights concerning the parameters ξ_g and $\{\beta_{gG}\}$ are provided by consideration of the logistic transformation of (45) to the linear model

$$\text{logit}(\theta_{ghi}) = \log_e \frac{\theta_{ghi}}{(1-\theta_{ghi})} = \xi_g + \sum_{G=1}^{u} \beta_{gG} x_{Ghi}. \tag{46}$$

In (46), the $\phi_{ghi} = \theta_{ghi}/(1-\theta_{ghi})$ represent the "odds" of favorable versus unfavorable response. Thus the $\{\exp(\beta_{gG})\}$ are interpretable as multipliers for the "odds" per unit change in the x_{Ghi}.

Estimates of the parameters ξ_g and $\{\beta_{gG}\}$ are usually obtained by maximum likelihood methods. More specifically, the likelihood (44) is expressed as a function of ξ_g and the $\{\beta_{gG}\}$ by replacement of the θ_{ghi} with their model counterparts from (45); then its natural logarithm is differentiated with respect to ξ_g and the $\{\beta_{gG}\}$. The nonlinear equations that result from setting these derivatives equal to 0 are then solved for the maximum likelihood estimates $\hat{\xi}_g$ and $\{\hat{\beta}_{gG}\}$ by an iterative procedure such as the Newton–Raphson method. When the sample sizes n_{hi} are sufficiently large, $\hat{\xi}_g$ and the $\{\hat{\beta}_{gG}\}$ approximately have a multivariate normal distribution for which the covariance matrix can be consistently estimated by

$$\hat{V}_{g,\mathbf{x}} = \mathbf{V}(\hat{\xi}_g, \{\hat{\beta}_{gG}\}) = \left[\sum_{h=1}^{2}\sum_{i=A}^{P} n_{ni}\hat{\theta}_{ghi}(1-\hat{\theta}_{ghi})\mathbf{x}_{*hi}\mathbf{x}'_{*hi}\right]^{-1}, \tag{47}$$

where $\mathbf{x}_{*hi} = (1, x_{1hi}, \ldots, x_{uhi})'$ and

$$\hat{\theta}_{ghi} = \left[1 + \exp\left(-\hat{\xi}_g - \sum_{G=1}^{u} \hat{\beta}_{gG} x_{Ghi}\right)\right]^{-1};$$

a supportive condition for approximate normality of $\hat{\xi}_g$ and the $\{\hat{\beta}_{gG}\}$ for situations with a small number of strata (e.g., ≤ 30) is that nearly all of the N_{ghi*} and their complements $(n_{hi} - N_{ghi*})$ are ≥ 5; more generally, the relevant consideration is whether the sample size is sufficiently large to support approximate normality for the linear statistics $\sum_{h=1}^{2}\sum_{i=A}^{P} N_{ghi*}x_{Ghi}$ [see Cox (1970), Imrey et al. (1981, 1982), McCullagh and Nelder (1983), and Koch and Edwards (1985) for further discussion].

Two asymptotically equivalent criteria for evaluating the goodness of fit of the logistic model (45) for situations where the sample sizes within the strata are not excessively small (e.g., nearly all $n_{hi} \geq 5$) are the log-likelihood ratio chi-square statistic $Q_{L,g}$ and the Pearson chi-square statistic $Q_{P,g}$. Their definitions are

$$Q_{L,g} = \sum_{h=1}^{2}\sum_{i=A}^{P}\left[N_{ghi*}\log_e \frac{N_{ghi*}}{\hat{M}_{ghi*}} + (n_{hi} - N_{ghi*})\log_e \frac{(n_{hi} - N_{ghi*})}{(n_{hi} - \hat{M}_{ghi*})}\right], \tag{48}$$

$$Q_{P,g} = \sum_{h=1}^{2} \sum_{i=A}^{P} \left[\frac{(N_{ghi*} - \hat{M}_{ghi*})^2}{\hat{M}_{ghi*}} + \frac{(N_{ghi*} - \hat{M}_{ghi*})^2}{n_{hi} - \hat{M}_{ghi*}} \right]$$
$$= \sum_{h=1}^{2} \sum_{i=A}^{P} \frac{n_{hi}(N_{ghi*} - \hat{M}_{ghi*})^2}{\hat{M}_{ghi*}(n_{hi} - \hat{M}_{ghi*})}, \tag{49}$$

where $\hat{M}_{ghi*} = n_{hi}\hat{\theta}_{ghi}$ is the model predicted frequency of good or excellent response for the hth center and ith treatment (also, for $Q_{L,g}$, $0\{\log_e(0)\}$ is defined to be 0). The test statistics $Q_{L,g}$ and $Q_{P,g}$ approximately have chi-square distributions with d.f. = [(number of strata)-(number of parameters)] = $4 - (u + 1)$ when the sample sizes within the strata are sufficiently large [e.g., all $\hat{M}_{ghi*} \geq 5$ and all $(n_{hi} - \hat{M}_{ghi*}) \geq 5$; or equivalently, $5 \leq \hat{M}_{ghi*} \leq (n_{hi} - 5)$ for all strata]. Applicability of chi-square approximations to $Q_{P,g}$ have also been found through numerical studies [e.g., Larntz (1978)] to be reasonable for many situations with small or moderate sample sizes (e.g., $2 < \hat{M}_{ghi*} < n_{hi} - 2$ for most strata and only a few strata with $\hat{M}_{ghi*} < 1$ or $\hat{M}_{ghi*} > n_{hi} - 1$).

For the dichotomous response variables at visits 1 to 4, results for a logistic regression model with explanatory variables for treatment and center are given in Table 8. The model specification in these analyses for the probability of good or excellent response at the gth visit is

$$\theta_{ghi} = [1 + \exp(-\xi_g - \beta_{g1}x_{1hi} - \beta_{g2}x_{2hi})]^{-1}, \tag{50}$$

where $x_{1hi} = 1$ if $i = A$ and $x_{1hi} = 0$ if $i = P$ indicates treatment and $x_{2hi} = 1$ if $h = 2$ and $x_{2hi} = 0$ if $h = 1$ indicates center; the parameters ξ_g, β_{g1}, and β_{g2} are the reference value (of the logit) for placebo in center 1, the effect for active treatment, and the effect for center 2, respectively. The maximum likelihood estimates of these parameters and their standard errors [from the square roots of the diagonal elements of (47)] are shown in Table 8. Since the sample sizes for the data in Table 1 are considered large enough to support approximately normal distributions for the maximum likelihood estimates $\hat{\xi}_g$, $\hat{\beta}_{g1}$, and $\hat{\beta}_{g2}$, statistical tests for whether their corresponding parameters are equal to 0 can be undertaken with Wald statistics. These criteria have the form

$$Q_W = \frac{(\text{maximum likelihood estimate})^2}{(\text{estimated standard error})^2}; \tag{51}$$

approximate p-values for Q_W are based on the chi-square distribution with d.f. = 1. These p-values are shown in Table 8 with the estimates to which they apply. For the estimated treatment effects $\hat{\beta}_{g1}$, they are significant ($p \leq 0.05$) at visits 1 to 3 and nearly significant at visit 4 ($p = 0.063$). These

Table 8 Maximum Likelihood Estimates, Standard Errors, and p-Values for Parameters in Logistic Regression Models for Probability of Good or Excellent Response at Visits 1, 2, 3, and 4 and Corresponding Goodness-of-Fit Statistics[a]

Parameter	Statistic	Visit 1	Visit 2	Visit 3	Visit 4
Reference value for placebo in center 1	Estimate	−0.564	−0.814	−0.476	−0.894
	SE	0.341	0.351	0.338	0.354
	p-value	0.099	0.020[b]	0.16	0.012[b]
Effect for active treatment	Estimate	0.859	1.361	1.150	0.758
	SE	0.410	0.411	0.409	0.407
	p-value	0.036[b]	0.001[c]	0.005[c]	0.063
Effect for center 2	Estimate	1.072	0.685	0.603	1.268
	SE	0.410	0.409	0.406	0.407
	p-value	0.009[c]	0.094	0.14	0.002[c]
Goodness of fit statistic (treatment × center interaction)	Q_L (d.f. = 1)	1.52	0.82	0.53	0.23
	p-value	0.22	0.36	0.47	0.63
	Q_P (d.f. = 1)	1.50	0.82	0.53	0.23
	p-value	0.22	0.37	0.47	0.63

[a]The logistic model has the specification in (50); that is, (probability of good or excellent response) $= [1 + \exp(-\xi - \beta_1 x_1 - \beta_2 x_2)]^{-1}$, where $x_1 = 1$ if active or $x_1 = 0$ if placebo indicates treatment, $x_2 = 1$ if center 2 or $x_2 = 0$ if center 1 indicates center, and ξ, β_1, β_2 are unknown parameters corresponding to reference value for placebo in center 1, effect for active treatment, and effect for center 2. Estimates for ξ, β_1, β_2 are from maximum likelihood methods; their standard errors are from square roots of the diagonal elements of (47); and their p-values are from Wald statistics Q_W in (51); goodness-of-fit statistics are the log-likelihood ratio statistic Q_L in (48) and the Pearson statistic Q_P in (49). Both have one degree of freedom and pertain to treatment × center interaction. Computations were performed with the CATMOD and LOGIST Procedures in the SAS System (1985).

[b]Results with $p \le 0.05$.

[c]Results with $p \le 0.01$.

results agree very well with those from the Mantel–Haenszel statistic in Table 4; indeed, they appear to be virtually the same. The principal reason for this is that the Mantel–Haenszel statistic is asymptotically equivalent to test statistics for treatment effects in a logistic regression model like (50) with additive effects for center and treatment for the $\{\text{logit}(\theta_{ghi})\}$ [see Birch (1964, 1965) and Breslow and Day (1980) for further discussion]. Moreover, the compatibility of the θ_{ghi} with this type of model is supported for the dichotomous response variables at visits 1 to 4 by the nonsignificance of the goodness-of-fit statistics $Q_{L,g}$ and $Q_{P,g}$. The approximate p-values for these criteria are shown in Table 8; they are based on the chi-square distribution with d.f. $= 4-(u+1) = 1$, and all of them have ≥ 0.10 status. The remaining results in Table 8 that merit a comment are the p-values for the center effects $\hat{\beta}_{g2}$; those at visits 1 and 4 are significant ($p \leq 0.05$) and that at visit 2 is suggestive ($p = 0.094$). Thus center effects need to be maintained in the logistic model (50) for the θ_{ghi} so that variation across centers as well as between treatments is described appropriately.

Another logistic model that is of potential interest for the θ_{ghi} is the expansion of (50) to include a component for treatment × center interaction; the specification for this expanded model is

$$\theta_{ghi} = [1 + \exp(-\xi_g - \beta_{g1}x_{1hi} - \beta_{g2}x_{2hi} - \beta_{g3}x_{3hi})]^{-1}, \tag{52}$$

where $x_{3hi} = x_{1hi}x_{2hi}$ and β_{g3} is the effect for treatment × center interaction. For the expanded model (52), the extent to which the odds of favorable versus unfavorable response is greater for active treatment than for placebo at the hth center is expressed through the "odds ratios"

$$\psi_{gh} = \frac{\phi_{ghA}}{\phi_{ghP}} = \frac{\theta_{ghA}(1-\theta_{ghP})}{\theta_{ghP}(1-\theta_{ghA})} = \exp(\beta_{g1} + \beta_{g3}x_{*h*}), \tag{53}$$

where $x_{*h*} = 1$ if $h = 2$ and $x_{*h*} = 0$ if $h = 1$ (i.e., the "odds ratios" are measures of treatment effects within the respective centers). When $\beta_{g3} = 0$, the "odds ratios" for the respective centers are all equal to $\exp(\beta_{g1})$, so treatment effects are homogeneous across centers in this sense. On this basis, a statistical test of whether β_{g3} is 0 is a test of homogeneity of treatment effects across centers. However, when $\beta_{g3} = 0$, the model (52) simplifies to the model (50). For this reason, the goodness-of-fit statistics $Q_{L,g}$ and $Q_{P,g}$ in Table 8 for the model (50) are also test statistics for $\beta_{g3} = 0$ in the model (52); as tests of treatment × center interaction, they are also tests of homogeneity of treatment effects across centers. Thus the nonsignificance of the results of the goodness-of-fit tests in Table 8 enables treatment effects to be interpreted as homogeneous across centers, and this supports their generalizability for the target population.

The estimated treatment effect that corresponds to the homogeneous "odds ratios" for the respective centers is $\hat{\psi}_{g**} = \exp(\hat{\beta}_{g1})$. At visit 1, $\hat{\psi}_{1**} = \exp(0.859) = 2.36$; so the odds of favorable versus unfavorable response is 2.36 times greater for active than for placebo. Also, since $\{\hat{\beta}_{g1} \pm 1.96[\text{SE}(\hat{\beta}_{g1})]\}$ is an approximately 95% confidence interval for β_{g1}, its exponential transformation is an approximately 95% confidence interval for ψ_{g**}. On this basis, $\exp(0.055, 1.663) = (1.06, 5.28)$ is an approximately 95% confidence interval for ψ_{1**}. When sample sizes are not considered large enough to support the approximate normality of $\hat{\beta}_{g1}$ in a logistic model with a no-interaction structure such as (50), methods are available for determining an exact confidence interval for the homogeneous odds ratio ψ_{g**} that applies across a set of strata [for their discussion, see Gart (1971), Thomas (1975), Breslow and Day (1980), and Mehta et al. (1985)].

Another noteworthy feature of logistic regression analysis is the description that its predicted values $\hat{\theta}_{ghi}$ provide for the variation of the probabilities of favorable response across treatments and centers. These predicted values [which are defined following (47)] and their standard errors are shown in Table 9; the standard errors were obtained via

$$\begin{aligned}\text{SE}(\hat{\theta}_{ghi}) &= \hat{\theta}_{ghi}(1-\hat{\theta}_{ghi})[\text{SE}(\hat{\xi}_g + \sum_{G=1}^{u} \hat{\beta}_{gG} x_{Ghi})] \\ &= \hat{\theta}_{ghi}(1-\hat{\theta}_{ghi})(\mathbf{x}'_{*hi}\hat{V}_{g,\mathbf{x}}\mathbf{x}_{*hi})^{1/2}, \qquad (54)\end{aligned}$$

where $\hat{\mathbf{V}}_{g,x}$ and the $\mathbf{x}_{*hi}$ are defined via (47). There is agreement between the $\hat{\theta}_{ghi}$ in Table 9 and their counterparts from Table 4 for the actual proportions of patients with good or excellent responses for the respective center × treatment × visit combinations [i.e., the $p_{ghi} = (\%)_{ghi}/100$, where the $(\%)_{ghi}$ are defined in (27)]. This finding is compatible with the previously stated support provided for the model by the nonsignificance of the goodness-of-fit statistics $Q_{L,g}$ and $Q_{P,g}$. An important descriptive advantage of the predictive values $\hat{\theta}_{ghi}$ is that they tend to have smaller estimated standard errors than the actual proportions p_{ghi}. This property is a consequence of their structure not involving the extraneous variability for factors not included in the model (i.e., treatment × center interaction).

As discussed in Section 3.1, the integer score means $\bar{y}_{ghi}$ in (31) describe the distributions of the ordinal response variables for each center × treatment × visit. These statistics are unbiased estimates for the subpopulation means $\eta_{ghi} = \sum_{j=0}^{4} j\pi_{ghij}$ of the multinomial distribution (43) for the response at the gth visit by patients receiving the ith treatment at the hth center. Relative to the means η_{ghi}, the difference between active and placebo treatments for the hth center is $\delta_{gh} = (\eta_{ghA} - \eta_{ghP})$; so ho-

Table 9 Predicted Values and Standard Errors from Logistic Regression Model for Probability of Good or Excellent Response and Linear Model for Integer Score Mean Response

Response variable	Treatment	Statistic	Probability good or excellent response[a]		Integer score mean response[b]	
			Center 1	Center 2	Center 1	Center 2
Visit 1	Active	Pred. val.	0.573	0.797	2.57	3.30
		SE	0.084	0.063	0.16	0.14
	Placebo	Pred. val.	0.363	0.624	2.15	2.87
		SE	0.079	0.081	0.19	0.16
Visit 2	Active	Pred. val.	0.633	0.774	2.90	3.36
		SE	0.081	0.067	0.17	0.17
	Placebo	Pred. val.	0.307	0.468	1.91	2.37
		SE	0.075	0.084	0.20	0.20
Visit 3	Active	Pred. val.	0.662	0.782	2.92	3.22
		SE	0.079	0.065	0.20	0.17
	Placebo	Pred. val.	0.383	0.532	2.09	2.39
		SE	0.080	0.084	0.22	0.23
Visit 4	Active	Pred. val.	0.466	0.756	2.54	3.18
		SE	0.085	0.069	0.18	0.20
	Placebo	Pred. val.	0.290	0.592	1.95	2.60
		SE	0.073	0.082	0.21	0.24

[a] Results are based on (47) and (54) for the logistic regression model with specification given in Table 8.
[b] Results are based on (61) for the linear model with specification given in Table 10.

mogeneity of treatment differences across centers applies when there is no treatment × center interaction in the sense that

$$\delta_{g1} - \delta_{g2} = \eta_{g1A} - \eta_{g1P} - \eta_{g2A} + \eta_{g2P} = 0. \tag{55}$$

However, the constraint (55) for the η_{ghi} corresponds to the compatibility of the η_{ghi} with the linear model

$$\eta_{ghi} = \xi_g + \beta_{g1} x_{1hi} + \beta_{g2} x_{2hi}, \tag{56}$$

where ξ_g, β_{g1}, β_{g2}, the x_{1hi}, and the x_{2hi} have definitions like those stated for (50). As a consequence of this consideration, statistical tests for the goodness of fit of the linear model (56) are also tests for the homogeneity of treatment effects across centers for the η_{ghi}.

Since the sample sizes n_{hi} are sufficiently large (e.g., $n_{hi} \geq 25$) to support approximately normal distributions for the $\bar{y}_{ghi}$, an effective way to assess the goodness of fit of the linear model in (56) is through the weighted least squares methods discussed in Grizzle et al. (1969) and Koch et al. (1977, 1985a). For such analysis, estimates $\hat{\xi}_g$, $\hat{\beta}_{g1}$, and $\hat{\beta}_{g2}$ are determined so as to minimize the weighted residual sum of squares

$$Q_{W,g} = \sum_{h=1}^{2} \sum_{i=A}^{P} \left\{ (\bar{y}_{ghi} - \hat{\xi}_g - \hat{\beta}_{g1} x_{1hi} - \hat{\beta}_{g2} x_{2hi})^2 / v_{ghi,y} \right\}, \tag{57}$$

where the $v_{ghi,y} = \{\sum_{k=1}^{n_{hi}} (y_{ghik} - \bar{y}_{ghi})^2 / n_{hi}^2\}$ are estimated variances for the $\bar{y}_{ghi}$. This process involves the solution of a set of linear equations, so matrix notation provides a concise expression for the estimates that result from it. More specifically, let $\hat{\boldsymbol{\beta}}_{g*} = (\hat{\xi}_g, \hat{\beta}_{g1}, \hat{\beta}_{g2})'$ denote the vector of weighted least squares estimates, let $\bar{\mathbf{y}}_{g**} = (\bar{y}_{g1A}, \bar{y}_{g1P}, \bar{y}_{g2A}, \bar{y}_{g2P})'$ denote the vector of mean scores, let $\mathbf{V}_{g,y}$ denote the estimated covariance matrix for $\bar{\mathbf{y}}_{g**}$ with diagonal elements equal to the $v_{ghi,y}$ and all off-diagonal elements equal to 0, and let

$$\mathbf{X} = \begin{bmatrix} 1 & 1 & 0 \\ 1 & 0 & 0 \\ 1 & 1 & 1 \\ 1 & 0 & 1 \end{bmatrix} \tag{58}$$

denote the specification matrix for the model (56); then the matrix expression for the weighted least squares estimates is

$$\hat{\boldsymbol{\beta}}_{g*} = (\mathbf{X}'\mathbf{V}_{g,y}^{-1}\mathbf{X})^{-1}\mathbf{X}'\mathbf{V}_{g,y}^{-1}\bar{\mathbf{y}}_{g**}; \tag{59}$$

also, a consistent estimate for their corresponding covariance matrix is

$$\hat{\mathbf{V}}_{g,\beta} = (\mathbf{X}'\mathbf{V}_{g,y}^{-1}\mathbf{X})^{-1}. \tag{60}$$

The minimized weighted residual sum of squares $Q_{W,g}$ from the substitution of the weighted least squares estimates $\hat{\boldsymbol{\beta}}_{g*}$ from (59) into (57) is a goodness-of-fit statistic for the linear model (56). This test statistic approximately has the chi-square distribution with d.f. = (number of strata) − (number of parameters) = 4 − 3 = 1 when the sample sizes are sufficiently large for the $\bar{y}_{ghi}$ to have approximately normal distributions. Also, for such large-sample situations, $\hat{\xi}_g$ and the $\{\hat{\beta}_{gG}\}$ approximately have normal distributions, so p-values for tests of whether their corresponding parameters are equal to 0 can be based on chi-square approximations for Wald statistics such as (51).

Table 10 Weighted Least Squares Estimates, Standard Errors, and p-Values for Parameters in Linear Models for Integer Scores Mean Response at Visit 1, 2, 3, and 4 and Corresponding Goodness-of-Fit Statistics[a]

Parameter	Statistic	Visit 1	Visit 2	Visit 3	Visit 4
Reference value for placebo in center 1	Estimate	2.15	1.91	2.09	1.95
	SE	0.19	0.20	0.22	0.21
	p-value	< 0.001[b]	< 0.001[b]	< 0.001[b]	< 0.001[b]
Effect for active treatment	Estimate	0.42	0.99	0.83	0.59
	SE	0.19	0.22	0.24	0.24
	p-value	0.026[c]	< 0.001[b]	0.001[b]	0.014[c]
Effect for center 2	Estimate	0.72	0.46	0.29	0.64
	SE	0.19	0.21	0.23	0.24
	p-value	< 0.001[b]	0.028[c]	0.20	0.007[b]
Goodness of fit statistic (treatment × center interaction)	Q_W (d.f. = 1)	0.36	0.39	1.12	0.51
	p-value	0.55	0.53	0.29	0.48

[a]The linear model has the specification in (56); that is, (integer score mean response) = $\xi + \beta_1 x_1 + \beta_2 x_2$, where $x_1 = 1$ if active or $x_1 = 0$ if placebo indicates treatment, $x_2 = 1$ if center 2 or $x_2 = 0$ if center 1 indicates center, and ξ, β_1, β_2 are unknown parameters corresponding to reference value for placebo in center 1, effect for active treatment, and effect for center 2. Estimates for ξ, β_1, β_2 are from weighted least squares methods via (59); their standard errors are square roots of the diagonal elements of (60); and their p-values are from Wald statistics such as (51). The goodness-of-fit statistic is the weighted sum of squares (57) due to the residuals from the model's predicted values for (integer score mean response); it has one degree of freedom and is the same as the Wald statistic (62) for the treatment × center interaction. Computations were performed with the CATMOD Procedure in the SAS System (1985).

[b]Results with $p \leq 0.01$.

[c]Results with $p \leq 0.05$.

Results from the weighted least squares analysis for the linear model (56) are given in Table 10 for the ordinal responses at visits 1 to 4. They include estimates from (59) for the predicted mean response for placebo at center 1, the effect for active treatment, and the effect for center 2 together with the standard errors of these estimates [from square roots of the diagonal elements of the estimated covariance matrix in (60)] and p-values for tests of zero values from Wald statistics.

For the differences between treatments, the estimates, standard errors, and p-values in Table 10 for weighted least squares analyses are very similar to their counterparts in Table 5 from analyses through the extended Mantel–Haenszel statistic. A reason for this is the across-center homogeneity of the differences between the integer mean scores for the treatments. In this regard, such homogeneity is supported by the nonsignificance of the goodness-of-fit statistics $Q_{W,g}$ in (57) for the model (56); the p-values from these tests are shown in Table 10, and all have ≥ 0.25 status relative to their approximate chi-square distribution with d.f. = 1.

Some other results from weighted least squares analysis merit attention. For visits 1, 2, and 4, the p-values for center effects $\hat{\beta}_{g2}$ are significant ($p \leq 0.05$); so center effects need to be maintained in the linear model. Predicted values $\hat{\eta}_{ghi}$ from the linear model (56) and their standard errors are given for the integer mean scores η_{ghi} in Table 9. These results were obtained via

$$\hat{\eta}_{ghi} = \hat{\xi}_g + \hat{\beta}_{g1}x_{1hi} + \hat{\beta}_{g2}x_{2hi} = \mathbf{x}'_{*hi}\hat{\boldsymbol{\beta}}_{g*},$$
$$\text{SE}(\hat{\eta}_{ghi}) = \mathbf{x}'_{*hi}\hat{\mathbf{V}}_{g,\beta}\mathbf{x}_{*hi}. \tag{61}$$

Since usage of the linear model (56) was supported by the nonsignificance of the goodness-of-fit statistics $Q_{W,g}$ in (57), the predicted values $\hat{\eta}_{ghi}$ in Table 9 agree well with the actual mean scores $\bar{y}_{ghi}$ for the respective center × treatment × visit combinations. Also, by having a structure that does not involve sources of extraneous variation, the $\hat{\eta}_{ghi}$ tend to have smaller standard errors than the $\bar{y}_{ghi}$.

The weighted least squares analyses for the linear model (56) have some noteworthy theoretical properties. The goodness-of-fit statistic $Q_{W,g}$ in (57) is identical to the Wald statistic for the constraint (55) which corresponds to the model; that is,

$$Q_{W,g} = \frac{(\bar{y}_{g1A} - \bar{y}_{g1P} - \bar{y}_{g2A} + \bar{y}_{g2P})^2}{\sum_{h=1}^{2}\sum_{i=A}^{P} v_{ghi,y}}. \tag{62}$$

For models with linear constraints such as (55) for the parameters π_{ghij}, Bhapkar (1966) showed generally that the Wald statistic (Wald, 1943) was identical to the Neyman minimum modified chi-square statistic for goodness of fit. Thus, from Neyman (1949), $Q_{W,g}$ is asymptotically equivalent to the log-likelihood ratio statistic for the goodness of fit of the model (56) in the sense that the probability that the two methods contradict each other tends to zero as the sample sizes n_{hi} become large. Also, the weighted least squares estimates $\hat{\beta}_{g*}$ belong to the class of *best asymptotic normal* (BAN) estimates; so they are asymptotically unbiased, efficient, and equivalent to maximum likelihood estimates. For additional discussion of theoretical properties of weighted least squares methods for categorical data, see Koch et al. (1985a).

In summary, homogeneity of treatment effects across centers was evaluated in this section through the goodness of fit of statistical models which included explanatory variables for treatment and center. For the dichotomous variables of good or excellent response at each visit, logistic regression models were used; and for the ordinal response variables at each visit, linear models for integer mean scores were used. The goodness-of-fit statistics for these models corresponded to test statistics for treatment × center interaction. Although attention here was focused on an example with two centers and two treatments, the same principles and methods are applicable to studies with q centers and s treatments. The models for these situations would include $(s-1)$ indicator variables for treatment and $(q-1)$ indicator variables for center in addition to the reference value; and the statistical test for treatment × center interaction would be based on chi-square approximations with d.f. $= (q-1)(s-1)$ for the appropriate extensions of $Q_{L,g}$ in (48), $Q_{P,g}$ in (49), and $Q_{W,g}$ in (57). For the example, the results of the statistical tests for treatment × center interaction were nonsignificant; so they supported the conclusion that treatment effects were homogeneous across centers and, in this sense, were generalizable.

3.4 Evaluation of Treatment × Background Variable Interaction

Conclusions concerning treatment effects in a clinical trial are generalizable throughout a target population if they apply to all subgroups based on background variables such as age, sex, and baseline status. Generalizability in this sense requires homogeneity of treatment effects across these subgroups. Such homogeneity is evaluated in this section through analyses which are similar in spirit to those in Section 3.3 for homogeneity of treatment effects across centers. For these analyses, statistical models are used to describe the relationship between the response variables at each visit and center, treatment, and background variables. Confirmation that these models do not need to include components for treatment × background variable interaction or for treatment $\times$ center interaction supports the interpretation that treatment effects are homogeneous and hence generalizable throughout the target population.

Statistical models for the analysis of the homogeneity of treatment effects across subgroups based on background variables and centers for a multicenter clinical trial require an assumption for how the patients in the study population represent their counterparts in the target population. As discussed in Section 3.3, the perspective that the target population contains patients like those in the study population (e.g., younger persons, older persons, females, males, etc.) supports its representation in terms of conditional distributions of response variables given center, treatments, and background variables. This reasonable (but not provable) assumption is more formally expressed as the equivalence of the study population to a stratified simple random sample from the target population where the strata correspond to the cross-classification of center, treatment, and background variables. A lenient feature of this assumption is that the background variables themselves can possibly have different distributions in the study population than in the target population (i.e., the sampling rates can vary across the totality of possible strata).

The assumption that the patients in the study population represent those in the target population in a sense equivalent to stratified simple random sampling implies that their responses at the gth visit have the product multinomial distribution

$$\Pr(\{y_{ghijk}\}) = \prod_{h=1}^{2}\prod_{i=A}^{P}\prod_{k=1}^{n_{hi}}\left(\prod_{j=0}^{4}\pi_{ghijk}^{y_{ghijk}}\right), \tag{63}$$

where $y_{ghijk} = 1$ if the kth patient with the ith treatment at the hth center is classified into the jth response category at the gth visit and $y_{ghijk} = 0$ if otherwise; also, $\pi_{ghijk} = E\{y_{ghijk}\}$ denotes the probability that a randomly selected patient from the stratum corresponding to the hth center, ith treatment, and the same profile of background variables as the (hik)th patient (e.g., the same age, sex, and baseline status) is observed to have the jth response category at the gth visit; finally, $\sum_{j=0}^{4} y_{ghijk} = 1$ since the response at the gth visit is classified into one category.

As a consequence of the structure in (63), the dichotomous response variables $Y_{ghi*k} = y_{ghi3k} + y_{ghi4k}$ for good or excellent classifications have the product binomial distribution

$$\Pr(\{Y_{ghi*k}\}) = \prod_{h=1}^{2}\prod_{i=A}^{P}\prod_{k=1}^{n_{hi}}\theta_{ghik}^{Y_{ghi*k}}(1-\theta_{ghik})^{1-Y_{ghi*k}}; \tag{64}$$

here $\theta_{ghik} = \pi_{ghi3k} + \pi_{ghi4k}$ denotes the probability of good or excellent response at the gth visit for a randomly selected patient from the stratum corresponding to the hth center, ith treatment, and the same profile of background variables as the (hik)th patient. In accordance with the discussion in Section 3.3, logistic regression is a useful method for analyzing the relationship between the response variable at the gth visit and explanatory variables for center, treatment, and background characteristics such as age, sex, and baseline status. A specific model that is of interest for this purpose is

$$\theta_{ghik} = \left[1 + \exp\left(-\xi_g - \sum_{G=1}^{5} \beta_{gG} x_{Ghik}\right)\right]^{-1} ; \tag{65}$$

for this model, $x_{1hik} = 1$ if $i = A$ and $x_{1hik} = 0$ if $i = P$ indicates treatment; $x_{2hik} = 1$ if $h = 2$ and $x_{2hik} = 0$ if $h = 1$ indicates center, $x_{3hik} = 1$ if the (hik)th patient is male and $x_{3hik} = 0$ if female, x_{4hik} = baseline status for (hik)th patient, and x_{5hik} = age/10 for (hik)th patient; the parameters ξ_g, β_{g1}, β_{g2}, β_{g3}, β_{g4}, and β_{g5} are unknown parameters corresponding to a reference value, the effect for active treatment, the effect for center 2, the effect for males, the rate of change per category of baseline status, and the rate of change per 10 years of age, respectively. For models such as (65), the x_{Ghik} need to be nonredundant in the sense that none of them is expressible as a linear function of the others and a constant.

A noteworthy feature of the logistic model (65) is that it applies to the responses of individual patients and that it includes both categorical and continuous explanatory variables. In contrast, the logistic models (50) and (52) were specified for strata with a moderately large number of patients and included only categorical explanatory variables. However, even though the logistic model in (65) has a relatively general structure, the principles and procedures for estimating its parameters through maximum likelihood methods are essentially the same as those discussed in Section 3.3 for the much simpler models (50) and (52). The maximum likelihood estimates $\hat{\xi}_g$ and the $\{\hat{\beta}_{gG}\}$ approximately have a multivariate normal distribution when the sample sizes n_{hi} are sufficiently large to support approximately normal distributions for the linear statistics $\sum_{h=1}^{2} \sum_{i=A}^{P} \sum_{k=1}^{n_{hi}} x_{Ghik} Y_{ghi*k}$. A consistent estimate of the covariance matrix for these estimates is

$$\begin{aligned}\hat{\mathbf{V}}_{g,\mathbf{x}} &= \mathbf{V}(\hat{\xi}_g, \{\hat{\beta}_{gG}\}) \\ &= \left[\sum_{h=1}^{2} \sum_{i=A}^{P} \sum_{k=1}^{n_{hi}} \hat{\theta}_{ghik}(1 - \hat{\theta}_{ghik}) \mathbf{x}_{*hik} \mathbf{x}'_{*hik}\right]^{-1} ,\end{aligned} \tag{66}$$

where $x_{*hik} = (1, x_{1hik}, x_{2hik}, x_{3hik}, x_{4hik}, x_{5hik})'$ is the vector of explanatory variables for the (hik)th patient and $\hat{\theta}_{ghik} = [1 + \exp(-\hat{\xi}_g - \sum_{G=1}^{5} \hat{\beta}_{gG} x_{Ghik})]^{-1}$ is the predicted probability of good or excellent response at the gth visit for the (hik)th patient.

The maximum likelihood estimates for the parameters in the model (65) and their estimated standard errors [from square roots of the diagonal elements of (66)] are given in Table 11. Approximate p-values from Wald statistics such as (51) are also given there for tests of whether model parameters are equal to 0. In this regard, the sample size is considered to be sufficiently large to support approximately normal distributions for $\hat{\xi}_g$ and the $\{\hat{\beta}_{gG}\}$ and hence approximately chi-square distributions (with d.f. = 1) for the corresponding Wald statistics Q_W. The principal conclusions from the statistical tests in Table 11 for the parameters in the logistic model (65) are that the probability of good or excellent response at visits 1 to 4 is significantly ($p \leq 0.05$) higher for active treatment than for placebo and significantly ($p \leq 0.01$) increases with the extent to which baseline status is favorable. Also, the effects of sex are clearly nonsignificant (all p's ≥ 0.25). For center and age, there are mixed results across visits; the p-values for the center effects at visits 1 to 3 are clearly nonsignificant (all p's ≥ 0.25) while that for visit 4 is suggestive ($p = 0.025$); and for age, the p-values at visits 1 and 2 are clearly nonsignificant ($p \geq 0.25$) while those at visits 3 and 4 are suggestive ($p = 0.040, 0.055$). An interesting aspect of the results in Table 11 is that they indicate significantly more favorable response for active treatment than placebo in a stronger way than their counterparts in Table 8 for the logistic model (50) or in Table 4 from Mantel–Haenszel analyses. A reason for this is that the logistic model (65) provides covariance adjustment for baseline status which has a strong association with the response variables at visits 1 to 4 (see Table 3). Moreover, since the descriptive results in Table 2 suggest that baseline status was somewhat less favorable for patients at center 1 than those at center 2, adjustment for it might partly account for center effects; this consideration provides a reason why the results in Table 11 did not indicate differences between centers as strongly as those in Table 8.

Since the strata for a cross-classification of center, treatment, and background variables usually have very small sample sizes (e.g., essentially all can be 0 or 1 when the model includes continuous background variables), chi-square approximations are not applicable to goodness-of-fit statistics such as the log-likelihood ratio chi-square statistic $Q_{L,g}$ in (48) or the Pearson chi-square statistic $Q_{P,g}$ in (49). This consideration implies that these criteria can at most serve a descriptive role. Thus, other methods are necessary for the evaluation of the goodness of fit of models like (65). A

Table 11 Maximum Likelihood Estimates, Standard Errors, and p-Values for Parameters in Logistic Regression Model for Relationship Between Probability of Good or Excellent Response and Treatment, Center, Sex, Baseline Status, and Age and p-Values for Goodness of Fit Through Pairwise Interactions Not Included in Models[a]

Parameter	Statistic	Visit 1	Visit 2	Visit 3	Visit 4
Reference value	Estimate	−5.57	−2.37	−2.51	−2.38
	SE	1.43	1.09	1.14	1.12
	p-value	< 0.001[b]	0.029[c]	0.028[c]	0.033[c]
Effect for active treatment	Estimate	1.31	1.58	1.46	0.99
	SE	0.53	0.46	0.49	0.47
	p-value	0.013[c]	< 0.001[b]	0.003[b]	0.035[c]
Effect for center 2	Estimate	0.53	0.38	0.29	1.08
	SE	0.51	0.47	0.50	0.48
	p-value	0.30	0.42	0.56	0.025[c]
Effect for males	Estimate	−0.02	−0.27	−0.14	−0.48
	SE	0.64	0.57	0.59	0.60
	p-value	0.98	0.64	0.82	0.42
Baseline status	Estimate	1.54	0.72	1.04	0.90
	SE	0.33	0.23	0.26	0.25
	p-value	< 0.001[b]	0.002[b]	< 0.001[b]	< 0.001[b]
Age/10	Estimate	0.01	−0.18	−0.38	−0.35
	SE	0.19	0.17	0.18	0.18
	p-value	0.94	0.29	0.040[c]	0.055

Goodness-of-fit Tests	Statistic	Visit 1	Visit 2	Visit 3	Visit 4
Treatment × center	Q_S (d.f. = 1)	1.20	0.49	0.17	0.05
	p-value	0.27	0.49	0.68	0.82
Treatment × sex	Q_S (d.f. = 1)	0.02	0.76	5.80	2.09
	p-value	0.89	0.38	0.016[c]	0.15
Treatment × baseline	Q_S (d.f. = 1)	2.99	0.01	0.22	0.38
	p-value	0.084	0.94	0.64	0.54
Treatment × age	Q_S (d.f. = 1)	1.08	0.96	0.67	2.36
	p-value	0.30	0.33	0.41	0.12
All pairwise interactions with treatment	Q_S (d.f. = 4)	5.35	1.54	6.18	3.85
	p-value	0.25	0.82	0.19	0.43
All pairwise interactions	Q_S (d.f. = 10)	18.20	11.10	13.27	9.28
	p-value	0.052	0.35	0.21	0.51

reasonable principle on which to base such methods is a correspondence of lack of fit of a model to the need for the model to include one or more variables. Conversely, if statistical tests for the contribution of these additional variables are non-significant, then the goodness of fit of the model is supported. Evaluation of whether a logistic model needs to include additional explanatory variables can be undertaken effectively with the Rao score statistic. This criterion is directed at the extent to which the residuals $(Y_{ghi*k} - \hat{\theta}_{ghik})$ from the model are linearly associated with the additional explanatory variables. More specifically, let $w_{1hik}, w_{2hik}, \ldots, w_{whik}$ denote a set of w additional explanatory variables; let

$$f_{G'} = \sum_{h=1}^{2} \sum_{i=1}^{2} \sum_{k=1}^{n_{hi}} w_{G'hik}(Y_{ghi*k} - \hat{\theta}_{ghik}), \tag{67}$$

where $G' = 1, 2, \ldots, w$; and let $\mathbf{f} = (f_1, f_2, \ldots, f_w)'$. Then the Rao score statistic has the general form

$$Q_S = \mathbf{f}'\mathbf{V}_f^{-1}\mathbf{f} = \mathbf{f}'\{\mathbf{W}'[\mathbf{D}_{\hat{V}} - \mathbf{D}_{\hat{V}}\mathbf{X}\hat{\mathbf{V}}_{g,\mathbf{x}}\mathbf{X}'\mathbf{D}_{\hat{V}}]\mathbf{W}\}^{-1}\mathbf{f}, \tag{68}$$

for which $\mathbf{V}_f$ is the estimated covariance matrix for the linear functions of residuals $\mathbf{f}$. Also, $\mathbf{X}$ is the model specification matrix and has rows $\{\mathbf{x}'_{*hik}\}$, $\mathbf{W}$ is the specification matrix for the additional variables and has rows $\{\mathbf{w}'_{*hik} = (w_{1hik}, w_{2hik}, \ldots, w_{whik})\}$, $\mathbf{D}_{\hat{V}}$ is a diagonal matrix with the $\{\hat{v}_{ghik} = \hat{\theta}_{ghik}(1-\hat{\theta}_{ghik})\}$ on the diagonal, and $\hat{\mathbf{V}}_{g,x}$ is the estimated covariance matrix for $\hat{\xi}_g$ and the $\{\hat{\beta}_{g,G}\}$ from (66). The Rao score statistic Q_S in (67) approximately has the chi-square distribution with d.f. $= w$ when the sample sizes are sufficiently large; that is, the n_{hi} are large enough to support approximately normal distributions for the maximum likelihood

---

[a]The logistic model has the specification in (65); that is, probability of good or excellent response $= [1 + \exp(-\xi - \beta_1 x_1 - \beta_2 x_2 - \beta_3 x_3 - \beta_4 x_4 - \beta_5 x_5)]^{-1}$, where $x_1 = 1$ if active or $x_1 = 0$ if placebo indicates treatment, $x_2 = 1$ if center 2 or $x_2 = 0$ if center 1 indicates center, $x_3 = 1$ if male or $x_3 = 0$ if female indicates sex, $x_4 =$ baseline status, $x_5 = (\text{age}/10)$, and $\xi, \beta_1, \beta_2, \beta_3, \beta_4, \beta_5$ are unknown parameters corresponding to reference value, effect for active treatment, effect for center 2, effect for males, rate of change per category of baseline status, and rate of change per 10 years of age. Estimates for $\xi, \beta_1, \beta_2, \beta_3, \beta_4, \beta_5$ are from maximum likelihood methods; their standard errors are from square roots of the diagonal elements of (66); and their p-values are from Wald statistics like (51). The p-values for goodness of fit through pairwise interactions not in model are based on score statistics via (68). Computations were performed with the LOGIST Procedure in the SAS System (1985).

[b]Results with $p \leq 0.01$.

[c]Results with $p \leq 0.05$.

estimates of the parameters in the expanded model which includes both the specific variables of interest x_{Ghik} and the additional variables $w_{G'hik}$. Also, the $w_{G'hik}$ need to be nonredundant in the sense that the specification matrix $[\mathbf{X}, \mathbf{W}]$ for the expanded model has full rank $(1 + u + w)$. The Rao score statistic in (68) has two noteworthy properties. One is its asymptotic equivalence to the log-likelihood ratio chi-square statistic for testing whether the parameters for the $w_{G'hik}$ in the expanded model are zero. Since the latter criterion is obtained as the difference between the $Q_{L,g}$ in (48) for the model of interest and that for the expanded model, its determination requires the fitting of both models, whereas the determination of Q_S is more convenient in the sense of only involving results for the model of interest. This computational advantage is the other noteworthy property of the Rao score statistic.

Approximate p-values for Q_S are given in Table 11 for several types of additional variables that might be included in the logistic model (65). These correspond to the treatment × center interaction via $w_{1hik} = x_{1hik}x_{2hik}$, the treatment × sex interaction via $w_{2hik} = x_{1hik}x_{3hik}$, the treatment × baseline status interaction via $w_{3hik} = x_{1hik}x_{4hik}$, the treatment × age interaction via $w_{4hik} = x_{1hik}x_{5hik}$, all pairwise interactions with treatment via $(w_{1hik}, w_{2hik}, w_{3hik}, w_{4hik})$, and all pairwise interactions via $(w_{1hik}, \ldots, w_{10,hik})$, where the $w_{G'hik}$ encompass all pairwise products of the x_{Ghik}. Among the 16 statistical tests in Table 11 for the separate interactions of treatment with center and each of the background variables, only that for treatment × sex at visit 3 had ≤ 0.05 status, and only that for treatment × baseline status at visit 1 had $0.05 \leq p \leq 0.10$ status; all of the others were nonsignificant with $p \geq 0.10$. Moreover, the overall statistical tests for all pairwise interactions with treatment were nonsignificant $(p \geq 0.10)$ at all four visits. Since this pattern of results is compatible with chance for the situation of no association between the residuals of the model (65) and the w_{1hik}, w_{2hik}, w_{3hik}, and w_{4hik}, it is interpreted as indicating that the model does not need to include the interactions of treatment with center and background variables. Thus treatment effects are concluded to be homogeneous.

The goodness of fit of the model (65) is also reasonably supported by the results of the statistical tests for all pairwise interactions. At visits 2 to 4, the p-values for these tests are nonsignificant $(p \geq 0.10)$; but at visit 1, some departure from the model is suggested by $p = 0.052$. By further analysis, this departure was identified as due largely to center × baseline status interaction in the sense of a stronger association between the response at visit 1 and baseline status for center 1 than for center 2. Such interaction is considered here to be ignorable since it seems to be more an atypical feature of the study population than a meaningful source of variation. Thus, for each visit, the model (65) is concluded to provide a satisfactory description of the relationship of the probabilities of good or excellent response to treatment, center, sex, baseline status, and age. Moreover, it does this in a way that expresses the generalizability of treatment effects in terms of odds ratios. The estimates for these odds ratios are $\exp(\hat{\beta}_{g1}) = 3.71, 4.85, 4.31, 2.69$ for visits 1 to 4, respectively. As discussed in Section 3.3, they reflect the extent to which the odds of more favorable response is greater for active treatment than for placebo; and they apply in a homogeneous way to all subgroups of the target population (with respect to center, sex, age, and baseline status).

The probabilities of good or excellent response for different types of patients can be described further with predicted values from (65); in their determination, the range of a continuous variable such as age should be restricted to that for the study population. In other words, prediction from a model should not be extrapolated beyond the types of patients from whom the estimates for its parameters were obtained.

For purposes of completeness, a few additional comments about the goodness of fit of the model (65) merit attention. First, even though the $p = 0.016$ result for treatment $\times$ sex at visit 3 was interpreted as compatible with chance, consideration of its implications to generalizability is still of interest. The issue here is that the objective of analyses of interactions involving treatment effects is usually to confirm their absence because their presence might suggest that the generalizability of treatment effects is limited to a particular subgroup. For this reason, these analyses need to be reasonably comprehensive in exploring possibilities for interactions even though many of them may be for chance patterns of variation. The findings from such evaluation of the treatment $\times$ sex interaction at visit 3 indicated substantially more favorable responses for active treatment for both sexes and a stronger tendency of this type for the 23 females than the 88 males. This pattern of variation is interpreted as not suggesting any limitation of generalizability.

Another issue for the treatment $\times$ sex interaction at visit 3 is that 100% of the females on active treatment had good or excellent response; this aspect of its structure is contrary to its analysis in an expansion of the model (65) because it leads to computational anomalies (i.e., infinite estimates for one or more parameters may be forlornly sought by iterative estimation procedures). Also, it can undermine the large-sample properties which are principal reasons for the use of logistic regression. A rough rule that usually enables the avoidance of this awkward practical problem is the requirement that no linear combination of the columns of the model specification matrix $\mathbf{X}$ correspond to a set of strata for which all patients have the same response status (i.e., either 0% or 100% applies to an outcome such as good or excellent response). For the treatment × sex interaction at visit 3, this rule is not satisfied, so logistic regression analysis is not applicable to an expansion of the model (65) with this variable. A more formal discussion of conditions for the applicability of logistic regression is given in Silvapulle (1981). A third issue for the model (65) is that it only includes the linear components for age and baseline status. The need to include higher-order components (e.g., quadratic) also could be evaluated through Rao score statistics. Such analysis was not undertaken here because the role of the model (65) was more to provide a reasonable framework for the evaluation of generalizability than to seek an as complete as possible specification for the relationships between the dichotomous response variables and center, treatment, and background variables. The latter objective is also worthwhile and can identify additional models of interest. Since many aspects of the search for such models are subjective, use of a straightforward model such as (65) can be argued as appropriate on practical grounds.

For the ordinal response variables at each visit, the evaluation of treatment × background variable interaction cannot be based on weighted least squares methods (like those discussed for treatment × center interaction in Section 3.3) because the sample sizes for the strata in a cross-classification of center, treatment, and background variables are too small. An alternative strategy for the analysis of the relationships between an ordinal response variable and center, treatment, and background variables is based on maximum likelihood methods for the extension of the logistic regression model to what is often called the proportional odds model. Its applicability has the less stringent sample size requirement of sufficiently large numbers of patients for all treatments at all centers (e.g., $\sum_{h=1}^{2}\sum_{i=A}^{P} n_{hi} \geq 40$). The structure of the proportional odds model for the parameters π_{ghijk} in the product multinomial distribution (63) is applied through the probabilities $\theta_{ghijk} = \sum_{j'=j}^{4} \pi_{ghij'k}$ of response at least as favorable as the jth category for the gth visit and the (hik)th patient. For j = 1, 2, 3, 4, its specification consists of a parallel set of logistic models with the form

$$\theta_{ghijk} = \left[1 + \exp\left(-\xi_{gj} - \sum_{G=1}^{u} \beta_{gG} x_{Ghik}\right)\right]^{-1}, \tag{69}$$

where the x_{Ghik} are the values of u explanatory variables for the (hik)th patient, the $\{\beta_{gG}\}$ are corresponding regression parameters, and the ξ_{gj} are intercept parameters. The x_{Ghik} can correspond to either categorical or continuous variables; the parameters $\{\xi_{gj}\}$ and $\{\beta_{gG}\}$ can have any value in $(-\infty, \infty)$ since the θ_{ghijk} and the π_{ghijk} determined from them are always in (0,1). The proportional odds model (69) implies that the odds ratios for the (hik)th patient versus the $(h'i'k')$th patient have the same value

$$\frac{\theta_{ghijk}(1-\theta_{gh'i'jk'})}{(1-\theta_{ghijk})\theta_{gh'i'jk'}} = \exp\left[\sum_{G=1}^{u} \beta_{gG}(x_{Ghik} - x_{Gh'i'k'})\right] \tag{70}$$

for $j = 1, 2, 3, 4$. Thus the $\exp(\beta_{gG})$ are interpretable as multipliers for the odds of more favorable response versus less favorable response per unit change in the x_{Ghik} for each of the four partitions of the five response categories into unfavorable and favorable subsets. Also, by expressing the extent to which more favorable responses are more likely for the (hik)th patient than the $(h'i'k')$th patient, the $\exp(\beta_{gG})$ are indicative of location shifts for the corresponding distributions.

Aspects of statistical analysis for the proportional odds model are similar to those for a general logistic model like (65). Maximum likelihood methods can be used to obtain estimates of its parameters and an estimate of their covariance matrix. Statistical tests for whether model parameters are equal to zero can then be undertaken with Wald statistics like (51). Evaluation of whether additional explanatory variables like those for treatment × background variable interaction need to be included in the model can be based on Rao score statistics which are analogous to (67). Discussion of these methods for the proportional odds model is given in Harrell (1986), McCullagh (1980), McCullagh and Nelder (1983), and Walker and Duncan (1967).

Another consideration for the analysis of the goodness of fit of the proportional odds model is the compatibility of the data with its underlying assumption that the odds ratios in (70) for the four partitions of the five response categories are equal to one another for any pair of patients. Some insight for addressing this question about the appropriateness of the proportional odds model can be obtained by fitting separate logistic regression models to each response partition $j = 1, 2, 3, 4$. Similarity of the four estimated parameters for these separate analyses for the coefficients of each explanatory variable would tend to support the goodness of fit of the proportional odds model (69). Other methods for evaluating the compatibility of ordinal data with the proportional odds assumption are discussed in Genter and Farewell (1985), Harrell (1986), Koch et al. (1985b), McCullagh and Nelder (1983), and Peterson (1986). Since the proportional odds model provides an effective way to describe the relationship between an ordinal response variable and a set of explanatory variables, its use for exploratory analysis of treatment × center interaction and treatment × background variable interaction may be reasonable even when its goodness of fit may seem questionable. However, when usage of the proportional odds model seems clearly inappropriate, analyses of homogeneity of treatment effects across centers and subgroups based on background variables would need to be based on other methods for ordinal data. Some references concerning such methods are Agresti (1984), Clogg (1982), Cox and Chuang (1984), Koch and Edwards (1987), and McCullagh and Nelder (1983).

For the example considered in this chapter, the proportional odds model that was used for analysis of the relationship between the ordinal responses at each visit and center, treatment, sex, baseline status, and age had the specification

$$\theta_{ghijk} = \left[1 + \exp\left(-\xi_{gj} - \sum_{G=1}^{5} \beta_{gG} x_{Ghik}\right)\right]^{-1}; \tag{71}$$

the x_{Ghik} and the $\{\beta_{gG}\}$ have the same definitions as for the analogous logistic model in (65); and the $\{\xi_{gj}\}$ are intercept parameters for the respective partitions of the five response categories into unfavorable and favorable; also, ξ_{g3} is analogous to ξ_g in (65) since both correspond to good or excellent response. The maximum likelihood estimates for the parameters in the model (71), their standard errors, and approximate p-values for tests of 0 values from Wald statistics such as (51) are given in Table 12. The conclusions from these results are similar to those from Table 11 for the logistic model (65). At visits 1 to 4, the odds of more favorable response is significantly ($p \leq 0.05$) higher for active treatment than placebo and significantly increases with the extent to which baseline status is favorable. The p-values from the statistical tests for center and sex are nonsignificant at all visits (all p's ≥ 0.10), and those for age have a mixed nature; at visits 1, 2, and 4, the p-values for age are nonsignificant (all p's ≥ 0.10) while that at visit 3 is suggestive. For the comparisons between treatments, the results in Table 12 [from analyses of ordinal response variables at each visit with the proportional odds model (71)] indicate significantly more favorable response for active treatment than placebo in a similar way to those in Table 7 (from randomization covariance analyses), and in a stronger way than those in Table 10 for the analyses of the integer score means with the linear model (56) or in Table 5 from extended Mantel–Haenszel analyses. As discussed for Table 11 relative to Tables 4 and 8, the methods for Tables 7 and 12 have the advantage of involving covariance adjustment for baseline status and hence provide a more effective analysis in the sense of accounting for the strong association between baseline status and the response variables at visit 1 to 4.

The need for the proportional odds model (71) to include additional variables for the interaction of treatment with center, sex, baseline status, and age or for all pairwise interactions of its explanatory variables is eval-

Table 12 Maximum Likelihood Estimates, Standard Errors, and p-Values for Parameters in Proportional Odds Model for Relationship Between Ordinal Response and Treatment, Center, Sex, Baseline Status, and Age and p-Values for Goodness of Fit Through Pairwise Interactions Not Included in Models[a]

Parameter	Statistic	Visit 1	Visit 2	Visit 3	Visit 4
Reference value for $\geq$ poor	Estimate	−0.73	−0.22	0.44	−0.43
	SE	0.97	0.92	0.88	0.91
	p-value	0.45	0.81	0.61	0.64
Reference value for $\geq$ fair	Estimate	−2.04	−1.28	−0.24	−1.23
	SE	0.92	0.91	0.87	0.90
	p-value	0.027[b]	0.16	0.79	0.17
Reference value for $\geq$ good	Estimate	−4.22	−3.00	−1.52	−2.69
	SE	0.98	0.95	0.89	0.93
	p-value	< 0.001[c]	0.002[c]	0.085	0.004[c]
Reference value for excellent	Estimate	−5.89	−4.10	−2.71	−3.56
	SE	1.05	0.98	0.91	0.95
	p-value	< 0.001[c]	< 0.001[c]	0.003[c]	< 0.001[c]
Effect for active treatment	Estimate	0.98	1.75	1.30	0.98
	SE	0.39	0.39	0.38	0.37
	p-value	0.011[b]	< 0.001[c]	0.001[c]	0.009[c]
Effect for Center 2	Estimate	0.60	0.32	0.02	0.61
	SE	0.41	0.41	0.39	0.40
	p-value	0.14	0.42	0.97	0.12
Effect for males	Estimate	−0.33	−0.13	−0.45	−0.33
	SE	0.49	0.48	0.49	0.49
	p-value	0.50	0.79	0.35	0.51
Baseline status	Estimate	1.29	0.89	0.76	0.81
	SE	0.22	0.21	0.19	0.20
	p-value	< 0.001[c]	< 0.001[c]	< 0.001[c]	< 0.001[c]
Age/10	Estimate	−0.06	−0.19	−0.27	−0.11
	SE	0.14	0.14	0.14	0.14
	p-value	0.67	0.18	0.051	0.45

Table 12 (*continued*)

Goodness-of-fit tests	Statistic	Visit 1	Visit 2	Visit 3	Visit 4
Treatment × center	Q_S (d.f. = 1)	0.62	0.58	1.15	0.73
	p-value	0.43	0.44	0.28	0.39
Treatment × sex	Q_S (d.f. = 1)	0.01	0.20	5.44	4.74
	p-value	0.94	0.66	0.020[b]	0.029[b]
Treatment × baseline	Q_S (d.f. = 1)	0.11	0.06	0.10	0.38
	p-value	0.74	0.81	0.75	0.54
Treatment × age	Q_S (d.f. = 1)	0.86	0.02	0.01	3.75
	p-value	0.35	0.89	0.99	0.053
All pairwise interactions with treatment	Q_S (d.f. = 4)	2.48	0.70	6.90	7.13
	p-value	0.65	0.95	0.14	0.13
All pairwise interactions	Q_S (d.f. = 10)	17.73	12.51	14.23	16.95
	p-value	0.060	0.25	0.16	0.076

[a]The proportional odds model has the specification in (71); that is, probability of response $\geq j = [1 + \exp(-\xi_j - \beta_1 x_1 - \beta_2 x_2 - \beta_3 x_3 - \beta_4 x_4 - \beta_5 x_5]^{-1}$, where $x_1 = 1$ if active or $x_1 = 0$ if placebo indicates treatment, $x_2 = 1$ if center 2 or $x_2 = 0$ if center 1 indicates center, $x_3 = 1$ if male or $x_3 = 0$ if female indicates sex, x_4 = baseline status, x_5 = age/10. The ξ_j are unknown parameters corresponding to the reference distribution, β_1 is the effect for active treatment, β_2 is the effect for center 2, β_3 is the effect for male sex, β_4 is the rate of change per category for baseline status, β_5 is the rate of change per 10 years of age. Estimates for $\xi_1, \xi_2, \xi_3, \xi_4, \beta_1, \beta_2, \beta_3, \beta_4, \beta_5$ are from maximum likelihood methods. The p-value for parameters in model are based on Wald statistics; the p-values for goodness of fit through pairwise interactions not in model are based on score statistics. Computations were performed with the LOGIST Procedure in the SAS System (1985).
[b]Results with $p \leq 0.05$.
[c]Results with $p \leq 0.01$.

uated with Rao score statistics in a manner similar to that discussed for the logistic model (65). Approximate p-values from these statistical tests are given in Table 12. As was the case for their counterparts in Table 11, they tend to support the conclusion that treatment effects are homogeneous across centers and subgroups based on sex, baseline status, and age. In this regard the statistical tests for all pairwise interactions with treatment were nonsignificant ($p \geq 0.10$) at all four visits; also 13 of the 16 separate tests for such interactions were nonsignificant. The departures from this pattern were ≤ 0.05 p-values for treatment $\times$ sex interaction at visits 3 and 4 and $p = 0.053$ for treatment $\times$ age at visit 4. Since both females and males as well as patients of all ages tended to have more favorable responses for active treatment than placebo at each visit, these possible interactions are interpreted as not suggesting any limitation to the generalizability of treatment effects for the target population.

There is also reasonable support for the model (71) from the statistical tests for all pairwise interactions. The p-values for these tests are nonsignificant ($p \geq 0.10$) for visits 2 and 3, but suggest some departure from the model at visits 1 and 4 ($p = 0.060, 0.076$). This departure was found by additional analysis to be due to center $\times$ baseline status interaction, so it was considered to be an ignorable, atypical feature of the study population. On the basis of the interpretation given here for the Rao score statistics in Table 12, the proportional odds model (71) is concluded to provide a satisfactory description of the relationship between the distributions of the ordinal response variable at each visit and the effects of treatment, center, sex, baseline status, and age. Through this model, the extent to which the odds of more favorable response is greater for active treatment than for placebo is expressed by the estimated odds ratios $\exp(\hat{\beta}_{g1}) = 2.66$, 5.75, 3.67, 2.66 for visits 1 to 4, respectively. Also, treatment effects are homogeneous in this sense across subgroups of the target population (with respect to center, sex, age, and baseline status).

In summary, statistical models provide a useful framework for the analysis of the relationship between response variables in a clinical trial and treatment, center, and background variables. They also enable the evaluation of generalizability of treatment effects through statistical tests for whether a model needs to include components for treatment $\times$ center interaction or treatment $\times$ background variable interaction. The logistic regression model is of interest for such analyses of dichotomous response variables and its extension to the proportional odds model is of interest for ordinal response variables. Estimates of parameters and statistical tests of goodness of fit can be obtained for both of these types of models with maximum likelihood methods.

3.5 Computations

The p-values in Tables 4 to 6 were obtained with the FREQ Procedure in the SAS System (1985). The MEANS Procedure was used to determine the descriptive statistics for the separate centers in Tables 4 and 5, and algorithms in the IML Procedure were used to determine descriptive statistics for the combined centers. The computations for the p-values in Table 7 from randomization covariance analyses were performed with the procedures documented in Amara and Koch (1980); they could also be obtained with algorithms in the IML Procedure. The CATMOD Procedure in the SAS System (1985) and the LOGIST Procedure of Harrell (1986) were used to obtain the results in Tables 8 to 10; also the analyses for Table 11 and 12 were undertaken with the LOGIST Procedure.

4 MULTIVARIATE METHODS FOR RESPONSE VARIABLES

For studies with more than one visit, there is often interest in analyses that encompass the data for all visits simultaneously as well as those for each of the separate visits. The need for such multivariate analyses arises from the tendency for the differences between treatments to vary across visits. Such variation is of particular concern when it corresponds to results of statistical tests for treatment comparisons seeming inconsistent in the sense of being significant at some visits but not at others. Moreover, the multiplicity of statistical tests across visits can make such concern become greater by increasing the probability that observed patterns of apparently significant differences for the respective visits are due to chance. This issue can be addressed for some studies by formally indicating (in the protocol) that the response at one particular visit (e.g., the last visit) is the primary criterion for analysis and those at all others are supportive. For other situations, the data from all visits are considered informative, so alternative strategies are needed. One of these involves methods through which treatment differences are combined across visits in a similar spirit to how they are combined across centers for each visit separately. Aspects of its application are discussed in Section 4.1 in the context of multivariate extensions of the randomization covariance analyses in Section 3.2. The other strategy involves statistical models that describe the variation of response distributions across treatments, centers, and visits. Confirmation that such models do not need to include components for treatment $\times$ visit interaction supports the conclusion that treatment effects are homogeneous across visits and hence are interpretable in a unified way for all visits. Analyses along these lines are discussed in Section 4.2 in the context of multivariate extensions of the weighted least squares methods for fitting linear models in Section 3.3.

4.1 Randomization Covariance Analysis

Multivariate extensions of nonparametric methods such as the randomization covariance statistics in Section 3.2 enable comparisons between treatments to encompass the responses at all visits in a study under minimal assumptions. One family of these test statistics is directed at all visits simultaneously. When covariance adjustment is applied to a background variable such as baseline status and stratification adjustment is applied to center, the multivariate consideration of the residuals z_{ghik} in (38) in an extended Mantel–Haenszel sense such as (12) for the combined centers leads to the multivariate randomization covariance statistic

$$Q_{\mathbf{z}} = \left(\sum_{h=1}^{q}\sum_{k=1}^{n_{hA}} \mathbf{z}_{*hAk}\right)' \left[\text{var}\left(\sum_{h=1}^{q}\sum_{k=1}^{n_{hA}} \mathbf{z}_{*hAk}\right)\right]^{-1} \left(\sum_{h=1}^{q}\sum_{k=1}^{n_{hA}} \mathbf{z}_{*hAk}\right); \tag{72}$$

here $\mathbf{z}_{*hik} = (z_{1hik}, z_{2hik}, z_{3hik}, z_{4hik})'$ is the vector of residuals from the least squares prediction of the response at each of the respective visits as a linear function of baseline status,

$$\text{var}\left\{\sum_{h=1}^{q}\sum_{k=1}^{n_{hA}} \mathbf{z}_{*hAk}\right\} = \sum_{h=1}^{q} \frac{n_{hi}(n_h - n_{hi})}{n_h(n_h - 1)} \left(\sum_{i=A}^{P}\sum_{k=1}^{n_{hi}} \mathbf{z}_{*hik}\mathbf{z}'_{*hik}\right) \tag{73}$$

is the randomization based covariance matrix for the sum

$$\sum_{h=1}^{q}\sum_{k=1}^{n_{hA}} \mathbf{z}_{*hAK}$$

of all the residual vectors for active treatment, and $q = 2$ is the number of centers. The test statistic $Q_{\mathbf{z}}$ approximately has the chi-square distribution with d.f. = (number of visits) = 4 for situations where the two treatment groups have sufficiently large sample sizes n_{+i} for the combined centers (e.g., $n_{+i} \geq 40$ if number of visits ≤ 6).

From (72), the structure of multivariate test statistics that do not involve covariance adjustment or stratification adjustment is reasonably apparent. If there is no covariance adjustment, the z_{ghik} in (38) are simplified to $y_{ghik} - \bar{y}_{gh*}$ in (72); and if there is no stratification adjustment, summation over h is not needed since only $h = 1 = q$ applies. Alternatively, more general versions of $Q_{\mathbf{z}}$ can be specified for situations with more than two treatments and covariance adjustment for more than one background variable; for their discussion, see Amara and Koch (1980), Koch and Bhapkar (1982), and Koch et al. (1982).

Another strategy for the usage of responses at all visits in treatment comparisons is based on the univariate analysis of the average responses $\bar{y}_{*hik} = (\sum_{g=1}^{4} y_{ghik}/4)$ over visits. The nonparametric methods that are applicable to this summary measure are the same as those discussed in Sections 3.1 and 3.2 for the responses at each visit separately. In particular, the counterpart to (72) for the covariance and stratification adjusted comparison between the two treatment groups with respect to the average responses over visits has the same form as (42), but with the gth visit residuals z_{ghik} from (38) replaced by the average residuals $\mathbf{z}_{*hik} = (\sum_{g=1}^{4} z_{ghik}/4)$. The resulting test statistic $Q_{\bar{z}}$ approximately has the chi-square distribution with d.f. = 1 when the two treatment groups have sufficiently large sample sizes n_{+i} for the combined centers (e.g., $n_{+i} \geq 20$). An important property of $Q_{\bar{z}}$ and other methods based on the average responses over visits is their greater effectiveness than their multivariate counterparts such as (72) for detecting consistent tendencies for one treatment group to have more favorable responses than the other across visits. The reason for this is that such patterns of treatment differences for the respective visits are reinforced in their average. In this sense, the advantage of $Q_{\bar{z}}$ over $Q_{\mathbf{z}}$ is analogous to that discussed for the extended Mantel–Haenszel statistic Q_{EMH} relative to the total association statistic $Q_{S,T}$ in (17). Moreover, $Q_{\bar{z}}$ has the noteworthy virtue of being specifiable as the primary method of analysis at the time the protocol for a study is prepared. This analysis strategy enables the issue of multiple comparisons (over center or visits) to be avoided in the sense that its basis is one test statistic that encompasses all visits by all patients at all centers. In this setting, the test statistics for the separate centers or separate visits would tend to serve a supportive and descriptive role.

Results from randomization covariance analysis for the responses at all visits of the study in the example are shown in the last two rows of Table 7. The responses in these analyses were expressed in terms of within-center, standardized midranks, and covariance adjustment was based on within-center, standardized midranks for baseline. The strata corresponded to the centers for the analyses in columns 3 to 5 and the center×sex groups for that in column 6. For the multivariate statistic (72), all p-values in the next-to-last row of Table 7 are significant ($p \leq 0.05$). The difference between treatment groups is more strongly indicated by the significance ($p \leq 0.005$) of the test statistics $Q_{\bar{z}}$ for the average of the within-center, standardized midranks over visits. Thus, these multivisit analyses clearly provide overall support for the conclusion that the responses to active treatment are more favorable than those to placebo.

4.2 Weighted Least Squares Analysis

Methods for fitting statistical models to describe the relationship between the response variables at each of the respective visits of a clinical trial and treatment, center, and background variables were discussed in Sections 3.3 and 3.4. For any of these models, the variation of the corresponding parameters across visits expresses the effects of visits. Such variation for the treatment effect constitutes treatment $\times$ visit interaction; so confirmation that treatment $\times$ visit interaction is negligible enables treatment effects to be interpretable as homogeneous across visits. Similar considerations apply to interactions between visits and other components of within-visit models.

A general strategy for analyzing the across-visits variation of the parameters of within-visit models has the following three stages:

i. Univariate methods such as those in Sections 3.3 and 3.4 are applied to fit models for each visit separately.
ii. A consistent estimate for the covariance matrix for the estimated parameters corresponding to all visits is constructed in a manner that accounts appropriately for the multivariate structure of the responses at the respective visits.
iii. Hypotheses concerning model parameters from stage (i) for all visits are tested with Wald statistics such as (51) or (62) or equivalent methods; also, simplified linear models can be fit to the parameters of within-visit models by weighted least squares methods in order to describe the effects of visits and the interactions between visits and treatments, centers, and background variables.

Aspects of the strategy in (i)–(iii) are described by Stram et al. (1988) for situations where maximum likelihood methods are used to fit logistic models to dichotomous response variables at the respective visits or proportional odds models to ordinal response variables. However, the application of such analysis to the data in Table 1 is beyond the scope of this chapter since the construction of an appropriate estimated covariance matrix for stage (ii) is conceptually and computationally complicated.

A relatively straightforward framework for the application of the strategy in (i)–(iii) is based on the multivisit extension of the weighted least squares methods outlined in (56)–(61) for the fitting of linear models. For such analysis, a noteworthy requirement is the availability of moderately large sample sizes for the subpopulations that correspond to the cross-classification of the explanatory variables in the model. Thus it has the limitation of only being able to account for a small number of categorical explanatory variables. In view of this consideration, its illustration here is directed primarily at the effects of treatment and center on the integer score means η_{ghi} through linear models like (56); such analysis is also provided for the probabilities of good or excellent response θ_{ghi} in (44).

Weighted least squares analysis of linear models for the η_{ghi} is applied to the corresponding estimates $\bar{y}_{ghi}$ in (32). Let $\bar{\mathbf{y}}_{*hi} = (\bar{y}_{1hi}, \bar{y}_{2hi}, \bar{y}_{3hi}, \bar{y}_{4hi})'$ denote the vector of estimated means at the respective visits for the patients who received the ith treatment at the hth center. A consistent estimate for the covariance matrix of $\bar{\mathbf{y}}_{*hi}$ is

$$\mathbf{V}_{hi,y} = \frac{\sum_{k=1}^{n_{hi}} (\mathbf{y}_{*hik} - \bar{\mathbf{y}}_{*hi})(\mathbf{y}_{*hik} - \bar{\mathbf{y}}_{*hi})'}{n_{hi}^2}, \tag{74}$$

where $\bar{\mathbf{y}}_{*hik} = (y_{1hik}, y_{2hik}, y_{3hik}, y_{4hik})'$ denotes the vector of responses at the respective visits by the kth patient with the ith treatment at the hth center. The compound vector $\bar{\mathbf{y}} = (\bar{\mathbf{y}}'_{*1A}, \bar{\mathbf{y}}'_{*1P}, \bar{\mathbf{y}}'_{*2A}, \bar{\mathbf{y}}'_{*2P})'$ concisely expresses all means in the $(2\times2\times4)$ cross-classification of center, treatment, and visit. A consistent estimate for its covariance matrix is the block diagonal matrix $\mathbf{V}_y$ with the $\mathbf{V}_{hi,y}$ in (74) as the diagonal blocks; that is,

$$\mathbf{V}_y = \begin{bmatrix} \mathbf{V}_{1A,y} & \mathbf{0}_{44} & \mathbf{0}_{44} & \mathbf{0}_{44} \\ \mathbf{0}_{44} & \mathbf{V}_{1P,y} & \mathbf{0}_{44} & \mathbf{0}_{44} \\ \mathbf{0}_{44} & \mathbf{0}_{44} & \mathbf{V}_{2A,y} & \mathbf{0}_{44} \\ \mathbf{0}_{44} & \mathbf{0}_{44} & \mathbf{0}_{44} & \mathbf{V}_{2P,y} \end{bmatrix} \tag{75}$$

where $\mathbf{0}_{44}$ denotes a (4×4) matrix of 0's. A linear model that describes the variation among the $\eta_{ghi} = E(\bar{y}_{ghi})$ across centers, treatments, and visits, can be concisely expressed as

$$E\{\bar{\mathbf{y}}\} = \boldsymbol{\eta} = \mathbf{X}\boldsymbol{\beta}, \tag{76}$$

where $\mathbf{X}$ is the specification matrix with full rank u, and $\boldsymbol{\beta}$ is the $(u \times 1)$ vector of unknown coefficients. The weighted least squares estimates $\hat{\boldsymbol{\beta}}$ for $\boldsymbol{\beta}$ are given by

$$\hat{\boldsymbol{\beta}} = (\mathbf{X}'\mathbf{V}_y^{-1}\mathbf{X})^{-1}\mathbf{X}'\mathbf{V}_y^{-1}\bar{\mathbf{y}}. \tag{77}$$

Since the sample sizes n_{hi} are considered sufficiently large for $\bar{\mathbf{y}}$ to have an approximately multivariate normal distribution, $\hat{\boldsymbol{\beta}}$ has an approximately multivariate normal distribution for which the covariance matrix is consistently estimated by

$$\hat{\mathbf{V}}_{\beta} = (\mathbf{X}'\mathbf{V}_{y}^{-1}X)^{-1}. \tag{78}$$

A goodness-of-fit statistic for the model (76) is the weighted residual sum of squares

$$Q_W = (\bar{\mathbf{y}} - \mathbf{X}\hat{\beta})'\mathbf{V}_{y}^{-1}(\bar{\mathbf{y}} - \mathbf{X}\hat{\beta}). \tag{79}$$

When $\bar{\mathbf{y}}$ is compatible with (76), Q_W approximately has the chi-square distribution with d.f. = (dimension $\bar{\mathbf{y}}$) – (dimension $\boldsymbol{\beta}$) = $16 - u$. Further analysis of models with satisfactory goodness of fit is often undertaken through tests of linear hypotheses $H_0 : \mathbf{C}\boldsymbol{\beta} = \mathbf{0}$, where $\mathbf{C}$ is a corresponding $(c \times u)$ specification matrix. For such hypotheses, the Wald statistic

$$Q_C = \hat{\beta}'\mathbf{C}'\{\mathbf{C}\hat{\mathbf{V}}_{\beta}\mathbf{C}'\}^{-1}\mathbf{C}\hat{\beta} \tag{80}$$

approximately has the chi-square distribution with d.f. $= c$.

The weighted least squares methods described in (74)–(80) for the integer score means $\bar{y}_{ghi}$ in (32) are also applicable to the analysis of the linear models for the proportions of good or excellent response p_{ghi} in (27). In fact, the p_{ghi} are means of indicator variables that have the value 1 if the response of a subject is good or excellent (i.e., $y_{ghik} = 3, 4$) and the value 0 if otherwise. For both the p_{ghi} and the $\bar{y}_{ghi}$, the weighted least squares methods in (74)–(80) have the same advantageous theoretical properties which were discussed in Section 3.3 for their counterparts (55)–(62) for the separate visits. These include the BAN property for the estimates $\hat{\boldsymbol{\beta}}$ and asymptotic equivalence of Q_W and Q_C to log-likelihood ratio test statistics.

A convenient model for the preliminary evaluation of sources of variation for the means $\bar{y}_{ghi}$ or the proportions of good or excellent response p_{ghi} has $\mathbf{X} = \mathbf{I}_{16}$, where $\mathbf{I}_{16}$ denotes the (16×16) identity matrix. It is usually called the cell means (or identity) model. Since $\boldsymbol{\beta} = \boldsymbol{\eta}$, $\hat{\boldsymbol{\beta}} = \bar{\mathbf{y}}$, and $\hat{\mathbf{V}}_{\beta} = \mathbf{V}_{y}$ for this model, the Wald statistic Q_C in (80) applies to tests of hypotheses H_0: $\mathbf{C}\boldsymbol{\eta} = \mathbf{0}$. Results from tests of this type for the effects of treatment, center, visit, and their interactions are shown in Table 13 for the model O heading. The corresponding $\mathbf{C}$ matrix for some of these tests are

$$\mathbf{C}_T = [\mathbf{1}_4', -\mathbf{1}_4', \mathbf{1}_4', -\mathbf{1}_4'] \text{ for treatment,} \tag{81}$$

$$\mathbf{C}_V = [\mathbf{I}_3, -\mathbf{1}_3, \mathbf{I}_3, -\mathbf{1}_3, \mathbf{I}_3, -\mathbf{1}_3, \mathbf{I}_3, -\mathbf{1}_3] \text{ for visit,} \tag{82}$$

$$\mathbf{C}_{TV} = [\mathbf{I}_3, -\mathbf{1}_3, -\mathbf{I}_3, \mathbf{1}_3, \mathbf{I}_3, -\mathbf{1}_3, -\mathbf{I}_3, \mathbf{1}_3] \text{ for treatment} \times \text{visit,} \tag{83}$$

where $\mathbf{I}_3$ denotes the (3×3) identity matrix and $\mathbf{1}_3 = (1, 1, 1)'$. For both the p_{ghi} and the $\bar{y}_{ghi}$, the tests for treatment × center interaction and treatment × center × visit interaction had clearly nonsignificant p-values

Table 13 *p*-Values for Effects of Treatment, Center, Visit, and Their Interactions in Linear Models to Describe the Variation of Probability of Good or Excellent Response and Integer Score Mean Response at Visit 1, 2, 3, and 4[a]

Source of variation	Statistic	Probability good or excellent response		Integer score mean response	
		Model 0	Model 1	Model 0	Model 1
Treatment	Q_W (d.f. = 1)	11.72	13.18	13.76	15.73
	p-value	0.001[b]	< 0.001[b]	< 0.001[b]	< 0.001[b]
Center	Q_W (d.f. = 1)	9.07	9.80	6.53	9.20
	p-value	0.003[b]	0.002[b]	0.011[c]	0.002[b]
Treatment × center	Q_W (d.f. = 1)	0.77	Not in	0.80	Not in
	p-value	0.38	model	0.37	model
Visit	Q_W (d.f. = 3)	3.52	4.67	2.40	2.57
	p-value	0.32	0.20	0.49	0.46
Treatment × visit	Q_W (d.f. = 3)	3.34	3.79	12.60	12.01
	p-value	0.34	0.29	0.006[b]	0.007[b]
Center × visit	Q_W (d.f. = 3)	4.49	5.30	8.13	10.16
	p-value	0.21	0.15	0.043[c]	0.017[c]
Treatment × center × visit	Q_W (d.f. = 3)	0.34	Not in	0.58	Not in
	p-value	0.95	model	0.90	model
Goodness of fit (i.e., sources not in model)	Q_W (d.f. = 4)	Does not	1.18	Does not	1.18
	p-value	apply	0.88	apply	0.88

[a]Model 0 is the cell mean model with $\mathbf{X} = \mathbf{I}_{16}$, where $\mathbf{I}_{16}$ is the 16×16 identity matrix; model 1 is the reduced model in (84) with the treatment × center interaction and the treatment × center × visit interaction excluded. The *p*-values are based on Wald statistics from (80) with specifications such as (81)–(83) for model 0. Computations were performed with the CATMOD Procedure in the SAS System (1985).
[b]Results with $p \leq 0.01$.
[c]Results with $p \leq 0.05$.

(i.e., $p > 0.25$). This finding suggested that a reduced model which did not include these sources of variation might be appropriate. This reduced model has the specification

$$
\begin{aligned}
\mathrm{E}\{\bar{\mathbf{y}}\} &= \boldsymbol{\eta} \\
&= \begin{bmatrix}
1 & 1 & 1 & 1 & 0 & 0 & 1 & 0 & 0 & 1 & 0 & 0 \\
1 & 1 & 1 & 0 & 1 & 0 & 0 & 1 & 0 & 0 & 1 & 0 \\
1 & 1 & 1 & 0 & 0 & 1 & 0 & 0 & 1 & 0 & 0 & 1 \\
1 & 1 & 1 & -1 & -1 & -1 & -1 & -1 & -1 & -1 & -1 & -1 \\
1 & -1 & 1 & 1 & 0 & 0 & -1 & 0 & 0 & 1 & 0 & 0 \\
1 & -1 & 1 & 0 & 1 & 0 & 0 & -1 & 0 & 0 & 1 & 0 \\
1 & -1 & 1 & 0 & 0 & 1 & 0 & 0 & -1 & 0 & 0 & 1 \\
1 & -1 & 1 & -1 & -1 & -1 & 1 & 1 & 1 & -1 & -1 & -1 \\
1 & 1 & -1 & 1 & 0 & 0 & 1 & 0 & 0 & -1 & 0 & 0 \\
1 & 1 & -1 & 0 & 1 & 0 & 0 & 1 & 0 & 0 & -1 & 0 \\
1 & 1 & -1 & 0 & 0 & 1 & 0 & 0 & 1 & 0 & 0 & -1 \\
1 & 1 & -1 & -1 & -1 & -1 & -1 & -1 & -1 & 1 & 1 & 1 \\
1 & -1 & -1 & 1 & 0 & 0 & -1 & 0 & 0 & -1 & 0 & 0 \\
1 & -1 & -1 & 0 & 1 & 0 & 0 & -1 & 0 & 0 & -1 & 0 \\
1 & -1 & -1 & 0 & 0 & 1 & 0 & 0 & -1 & 0 & 0 & -1 \\
1 & -1 & -1 & -1 & -1 & -1 & 1 & 1 & 1 & 1 & 1 & 1
\end{bmatrix}
\begin{bmatrix} \xi \\ \beta_1 \\ \beta_2 \\ \beta_3 \\ \beta_4 \\ \beta_5 \\ \beta_6 \\ \beta_7 \\ \beta_8 \\ \beta_9 \\ \beta_{10} \\ \beta_{11} \end{bmatrix} \\
&= \mathbf{X}_1 \boldsymbol{\beta},
\end{aligned}
\tag{84}
$$

where ξ represents the average of the η_{ghi}, β_1 corresponds to treatment, β_2 corresponds to center, β_3, β_4, β_5 correspond to visits, β_6, β_7, β_8 correspond to treatment $\times$ visit and β_9, β_{10}, β_{11} correspond to center $\times$ visit. Results from statistical tests concerning the model in (84) are shown in Table 13 under the model 1 heading. The ones for goodness of fit supported use of the model (84) by their nonsignificance. Among the tests concerning model parameters, those for treatment $\times$ visit and center $\times$ visit were significant ($p \leq 0.050$) for the integer mean scores $\bar{y}_{ghi}$ but nonsignificant for the p_{ghi}. On the basis of these findings, final descriptive models for the p_{ghi} and the $\bar{y}_{ghi}$ were formulated. The specification matrices for these models were represented as follows:

$$
\mathbf{X}_{2P} = \begin{bmatrix}
1\,1\,1\,1 & 1\,1\,1\,1 & 1\,1\,1\,1 & 1\,1\,1\,1 \\
1\,1\,1\,1 & 0\,0\,0\,0 & 1\,1\,1\,1 & 0\,0\,0\,0 \\
0\,0\,0\,0 & 0\,0\,0\,0 & 1\,1\,1\,1 & 1\,1\,1\,1
\end{bmatrix}' \tag{85}
$$

$$\mathbf{X}_{2y} = \begin{bmatrix} 1111 & 1111 & 1111 & 1111 \\ 1111 & 0000 & 1111 & 0000 \\ 0000 & 0000 & 1111 & 1111 \\ 0000 & 0000 & 0110 & 0110 \\ 0110 & 0000 & 0110 & 0000 \end{bmatrix}' . \qquad (86)$$

For the model $\mathbf{X}_{2y}$, the fourth column accounts for the center $\times$ visit interaction's correspondence to somewhat smaller differences between centers at visits 2 and 3 than at visits 1 and 4; and the fifth column accounts for the treatment $\times$ visit interaction's correspondence to somewhat larger differences between treatments at visits 2 and 3 than at visits 1 and 4. Estimated parameters, standard errors, and p-values from statistical tests are shown in Table 14 for the final models in (85) and (86). For the p_{ghi}, these results indicate that treatment effects are significant ($p \leq 0.001$) and that the proportion of patients with good or excellent response for active treatment homogeneously exceeds that for placebo by 0.268 at all visits for each center. The interpretation of treatment effects for the $\bar{y}_{ghi}$ is somewhat more complicated because their variation involved significant treatment $\times$ visit interaction. One way to address this matter is through consideration of the predicted values $\hat{\eta} = \mathbf{X}_{2y}\hat{\boldsymbol{\beta}}$ from the model (86). These predicted values and their corresponding standard errors (from square roots of the diagonal elements of $\hat{\mathbf{V}}_{\eta} = \mathbf{X}_{2y}\hat{\mathbf{V}}_{\beta}\mathbf{X}'_{2y}$) are given in Table 15; their counterparts for the p_{ghi} are also given there. The pattern of variation among the predicted values $\hat{\eta}_{ghi}$ for both centers indicates that the integer mean score for active treatment exceeds that for placebo by 0.54 at visits 1 and 4 and by 0.89 at visits 2 and 3. Also, in view of the results in Table 14, each is significant ($p < 0.01$) in its own right, and the difference between them is significant ($p < 0.01$). Thus the conclusion of more favorable response for active treatment than placebo is generalizable across both centers and visits even though the extent of treatment differences is heterogeneous across visits.

In summary, weighted least squares methods are useful for analyzing the variation of linear summary statistics such as the p_{ghi} or the $\bar{y}_{ghi}$ across the treatments, centers, and visits of a multicenter, multivisit study. An important aspect of their application is the evaluation of the generalizability of conclusions concerning treatment effects across visits through statistical tests of treatment $\times$ visit interaction. Additional discussion of the usage of weighted least squares methods for the multivariate analysis of categorical data from multivisit studies is given in Koch et al. (1977, 1980a, 1983, 1987, 1989), and Carr et al. (1989). These references provide examples which are directed at the pattern of variation of certain types of nonlinear summary

Table 14 Weighted Least Squares Estimates, Standard Errors, and p-Values for Parameters in Final Linear Models for Describing the Variation of Probability of Good or Excellent Response and Integer Score Mean Response in Terms of Effects of Treatment, Center, Visit, and Their Interactions and p-values for Goodness of Fit of Model[a]

	Probability good or excellent response			Integer score mean response		
Parameter	Estimate	SE	p-value	Estimate	SE	p-value
Reference value for placebo in center 1 at visit 1	0.300	0.060	< 0.001[b]	1.97	0.17	< 0.001[b]
Effect for active treatment	0.268	0.067	< 0.001[b]	0.54	0.17	0.002[b]
Effect for center 2	0.239	0.067	< 0.001[b]	0.80	0.17	< 0.001[b]
Interaction effect for active treatment at visits 2 and 3	Does not apply	Does not apply	Does not apply	0.35	0.10	< 0.001[b]
Interaction effect for visits 2 and 3 at Center 2	Does not apply	Does not apply	Does not apply	−0.30	0.10	0.002[b]
Goodness of fit	Q_W (d.f. = 13) = 15.35, $p = 0.29$			Q_W (d.f. = 11) = 8.79, $p = 0.64$		

[a]The linear models have the specifications shown in (85) and (86); that is, probability of good or excellent response $= \xi + \beta_1 x_1 + \beta_2 x_2$ and integer score mean response $= \xi + \beta_1 x_1 + \beta_2 x_2 + \beta_3 x_3 + \beta_4 x_4 + \beta_5 x_5$. For these models, $x_1 = 1$ if active or $x_1 = 0$ if placebo indicates treatment, $x_2 = 1$ if center 2 or $x_2 = 0$ if center 1 indicates center, $x_3 = 1$ if visit 2 or visit 3 for center 2 or $x_3 = 0$ if otherwise indicates (center × visit) interaction, and $x_4 = 1$ if visit 2 or visit 3 and active or $x_4 = 0$ if otherwise indicates (treatment × visit) interaction, and ξ, β_1, β_2, β_3, β_4 are unknown parameters as applicable. Estimates for the unknown parameters are from weighted least squares methods via (77); their standard errors are square roots of the diagonal elements of (78); and their p-values are from Wald statistics such as (80). The goodness-of-fit statistic is the weighted sum of squares (79) due to residuals from the model's predicted values. Computations were performed with the CATMOD Procedure in the SAS System (1985).
[b]Results with $p \leq 0.01$.

Table 15 Predicted Values and Standard Errors from Final Linear Models for Describing the Variation of Probability of Good or Excellent Response and Integer Score Mean Response in Terms of Effects of Treatment, Center, Visit, and Their Interactions[a]

Response variable	Treatment	Statistic	Probability good or excellent response: Center 1	Probability good or excellent response: Center 2	Integer score mean response: Center 1	Integer score mean response: Center 2
Visit 1	Active	Estimate	0.568	0.807	2.50	3.30
		SE	0.061	0.051	0.14	0.14
	Placebo	Estimate	0.300	0.539	1.97	2.76
		SE	0.060	0.059	0.17	0.15
Visit 2	Active	Estimate	0.568	0.807	2.86	3.36
		SE	0.061	0.051	0.15	0.15
	Placebo	Estimate	0.300	0.539	1.97	2.47
		SE	0.060	0.059	0.17	0.16
Visit 3	Active	Estimate	0.568	0.807	2.86	3.36
		SE	0.061	0.051	0.15	0.15
	Placebo	Estimate	0.300	0.539	1.97	2.47
		SE	0.060	0.059	0.17	0.16
Visit 4	Active	Estimate	0.568	0.807	2.50	3.30
		SE	0.061	0.051	0.14	0.14
	Placebo	Estimate	0.300	0.539	1.97	2.76
		SE	0.060	0.059	0.17	0.15

[a]Results are based on the linear models with specifications given in Table 14.

statistics as well as linear ones; such nonlinear statistics include estimates for logits (e.g., the $\log_e[p_{ghi}/(1-p_{ghi})]$) and rank measures of association such as those considered in Semenya et al. (1983).

4.3 Computations

The computations for the p-values in Table 7 from randomization covariance analyses were performed with the procedures documented in Amara and Koch (1980); they could also be obtained with algorithms in the IML Procedure of the SAS System (1985). The CATMOD Procedure in the SAS System (1985) was used to obtain the results in Tables 13 to 15.

5 SUMMARY OF ROLES OF ALTERNATIVE METHODS

In this chapter we have methods for the analysis of categorical response variables from studies in the pharmaceutical sciences. These methods addressed the following underlying components of situations in statistical practice.

1. Measurement scale (dichotomous and ordinal response variables)
2. Data structure [case records as in Table 1 and contingency tables as in (5) and (20)]
3. Dimension (univariate consideration of the response at each visit separately and multivariate consideration of the responses at all visits simultaneously)
4. Extent of assumptions and their implications to the scope of inference (design-based inference for the study population and model-based inference for a conceptual target population)
5. Management of explanatory variables for center and background characteristics of patients (stratification adjustment and covariance adjustment)

Analyses that corresponded to appropriate combinations of the features encompassed by the components 1–5 were illustrated for data from a multicenter, multivisit clinical trial. These included nonparametric statistical tests for design-based inferences concerning the existence of differences between treatments and the fitting of statistical models for the description of the relationship between response variables and treatment, center, and background variables. Also, the statistical models provided a framework for the evaluation of the generalizability of treatment differences through statistical tests of treatment × center interaction and treatment × background variable interaction.

APPENDIX: USAGE OF THE SAS SYSTEM (1985) TO GENERATE RESULTS FROM ANALYSIS

The following discussion assumes that the reader has a working knowledge of the SAS System, particularly the basic concepts of the data and proc steps.

A.1 FREQ Procedure

The FREQ procedure was used to obtain the results displayed in Tables 1 to 5 and discussed in Sections 2, 3.1, 3.2. FREQ performs statistical tests and computes measures of association for contingency tables; it also calculates the extended Mantel–Haenszel statistic. The input for the procedure consists of observations with variables containing information pertaining to treatment, background, and response outcomes. FREQ produces the appropriate cross-tabulation or tables based on the specified variables, and then calculates the desired statistics. In the following illustrations, SEX refers to the variable for sex, CENTER indicates center 1 or center 2, TRTMENT indicates treatment category (active or placebo), AGE means age in years, BASE represents baseline status, and DBASE represents the dichotomous baseline response outcome. The following statements produce many of the results displayed in Table 2.

```
PROC FREQ:
TABLES CENTER*TRTMENT*(SEX BASE DBASE)/SCORES
     =MODRIDIT CHISQ CMH:
```

The TABLES statement request that three sets of two way tables be formed. Each set has two tables for the two centers, and each table has TRTMENT as the rows and SEX, BASE, or DBASE as the columns. The resulting sets of two-way tables have a three-way structure [e.g., a $(2\times2\times2)$ table applies to (CENTER $\times$ TRTMENT $\times$ SEX)]. The CHISQ option requests that Fisher's exact test, the Pearson chi-square, and other test statistics be calculated for each two-way table in each set. Measures of association based on chi-square are also printed. The CMH option requests that extended Mantel–Haenszel statistics be computed for the association of SEX with TRTMENT adjusting for CENTER. SCORES=MODRIDIT specifies that standardized ranks are to be used as scores. This is how the p-values for BASE in Table 2 for the combined centers were obtained. The default scores used by PROC FREQ are TABLE scores, which are the row and column heading values for numeric classification variables, and the integers for character-valued variables. They were used for SEX and DBASE.

The following statements allow one to produce Wilcoxon rank sum statistics for center 1 and center 2 for the association of treatment with age and also the extended Mantel–Haenszel statistic for the combined centers.

```
PROC FREQ:
BY CENTER:
TABLES TRTMENT*AGE/SCORES=MODRIDIT CMH NOPRINT:
```

```
PROC FREQ;
TABLES CENTER*TRTMENT*AGE/SCORES
      =MODRIDIT CMH NOPRINT:
```

The resulting mean score statistic printed for each center by the first invocation of PROC FREQ can be shown to be equivalent to Wilcoxon rank sum statistics. Note that since age is continuous, and has many levels, the NOPRINT option is employed to suppress printing of the tables. The second invocation of PROC FREQ requests the extended Mantel–Haenszel statistic for the combined centers.

An alternative way in which to obtain the Wilcoxon rank sum statistic for the separate centers would have been to employ the NPAR1WAY procedure of the SAS System. The following statements generate the appropriate results:

```
PROC NPAR1WAY WILCOXON;
    BY CENTER;
    CLASS TRTMENT;
    VAR AGE;
```

The chi-square approximation for the Kruskal–Wallis test is equivalent to the mean score statistic from PROC FREQ discussed previously.

Table 3 contains results of analyses to assess the association of SEX with the responses at visits 1 to 4. PROC FREQ was used to obtain the extended Mantel–Haenszel statistic for this association while adjusting for the effect of CENTER. The following statements illustrate how the FREQ procedure would be used for this purpose:

```
PROC FREQ;
  TABLES CENTER*SEX*(VISIT1 VISIT2 VISIT3 VISIT4)/CMH
      SCORES=MODRIDIT;
```

These statements produce the extended Mantel–Haenszel statistic with standardized ranks (the van Elteren statistic) for the association of sex with the response variables, adjusting for center. Also generated are the Spearman rank correlation chi-square statistic, and its extended Mantel–Haenszel counterpart. The CMH option produces three extended Mantel–Haenszel statistics: a mean score statistic, a correlation statistic, and a general association statistic; some of these may not be appropriate for the data under analysis. One can restrict the analysis to the correlation statistic by specifying the 'CMH1' option instead; similarly, the 'CMH2' option requests both the mean score and correlation statistic.

A.2 CATMOD Procedure

The CATMOD procedure performs weighted least squares analysis for categorical data. It fits linear models to functions of response probabilities. It also can perform maximum likelihood analysis for logistic regression. Table 8 contains parameter estimates, standard errors, and p-values for the logistic regression models for good or excellent response. The following statements were used to obtain these results:

```
PROC CATMOD ORDER=DATA;
POPULATION CENTER TRTMENT;
RESPONSE LOGIT;
MODEL BWK1 = (1 1 0,
              1 0 0,
              1 1 1,
              1 0 1)/ML PRED NOGLS;
```

The input for PROC CATMOD consists of data observations containing the values (0,1) for BWK1, where 1 indicates good or excellent response at visit 1 and 0 other; the variable CENTER takes the value 1 or 2, and TRTMENT is the variable for treatment and takes the values 'active' or 'placebo.' The model specification matrix is direct input in this application of CATMOD since a reference cell model is desired. The default parameterization which CATMOD uses has a centerpoint structure such as (84), in which case the necessary MODEL statement is similar to that employed in the GLM procedure:

```
MODEL BWK1=CENTER TRTMENT/ML PRED NOGLS;
```

As noted previously, CATMOD does include the capacity for users to input their own model specification matrices for greater flexibility.

The POPULATION statement indicates which variables are to be used to determine the subpopulations under investigation. ML is the option used to request maximum likelihood analysis, PRED requests that the predicted and observed response functions be printed for each subpopulation, and NOGLS requests that the standard weighted least squares analysis be suppressed. Note the inclusion of the ORDER=DATA option in the PROC statement. Since it was desired to have center 1, placebo as the reference value, it was necessary to sort the data by CENTER and descending TRTMENT before PROC CATMOD was invoked and then to request CATMOD to create subpopulations based on the order in which it encountered variable values, rather than by the standard sort order. The parameter estimates produced by CATMOD are the same as those that would be produced by a logistic regression procedure except that the signs are reversed. CATMOD normalizes on the '0' response rather than the '1' response.

Table 10 contains weighted least squares estimates and standard errors for a linear model for integer score mean response at visits 1 to 4. These estimates were also produced with the CATMOD procedure, by using the following statements:

```
PROC CATMOD ORDER= DATA;
  POPULATION CENTER TRTMENT;
  RESPONSE 0 1 2 3 4;
  MODEL WK1 = (1 1 0,
               1 0 0
               1 1 1,
               1 0 1)/PRED COV;
```

The RESPONSE statement serves to specify the type of response function desired. In this case, there will be four response functions, one for each combination of center and treatment. Each response function is the mean response generated by scoring the five possible response outcome categories by 0, 1, 2, 3, 4. WK1 is the variable corresponding to the response for week 1. Similar computer analyses were performed for WK2, WK3, and WK4.

A.3 LOGIST Procedure

Table 12 contains results generated with the LOGIST procedure of Harrell (1986), also available with the SAS system. This procedure fits the logistic multiple regression model to either a binary response or an ordinal dependent variable. Proportional odds models can be fit with the LOGIST procedure. Variables may have to be coded beforehand in order to represent interaction terms. Following are the statements used to compute some of the results presented in Table 12:

```
PROC LOGIST K=4 PRINTC;
  MODEL WK2 =
       ITRT ISEX AGE ICLINIC BASE TRTSEX
            TRTCLIN TRTBASE AGETRT /
       STEPWISE INCLUDE=5 PRINTI PRINTQ
            SLENTRY=0.001 SLSTAY=0.10;
```

Many of the variables were created in a previous data step by statements such as AGEBASE=AGE*BASE in order to represent interaction effects. The dependent variable here is WK2, or the response outcome at the second week, with possible values from 0 to 4. $K = 4$ on the PROC statement specifies that the value '4' is the largest value allowable for the ordinal dependent variable. The stepwise mode of model building is specified by the STEPWISE option on the MODEL statement; INCLUDE= 5 indicates that the first five independent variables listed are to be included in every model. Other options used on the MODEL statement specify what type of criteria to use for a variable to be entered or retained in a model, as well as what types of parameter estimates and statistics to print out; in particular, PRINTQ indicates that score statistics analogous to (68) are to be printed.

This appendix is intended to give an overview of the types of computational strategies employed to generate the results of the analyses in this chapter. Additional details can be found in the appropriate documentation for the SAS software used.

Acknowledgments. The research for this chapter was supported in part by the U.S. Bureau of the Census through Joint Statistical Agreement JSA–84–5. The authors would like to thank Donald Berry, Myra Carpenter, Suzanne Edwards, Amy Goulson, James Grady, William Sollecito, and Kenneth Williams for helpful comments with respect to the preparation of the manuscript. They would also like to thank Ans Janssens for editorial assistance.

REFERENCES

Agresti, A. (1984). *Analysis of Ordinal Categorical Data.* Wiley, New York.

Amara, I. A., and G. G. Koch (1980). A macro for multivariate randomization analyses of stratified sample data. *Proceedings of the Fifth Annual SAS Users Group International Conference*, pp. 134–144.

Bhapkar, V. P. (1966). A note on the equivalence of two test criteria for hypotheses in categorical data. *J. Amer. Statist. Assoc. 61*, 228–235.

Birch, M. W. (1964). The detection of partial association: I. The 2×2 case. *J. Roy. Statist. Soc. B 26*, 313–324.

Birch, M. W. (1965). The detection of partial association: II. The general case. *J. Roy. Statist. Soc. B 27*, 111–124.

Bishop, Y. M. M., S. E. Fienberg, and P. W. Holland (1975). *Discrete Multivariate Analysis: Theory and Practice.* MIT Press, Cambridge, Mass.

Breslow, N. E., and N. E. Day (1980). *Statistical Methods in Cancer Research*, Vol. I: *The Analysis of Case-Control Studies*, International Agency for Research on Cancer, Lyon.

Carr, G. J., K. B. Hafner, and G. G. Koch (1989). Analysis of rank measures of association for ordinal data from longitudinal studies. *J. Amer. Statist. Assoc. 84*, in press.

Clogg, C. C. (1982). Some models for the analysis of association in multiway cross-classifications having ordered categories. *J. Amer. Statist. Assoc. 77*, 803–815.

Cochran, W. G. (1977). *Sampling Techniques*. Wiley, New York

Cox, C., and C. Chuang (1984). A comparison of chi-square partitioning and two logit analyses of ordinal pain data from a pharmaceutical study. *Statist. Med. 3*, 273–285.

Cox, D. R. (1970). *The Analysis of Binary Data*. Chapman & Hall, London.

Everitt, B. S. (1977). *The Analysis of Contingency Tables*. Chapman & Hall, London.

Fienberg, S. E. (1980). *The Analysis of Cross-Classified Categorical Data*. MIT Press, Cambridge, Mass.

Fleiss, J. L. (1981). *Statistical Methods for Rates and Proportions*. Wiley, New York.

Fleiss, J. L. (1986). *The Design and Analysis of Clinical Experiments*. Wiley, New York.

Forthofer, R. N., and R. G. Lehnen (1981). *Public Program Analysis: A New Categorical Data Approach*, Wadsworth, Belmont, Calif.

Freeman, D. H., Jr. (1987). *Applied Categorical Data Analysis*, Marcel Dekker, New York.

Friedman, L. M., C. D. Furberg, and D. L. DeMets (1981). *Fundamentals of Clinical Trials*. John Wright-PSG, Littleton, Mass.

Gart, J. J. (1971). The comparison of proportions: a review of significance tests, confidence intervals, and adjustments for stratification. *Internat. Statist. Rev. 39*, 148–169.

Genter, F. C., and V. T. Farewell (1985). Goodness-of-link testing in ordinal regression models. *Canad. J. Statist. 13(1)*, 37–44.

Grizzle, J. E., C. F. Starmer, and G. G. Koch (1969). Analysis of categorical data by linear models. *Biometrics 25*, 489–504.

Harrell, F. E. (1986). LOGIST. *SUGI Supplementary Library User's Guide*. SAS Institute, Cary, N. C. pp. 269–292.

Holford, T. R. (1980). The analysis of rates and survivorship using log-linear models. *Biometrics 36*, 299–305.

Huitema, B. E. (1980). *The Analysis of Covariance and Alternatives*. Wiley, New York.

Imrey, P. B., G. G. Koch, M. E. Stokes, J. N. Darroch, D. H. Freeman, Jr. and H. D. Tolley (1981). Categorical data analysis: some reflections on the log linear model and logistic regression: p. I. *Internat. Statist. Rev. 49*, 265–283.

Imrey, P. B., G. G. Koch, M. E. Stokes, J. N. Darroch, D. H. Freeman, Jr. and H. D. Tolley (1982). Categorical data analysis: some reflections on the log linear model and logistic regression: p. II. *Internat. Statist. Rev. 50*, 35–64.

Koch, G. G., and V. P. Bhapkar (1982). Chi-square tests. In *Encyclopedia of Statistical Sciences*, Vol. 1 (N. L. Johnson and S. Kotz, eds.). Wiley, New York, pp. 442–457.

Koch, G. G., and S. Edwards (1985). Logistic regression. In *Encyclopedia of Statistical Sciences*, Vol. 5 (N. L. Johnson and S. Kotz, eds.). Wiley, New York, pp. 128–132.

Koch, G. G., and S. Edwards (1987). Clinical efficacy trials with categorical data. In *Handbook of Biopharmaceutical Statistics in Human Drug Development* (Karl E. Peace, ed.). Marcel Dekker, New York, Chap. 9, pp. 403–457.

Koch, G. G., and D. B. Gillings (1983). Inference, design based vs. model based. In *Encyclopedia of Statistical Sciences*, Vol. 4 (N. L. Johnson and S. Kotz, eds.). Wiley, New York, pp. 84–88.

Koch, G. G., and W. A. Sollecito (1984). Statistical considerations in the design, analysis, and interpretation of comparative clinical studies: an academic perspective. *Drug Inform. J. 18*, 131–151.

Koch, G. G., J. R. Landis, J. L. Freeman, D. H. Freeman, Jr. and R. G. Lehnen (1977). A general methodology for the analysis of experiments with repeated measurement of categorical data. *Biometrics 33*, 133–158.

Koch, G. G., J. E. Grizzle, K. Semenya, and P. K. Sen (1978). Statistical methods for evaluation of mastitis treatment data. *J. Dairy Sci. 61*, 829–847.

Koch, G. G., I. A. Amara, M. E. Stokes, and D. B. Gillings (1980a). Some views on parametric and non-parametric analysis for repeated measurements and selected bibliography. *Internat. Statist. Rev. 48*, 249–265.

Koch, G. G., D. B. Gillings, and M. E. Stokes (1980b). Biostatistical implications of design, sampling, and measurement to health science data analysis. *Annual Rev. Public Health 1*, 163–225.

Koch, G. G., I. A. Amara, G. W. Davis, and D. B. Gillings (1982). A review of some statistical methods for covariance analysis of categorical data. *Biometrics 38*, 563–595.

Koch, G. G., S. L. Gitomer, L. Skalland, and M. E. Stokes (1983). Some non-parametric and categorical data analyses for a change-over design study and discussion of apparent carry-over effects. *Statist. Med. 2*, 397–412.

Koch, G. G., P. B. Imrey, J. M. Singer, S. S. Atkinson, and M. E. Stokes (1985a). *Analysis of Categorical Data.* Les Presses de l'Université de Montréal, Montreal.

Koch, G. G., J. M. Singer, and I. A. Amara (1985b). A two-stage procedure for the analysis of ordinal categorical data. In *Biostatistics: Statistics in Biomedical, Public Health and Environmental Sciences*, The Bernard G. Greenberg Volume (P. K. Sen, ed.). North-Holland, New York, pp. 357–387.

Koch, G. G., S. S. Atkinson, and M. E. Stokes (1986). Poisson regression, In *Encyclopedia of Statistical Sciences*, Vol. 7 (N. L. Johnson and S. Kotz, eds.). Wiley, New York, pp. 32–42.

Koch, G. G., J. D. Elashoff, and I. A. Amara (1987). Repeated measurements studies, design and analysis. In *Encyclopedia of Statistical Sciences*, Vol. 8 (N. L. Johnson and S. Kotz, eds.). Wiley, New York, pp. 46–73.

Koch, G. G., J. M. Singer, M. E. Stokes, G. J. Carr, S. B. Cohen, and R. N. Forthofer (1989). Some aspects of weighted least squares analysis for longitudinal categorical data. In *Statistical Models for Longitudinal Studies of Health* (J. H. Dwyer, ed.). Oxford University Press, Oxford, in press.

Kruskal, W. H., and W. A. Wallis (1953). Use of ranks in one criterion variance analysis. *J. Amer. Statist. Assoc. 46*, 583–621.

Landis, J. R., E. R. Heyman, and G. G. Koch (1978). Average partial association in three-way contingency tables: a review and discussion of alternative tests. *Internat. Statist. Rev. 46*, 237–254.

Landis, J. R., M. M. Cooper, T. Kennedy, and G. G. Koch, (1979). A computer program for testing average partial association in three-way contingency tables (PARCAT). *Comput. Programs Biomed. 9*, 223–246.

Larntz, K. (1978). Small sample comparisons of exact levels for chi-squared goodness of fit statistics. *J. Amer. Statist. Assoc.*, *73*, 253–263.

Lehmann, E. L. (1975). *Nonparametrics: Statistical Methods Based on Ranks.* Holden–Day, San Francisco.

Mantel, N. (1963). Chi-square tests with one degree of freedom: extensions of the Mantel–Haenszel procedure. *J. Amer. Statist. Assoc. 58*, 690–700.

Mantel, N. (1966). Evaluation of survival data and two new rank order statistics arising in its consideration. *Cancer Chemother. Rep. 50*, 163–170.

Mantel, N., and J. Fleiss (1980). Minimum expected cell size requirements for the Mantel–Haenszel one-degree-of-freedom chi-square test and a related rapid procedure. *Amer. J. Epidemiol. 112*, 129–134.

Mantel, N., and W. Haenszel (1959). Statistical aspects of the analysis of data from retrospective studies of disease. *J. Nat. Cancer. Inst. 22*, 719–748.

McCullagh, P. (1980). Regression models for ordinal data (with discussion). *J. Roy. Statist. Soc. B 42*, 109–142.

McCullagh, P., and J. A. Nelder (1983). *Generalized Linear Models*. Chapman & Hall, New York.

Mehta, C. R., N. R. Patel, and A. A. Tsiatis (1984). Exact significance testing to establish treatment equivalence with ordered categorical data. *Biometrics 40*, 819–825.

Mehta, C. R., N. R. Patel, and R. Gray (1985). Computing an exact confidence interval for the common odds ratio in several 2×2 contingency tables. *J. Amer. Statist. Assoc. 80*, 969–973.

Neyman, J. (1949). Contributions to the theory of the χ^2-test. *Proceedings of the Berkeley Symposium on Mathematical Statistics and Probability* (J. Neyman ed.). University of California Press, Berkeley, pp. 239–273.

Owen, D. B. (1962). *Handbook of Statistical Tables*. Addison–Wesley, Reading, Mass.

Peterson, B. L. (1986). Proportional odds and partial proportional odds models for ordinal response variables. Dissertation submitted to the Department of Biostatistics, University of North Carolina, Chapel Hill.

Puri, M. L., and P. K. Sen, (1971). *Non-parametric Methods in Multivariate Analysis*. Wiley, New York.

Quade, D. (1967). Rank analysis of covariance. *J. Amer. Statist. Assoc. 62*, 1187–1200.

Quade, D. (1982). Nonparametric analysis of covariance by matching. *Biometrics 38*, 597–611.

SAS Institute, Inc. (1985). *SAS User's Guide: Statistics Version, 5th ed.* SAS Institute, Cary N. C.

Semenya, K. A., G. G. Koch, M. E. Stokes, R. N. Forthofer (1983). Linear models methods for some rank function analyses of ordinal categorical data. *Comm. Statist. 12*, 1277–1298.

Shapiro, S. H., and T. A. Louis, eds. (1983). *Clinical Trials: Issues and Approaches*. Marcel Dekker, New York.

Silvapulle, M. J. (1981). On the existence of maximum likelihood estimators for the binomial response models. *J. Roy. Statist. Soc. B 43*, 310–313.

Stram, D. O., L. J. Wei, and J. H. Ware (1988). Analysis of repeated ordered categorical outcomes with possibly missing observations and time dependent covariates. *J. Amer. Statist. Assoc. 83*, 631–637.

Thomas, D. G. (1975). Exact and asymptotic methods for the combination of 2×2 tables. *Comput. Biomed. Res. 8*, 423–446.

Tygstrup, N., J. M. Lachin, and E. Juhl (1982). *The Randomized Clinical Trial and Therapeutic Decisions.* Marcel Dekker, New York.

van Elteren, P. H. (1960). On the combination of independent two-sample tests of Wilcoxon. *Bull. Internat. Statist. Inst.* *37*, 351–361.

Wald, A. (1943). Tests of statistical hypotheses concerning several parameters when the number of observations is large. *Trans. Amer. Math. Soc.* *54*, 426–482.

Walker, S. H., and D. B. Duncan (1967). Estimation of the probability of an event as a function of several independent variables. *Biometrika* *54*, 167–179.

14

Causality Assessment For Adverse Drug Reactions

DAVID A. LANE University of Minnesota, Minneapolis, Minnesota

A patient takes a drug and subsequently experiences an adverse clinical event. Did the drug cause the event to happen? Answering this question is the goal of causality assessment. Causality assessment plays a role in clinical decision making, in the discovery of previously unsuspected adverse reactions to drugs, in pharmacoepidemiology, and in liability litigation. General discussions of causality assessment and its applications can be found in Venulet et al. (1982), Herman (1984), Jones and Herman (1986), Stephens (1985), and Lane (1987).

The purpose of this chapter is to present the elements of a quantitative approach to causality assessment, based on the use of subjective probability. This approach is introduced, discussed, and illustrated in Auriche (1985), Lane et al. (1986. 1987), Jones and Herman (1986), and Lane (1987).

To appreciate the advantages of the probabilistic approach to causality assessment, it is important first to consider what makes causality assessment problems difficult and then to see that alternative existing methods of causality assessment fail to come to grips with these difficulties. These topics are discussed in Sections 1 and 2. In Section 3 we explain the role that subjective probability can play in causality assessment, and in Section 4 we outline a method of probabilistic causality assessment and apply it to a particular case. Finally, in Section 5 we consider several technical issues that arise in implementing the method.

1 WHY IS CAUSALITY ASSESSMENT DIFFICULT?

There are two features of causality assessment problems that contribute substantially to their difficulty: they are typically complex and they are fraught with uncertainty. Consider the following example, paraphrased from a report submitted to the manufacturer of one of the drugs [this case is analyzed in Kramer (1986b)].

1.1 Example 1

A 42-year-old woman was found dead in her home in the evening following a 1 P.M. appointment with her dentist for a wisdom tooth extraction. The woman had been taking propranolol for high blood pressure, but was reportedly otherwise in good health. The dentist related that she had given a history of heart murmur on her previous visit and that he had instructed her to take two penicillin V tablets 1 hour before her appointment. She gave no history of drug allergy. Prior to the oral surgery, she had an injection of xylocaine. The extraction procedure lasted 40 minutes. She was instructed to go home and rest and was given a prescription for five zomepirac tablets, 100 mg, every 4 to 6 hours for pain, as needed. She was also instructed to continue the penicillin for 1 day.

Filled prescriptions for zomepirac, penicillin V, and propranolol were found in her home. Autopsy revealed pulmonary congestion and some hyperinflation, along with evidence of laryngeal edema and swelling of the extremities. An analysis of the stomach contents revealed no drugs associated with abuse, such as narcotics, amphetamines, or barbiturates. The coroner estimated the time of death as 4:00 P.M. $\pm$ 2 hours.

1.2 Complexity

Was the woman's death caused by a drug—and if so, which one? Several factors have evidentiary significance for this causality assessment problem. First, there are several possible causes of the woman's death to consider, including the fact that three of the drugs mentioned in the report can cause sudden death from anaphylaxis (xylocaine, penicillin, and zomepirac). Second, there are details of the patient's history (her high blood pressure and history of heart murmur) that may have placed her at special risk for possible nondrug causes of death; and the fact that she was taking propranolol may have increased the chance that she suffered an immunologic reaction to the other drugs. The relation between the time at which she took the various drugs and when she died may also provide evidence about what killed her, as may the autopsy findings.

To interpret the evidence provided by each of these factors, the assessor can access relevant information obtained from many different sources: observations and findings for the particular case at hand, his or her own previous clinical experience, other case reports and epidemiological studies, and facts and theories derived from pharmacology and other basic sciences. The quality of the data derived from these different sources can vary enormously, from "relatively hard" to "very soft."

1.3 Uncertainty

The assessor cannot know all the relevant information with certainty. In particular, this report leaves out some of the most important facts of the case: Did the woman actually take the zomepirac (nobody seems to have counted how many pills were left)? If so, when? When exactly did she die? In addition, the assessor may be uncertain about background information that affects how the facts of the case are interpreted. For example, what is the incidence of anaphylaxis due to penicillin? to zomepirac? to xylocaine? Is there any mechanism other than anaphylaxis whereby any of the drugs could cause sudden death? What other causes of sudden death are consistent with the findings in this case?

In summary, then, to solve causality assessment problems, it is necessary to weigh information about a variety of factors, coming from a variety of sources, in the presence of a large amount of residual uncertainty, to arrive at an overall measure of how plausible it is that a particular drug caused the adverse event in question.

2 QUALITATIVE CAUSALITY ASSESSMENT METHODS

2.1 Global Introspection

The usual approach to a causality assessment problem is to refer it to an expert, who solves it by an act of global introspection. That is, the expert collects all the facts that he or she thinks are relevant to the problem at hand, mixes them together, and then just decides what the answer is. In the causality assessment context, this answer is usually expressed in terms of a qualitative probability scale: for example, "definite," "probable," "possible," "doubtful," or "unrelated."

Unfortunately, global introspection does not work well. Cognitive psychologists have shown that the ability of the human brain to make unaided assessments of uncertainty in complicated situations is poor, especially when assessing the probability of a cause given an effect, precisely the task of causality assessment (Kahneman et al., 1982). In fact, several groups of clinical pharmacologists have demonstrated how unreliable global introspection is as a causality assessment method, by comparing their individual evaluations of a series of suspected adverse drug reactions and documenting the extent of their disagreement (Karch et al., 1976; Koch-Weser et al., 1977; Dangomau et al., 1980). Another problem with global introspection is that it is uncalibrated: one assessor's "possible" might mean the same thing as another assessor's "probable." Other shortcomings of global introspection as a causality assessment method are discussed in Lane (1984) and Kramer (1986a).

2.2 Standardized Assessment Methods

Because of these difficulties with global introspection, during the past decade much effort has been devoted to developing decision aids for causality assessment. Physicians from industry, regulatory agencies, and academia have now published more than a dozen standardized assessment methods (SAM) [see Venulet et al. (1982), Herman (1984), and Stephens (1985, 1987), for reviews and examples of these methods].

The SAM range from simple flowcharts posing 10 or fewer questions to lengthy questionnaires containing up to 84 items. However, they share a common basic structure. They divide the considerations that bear on causality assessment into a number of factors or axes: for example, the timing of the adverse event in relation to administration of the drug; alternative etiological candidates; previous recognition of the event as a possible adverse reaction to the drug; the response when the drug is discontinued (dechallenge) and when the drug is subsequently readministered (rechallenge). Information relevant to each factor is elicited by a series of questions, the answers to which are restricted to yes/no/(and for some methods) don't know. The answers to these questions are then converted to a score for each factor, the factor scores are summed, and this overall score is converted into a value on a qualitative probability scale.

Although SAM have advantages compared to global introspection (Lane, 1984), they are not free from criticism. Some experts in adverse reactions complain that SAM, with their preset series of questions and limited range of possible answers, are too inflexible to deal with all the kinds of evidence that may differentiate between drug and nondrug causation (Dukes, 1984). In particular, SAM cannot handle uncertainty about the facts of a case, such as whether or not the woman in Example 1 actually took zomepirac. Moreover, even adherents of SAM agree that their procedures for converting answers into probability ratings are arbitrary.

The following artificial example points out a more serious difficulty with SAM: in situations in which quantitative probability calculations are appropriate, the methods give answers that contradict the results of these calculations.

2.3 Example 2

An analgesic (D) is commonly taken to relieve pain associated with flu (M). Data from a large epidemiological study indicate that about 1 in 8 of patients who take D subsequently experience nausea (E), while 1 in 10 flu patients who do not take D experience nausea due to their flu. The mechanism of D-induced nausea is well understood, and it implies that such nausea always occurs within 1 hour of administration of D. On the other hand, M-caused nausea may occur any time within 2 days following the onset of M.

PROBLEM: A patient takes D as soon as the symptoms of M begin and becomes nauseated with 45 minutes. What is the chance that the nausea is D-induced?

Solution: Bayes' theorem can be applied to solve this problem. Let B represent the background incidences reported above, and Ti the fact that the nausea occurred in the first hour after administration of D. Then

$$\begin{aligned}\frac{P(\text{D caused E} \mid \text{B}, \text{Ti})}{P(\text{M caused E} \mid \text{B}, \text{Ti})} &= \frac{P(\text{D caused E} \mid \text{B})}{P(\text{M caused E} \mid \text{B})} \cdot \frac{P(\text{Ti} \mid \text{D caused E}, \text{B})}{P(\text{Ti} \mid \text{M caused E}, \text{B})} \\ &= \frac{1/5}{4/5} \cdot \frac{1}{1/48} \\ &= 12; \qquad (1)\end{aligned}$$

that is,

$$P(\text{D caused E} \mid \text{B}, \text{Ti}) = \frac{12}{13} = 0.92.$$

The evaluations of $P(\text{D caused E} \mid \text{B})$ and $P(\text{M caused E} \mid \text{B})$ follow from the epidemiological data. That is, assuming that the incidence of M-caused nausea is the same among those patients who take D and those who do not, $1/8 - 1/10 = 1/40$ of the flu patients taking D suffer from D-induced nausea, while 1/10 suffer from M-caused nausea. Thus 1/5 of the nausea suffered by flu patients taking D is caused by D. The evaluations of $P(\text{Ti} \mid \text{M caused E, B})$ and $P(\text{Ti} \mid \text{M caused E, B})$ follow from the given timing information. All D-induced nausea begins in the first hour after administration, so $P(\text{Ti} \mid \text{D caused E, B}) = 1$. Assuming a uniform distribution for onset of M-caused nausea over the assumed 2-day vulnerable period, only 1/48 of the M-caused nausea begins in the first hour, so $P(\text{Ti} \mid \text{M caused E, B}) = 1/48$.

2.4 Inconsistency Between SAM and Bayes' Theorem

When SAM are applied to this case, they yield answers ranging from "doubtful" to "possible," much too conservative to characterize a quantitative probability of 0.92. There are several reasons for this inconsistency. First, SAM do not allow sharp information about a single factor (in this case, timing) to override neutral or weakly negative data relating to other factors (e.g., the absence of dechallenge and rechallenge information, or the existence of an alternative etiologic candidate, M). Second, SAM do not directly compare how consistent the observed data are with each alternative etiology, while Bayes' theorem measures the evidence in each piece of data by its relative plausibility, given each competing etiological hypothesis. Finally, SAM do not process quantitative evidence directly, so that the strength of the evidence about timing and about background incidences in the example cannot be adequately assessed.

3 THE ROLE OF SUBJECTIVE PROBABILITY

3.1 Probability, Frequencies, and Coherence

The key to the solution of Example 2 is the use of Bayes' theorem, which isolates the separate effects of the two sources of evidence, B and Ti, and determines how the given information from each of these sources gets converted into the appropriate measure of evidence for (or against) D-causation. What justifies this use of Bayes' theorem? The axioms of probability theory and hence Bayes' theorem hold for relative frequencies in finite populations, and at first glance, the calculation seems to be about such frequencies: the calculation just determines what fraction of patients suffer D-induced nausea among all patients with flu who take D and become nauseated within 1 hour.

However, a closer look makes it clear that more than information about frequencies is involved in assessing and interpreting the probabilities that appear in equation (1). First, the probabilities for Ti are calculated conditionally on unobserved causes, so they could not be based directly on observed frequencies; in fact, the probability given D-causation derives from a model for the mechanism whereby D causes nausea. Second, the probabilities appearing on the left-hand side of equation (1) refer only to the individual patient at hand. The relevance of the given frequency information [used in evaluating the first ratio on the right of equation (1)] follows from a judgment by the assessor that this patient is fungible with those on whom the frequency information is available. If, for example, the assessor learns that this patient had had nausea within 2 hours of his five previous flu attacks when he did not take D, the questions posed by the probabilities on the left of (1) still have meaning, but the frequencies given by the background incidence figures are no longer directly relevant. In fact, all the probabilities that appear in (1) really refer to the individual case at hand, and they can be reasonably interpreted only as measures of the assessor's degree of belief, even though frequencies may be used to help assess some of them.

To understand why the solution to Example 2 has prescriptive force, and to extend the idea behind the solution to more general causality assessment problems, it is first necessary to answer two questions:

1. What does it mean to interpret probability as a measure of degree of belief?
2. Why do the axioms of probability theory (and hence Bayes' theorem) apply to probabilities so interpreted?

The Italian mathematician Bruno de Finetti answered these questions by means of an economic metaphor: he "operationalized" an assessor's degree of belief in the truth of the proposition A as the number p such that the assessor is neutral between buying and selling for $\$p$ a ticket that will be worth \$1 if A is true, and otherwise it will be worth nothing [see de Finetti (1974) and Lane (1981)]. (Note: It is easy to argue that such a p exists, even if it may be difficult to assess it.) Similarly, the conditional probability $p(\mathrm{A} \mid \mathrm{B})$ is interpreted as a price for a ticket worth \$1 of A is true and otherwise worthless, with the proviso that the price is refunded and no money changes hands unless the conditioning proposition B is true.

With these definitions, it is possible to give a precise meaning to consistent (and inconsistent) reasoning in the face of uncertainty. Suppose that an assessor simultaneously measures her belief in a number of different propositions, so that she has set the price for many different tickets. Is it possible that someone could then transact with her for some of these, at the assessor's prices, in such a way that the assessor must pay out more than she receives, no matter which of the propositions are true and which are false? If so, in her assessments she has in effect made economic decisions with unacceptable economic consequence: certain financial loss. The possibility of such loss is a concretization of the inconsistent reasoning that underlies it.

A set of assessments is called incoherent if it can result in sure loss as described above; otherwise, it is coherent. De Finetti proved the following fundamental result: A set of assessments is coherent if and only if the assessments satisfy the usual axioms of probability theory (the familiar addition and multiplication laws). Thus the relations between probability assessments that follow from the axioms (including Bayes' theorem) must obtain, or the assessor is committing herself to opinions that are as inconsistent as is the behavior of someone who claims to value money and yet gives it away with no benefit (material or psychological) to herself.

We can now interpret equation (1) as a statement of subjective probability. The ratio on the left-hand side of (1) represents the assessor's odds in favor of D-causation for the case at hand, which is what the assessor must evaluate to solve the causality assessment problem. The first ratio on the right-hand side of (1) represents the assessors' odds in favor of D-causation, not taking into account just when the nausea occurred; the second represents the ratio between her probability that D-induced nausea would happen in the first hour and her evaluation of the same probability for M-induced nausea. Now the probabilities in the latter two ratios are easy for her to evaluate, using the given information (and her judgment of fungibility between this patient and the patients to whom the frequency information refers). De Finetti's result tells the assessor that there is only one coherent relationship between the opinions that are expressed in the two ratios that are easy to evaluate and the ratio she wants, her odds in favor of D-causation taking into account when the nausea occurred. That relationship follows from Bayes' theorem and is given by (1). Thus, if she wants to be coherent in her opinions, the assessor should use (1) to determine her solution to the causality assessment problem. If she evaluates it differently, she is in effect expressing an opinion that contradicts her own, better-founded beliefs.

Even though de Finetti's definition gives a meaning to probability, it does not imply that all probabilities are easy to assess (after all, it is generally difficult to determine just what you would be willing to pay for anything!). On the other hand, as the solution to Example 2 indicates, some probabilities are easy to assess. For example, it is a consequence of another famous result of de Finetti that in the presence of sufficient frequency information and the right judgments of fungibility, a coherent probability appraiser will evaluate his probabilities very close to the relevant observed frequencies. The advantage of a probabilistic approach to problems like causality assessment is that the rules of probability theory can be used to relate the probabilities you want to assess to probabilities that available information makes it possible (even easy) for you to assess.

3.2 Coherence and Causality Assessment

These considerations suggest the following strategy for a solution to the causality assessment problem based on subjective probability:

1. Decompose the causality assessment problem into subproblems, each of which is accessible to the knowledge and experience of the assessor.
2. Express the assessor's uncertainty about the solutions to the subproblems in quantitative from, as subjective probabilities.
3. Use the rules of probability theory to merge the solutions to these subproblems into a coherent solution to the overall causality assessment problem.

The first step in implementing this strategy is to define the goal of causality assessment in probabilistic terms. This is accomplished by the following expression, called the posterior odds in favor of D-causation:

$$\frac{P(\mathrm{D} \to \mathrm{E} \mid \mathrm{B}, \mathrm{C})}{P(\mathrm{D} \not\to \mathrm{E} \mid \mathrm{B}, \mathrm{C})}. \tag{2}$$

In this expression, E is an adverse event suffered by a particular patient, and D is a drug suspected of causing E. The proposition "D $\to$ E" (D caused E) means that E would not have happened as and when it did had D not been administered (i.e., D is a necessary, but not necessarily sufficient, cause of E). "D $\not\to$ E" denies that D $\to$ E. B represents background information, including everything the assessor knows about the connection between the drug D and events similar to E (from his own clinical experience, published case series and epidemiological studies, facts and theories from pharmacology, and other basic sciences). The only case-specific information in B is the proposition that a patient with a specified clinical condition M who has been administered drug D in a specified way subsequently develops an adverse event of type E_t. (M and E_t, discussed in the next section, are generic characterizations describing essential elements of the patient's condition and the event E, respectively.) C represents case information: details about the particular patient and his adverse event E.

Just as in the solution to Example 2, Bayes' theorem can be applied to the posterior odds to yield the following equation:

$$\underset{\text{posterior odds}}{\frac{P(\mathrm{D} \to \mathrm{E} \mid \mathrm{B}, \mathrm{C})}{P(\mathrm{D} \not\to \mathrm{E} \mid \mathrm{B}, \mathrm{C})}} = \underset{\text{prior odds}}{\frac{P(\mathrm{D} \to \mathrm{E}_t \mid \mathrm{B})}{P(\mathrm{D} \not\to \mathrm{E}_t \mid \mathrm{B})}} \cdot \underset{\text{likelihood ratio}}{\frac{P(\mathrm{C} \mid \mathrm{D} \to \mathrm{E}, \mathrm{B})}{P(\mathrm{C} \mid \mathrm{D} \not\to \mathrm{E}, \mathrm{B})}}. \tag{3}$$

Both the posterior and prior odds are calculated conditionally on B and so refer to a patient with clinical condition M who has been administered D and experienced an event of type E_t. However, the identity of the patient to whom the two terms refer is different. In the posterior odds, it is the particular patient under review; while in the prior odds, it is a "generic" patient (perhaps the "next" patient) with the three defining characteristics M, D, and E_t. Thus the prior odds can be regarded epidemiologically, as will be discussed in Sections 4 and 5; on the other hand, the probabilities in the likelihood ratio involve thinking in terms of mechanism, arguing from cause to effect.

It is helpful to consider the information in *C* in chronological order. A typical chronological sequence is illustrated in Figure 1. The categories of

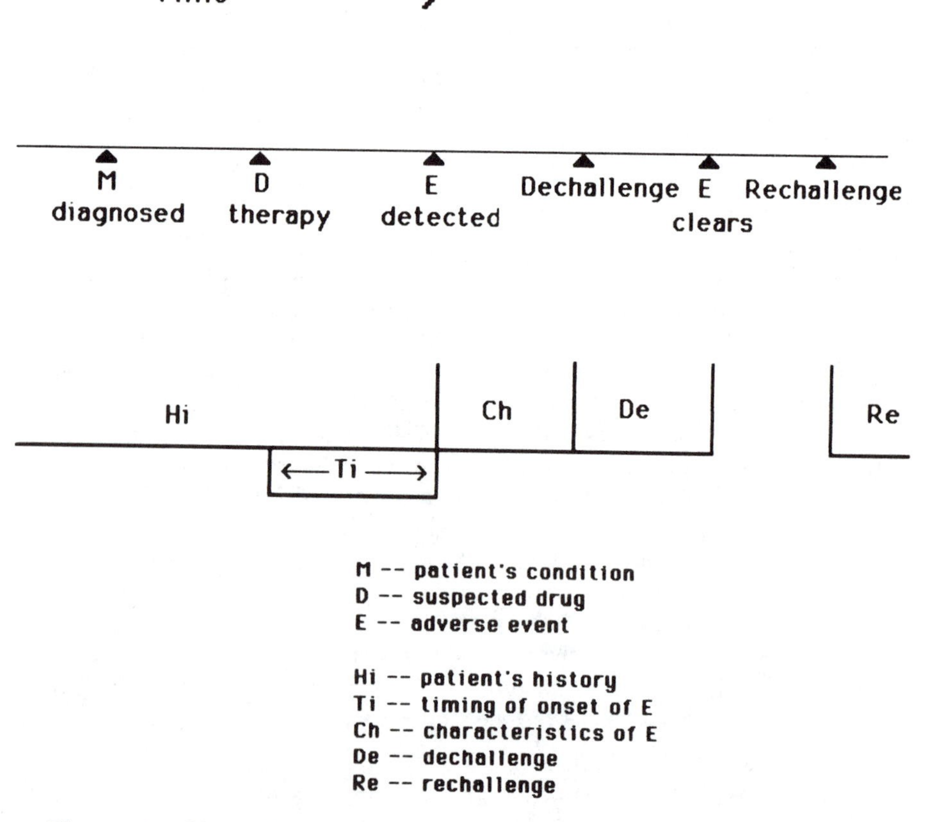

Figure 1 Chronological sequence of an adverse event.

case information include Hi, the patient's history antedating the onset of E; Ti, the timing of the onset of E in relation to the administration of D; Ch, characteristics of the event from time of onset to time of dechallenge, which can include information about duration, severity, evolution, and laboratory tests; De, response to dechallenge; and Re, response to rechallenge. The likelihood ratio (LR) is decomposed into factors, corresponding to these chronological categories of case information:

$$\mathrm{LR} = \mathrm{LR(Hi)} \times \mathrm{LR(Ti)} \times \mathrm{LR(Ch)} \times \mathrm{LR(De)} \times \mathrm{LR(Re)}, \qquad (4)$$

where, for example,

$$\mathrm{LR(Ti)} = \frac{P(\mathrm{Ti} \mid \mathrm{D} \rightarrow \mathrm{E,B,Hi})}{P(\mathrm{Ti} \mid \mathrm{D} \not\rightarrow \mathrm{E,B,Hi})}.$$

Note that the probabilities that appear in each likelihood ratio factor are evaluated conditionally on B and all chronologically preceding case information.

In summary, then, the probabilistic approach to causality assessment is designed to calculate the posterior odds in favor of D-causation, by evaluating the subjective probabilities that appear in the prior odds and a series of likelihood ratio factors corresponding to chronological categories of case information.

4 IMPLEMENTING THE PROBABILISTIC APPROACH

The probabilistic causality assessment method outlined in this section is designed to elicit and process the opinions of assessors with medical or pharmacological expertise. The method is illustrated here by an analysis of a fairly simple case (Example 3), based on assessments provided by Michael Kramer and Tom Hutchinson of the Departments of Pediatrics, Medicine, and Epidemiology and Biostatistics, McGill University. Further technical aspects of the method are discussed in Section 5; more details and examples can be found in Jones and Herman (1986).

4.1 Example 3

B.L. is a 17-month-old male day-care-center attendee who on December 10 developed signs and symptoms of an upper respiratory tract infection with rhinorrhea and cough, but without fever or gastrointestinal symptoms. On December 12, his temperature rose to 39.4°C, he became irritable, and he began to pull at his ears. He was seen by his pediatrician on that day and was diagnosed as having bilateral otitis media. Treatment was initiated with amoxicillin suspension in a dose of 125 mg three times per day. Over the next 24 hours (December 13), B.L. had three watery bowel movements. By December 14, he was afebrile, and the diarrhea continued without exacerbation. The pediatrician suggested continuing the amoxicillin therapy as prescribed. From December 15 to 21, B.L. remained afebrile and became less irritable and more playful, but the diarrhea persisted. On December 21, the amoxicillin was discontinued, and by December 23 the diarrhea had resolved.

4.2 Implementation Step 1: Determine the Case Parameters (M, E_t, Cause List, Time Horizon)

The case parameters establish the context in which the assessment is carried out. M and E_t create an epidemiological reference set for the patient under consideration; the cause list specifies the alternative etiological candidates; and the time horizon determines a period of time to which all considerations about drug-event connection are restricted.

M and E_t

E_t specifies the general type of the adverse event E, and M abstracts out the most important aspects of the patient's condition that determine his risk for events of type E_t from causes other than the drug under consideration. It is important to define these parameters as explicitly as possible.

Sometimes, there will be a question about whether to include certain aspects of the patient's condition or the event in the definitions of these parameters or in the appropriate chronological category of case information. The choice should be guided by the ease of the ensuing assessments and so depends on the assessor's experience and information; roughly, the assessor should choose definitions for M and E_t that make it easiest for him to "think epidemiologically" about the class determined by these definitions. The essential thing is consistency in the course of the assessment: M and E_t are included in B, the background information, and are part of the reference set for every calculation.

Cause List

The cause list consists of a set of mutually exclusive propositions about the possible causes of E. Typically, there are a number of possible hypotheses specifying drug causal candidates—say, $D_1, \ldots, D_n$—followed by a number of hypotheses specifying nondrug causes.

The requirement that the propositions on the cause list be mutually exclusive is somewhat artificial and requires a bit of care in defining and interpreting the propositions. For example, suppose the assessor believes that an interaction between drugs D_A and D_B may have caused E. Then he should have a separate entry on the cause list for this interaction; and if he also believes that either drug alone may also have caused E, he must include entries for "D_A alone" (i.e., "E would have happened as and when it did had D_A and not D_B been given, but not if D_B and not D_A had been given") and "D_B alone." Similarly, there is an asymmetry between drug and nondrug causes: because of the definition of the proposition "D caused E" for a possible drug cause D, if N is a possible nondrug cause, the proposition "N caused E" implies that "E would have happened as and when it did had none of the drugs mentioned in $D_1, \ldots, D_n$ been given." Finally, since causality assessment focuses on the question of drug responsibility, it is possible to lump together different nondrug causes, as long as they give the same probability to each case datum that distinguishes drug from nondrug causation.

Time Horizon

B includes the assertion that a patient with condition M experiences an event of type E_t. The time horizon puts an upper limit on the length of time after D-therapy begins in which it is asserted that the event occurs. To choose the time horizon, the assessor should think about the distribution for the onset of an event of type E_t that is caused by D; the time horizon should be about as long as the support of this distribution. It is easy to see that for a coherent assessor, the exact value selected will not affect the resulting posterior odds. The reason for specifying a time horizon at all is that doing so increases the accessibility of some of the assessment tasks (especially the prior odds and likelihood ratio for timing).

Case Parameters for Example 3

M: upper respiratory infection and otitis media in a 12-to 24-month-old child
E_t: Diarrhea
Cause list:
(1) Amoxicillin (D)
(2) Late-occurring GI symptoms secondary to the original infection (M)
(3) Coincidental infectious gastroenteritis (CG)
Time horizon: 1 week

4.3 Implementation Step 2: Collect the Case Information

All the information that can differentiate between drug and nondrug causation should be listed in the appropriate chronological category.

Case Information for Example 3

Hi: (1) Occurrence in December (the incidence of infectious gastroenteritis fluctuates seasonally, with highest rates in winter)
(2) Day-care-center attendance (the incidence of infectious gastroenteritis is higher among day-care-center attendees)
Ti: Onset 1 day following initiation of D
Ch: Diarrhea persisted 9 days until dechallenge
De: Diarrhea resolved within 48 hours after dechallenge

4.4 Implementation Step 3: Evaluate the Prior Odds

According to (3), the assessor can determine his value for the prior odds by answering the following question: Consider a class of patients with condition M who receive D and subsequently (within the time horizon) experience an event of type E_t; in what proportion of these patients is the event caused by D?

Alternatively, the assessor can consider the same problem from a prospective point of view, as follows. Imagine a large class of patients with M. Suppose that half of them are selected at random and receive D, while the rest receive some alternative therapy with the same beneficial effects as D, but which cannot cause events of type E_t. Let $P(E_t \mid D)$ represent the assessor's estimate of the proportion of the patients who receive D that experience events of type E_t, and $P(E_t \mid D^c)$, his corresponding estimate for the proportion of those who do not receive D. Then, for this assessor,

$$\text{prior odds} = \frac{P(E_t \mid D) - P(E_t \mid D^c)}{P(E_t \mid D^c)}. \tag{5}$$

Thus one strategy for assessing prior odds is to use what information is available to evaluate the two quantities $P(E_t \mid D)$ and $P(E_t \mid D^c)$ as defined above, and then use (5) to determine the prior odds. Often, the assessor's uncertainty about the incidences in this imaginary "clinical trial" is sufficiently diffuse that it is best to assess her subjective distributions for these quantities, and then evaluate the means of these distributions to plug into (5). These distributions are also helpful if the assessor should choose to carry out a sensitivity analysis at the conclusion of her assessment. Some other considerations bearing on the prior odds are discussed in Section 5.

Evaluating the Prior Odds for Example 3

The assessors employed the strategy based on (5), using observed frequencies obtained from a study monitoring antibiotic-associated gastrointestinal symptoms in pediatric outpatients in Montreal [some results from this study, but not the raw data we use, are presented in Kramer et al. (1985a, 1985b)]. In addition, we use data from diarrhea surveillance studies reported in Bartlett et al. (1985a, 1986b).

TO EVALUATE $P(\mathrm{E}_t \mid \mathrm{D})$ In the Montreal study about 10% of the more than 1300 patients receiving amoxicillin suffered from diarrhea within a week of beginning therapy. So the assessors evaluated: $P(\mathrm{E}_t \mid \mathrm{D}) = 0.10$.

TO EVALUATE $P(\mathrm{E}_t \mid \mathrm{D}^c)$ The assessors estimated this quantity in two different ways. First, in the Montreal study, the lowest incidence of diarrhea followed trimethoprim/sulfamethoxazole therapy, and was about 2.5% in the first week of therapy. This drug is not generally considered to be associated with diarrhea, but some of this incidence may represent drug-induced diarrhea, so the assessors considered it appropriate to adjust this figure downward slightly.

The assessors also developed a lower-bound estimate for the incidence of non-drug-induced diarrhea, by thinking about the spontaneous occurrence of diarrhea in children not taking drugs prior to their diarrhea. They assumed that 1- to 2-year old children experience approximately one such episode per year on average [this is based primarily on data in Bartlett et al. (1985a)], equivalent to an incidence (per child) of about 0.019 per week. This must be increased somewhat, since it does not condition on the children having an infection (M), which increases the probability of developing diarrhea.

So, their estimate for the incidence (per child) of non-drug-induced diarrhea among children with M, in the week following initiation of amoxicillin therapy, is between 0.019 and 0.025. They adopted a value of 0.022:

$$P(\mathrm{E}_t \mid \mathrm{D}c) = 0.022.$$

TO EVALUATE THE PRIOR ODDS By (5),

$$\begin{aligned}\text{prior odds} &= \frac{P(\mathrm{E}_t \mid \mathrm{D}) - P(\mathrm{E}_t \mid \mathrm{D}^c)}{P(\mathrm{E}_t \mid \mathrm{D}^c)} \\ &= \frac{0.01 - 0.022}{0.022} \\ &= 3.5.\end{aligned}$$

Here are some consequences of the assessments above that will be used below. Denote by $P(\mathrm{E_M} \mid \mathrm{B})$ and $P(\mathrm{E_{CG}} \mid \mathrm{B})$ the assessments for the incidence of diarrhea caused by M and by coincidental gastroenteritis, respectively. Then, from the assessments above, one can conclude that

$$0.022 = P(\mathrm{E}_t \mid \mathrm{D}^c) = P(\mathrm{E_M} \mid \mathrm{B}) + P(\mathrm{E_{CG}} \mid \mathrm{B});$$

and assuming that having M does not affect the chance of contracting a coincidental gastroenteritis,

$$0.019 = \{P(\mathrm{E_M} \mid \mathrm{B}) \cdot P(\mathrm{M})\} + P(\mathrm{E_{CG}} \mid \mathrm{B}).$$

Since $P(\mathrm{M})$, the weekly incidence of M among 1-to 2-year-old children, is relatively small (certainly less than 10%), the following relations hold (up to rounding error):

$$P(\mathrm{E_M} \mid \mathrm{B}) = 0.003,$$

$$P(\mathrm{E_{CG}} \mid \mathrm{B}) = 0.019,$$

$$P(\mathrm{M} \rightarrow \mathrm{E} \mid \mathrm{B}, \mathrm{D} \not\rightarrow \mathrm{E}) = \frac{P(\mathrm{E_M} \mid \mathrm{B})}{P(\mathrm{E}_t \mid \mathrm{D}^c)} = 0.14).$$

4.5 Implementation Step 4: Evaluate the Likelihood Ratio Factor for History, LR(Hi)

Information in Hi differs from the data in the other chronological categories in that it antedates the adverse event E and frequently the administration of D as well. Thus it is easier to evaluate LR(Hi) as an adjustment to the prior odds (by restricting the relevant reference class) than to evaluate the probabilities for the data in Hi given the possible causes of E.

Evaluating LR(Hi) for Example 3

Basing their evaluation on data in Bartlett et al. (1985b), the assessors estimated that day-care-center attendees are 1.4 times as likely to suffer from non-drug-induced diarrhea as the general pediatric population, because of their greater exposure rate to infections. On the other hand, they are at no greater risk for drug-induced diarrhea (given M). Also, again based on data in Bartlett et al. (1985b) and general pediatric experience, the incidence of non-drug-induced diarrhea is approximately twice as high in the winter as the yearly average, while there should be no seasonal effects for drug-caused diarrhea (again, given M).

To calculate LR(Hi), the assessors first modified (5) by conditioning on the data in Hi to compute the odds in favor of D-causation posterior to Hi. Neither the numerator, the incidence of D-caused diarrhea, nor

$P(\mathrm{E_M} \mid \mathrm{B})$ change, given M. However, $P(\mathrm{E_{CG}} \mid \mathrm{B})$ increases by a factor of $2 \times 1.4 = 2.8$. Thus

$$\begin{aligned} P(\mathrm{E}_t \mid \mathrm{B}, \mathrm{Hi}) &= (0.14)(0.003) + (0.86)(0.019)(2.8) \\ &= 0.046, \end{aligned}$$

so

$$\begin{aligned} \text{posterior odds given history} &= \frac{0.10 - 0.022}{0.046} \\ &= 1.7. \end{aligned}$$

Finally, we can compute LR(Hi) as the ratio of the posterior odds given history and the prior odds:

$$\mathrm{LR(Hi)} = \frac{1.7}{3.5} = 0.5.$$

4.6 Implementation Step 5: Evaluate the Remaining Likelihood Ratio Factors

The probability for each piece of case information must be evaluated, given each possible cause and all preceding data. Even though only the probability for the data actually observed plays a role in these likelihood ratio factors, to ensure meaningful and reliable results, it is important to evaluate these probabilities in their proper context. For example, for information that refers to timing (time to onset of E, duration of E before dechallenge, time of disappearance of E after dechallenge), it is best to construct entire timing distributions for the relevant events, as illustrated in the example below. Similar considerations hold for probabilities about the results of laboratory tests. Some formulas and techniques useful in assessing likelihood ratio factors are presented in Section 5.

Evaluating Likelihood Ratio Factors for Example 3

All the information in Ti, Ch, and De concerns timing. Moreover, to the assessors, all the relevant timing distributions were judged to be independent of one another (i.e., given the cause of the diarrhea, knowing how long it takes it to develop would not affect the assessors' opinions about how long it might persist) and to be independent of the information in Hi.

LR(Ti): To assess LR(Ti), the assessors evaluated their distributions for time to onset of diarrhea given each of the three listed causes. Recall that they are conditioning on the facts that no diarrhea was present until the amoxicillin was first administered and that diarrhea then appeared sometime with the next week (the time horizon). Their timing distribution given drug causation is shown in Figure 2; it is based on the assumption that the mechanism for D-induced diarrhea is initiated by dose-dependent effects on gut flora and mucosal absorptive function.

The timing distribution for onset of M-caused diarrhea is a little more complicated to assess, because the reasonable time origin for such a distribution is onset of M rather than administration of D. Thus the assessors evaluated their distribution from this natural time origin (Figure 3), and then obtained the relevant distribution (Figure 4) by conditioning on diarrhea onset occurring after D-initiation (i.e., by truncating at December 12 and rescaling). The distribution for onset of diarrhea due to coincidental gastroenteritis is of course uniform over the relevant time period and is pictured in Figure 5.

Using these distributions, LR(Ti) is evaluated as follows. Ti states that the diarrhea actually first occurred on the first day of D-therapy. So

$$P(\mathrm{Ti} \mid \mathrm{D} \rightarrow \mathrm{E}) = 0.33.$$

By the law of total probability,

$$\begin{aligned} P(\mathrm{Ti} \mid \mathrm{D} \not\rightarrow \mathrm{E}) &= P(\mathrm{Ti} \mid \mathrm{M} \rightarrow \mathrm{E}) \cdot P(\mathrm{M} \rightarrow \mathrm{E} \mid \mathrm{D} \not\rightarrow \mathrm{E}) \\ &\quad + P(\mathrm{Ti} \mid \mathrm{CG} \rightarrow \mathrm{E}) \cdot P(\mathrm{CG} \rightarrow \mathrm{E} \mid \mathrm{D} \not\rightarrow \mathrm{E}) \\ &= (0.33)(0.14) + (0.14)(.86) \\ &= 0.17. \end{aligned}$$

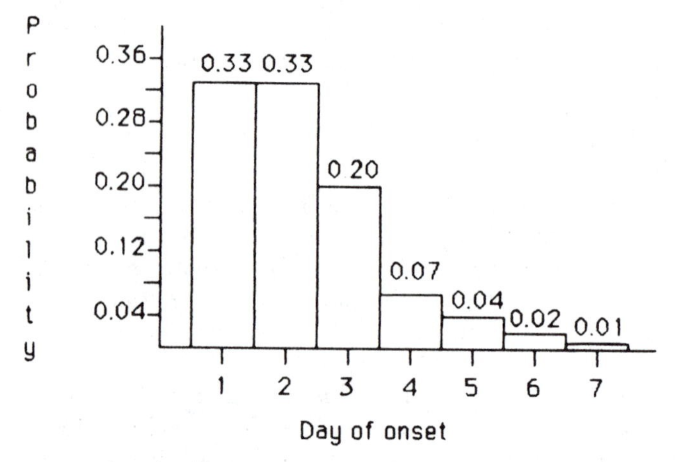

Figure 2 Time to onset of D-induced diarrhea.

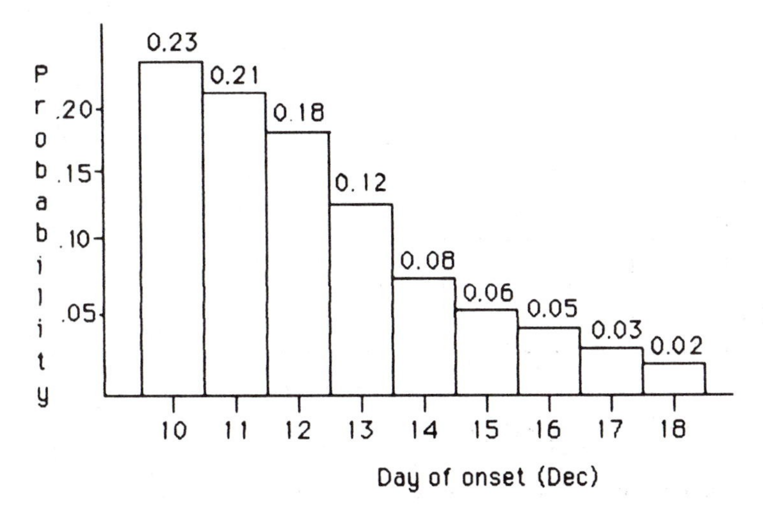

Figure 3 Time to onset of M-induced diarrhea (from December 10).

(Recall that the probability for M-causation given nondrug causation was calculated in the note following the evaluation of the prior.) So

$$\mathrm{LR(Ti)} = \frac{P(\mathrm{Ti} \mid \mathrm{D} \to \mathrm{E})}{P(\mathrm{Ti} \mid \mathrm{D} \not\to \mathrm{E})} = \frac{0.33}{0.17} = 2.$$

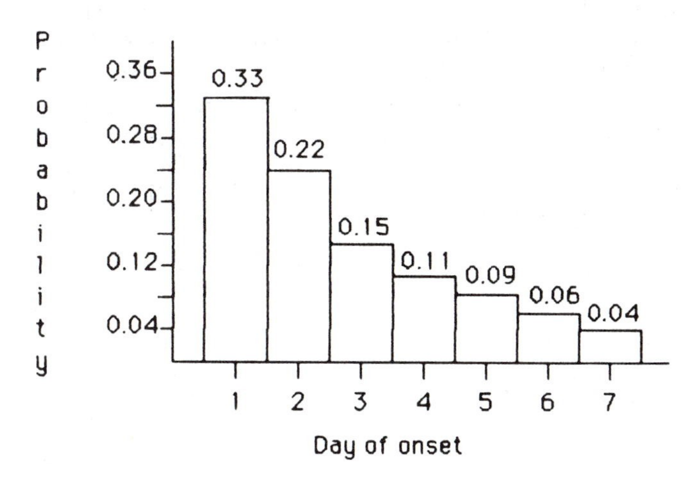

Figure 4 Time to onset of M-induced diarrhea.

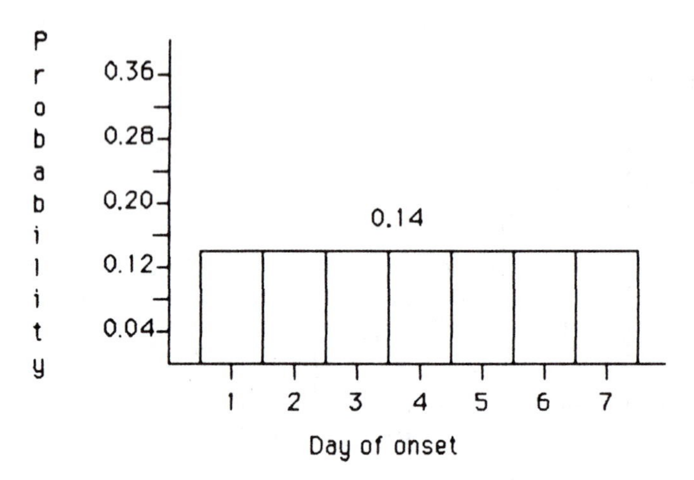

Figure 5 Time to onset of diarrhea caused by coincidental gastroenteritis.

LR(Ch): The information in Ch is that the diarrhea lasted until dechallenge (9 days). The assessors felt that most cases of D-caused diarrhea would last until the drug was withdrawn. More precisely, they evaluated

$$P(\text{Ch} \mid \text{D} \to \text{E}) = 0.70.$$

They also believed that the duration of non-drug-caused diarrhea would not depend on whether the diarrhea was a sequela to M or was caused by a coincidental gastroenteritis, so they evaluated a single distribution for the duration of non-drug-caused diarrhea (based on their clinical pediatric experience), as shown in Figure 6. (*Note*: The assessors assigned a probability of 0.7 to the first week, but since to do so would be irrelevant to their analysis, they made no attempt to subdivide this probability further.)

The probability assigned by the distribution pictured in Figure 6 to a duration of 9 or more days is 0.22. That is,

$$P(\text{Ch} \mid \text{D} \not\to \text{E}, \text{Ti}) = 0.22.$$

Thus

$$\begin{aligned}\text{LR(Ch)} &= \frac{P(\text{Ch} \mid \text{D} \to \text{E}, \text{Ti})}{P(\text{Ch} \mid \text{D} \not\to \text{E}, \text{Ti})} \\ &= \frac{0.70}{0.22} \\ &= 3.2.\end{aligned}$$

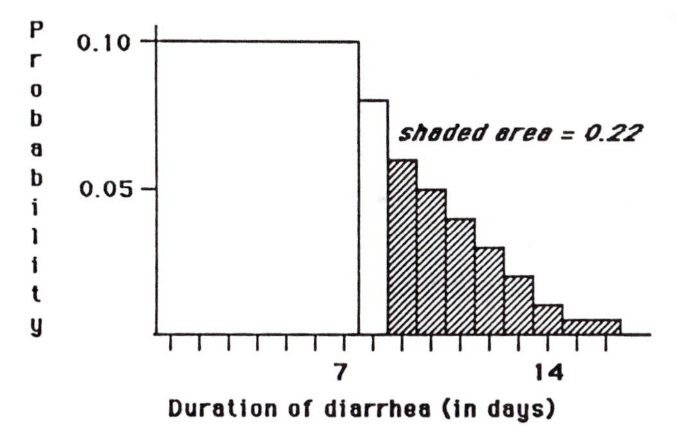

Figure 6 Duration of non-drug-induced diarrhea.

LR(De): The information in De is that the diarrhea resolved within 2 days of dechallenge (i.e., the drug was withdrawn on day 9, and the diarrhea had resolved by day 11). The assessors believed that the time to resolution for D-caused diarrhea had the same distribution as the time to onset, since resolution is a matter of reversing the two processes that determine the onset time, namely the time to accumulation of D in the gut and the time it takes for change in the gut flora and gastrointestinal mucosal function corresponding to the new, D-enriched environment. Hence

$$P(\mathrm{De} \mid \mathrm{D} \to \mathrm{E}, \mathrm{Ti}, \mathrm{Ch}) = 0.33 + 0.33 = 0.66.$$

(*Note*: Ch is included in the conditioning statement because it states that the diarrhea persisted at least until dechallenge.)

On the other hand, their assessment for the probability that resolution would occur within 2 days of dechallenge is determined by the distribution given in Figure 6: it is just the conditional probability of resolution of resolution on day 10 or 11 given that the diarrhea lasted at least 9 days. Thus

$$P(\mathrm{De} \mid \mathrm{D} \not\to \mathrm{E}, \mathrm{Ti}, \mathrm{Ch}) = 0.41,$$

so

$$\mathrm{LR}(\mathrm{De}) = \frac{0.66}{0.41} = 1.6.$$

4.7 Implementation Step 6: Calculate the Posterior Odds Favoring D-Causation

This step is now automatic. The answer is obtained by multiplying together the prior odds and the likelihood ratio factors.

Calculating the Posterior Odds for Example 3

$$\begin{aligned}\text{posterior odds} &= \text{prior odds} \times \text{LR(Hi)} \times \text{LR(Ti)} \times \text{LR(Ch)} \times \text{LR(De)}\\ &= 3.5 \times 0.5 \times 2 \times 3.2 \times 1.6\\ &= 17.2.\end{aligned}$$

Equivalently,

$$\text{posterior probability of D-causation} = \frac{17.2}{18.2} = 0.95.$$

5 IMPLEMENTING THE PROBABILISTIC APPROACH: SOME TECHNICAL ISSUES

5.1 Multiple Drugs

In Examples 2 and 3, there is only one drug on the cause list. Frequently, as in Example 1, there are many, and the problem of multiple drug causal candidates is one of the most difficult aspects of causality assessment. None of the SAM deals with this problem in a satisfactory way; for example, most of them make it possible to report many "probable" drug causes of a single event E.

On the other hand, the problem is easily handled probabilistically, by means of the "one-drug-at-a-time strategy" (Lane et al., 1986). This strategy works as follows. Suppose that $D_1, \ldots, D_n$ are the drug hypotheses on the cause list and that N is the union of all nondrug causes. Let A_i represent "D_i or N" (i.e., A_i is the hypothesis that if E was caused by a drug, the drug cause was D_i). Also, let $PO(D_i)$ represent odds in favor of cause D_i, and $PO(D_i \mid A_i)$ the posterior odds in favor of cause D_i, given A_i. That is, $PO(D_i \mid A_i)$ solves the causality assessment problem for a case otherwise identical to the one under consideration, except that there is only a single drug causal candidate, D_i.

The following formula, which is a consequence of the rules of coherence, gives $PO(D_i)$ in terms of the conditional posterior odds:

$$PO(D_i) = \frac{PO(D_i \mid A_i)}{1 + \sum_{j \neq i} PO(D_j \mid A_j)}. \tag{6}$$

Thus, when faced with a problem in which more than one drug candidate appears on the cause list, the assessor can solve the problem by first addressing a series of problems each of which has only a single drug candidate, and then amalgamating the solutions to these problems using equation (6). See Kramer (1986b) for an example of the application of this strategy.

It is certainly not necessary to use the "one-drug-at-a-time strategy" when carrying out a probabilistic causality assessment. However, assessors tend to become confused (and hence incoherent) when they try to compare directly the possible effects of many drugs. We have found that the strategy helps assessors achieve self-consistency by concentrating their attention on the effects of each drug candidate in turn.

5.2 Missing Information

Physicians who work for pharmaceutical companies or national monitoring agencies do not usually themselves observe suspected adverse drug reactions, but instead rely for their case information on spontaneous reports submitted by attending clinicians. Such reports are notorious for the incompleteness of the information they contain. Thus any causality assessment method should be able to take into account what information is not available, as well as that which is.

However, neither global introspection nor SAM do well in this regard. Experts who are asked to carry out causality assessments based on spontaneous reports frequently say they cannot do so, without the results of this test or the exact time at which that occurred; while others may base their assessments entirely on plausible but highly improbable scenarios that posit particular values to missing quantities and ignore the possibility that these assumptions are in error (Lane, 1984). SAM tend either to exclude missing information from consideration or to count it against the hypothesis of drug causation. How the probabilistic approach handles missing information will now be demonstrated, with respect to two important and common problems.

Noncompliance

A drug cannot cause an event if the patient did not take the drug. We generally know that a patient was prescribed a drug; our knowledge that he actually took the drug as prescribed is not usually so certain. Example 1 gives an extreme instance of this problem.

Here is the probabilistic solution to the problem of noncompliance, when only one particular administration of the drug is under consideration. Let

Com be the proposition that the patient was compliant: she took the drug D as prescribed. Let B be background information as defined previously; so B includes the statement that the patient took D (i.e., Com) and subsequently experienced an event of type E_t. Now let B_0 consist of the noncase information in B, plus the information that a patient with condition M who was prescribed (but did not necessarily take) D experienced an event of type E_t. That is, B is the intersection of B_0 and Com.

The following can then be derived from the rules of coherence:

$$\frac{P(\mathrm{D} \to \mathrm{E} \mid \mathrm{B}_0, C)}{P(\mathrm{D} \not\to \mathrm{E} \mid \mathrm{B}_0, C)} = P(\mathrm{Com} \mid \mathrm{M}) \times \frac{P(\mathrm{D} \to \mathrm{E} \mid \mathrm{B}, C)}{P(\mathrm{D} \not\to \mathrm{E} \mid \mathrm{B}, C)}. \tag{7}$$

In this expression, $P(\mathrm{Com} \mid \mathrm{M})$ is the probability that a "generic patient" with condition M prescribed D will comply with his prescription; it is not calculated conditionally on the patient experiencing an event of type E_t.

Thus (7) can be read as follows. First, evaluate the chance that a patient with condition M who is prescribed D would comply with this prescription. Next, evaluate the posterior odds in favor of D-causation for the particular case under consideration, assuming that the patient actually took D as prescribed. Finally, to calculate coherently the posterior odds that D caused E without assuming compliance, multiply the results of the previous two evaluations together.

For example, suppose that you believe, like Kramer (1986b) that about 80% of the patients who undergo a wisdom tooth extraction and are prescribed an analgesic to take as needed for postoperative pain will take the drug prescribed. Suppose also that you would give 20:1 odds that the zomepirac killed the woman in Example 1, if you knew that she had taken the drug. Then, according to (7), you should give 16:1 odds in favor of zomepirac, based on the actual information provided.

Note: At the conference in which Kramer (1986b) was presented, some eminent experts in adverse reactions expressed the view that their posterior probability that zomepirac caused the woman's death could not exceed their probability that someone would take zomepirac after a wisdom tooth extraction [see Jones and Herman (1986, p. 560)]. Their error, put right by equation (6), consists of mistaking $P(\mathrm{Com} \mid \mathrm{M})$ for $P(\mathrm{Com} \mid \mathrm{M}, \mathrm{E}_t)$. (In words, apparently healthy people who have their wisdom teeth extracted do not necessarily take a drug for pain; but almost no such people die suddenly—and for those who do, something had to kill them.) It is unrealistic to expect global introspection to produce coherent assessments, especially in the face of missing information.

Missing "Vital" Case Information

When an assessor must rely on secondhand case information (e.g., a spontaneous report), he may think of some item of missing information that, for him, would play a decisive role in his causality assessment were it available. In Example 1 there is no mention of whether or not the pathologist checked for a cerebral hemorrhage, which, if present, could provide a possible non-drug explanation for the woman's sudden death. Similarly, a spontaneous report of a case of suspected drug-induced pancreatitis fails to mention whether or not the patient was alcoholic or whether she was checked for gallstones (these are two of the most common causes of acute pancreatitis) (Begaud, 1984).

To state the problem generally, suppose that A is a case information proposition which, if known, would have differential diagnostic significance for the causality assessment. How should the fact that neither A nor A^c is specified in the given data affect the resulting assessment? Let A^* denote the information that neither A nor A^c is specified, and $LR(A^*)$ the contribution of A^* to the posterior odds. The problem, then, is to evaluate the quantity $LR(A^*)$.

At first sight it might seem that "negative information" such as A^* should have no effect on the causality assessment. However, the assessment would have a very different result if A were known to be true than if it were known to be false, and A^* should affect the assessor's opinions about how likely A is to be true. For suppose that whoever submits the report has some chance of appreciating the significance of the truth of A and may therefore have sought to ascertain it: then the chance that the report is submitted at all and given that it is, that neither A nor A^c is mentioned in it, depends to some extent on whether A or A^c is true. Thus A^* should affect the overall causality assessment.

The quantitative effect of A^* is given by the following formula, determined by the rules of coherence:

$$\mathrm{LR}(\mathrm{A}^*) = p + [(1-p) \times \mathrm{LR}(\mathrm{A}^c)], \tag{8}$$

where

$$p = \frac{a}{a+bc},$$

$$a = P(\mathrm{A}^* \mid \mathrm{A}), b = P(\mathrm{A}^* \mid \mathrm{A}^c) - P(\mathrm{A}^* \mid \mathrm{A}),$$

$$c = P(\mathrm{A}^c \mid \mathrm{B}, \mathrm{D} \not\rightarrow \mathrm{E}, \mathrm{S}).$$

Here S is the case information chronologically preceding A. Now c is just the denominator of $LR(A^c)$, and hence would be evaluated in the course of assessing this likelihood ratio factor. The quantities a and b measure the assessor's opinion of the process whereby the case information came to him: that is, for a, he has to decide how likely he thinks it is that the case report would not mention A, if A were actually true (and also, for b, if A were false).

Frequently, as in the two examples of missing case information cited above, A gives strong information in favor of one of the causal candidates (usually nondrug), while A^c gives weak evidence (by default) for the other candidates. In such cases it is reasonable to believe that the author of the case report is more likely not to mention anything about A when A is false than when it is true. From (8) it then follows that $LR(A^*)$ can be regarded as an average of two components: 1, which is the appropriate likelihood ratio factor for information that does not discriminate at all between drug and nondrug causation; and $LR(A^c)$, the likelihood ratio factor that would be appropriate if A were known to be false. The more likely there is to be no mention of A when A is false than when it is true, the more $LR(A^*)$ will resemble $LR(A^c)$. Note that if A is always mentioned when it is true, then $LR(A^*)$ equals $LR(A^c)$ (since A^* then implies A^c); while if there is no mention of A just as frequently when A is true as when it is false (so $b = 0$), then $LR(A^*)$ equals 1 (i.e., there is no information in A^*).

In summary, to evaluate the likelihood ratio corresponding to the fact that a potentially vital piece of case information, A, is simply not mentioned, do the following:

1. Evaluate $LR(A^c)$ [and its denominator, $P(A^c \mid B, D \not\to E, S)$].
2. Evaluate $P(A^* \mid A)$ and $P(A^* \mid A^c)$.
3. Calculate $LR(A^*)$ from equation (8).

5.3 Conditioning and Decomposition

Determining which probability assessment tasks are accessible is largely empirical and highly context dependent. Experts with some probability assessment experience can be queried to discover whether they "feel comfortable" carrying out particular types of assessment tasks. When they do not, they usually complain that they just "don't know" whether or not the proposition in question is true, rather than measure their uncertainty in it. Also, assessment tasks that pose questions that are insufficiently "local" often produce widely varying answers from assessors with similar expertise. It is frequently possible to probe for the sources of such disagreement in the form of information or posited mechanisms that some, but not all, of the disagreeing assessors have taken into consideration.

Once it is determined that an assessment task is too global, how can it be refined to increase accessibility? Two important techniques in this regard are decomposition and conditioning. Decomposition involves expressing a quantity as a series of component parts, each of which relates to a particular feature of the assessor's knowledge and experience. For example, the time to onset of a dose-dependent adverse drug reaction can often be assessed more easily when it is decomposed into three components: T_1, the time it takes the drug or its relevant metabolite to build up to toxic levels at the target organ (which depends primarily on the pharmacokinetics of D); T_2, the time from onset of toxicity until the injury is clinically detectable (which depends primarily on the nature of the event type E_t); and T_3, the time from clinical detectability until detection (which depends on M and E_t and the intensity of surveillance, as well as personal attributes of the patients expressed on Hi). The assessor then must determine what dependencies, if any, there are for him between the distributions for the components. It is often the case, as in this example, that he can regard these distributions as independent (since they will frequently depend on completely different aspects of the drug, event, patient, and surveillance system), in which case the distribution of their sum, the relevant time to onset, can be determined by convolution.

As as example of a situation in which conditioning is appropriate, suppose that an assessor wants to evaluate her distribution for time to onset of an adverse drug reaction, but is uncertain whether the mechanism for this reaction is immunologic or cytotoxic—and her timing distributions given these two possible mechanisms differ. She must then condition on each in turn, evaluate the relevant conditional distributions, determine her probability that each mechanism is actually the operative one, and then calculate the relevant timing distribution by the law of total probability.

To illustrate the use of both these techniques, here is the calculation for LR(Ti) in Example 1, with zomepirac as the drug causal candidate. As described in the preceding two subsections, for this calculation we may assume that zomepirac is the only drug candidate and that the woman actually took zomepirac. However, we do not know when she took the drug, and the only information in Ti is that the coroner placed the time of death at 4 P.M. $\pm$ 2 hours (recall that the surgery took place from 1 P.M. until 1:40 P.M.). Call this datum Ti.

To determine his probability for Ti, given that zomepirac was responsible for the woman's death, Kramer (1986b), first decomposed the time of death into two components: the time at which the zomepirac was taken, and the time between taking zomepirac and death. Kramer's distributions for these quantities are given in Figures 7 and 8. The first of these depends on how long it would take the xylocaine to wear off and the patient's pain threshold,

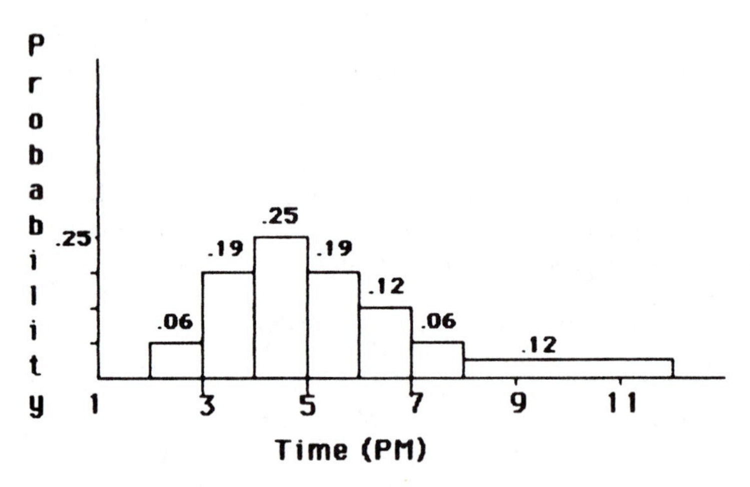

Figure 7 Time at which zomepirac is taken.

while the second depends on absorption time of oral zomepirac and the mechanism of anaphylaxis. Hence the distributions are independent, so their convolution, sketched in Figure 9, gives Kramer's distribution for the time of zomepirac-caused death.

Next, Kramer evaluated his probability for Ti, given that death actually occurred at hour j, for each possible hour j. He based this evaluation on

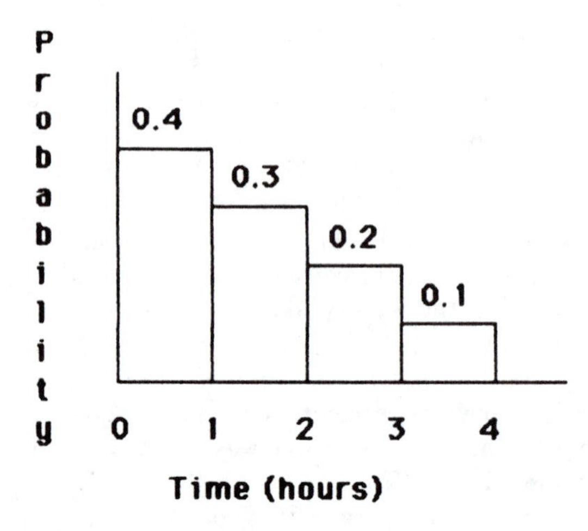

Figure 8 Time between taking zomepirac and zomepirac-caused death.

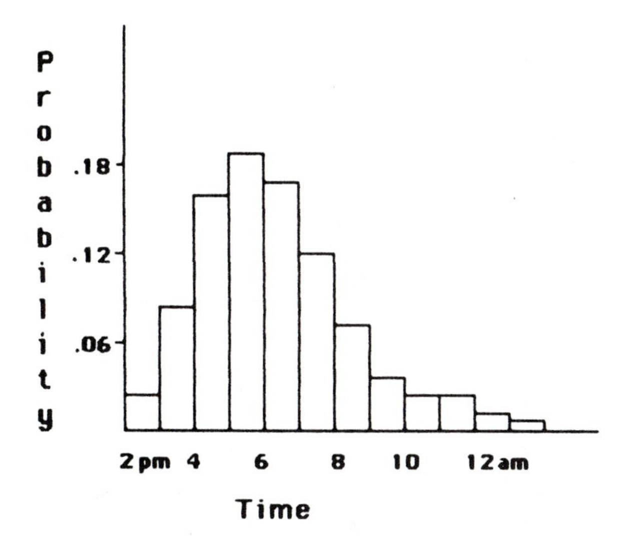

Figure 9 Time of zomepirac-caused death.

the assumption that the coroner's stated time of death would be off by an hour in either direction with probability 0.4, and would be off by 2 hours in either direction with probability 0.2. (This is, of course, a somewhat oversimplified summary of his opinions about the accuracy of pathological techniques for time-of-death determination.)

From the evaluations reported in the preceding two paragraphs, the following calculation follows by the law of total probability:

$$\begin{aligned} &P(\mathrm{Ti} \mid \mathrm{D} \rightarrow \mathrm{E}) \\ &\quad = \sum_j P(\mathrm{Ti} \mid \text{death at hour } j, \mathrm{D} \rightarrow \mathrm{E}) P(\text{death at hour } j \mid \mathrm{D} \rightarrow \mathrm{E}) \\ &\quad = \sum_j P(ti \mid \text{death at hour } j) P(\text{death at hour } j \mid \mathrm{D} \rightarrow \mathrm{E}) \\ &\quad = (0.2)(0.025) + (0.4)(0.094) + (0.4)(0.169) + (0.2)(0.194) \\ &\quad = 0.15. \end{aligned}$$

On the other hand, since given nondrug cause, the woman was judged equally likely to die at any time in the period determined by the time horizon, which was taken to be 24 hours,

$$P(\mathrm{Ti} \mid \mathrm{D} \not\rightarrow \mathrm{E}) = \frac{1}{24} = 0.04.$$

So with these assessments,

$$\mathrm{LR(Ti)} = \frac{0.15}{0.04} = 3.75.$$

5.4 The Prior Odds

Most serious adverse drug reactions are quite rare, with incidences in the range of 1 per 1000 to 1 per 1 million courses of therapy. As a result, few assessors can bring to bear much relevant personal clinical experience in assessing the prior odds. Moreover, there are not many reliable epidemiological data on the incidence of adverse events. Consequently, the prior odds present the most challenging of the assessment tasks required by the probabilistic method.

The factors that are relevant to the assessment of the prior odds are listed below. The order of the factors is determined by how much information about the factor can sharpen an assessor's distribution for the prior odds. Much work remains to be done to develop techniques for converting information about these factors into usable probability distributions for the prior odds.

Frequencies

When epidemiological data are available that allow the assessor to evaluate the quantities $P(\mathrm{E}_t \mid \mathrm{D})$ and $P(\mathrm{E}_t \mid \mathrm{D}^c)$ reliably, as in the analysis of Example 3, the strategy based on equation (5) is the best way to proceed. Usually, some subjective adjustments to published frequencies are necessary to accommodate these data to the appropriate reference set defined by M and E_t.

Sometimes, only indirect frequencies are available. For example, in the analysis of the sudden death case (Example 1), we knew that about 30 cases of fatal anaphylaxis associated with zomepirac had been reported to the Food and Drug Administration (FDA) prior to the receipt of the report on which this case was based. From sales data we estimated that at this time about 10 million patients had been exposed to the drug. To estimate $P(\mathrm{E}_t \mid \mathrm{D})$ from these data, we only needed to estimate the reporting fraction: the proportion of such events that were actually reported to the FDA. This fraction depends on such factors as the seriousness and etiological specificity of the adverse event, the amount of time the drug has been on the market, and the duration of the time interval between drug administration and event (i.e., exactly the factors that play a role in causality assessment). For this case, Judith Jones, who at the time this case was reported was in charge of the FDA's spontaneous reporting system, produced her distribution for the reporting fraction; this distribution had a mean of 20%. Thus the estimate used for $P(E_t \mid D)$ used in the analysis was 1.5 cases per 100,000 patients exposed. A distribution around this figure (for sensitivity analysis) could be generated by our uncertainty distributions for the reporting fraction and the total number of exposures.

Drug Similarity

Are drugs that are similar chemically or pharmacologically to the drug associated with the event?

Event Similarity

Is the drug associated with events that are predictably related to the event in question? (For example, the incidence of agranulocytosis caused by a drug may be predictable from the incidence with which it induces less severe neutropenia, which can be measured on a much smaller study population.)

Mechanism

How biologically plausible is the association?

Analogy of Uncertainty

How does the assessor's uncertain opinions about the strength of this drug-event association compare to his a priori opinions about other such associations, for which the risks have been qualified? [For example, because zomepirac had been withdrawn from the market due to its association with anaphylaxis, the assessor in Kramer (1986b) judged this association to be at least as strong as that of parenteral penicillin with anaphylaxis, which was reported in the literature to be 1:100,000.]

REFERENCES

Auriche, M. (1985). Approche Bayesienne de l'imputabilite des phénomènes indésirables aux médicaments. *Therapie 40*, 301–306.

Bartlett, A., M. Moore, G. Gary, K. Starko, J. Erben, and B. Meredith (1985a). Diarrheal illness among infants and toddlers in day care centers: I. Epidemiology and pathogens. *J. Pediatr. 107*, 495–502.

Bartlett, A., M. Moore, G. Gary, K. Starko, J. Erben, and B. Meredith (1985b). Diarrheal illness among infants and toddlers in day care centers: II. Comparison with day care homes and households *J. Pediatr. 107*, 503–509.

Begaud, B. (1984). Standardized assessment of adverse drug reactions: the method used in France. *Drug Inform. J. 18*, 275–282.

Dangomau, J., B. Begaud, A. Boisseau, and H. Albin (1980). Les effets indésirables des médicaments. *Nouv. Presse Med. 9*, 1607–1609.

de Finetti, B. (1974). *Theory of Probability.* Wiley, New York.

Dukes, M. (1984). Adverse reactions: a changing challenge. *Proceedings of the Second World Conference on Clinical Pharmacology and Therapeutics*, Bethesda, Md., pp. 223–232.

Herman, R., ed. (1984). Drug-event associations: perspectives, methods, and uses, Proceedings of the Drug Information Association Workshop, Arlington Va., Oct. 30-Nov. 2, 1983. *Drug Inform. J. 18*(3,4).

Jones, J., and R. Herman, eds. (1986). The future of adverse drug reaction diagnosis: computers, clinical judgment and the logic of uncertainty, Proceedings of the Drug Information Association Workshop, Arlington Va., Feb. 1–4, 1986. *Drug Inform. J. 20*(4).

Kahneman, D., P. Slovic, and A. Tversky (1982). *Judgement Under Uncertainty: Heuristics and Biases.* Cambridge University Press, Cambridge.

Karch, F., C. Smith, B. Kernzer, J. Mazullo, M. Weintraub, and L. Lasagna (1976). Adverse drug reactions—a matter of opinion. *Clin. Pharmacol. Ther. 19*, 489–492.

Koch–Weser, J., E. Sellers, and R. Zacest (1977). The ambiguity of adverse drug reactions. *European J. Clin. Pharmacol. 11*, 75–78.

Kramer, M. (1986a). Assessing causality of adverse drug reactions: global introspection and its limitations. *Drug Inform. J. 20*, 433–438.

Kramer, M. (1986b). A Bayesian approach to assessment of adverse drug reactions: evaluation of a case of fatal anaphylaxis. *Drug Inform. J. 20*, 505–518.

Kramer, M., T. Hutchinson, L. Naimark, R. Contardi, K. Flegel, and D. Leduc (1985a). Adverse drug reactions in general pediatric outpatients. *J. Pediatr. 106*, 305–310.

Kramer, M., T. Hutchinson, L. Naimark, R. Contardi, K. Flegel, and D. Leduc (1985b). Antibiotic-associated gastrointestinal symptoms in general pediatric outpatients. *Pediatrics 76*, 365–370.

Lane, D. (1981). Coherence and prediction. *Bull. Internat. Statist. Inst. 49*(1), 81–96.

Lane, D. (1984). A probabilist's view of causality assessment. *Drug Inform J. 18*, 323–330.

Lane, D. (1987). Causality assessment for adverse drug reactions: an application of subjective probability to medical decision making. In *Proceedings of the Fourth Purdue Symposium on Statistical Decision Theory and Related Topics* (J. Berger and S. Gupta, eds.), 1, 235–250.

Lane, D., T. Hutchinson, J. Jones, M. Kramer, and C. Naranjo (1986). A Bayesian approach to causality assessment, Tech. Rep. 472, University of Minnesota School of Statistics, Minneapolis.

Lane, D., M. Kramer, T. Hutchinson, J. Jones, and C. Naranjo (1987). The causality assessment of adverse drug reactions using a Bayesian approach. *Pharmaceutical Medicine 2*, 265–283.

Stephens, M. (1985). *The Detection of New Adverse Drug Reactions.* Plenum, London.

Stephens, M. (1987). The diagnosis of adverse medical events associated with drug treatment. *J. Adverse Drug React. Acute Poisoning Rev.* in press.

Venulet, J., G. D. Berneker, and A. G. Ciucci, eds. (1982). *Assessing Causes of Adverse Drug Reactions.* Academic Press, London.

15

Bayesian Metaanalysis

WILLIAM DuMOUCHEL BBN Software Products Corporation, Cambridge, Massachusetts

In this chapter we provide step-by-step instructions for setting up a Bayesian hierarchical model in order to combine statistical summaries from several studies into a single superanalysis which integrates the results from each study. A discussion of the data requirements of the methodology is followed by a specification of a particular Bayesian model designed to be both flexible and easy to use. A set of formulas define all the computations necessary to obtain the posterior distributions of the relevant parameters. An example metaanalysis shows how different specifications of the prior distribution can affect the results.

1 KINDS OF METAANALYSES

1.1 Qualitative Versus Quantitative

Metaanalysis refers to the compilation of a review or synthesis of several presumably related studies or experiments, performed by different researchers, to come to a single overall conclusion. Critical judgments about the accuracy, quality, and/or methodologies of the individual studies are necessary in order to combine them intelligently. Qualitative metaanalyses concentrate on reviewing a set of studies of a particular problem with emphasis on classifying them by qualitative characteristics, such as the kind of measurements taken, the potential biases they were subject to, and the degree to which the conclusions drawn by the original authors were justified, as well as what those conclusions were. The goal of such a research review may be to come to a general conclusion as to which of several competing hypotheses seem most supported by the preponderance of the evidence in the literature.

The focus of a quantitative metaanalysis is on using the specific statistical information from a set of studies in an overall statistical analysis to provide quantitative summary results. For this purpose it may be necessary to conduct an informal, qualitative metaanalysis of a larger set of studies first, in order to select that subset of studies deemed suitable for the quantitative metaanalysis. For example, one might only use studies thought to be free of serious and hard-to-quantify biases, and for which certain necessary statistical summaries are available. Because a quantitative metaanalysis concentrates on performing a single statistical analysis of data from all the selected studies at once, the term *superanalysis* might be a more appropriate term. The book by Light and Pillemer (1984) provides many examples and discussions of both qualitative and quantitative aspects of research reviews. This chapter is limited to discussion and explication of a particular class of quantitative metaanalyses: hierarchical Bayesian metaanalyses. Its purpose is to teach someone who is not a specialist in Bayesian statistics how to set up and use the Bayesian methodology in this important application.

1.2 Classical Versus Bayesian

The book by Hedges and Olkin (1985) surveys classical statistical methods of metaanalysis. The articles by Louis et al. (1985) and Sacks et al. (1987) each review many metaanalyses in the areas of public health and clinical trials. Most authors recommend that a review of the research literature be conducted much like any statistical survey: Define a protocol for inclusion into the review, document the search for studies and list those found and those excluded for various reasons, address questions of combinability and potential biases of the studies used, and define a recognized statistical methodology to be used to combine the results. Preliminary descriptive summaries and graphical displays comparing the studies' results should precede the formal statistical pooling methodology. Of particular concern is the so-called "file-drawer problem," which occurs if those studies which happen to show statistically significant effects have a much greater chance of being published than do studies without significant effects, which remain hidden in their investigators' file drawers.

In this chapter we focus on formal methods of quantitative synthesis, assuming that the important preliminary issues mentioned above, and discussed at length by the referenced authors, have been handled satisfactorily. Many classical statistical methods for combining studies have been used. They include merely counting the number of studies that find a significant result, computing an average effect size across all studies, and computing a single combined level of significance for a set of statistical hypothesis tests, one from each study. Unfortunately, methods for combining significance levels from different studies do not distinguish between small studies with large effects and large studies with small effects. An important distinction is whether the method of synthesis assumes that each study is measuring the same underlying parameter. A common recommendation is first to conduct a formal hypothesis test of between-study homogeneity; only if this test is not significant is one advised to estimate the supposedly common parameter uniting the studies. This recommendation ignores the distinction between failing to reject interstudy homogeneity and proving that it is present. Methods of synthesis that explicitly allow for a component of variance for study-to-study variation avoid this logical fallacy. Such methods usually require more detailed information from the primary studies than do other metaanalytic techniques, but they also usually provide more useful results for scientific and policy purposes.

The hierarchical Bayesian approach is distinguished by the construction and use of a formal statistical model at two levels. First, a parametric model is set up for each of the individual studies, in which a likelihood function relates the distribution of the sample statistics to one or more unknown parameters characterizing that study. Next, a second parametric statistical model is constructed which relates the parameters from the separate studies to each other. The computations involved in combining the two levels of the model are derived by the application of Bayes' formula for conditional probability.

The Bayesian approach is also usually distinguished by having little or no emphasis on hypothesis testing, as opposed to estimation. The Bayesian superanalysis provides a posterior distribution for each study-specific parameter; this will be a satisfying goal if the models are defined in terms of meaningful parameters. Research questions must be phrased as questions about the values of these parameters. The Bayesian model allows data from some studies to assist in the estimation of parameters characterizing the other studies. This notion of different studies "borrowing strength" from each other is a crucial one. However, in most realistic problems the degree to which different studies are relevant to each other is somewhat uncertain. Hence all but the simplest hierarchical Bayesian models also use the data to help decide *how related* the different studies are. Depending on whether or not the estimates from each study accord with the prior beliefs reflected in the model relating the different studies, the studies may or may not be able to borrow strength from each other.

This last fact leads to the conclusion that the model relating the study-specific parameters should embody as much knowledge as possible about the problem area. Knowledge about mechanisms known to relate the different parameters, as well as more subjective knowledge, should be used, as long as the uncertainty of such estimates can be fairly expressed and incorporated into the model. These somewhat abstract principles are illustrated in the example in Section 4, where it should be clear that the ability to incorporate such subjective knowledge into the analysis is a strength of the Bayesian methodology.

2 DATA REQUIREMENTS FOR A BAYESIAN METAANALYSIS

2.1 Estimates of Parallel Quantities from Each Study

To carry out a hierarchical Bayesian analysis on the data from many studies, the data available from each must have a certain commonality or comparability. The requirement of a second-level model relating parameters from the different studies implies that the estimates of these parameters, based on data within each study, have related meanings. This does not mean that the studies to be combined have to be exactly alike. Studies which have exactly the same design and differ only in that they were carried out in different but closely related populations are easily combined using traditional randomized block analyses. Bayesian and classical versions of these random-effects analyses will often have the feature that estimates of parameters from different populations borrow strength from each other to the degree that certain of the variance components are estimated to be small. Rubin (1980) analyzes law school admissions data from 82 law schools using such techniques.

The challenge in most research reviews is that the different studies are purportedly about the same problem but have somewhat different designs, or are based on quite dissimilar populations or treatment comparisons. However, it will often be possible to define analogous parameters to be estimated in each study. For example, a series of carcinogenesis studies may each estimate a relative risk or a standardized mortality ratio (SMR). Even though all the different SMRs might not reasonably be hypothesized to be equal, certain relationships between them may be plausible enough to allow a reasonable statistical model for them to be constructed.

In other situations, each study may estimate the slope of a dose-response curve or the size of a treatment effect. Even though the slopes or effects from different studies may be expressed in widely varying units, it may still be possible to hypothesize approximate relationships between the parameters, as in DuMouchel and Harris (1983), where the dose-response slopes from studies of human lung cancer, mouse skin papillomas, and in vitro cell transformations and mutation rates are used in a Bayesian analysis.

In the social and behavioral sciences, the term "effect size" often has a specific meaning related to a convenient way of relating the power of an hypothesis test to the sample size [see, e.g., Cohen (1977)]. In a comparison of means for treatment versus control groups, the effect size might be defined as the difference in means divided by the standard deviation of the response within the population. One question is whether different studies are more usefully compared by their effect sizes thus defined, or by the simple difference in means unscaled by the response standard deviation. The answer depends on whether it is reasonable to posit a consistent and predictable relationship between the standard deviation and the treatment difference, across studies. If not, the simple difference in means may be more useful and meaningful for the Bayesian superanalysis.

2.2 Variability Measures for Each Parallel Estimate

The second requirement which the data must satisfy is that each of the estimates must be accompanied by its (approximate) standard error. If more than one parameter estimate comes from a single study, one should have estimates of the covariances between estimates taken from the same study. If these estimates are known to be quite rough, as happens if error variances are estimated with few degrees of freedom, the metaanalyst should be able to quantify the uncertainty in the standard errors, in terms of how great the ratio between true and estimated standard errors is likely to be.

The formal Bayesian model presented in Section 3 assumes that the vector of estimates from all studies has a multivariate normal distribution, conditional on the true parameter values and standard errors from all studies. If the individual estimates are not based on very small samples, this assumption is likely to be a good one, and in any case moderate violations of this assumption will not seriously affect the analysis.

A more serious consideration is the fact that many published studies do not contain enough statistical detail to enable the parameter estimates and, especially, their standard errors, to be calculated. A particular author may have taken a different analysis tack than that required by the proposed metaanalysis, or even misanalyzed the data. To construct the needed set of parallel parameter estimates with associated standard errors it may be necessary to reanalyze many of the original data sets. This often requires the cooperation of the original researchers and involves much more time and effort than does the metaanalysis itself. In addition, the construction of the Bayesian model will often be severely constrained by the types of data available from the studies being reviewed.

3 BAYESIAN MODELS RELATING THE TRUE PARAMETERS

3.1 Hierarchical Bayesian Models

Specifying the statistical model relating the true parameters from the various studies, which involves only unobservables, is equivalent to specifying the prior distribution of these parameters. Prior distributions of a set of parameters, when represented as a statistical model conditional on the values of other parameters (hyperparameters), are called hierarchical prior distributions. The article of Lindley and Smith (1972) popularized these types of models; Good (1980) provides a history. A simple and very common example of a hierarchical prior distribution for a vector of parameters $\boldsymbol{\theta} = (\theta_1, \theta_2, \ldots, \theta_K)^T$ is defined by

$$(\boldsymbol{\theta} \mid \boldsymbol{\mu}) \sim N(\mathbf{X}\boldsymbol{\mu}, \mathbf{V}),$$
$$\boldsymbol{\mu} \sim N(\mathbf{m}, \mathbf{D}),$$

where "$\sim$" means "is distributed as," $\boldsymbol{\mu}$ is a vector of hyperparameters which has the normal prior distribution as specified above, the matrices $\mathbf{X}$, $\mathbf{V}$, and $\mathbf{D}$, and the vector $\mathbf{m}$ are specified by the user of the prior distribution. The use of $\boldsymbol{\mu}$ was not necessary to the specification of the distribution of $\boldsymbol{\theta}$; the unconditional distribution of $\boldsymbol{\theta}$ is found by integrating the $N(\mathbf{X}\boldsymbol{\mu}, \mathbf{V})$ distribution with respect to the normal distribution of $\boldsymbol{\mu}$. The result is that, unconditionally, $\boldsymbol{\theta}$ has a normal distribution with mean $\mathbf{Xm}$ and covariance matrix $(\mathbf{XDX}^T + \mathbf{V})$. The advantage of the hierarchical representation in terms of hyperparameters is its intuitive appeal, suggesting a possible mechanism or series of stages giving rise to the generation of $\boldsymbol{\theta}$. The scientist selects $\mathbf{X}$ and the other constants in accordance with the available knowledge of these possible mechanisms.

There are many variations on systems of hierarchical prior distributions, even when we restrict ourselves to those based on the normal distribution, as we do here. For more examples, see Efron and Morris (1973), Smith (1973), Harville (1977), Dempster et al. (1981), Laird and Ware (1982), DuMouchel and Harris (1983), DuMouchel (1987), and DuMouchel and

Groër (1987). Some of these hierarchical systems are only slight variations on each other, and differ from one another more in notation than in substance. But the different versions can be confusing to the nonspecialist, and the lack of a "standard" hierarchical model is perhaps one reason why they are not used more widely. The particular model to be proposed next is meant to be as simple as possible, while remaining flexible enough to be useful in a wide variety of situations.

3.2 A "Standard" Hierarchical Bayesian Model

Let $\mathbf{y}$ be a K-vector of observed statistics, and assume that conditional on $\boldsymbol{\theta}$ and τ, y has a multivariate normal distribution with mean vector $\boldsymbol{\theta}$ and covariance matrix $\tau^2\mathbf{C}$, where $\mathbf{C}$ is a known $K \times K$ matrix and the scalar parameter τ^{-2} has a χ^2/df_τ distribution with df_τ degrees of freedom. In symbols,

$$(\mathbf{y} \mid \boldsymbol{\theta}, \tau) \sim N(\boldsymbol{\theta}, \tau^2\mathbf{C}), \tag{1}$$

$$\tau^{-2} \sim \frac{\chi^2(\text{df}_\tau)}{\text{df}_\tau}. \tag{2}$$

We might assume that $\mathbf{C}$ includes as a factor a sample mean square having df_τ degrees of freedom, or, alternatively, that df_τ is chosen subjectively in accordance with the uncertainty in $\mathbf{C}$.

Further, let the distribution of $\boldsymbol{\theta}$ be represented hierarchically by

$$(\boldsymbol{\theta} \mid \boldsymbol{\mu}, \sigma) \sim N(\mathbf{X}\boldsymbol{\mu} + \mathbf{d}, \sigma^2\mathbf{V}), \tag{3}$$

$$(\boldsymbol{\mu} \mid \sigma) \sim N(\mathbf{0}, \mathbf{D} \longrightarrow \infty), \qquad \text{so } \boldsymbol{\mu} \text{ has a diffuse prior distribution,} \tag{4}$$

$$\sigma^{-2} \sim \frac{\chi^2(\text{df}_\sigma)}{\text{df}_\sigma}, \tag{5}$$

where the $K \times p$ matrix $\mathbf{X}$, the K-vector $\mathbf{d}$, the $K \times K$ matrix $\mathbf{V}$, and the number of degrees of freedom measuring uncertainty in $\mathbf{V}$, df_σ, is to be specified by the user. The interpretation of $\mathbf{X}$ and the diffuse prior distribution for $\boldsymbol{\mu}$ is that the user has virtually no information regarding the p-dimensional subspace of $\boldsymbol{\theta}$ spanned by the columns of $\mathbf{X}$, while in other dimensions of $\boldsymbol{\theta}$ the $N(\mathbf{d}, \sigma^2\mathbf{V})$ distribution describes the user's uncertainty.

This model includes the hyperparameters σ^2 and τ^2, which have prior distributions centered near the value 1. These particular prior distributions are chosen for mathematical convenience so that both the likelihood function for $\boldsymbol{\theta}$ based on $\mathbf{y}$ and the prior distribution of $\boldsymbol{\theta}$ (conditional on $\boldsymbol{\mu}$) are multivariate Student t-distributions. The posterior distribution of $\boldsymbol{\theta}$ given $\mathbf{y}$ can be derived by standard techniques [e.g., as in DuMouchel (1987)]. It turns out to be a mixture of multivariate Student t-distributions, each with degrees of freedom $\mathrm{df}_\sigma + \mathrm{df}_\tau + K - p$. Here we propose to use a multivariate normal approximation to this posterior distribution by computing the posterior mean vector and covariance matrix of $\boldsymbol{\theta}$. The posterior mean vector is

$$E(\boldsymbol{\theta} \mid \mathbf{y}) = \int E(\boldsymbol{\theta} \mid \phi, \mathbf{y}) p(\phi \mid \mathbf{y}) d\phi, \tag{6}$$

where

$$E(\boldsymbol{\theta} \mid \phi, \mathbf{y}) = \mathbf{d} + (\mathbf{I} + \phi \mathbf{V}\mathbf{C}^{-1})^{-1}[\mathbf{X}\mathbf{m}(\mathbf{y}, \phi) + \phi \mathbf{V}\mathbf{C}^{-1}(\mathbf{y} - \mathbf{d})], \tag{7}$$

$$\mathbf{m}(\mathbf{y}, \phi) = [\mathbf{X}^T\mathbf{W}(\phi)\mathbf{X}]^{-1}\mathbf{X}^T\mathbf{W}(\phi)(\mathbf{y} - \mathbf{d}), \tag{8}$$

$$\mathbf{W}(\phi) = (\phi\mathbf{V} + \mathbf{C})^{-1}, \tag{9}$$

and where $p(\phi \mid \mathbf{y})$, the posterior density of σ^2/τ^2, is

$$p(\phi \mid \mathbf{y}) \propto \phi^{-[\mathrm{df}_\sigma + 1]/2} |\mathbf{W}|^{0.5} |\mathbf{X}^T\mathbf{W}(\phi)\mathbf{X}|^{-0.5} \times \left\{ \mathrm{df}_\tau + \frac{\mathrm{df}_\sigma}{\phi} + S(\mathbf{y}, \phi) \right\}^{-[\mathrm{df}_\sigma + \mathrm{df}_\tau + K - p]/2}, \tag{10}$$

where "$|\cdot|$" denotes the determinant of a matrix, and where

$$S(\mathbf{y}, \phi) = (\mathbf{y} - \mathbf{d} - \mathbf{X}\mathbf{m}(\mathbf{y}, \phi))^T \mathbf{W}(\phi)(\mathbf{y} - \mathbf{d} - \mathbf{X}\mathbf{m}(\mathbf{y}, \phi)). \tag{11}$$

The integral in (6) extends from 0 to ∞, but in practice one first evaluates (10) in widening neighborhoods of $\phi = 1$ until $p(\phi \mid \mathbf{y})$ becomes small compared to its maximum value, then normalize $p(\phi \mid \mathbf{y})$ so that it integrates to 1, and approximate the integral in (6) by a summation. Usually, no more than 10 well-chosen values of ϕ are needed to provide sufficient accuracy for computation of $E(\boldsymbol{\theta} \mid \mathbf{y})$ and $\mathrm{cov}(\boldsymbol{\theta} \mid \mathbf{y})$. The latter matrix is computed from the formulas

$$\mathrm{cov}(\boldsymbol{\theta} \mid \mathbf{y}) = \int \{\mathrm{cov}(\boldsymbol{\theta} \mid \phi, \mathbf{y}) + [E(\boldsymbol{\theta} \mid \phi, \mathbf{y}) - E(\boldsymbol{\theta} \mid \mathbf{y})] \times [E(\boldsymbol{\theta} \mid \phi, \mathbf{y}) - E(\boldsymbol{\theta} \mid \mathbf{y})]^T\} p(\phi \mid \mathbf{y}) d\phi, \tag{12}$$

$$\mathrm{cov}(\boldsymbol{\theta} \mid \phi, \mathbf{y}) = c(\mathbf{y}, \phi)[\phi\mathbf{V}\mathbf{W}(\phi)\mathbf{C} + \mathbf{C}\mathbf{W}(\phi)\mathbf{X}(\mathbf{X}^T\mathbf{W}(\phi)\mathbf{X})^{-1}\mathbf{X}^T\mathbf{W}(\phi)\mathbf{C}], \tag{13}$$

$$c(\mathbf{y}, \phi) = \frac{[\mathrm{df}_\tau + \mathrm{df}_\sigma/\phi + S(\mathbf{y}, \phi)]}{\mathrm{df}_\sigma + \mathrm{df}_\tau + K - p - 2}. \tag{14}$$

Although the computational formulas (6)–(14) may seem rather forbidding for a "standard" method, this model has many advantages. First, the computations are readily programmed on a computer since no iterative computations are involved, and the one-dimensional integrals in (6) and

(12) are quite well behaved. (If $\mathbf{C}$ or $\mathbf{V}$ is diagonal, the computations simplify somewhat.) As will be seen in the following examples, the model is flexible enough to accommodate a wide variety of applications. Compared to simpler Bayesian models, the present model derives its flexibility, and its accompanying computational complexity, from the uncertainty associated with the three hyperparameters τ, μ, and σ, specified in (2), (4), and (5), respectively. Models that omit one or more of these hyperparameters are simpler, but are often overoptimistically simple, and ignore scientific uncertainties present in the problem to which they are applied. For example, this model has a desirable property which many simpler models do not: If the data disagree violently with the prior distribution, the variance of the posterior distribution of θ can become larger than $\mathbf{V}$ or $\mathbf{C}$, warning the scientist that the statistical model probably needs revision.

It may be helpful to contrast this hierarchical model with more traditional Bayesian models, as presented, for example, in Box and Tiao (1973). Chapter 9 of that text concerns estimation of common regression coefficients from different sources. The phrase "common regression coefficient" implies, using the notation of the present chapter, that the model assumes an exact relationship between the elements of $\boldsymbol{\theta}$, and that the parameter σ^2 in (3) is assumed to be zero. On the other hand, Box and Tiao (1973) do not assume that $\text{cov}(\mathbf{y} \mid \boldsymbol{\theta})$ is known up to a single scale parameter, as we do in (1). In developing various exact and approximate results for handling the situation when little is assumed known a priori about several sampling variances, each having possibly different degrees of freedom, these authors are led to formulas about as complicated as those presented above. So we see a trade-off in choosing whether to concentrate parametric complexity on the specification of $\mathbf{C}$ in (1) or in $\mathbf{V}$ of (3). The hierarchical model puts equal emphasis on each equation, allotting one parameter to each, while the traditional Bayesian analysis focuses more on uncertainty in the sampling variances in $\mathbf{C}$. [Box and Tiao (1973) do encourage the analyst to make formal and/or graphical checks of any assumptions about relationships between elements of $\boldsymbol{\theta}$.]

In the Bayesian approach, inferential questions involve the posterior distributions of $\boldsymbol{\theta}$ or $\boldsymbol{\mu}$. Such questions are readily answered once the multivariate normal approximation for these posterior distributions is formed. The posterior expectation and covariance matrix of $\boldsymbol{\mu}$ are

$$E(\boldsymbol{\mu} \mid \mathbf{y}) = \int \mathbf{m}(\mathbf{y}, \phi) p(\phi \mid \mathbf{y}) d\phi, \tag{15}$$

$$\begin{aligned}\text{cov}(\boldsymbol{\mu} \mid \mathbf{y}) = \int \{ & c(\mathbf{y}, \phi)[\mathbf{X}^T \mathbf{W}(\phi) \mathbf{X}]^{-1} + [\mathbf{m}(\mathbf{y}, \phi) - E(\boldsymbol{\mu} \mid \mathbf{y})] \\ & \times [\mathbf{m}(\mathbf{y}, \phi) - E(\boldsymbol{\mu} \mid \mathbf{y})]^T \} \, p(\phi \mid \mathbf{y}) d\phi.\end{aligned} \tag{16}$$

Some investigations may require estimates of the variance hyperparameters τ^2 and σ^2. Their posterior expectations are

$$E(\tau^2 \mid \mathbf{y}) = \int c(\mathbf{y}, \phi) p(\phi \mid \mathbf{y}) d\phi, \tag{17}$$

$$E(\sigma^2 \mid \mathbf{y}) = \int \phi c(\mathbf{y}, \phi) p(\phi \mid \mathbf{y}) d\phi, \tag{18}$$

which may be compared to the means of their prior distributions, namely $\mathrm{df}_\tau/(\mathrm{df}_\tau - 2)$ and $\mathrm{df}_\sigma/(\mathrm{df}_\sigma - 2)$, provided that these degrees of freedom are both greater than 2.

3.3 Formulating a Model by Defining y, X, and V

To apply the formulas of Section 3.2, the analyst must supply the quantities $\mathbf{y}$, $\mathbf{C}$, df_τ, $\mathbf{X}$, $\mathbf{d}$, $\mathbf{V}$, and df_σ. Of these, the choice of $\mathbf{y}$, $\mathbf{X}$, and $\mathbf{V}$ typically involve the most skill in the art of model formulation. Once $\mathbf{y}$ is defined, its sampling distribution will automatically determine $\mathbf{C}$ and df_τ. The value of $\mathbf{d}$ is defined as the scientist's best guess for $\boldsymbol{\theta}$ before seeing the data from the individual studies. Once $\mathbf{X}$ and $\mathbf{V}$ are defined, df_σ is determined by a relatively simple process of introspection concerning uncertainty about $\mathbf{V}$. But the specification of $\mathbf{y}$, $\mathbf{X}$, and $\mathbf{V}$ require the user to build in as many realistic components of the situation as possible so that an incisive model results.

For example, defining $\mathbf{y}$ means making a choice as to just which statistics from each study should be included in the metaanalysis. One might take the log of the odds ratio from a frequency table from each study, or the coefficients from a regression analysis from each study, or just simple means or medians. It often boils down to choosing what works or, frequently, what is available, and it may mean that a reanalysis of some of the data from some of the studies is necessary.

For a given definition of $\mathbf{y}$, $\boldsymbol{\theta}$ is defined as the expected or "true" value of $\mathbf{y}$ for each particular study. Defining $\mathbf{X}$ and $\mathbf{V}$ entails representing the connections between the elements of $\boldsymbol{\theta}$ as accurately as possible, while also faithfully representing the uncertainty as well as possible.

One simple example is the choice of $\mathbf{X} = (1, 1, \ldots, 1)^T$, $\mathbf{d} = (0, 0, \ldots, 0)^T$, $\mathbf{V} = v\mathbf{I}$, where $v > 0$, and $\mathbf{I}$ is the identity matrix of order K. Then $\boldsymbol{\mu} = \mu_1$, a scalar, and is the mean of the elements of $\boldsymbol{\theta}$. This prior specification would not place any prior constraints on $\boldsymbol{\mu}$, but would reflect a belief that every difference between two θ's has mean 0 and variance $2v\sigma^2$, conditional on σ. If $\sigma = 1$, then the user believes it very unlikely that θ_1 and θ_2 (or any other pair of θ's) are more than $2\sqrt{(2v)}$ apart, using the "± 2 standard deviations" interpretation of "very unlikely."

The value of df_σ is chosen to reflect the degree of belief that σ is near 1, or equivalently, that the assessment of v was accurate. One interpretation of df_σ is as the "equivalent sample size" measuring the accuracy of v. For example, if $df_\sigma = 3$, then, if the differences between three pairs of θ's were subsequently observed, a revised estimate of v would give equal weight to the original estimate of v and to the information from the three differences. An alternative interpretation of df_σ would focus on the percentiles of the distribution of σ, assuming that σ^{-2} has χ^2/df_σ distribution. Table 1 shows some percentiles of σ under that assumption.

Using Table 1, one sees that if $df_\sigma = 3$, then the "true" standard deviation of each contrast is assumed to lie between 56 and 370% of the nominally assessed value of $\sqrt{2v}$, with 95% probability. The choice of df_σ depends on how much confidence the assessor wants to place in the assessed value of $\mathbf{V}$. Values of $df_\sigma > 10$ are not recommended, since they would result in too great an emphasis on the prior distribution, and too little weight on information about σ present in the data, and summarized in the function $S(\mathbf{y}, \phi)$ of (11). $S(\mathbf{y}, \phi)$ is a quadratic form having $K - p$ degrees of freedom, and if $K - p$ is large (e.g., $K - p = 20$), we want the procedure to give substantially more weight to $S(\mathbf{y}, \phi)$ than to the prior estimate that $\sigma = 1$. (On the other hand, large values of df_τ may be appropriate, since df_τ describes uncertainty in $\mathbf{C}$, the covariance matrix of $\mathbf{y}$, which may be based on many degrees of freedom, depending on the details of the individual studies.)

In defining $\mathbf{V}$, it may be useful to represent $\boldsymbol{\theta}$ as the sum

$$\boldsymbol{\theta} = \mathbf{X}\boldsymbol{\mu} + \mathbf{Z}\boldsymbol{\beta} + \boldsymbol{\delta}, \tag{19}$$

where $\mathbf{Z}$ is a $K \times q$ matrix, $p + q < K$, $\boldsymbol{\beta} \sim N(\mathbf{b}, \mathbf{V}_\beta)$, and $\boldsymbol{\delta} \sim N(\mathbf{0}, v_\delta \mathbf{I})$, independently of $\boldsymbol{\beta}$. Depending on the structure of the problem incorporated into the definition of $\mathbf{Z}$, it may be easier to elicit the values of $\mathbf{b}$, $\mathbf{V}_\beta$,

Table 1 Percentiles of σ, Assuming That σ^{-2} Has a χ^2/df Distribution

df	1	2	3	5	10	50
$\sigma_{0.025}$	0.45	0.52	0.56	0.62	0.70	0.84
$\sigma_{0.1}$	0.61	0.66	0.69	0.74	0.79	0.89
$\sigma_{0.5}$	1.48	1.20	1.13	1.07	1.03	1.01
$\sigma_{0.9}$	8.0	3.1	2.3	1.76	1.43	1.15
$\sigma_{0.975}$	32	6.3	3.7	2.5	1.75	1.24

and v_δ rather than those of $\mathbf{d}$ and $\mathbf{V}$. Then we let

$$\mathbf{d} = \mathbf{Z}\mathbf{b}, \tag{20}$$

$$\mathbf{V} = \mathbf{Z}\mathbf{V}_\beta \mathbf{Z}^T + v_\delta \mathbf{I}. \tag{21}$$

In this situation, the formulas above allow us to compute the posterior means and covariance of $\boldsymbol{\theta}$ and $\boldsymbol{\mu}$, but more is needed to get the posterior moments of $\boldsymbol{\beta}$ and the covariances between $\boldsymbol{\mu}$ and $\boldsymbol{\beta}$. To that end, first define

$$\boldsymbol{\alpha} = \begin{bmatrix} \boldsymbol{\mu} \\ \boldsymbol{\beta} \end{bmatrix}, \qquad \mathbf{b}_0 = \begin{bmatrix} \mathbf{0} \\ \mathbf{b} \end{bmatrix}, \qquad \mathbf{A}(\phi) = \begin{bmatrix} \mathbf{0} & \mathbf{0} \\ \mathbf{0} & (\phi \mathbf{V}_\beta)^{-1} \end{bmatrix},$$

$$\mathbf{U} = \begin{bmatrix} \mathbf{X} & \mathbf{Z} \end{bmatrix}, \tag{22}$$

$$\mathbf{H}(\phi) = (\phi v_\delta \mathbf{I} + \mathbf{C})^{-1}, \tag{23}$$

where the compound vectors and matrices have total extents $p + q$ in accordance with the definitions of their components. Assuming that $\mathbf{U}$, $\mathbf{V}_\beta$, and $\mathbf{H}$ are of full rank, the equations

$$\mathbf{a}(\mathbf{y}, \phi) = [\mathbf{A}(\phi) + \mathbf{U}^T \mathbf{H}(\phi)\mathbf{U}]^{-1} [\mathbf{A}(\phi)\mathbf{b}_0 + \mathbf{U}^T \mathbf{H}(\phi)\mathbf{y}], \tag{24}$$

$$E(\boldsymbol{\alpha} \mid \mathbf{y}) = \int \mathbf{a}(\mathbf{y}, \phi) p(\phi \mid \mathbf{y}) d\phi, \tag{25}$$

$$\begin{aligned} \mathrm{cov}(\boldsymbol{\alpha} \mid \mathbf{y}) = \int \{ & c(\mathbf{y}, \phi)[\mathbf{A}(\phi) + \mathbf{U}^T \mathbf{H}(\phi)\mathbf{U}]^{-1} + [\mathbf{a}(\mathbf{y}, \phi) \\ & - E(\boldsymbol{\alpha} \mid \mathbf{y})][\mathbf{a}(\mathbf{y}, \phi) - E(\boldsymbol{\alpha} \mid \mathbf{y})]^T \} \, p(\phi \mid \mathbf{y}) d\phi, \end{aligned} \tag{26}$$

show how to compute the first two moments of $\boldsymbol{\alpha} = (\boldsymbol{\mu}, \boldsymbol{\beta})^T$. Note that the formulas (24)–(26) are exact matches for formulas (8), (15), and (16), respectively, with the substitutions $\boldsymbol{\alpha} \Leftrightarrow \boldsymbol{\mu}$, $\mathbf{b}_0 \Leftrightarrow \mathbf{0}$, $\mathbf{A} \Leftrightarrow \mathbf{0}$, $\mathbf{H} \Leftrightarrow \mathbf{W}$, $\mathbf{0} \Leftrightarrow \mathbf{d}$, $\mathbf{U} \Leftrightarrow \mathbf{X}$, and $\mathbf{a}(\mathbf{y}, \phi) \Leftrightarrow \mathbf{m}(\mathbf{y}, \phi)$.

Similar incorporation of structure into the elicitation of $\mathbf{V}$ is discussed in more detail in DuMouchel (1988) and DuMouchel and Groër (1987) and shown in the example of Section 4.2. DuMouchel (1988) also demonstrates an interactive computer graphical methodology for eliciting the components of $\mathbf{V}$.

4 AN EXAMPLE METAANALYSIS

4.1 Combining Studies Which Compare Proportions

Janicak et al. (1988) review the literature on the effectiveness of the drug S-adenosylmethionine (SAMe) in treating depression. In each of nine controlled clinical trials, patients were randomly assigned to either SAMe or a control drug, and the proportion in each group judged to have responded positively was recorded. In two of the trials the control drug was a placebo, in six of the trials the control group received a standard antidepressant, and in the ninth trial both types of control groups were used. Table 2 shows the proportion responding in each group in each trial.

Defining $\mathbf{y}$ and $\boldsymbol{\theta}$

For each comparison of a treatment and a control group, we define y to be the difference between the proportion responding to SAMe and the proportion responding in the control group. Other choices, such as the ratio of the two proportions, or the ratio of the odds of responding, might also be made. One reason for choosing the differences is that some of the observed proportions are exactly 0 or 1, making ratios or odds ratios harder to deal with. The parameter θ for each comparison is the "true" difference in proportion responding, measurable if a very large sample were obtained from the populations from which each trial drew. Although there are just nine trials, there are 10 values of y and $\boldsymbol{\theta}$, since the ninth trial involves two comparisons.

Table 2 Sample Size (N) and Proportion Responding (P) in Each Group for Nine Clinical Trials of SAMe

Trial	Type of control	SAMe N	SAMe P	Control N	Control P
1	Placebo	20	1.00	10	0.10
2	Placebo	10	0.40	10	0.00
3	Standard	16	0.69	15	0.60
4	Standard	19	0.53	10	0.80
5	Standard	14	0.36	14	0.29
6	Standard	46	0.78	41	0.73
7	Standard	10	0.90	10	0.90
8	Standard	9	0.78	9	0.67
9	Placebo	6	0.67	5	0.00
	Standard			4	0.75

Source: Adapted from Janicak et al. (1988).

Defining C

The variance of each difference is estimated to be $P_1(1 - P_1)/N_1 + P_2(1 - P_2)/N_2$, where N_1 and P_1 are the observed sample size and proportion responding in the SAMe group and N_2 and P_2 are the corresponding quantities for the control group of a comparison. The covariance between any two y-values is assumed to be 0 (conditional on $\boldsymbol{\theta}$) except for the two comparisons in trial 9, which share the same SAMe group; their covariance is estimated to be $P_1(1 - P_1)/N_1 = (0.67)(0.33)/6 = 0.037$. [It might be better practice to replace the products $P(1 - P)$ in the expressions above by a small number like 0.1 whenever a proportion is exactly 0 or 1, but doing so in this example would make a negligible difference in the outcome. Of course, an exact analysis would use binomial rather than normal likelihood functions, but one purpose in choosing this example was to show that the normal approximation works fine even for these small sample sizes.]

Defining df_τ

When working with binomial proportions, it is customary to assume that sampling variances are known, since they are a simple function of the proportions. So we use a large value for df_τ, namely $\mathrm{df}_\tau = 50$.

Defining X, μ, and d

We define a two-dimensional hyperparameter $\boldsymbol{\mu} = (\mu_1, \mu_2)^T$, where μ_1 is the average difference in proportion responding (over all potential populations of depressed patients) of SAMe groups versus placebo groups, and where μ_2 is the average difference between SAMe groups and groups treated with a standard antidepressant. (Since our model places a diffuse prior on $\boldsymbol{\mu}$ [see equation (4)] this definition of $\boldsymbol{\mu}$ implies that we have decided to ignore any prior information we may have on the values of μ_1 or μ_2 or any relation between them.) To accompany this definition of $\boldsymbol{\mu}$, we define $\mathbf{X}$ to be the 10×2 matrix with elements $X_{i1} = 1$ if the ith comparison involves placebo, 0 otherwise, and $X_{i2} = 1$ if the ith comparison involves a standard antidepressant, 0 otherwise. The parametric model for θ is thus

$$\boldsymbol{\theta} = \mathbf{X}\boldsymbol{\mu} + \boldsymbol{\delta}, \tag{27}$$

where $\boldsymbol{\delta}$ is a vector of 10 population-specific deviations of $\boldsymbol{\theta}$'s from the average over all populations. With no information that any one of the 10 populations has a specific bias for or against exhibiting an effect of SAMe, the elements of $\mathbf{d}$ are all taken to be 0.

Defining V

Using the available knowledge about the reactions typical of populations of depressed patients, it is thought to be very rare that any large populations of patients would differ from the overall average on any particular SAMe-minus-control comparison of proportion responding by more than 0.3. If "very rare" is taken to mean a two-standard-deviation limit, the standard deviation of each δ_i is 0.15. With no information to the contrary, the elements of $\boldsymbol{\delta}$ are assumed to be uncorrelated. Therefore, we define $\mathbf{V}$, the estimated covariance matrix of $\boldsymbol{\delta}$, to be 0.0225 $\mathbf{I}$.

Defining df_σ

The estimate of 0.15 for the standard deviation of each $\boldsymbol{\delta}_i$ was based on relatively little hard data. We would much prefer to have observed as many as 5 or 10 very large clinical trials involving SAMe and then take the sample variance of the resulting set of estimates. Thus we take df_σ to be rather smaller than 5 or 10, say $\text{df}_\sigma = 3$.

Obtaining and Interpreting the Posterior Distributions

Having defined all the parameters that the Bayesian model requires to be specified, one can use the equations in Section 3 to obtain the posterior means and variances of the parameters and hyperparameters. Table 3 displays the values of $\mathbf{y}$, $\mathbf{C}$, df_τ, $\mathbf{X}$, $\mathbf{d}$, $\mathbf{V}$, and df_σ specified above. Table 4 shows the values of the posterior means and standard deviations of θ and compares them to those of $\mathbf{y}$. (For now, ignore the last two columns of Table 4, which are discussed in Section 4.2.) The results under the heading "posterior based on prior from Section 4.1" in Table 4 should be thought of as adjustments to the estimates from the various trials, made in light of the results of the other trials. For example, in the fourth trial, the standard antidepressant had a response rate 0.27 greater than did SAMe. However, taking into account the sampling error and the typical variation from population to population, the value 0.11 (standard deviation 0.12) is a better estimate of the true difference in that trial.

In Table 5, the columns headed "posterior based on prior from Section 4.1" show the posterior means and standard deviations of $\boldsymbol{\mu}$ and the posterior means of τ^2 and of σ^2, computed from (15)–(18). The difference between the proportions responding to SAMe and placebo, averaged over all populations, is estimated to be 0.70 with a standard deviation of 0.12, while there is virtually no difference between the estimated proportions responding to SAMe and standard antidepressants. The posterior expectations of τ^2 and σ^2 are 1.01 and 1.06, respectively. Their prior expectations

Table 3 Values of Input Variables Used in the Analysis of Section 4.1

y ($\times 10^2$)	C ($\times 10^4$)										df_τ
90	90	0	0	0	0	0	0	0	0	0	50
40	0	240	0	0	0	0	0	0	0	0	
9	0	0	294	0	0	0	0	0	0	0	
−27	0	0	0	291	0	0	0	0	0	0	
7	0	0	0	0	310	0	0	0	0	0	
5	0	0	0	0	0	86	0	0	0	0	
0	0	0	0	0	0	0	180	0	0	0	
11	0	0	0	0	0	0	0	439	0	0	
67	0	0	0	0	0	0	0	0	370	370	
−8	0	0	0	0	0	0	0	0	370	839	

x	d	V ($\times 10^4$)										df_σ
1 0	0	225	0	0	0	0	0	0	0	0	0	3
1 0	0	0	225	0	0	0	0	0	0	0	0	
0 1	0	0	0	225	0	0	0	0	0	0	0	
0 1	0	0	0	0	225	0	0	0	0	0	0	
0 1	0	0	0	0	0	225	0	0	0	0	0	
0 1	0	0	0	0	0	0	225	0	0	0	0	
0 1	0	0	0	0	0	0	0	225	0	0	0	
0 1	0	0	0	0	0	0	0	0	225	0	0	
1 0	0	0	0	0	0	0	0	0	0	225	0	
0 1	0	0	0	0	0	0	0	0	0	0	225	

were df/(df − 2), or 1.04 and 3.00, respectively. Since df_τ was large, the expectation of τ^2 was hardly affected by the data, while that of σ^2 changed quite a bit, since there are $K - p = 8$ degrees of freedom in **y** available for estimating σ^2, while df_σ was only 3. The fact that σ^2 is estimated to be near 1 indicates that the data support the estimate of **V** elicited for the analysis.

4.2 Adding More Specific Prior Information

The analysis above did not use any knowledge relating the two control treatments to each other. In fact, there is much accumulated evidence on the proportion of depressed patients who respond to the standard antide-

Table 4 Comparison of Estimates and Standard Deviations: Original Data Versus Posterior Distributions Arising from Two Different Prior Specifications

				Posterior based on prior from:			
		Original data		Section 4.1		Section 4.2	
Trial	Type of control	Est.	(SD)	Est.	(SD)	Est.	(SD)
1	Placebo	0.90	(0.09)	0.84	(0.09)	0.81	(0.09)
2	Placebo	0.40	(0.15)	0.56	(0.13)	0.45	(0.12)
3	Standard	0.09	(0.17)	0.04	(0.12)	0.09	(0.13)
4	Standard	−0.27	(0.17)	−0.11	(0.12)	−0.10	(0.14)
5	Standard	0.07	(0.18)	0.03	(0.12)	0.09	(0.13)
6	Standard	0.05	(0.09)	0.03	(0.08)	−0.01	(0.08)
7	Standard	0.00	(0.13)	0.00	(0.10)	0.01	(0.11)
8	Standard	0.11	(0.21)	0.04	(0.13)	0.13	(0.14)
9	Placebo	0.67	(0.19)	0.70	(0.12)	0.68	(0.13)
	Standard	−0.08	(0.29)	−0.02	(0.14)	0.05	(0.16)

pressants, compared to a placebo. This information can be used to sharpen the analysis relating SAMe to the two types of controls.

The best way to do this would be to integrate data from studies comparing the standard antidepressants to placebos directly into the metaanalysis.

Table 5 Estimates of Hyperparameters for the Analysis of Nine Clinical Trials Involving SAMe

	Posterior based on prior from:			
	Section 4.1		Section 4.2	
Hyperparameter	Mean	(SD)	Mean	(SD)
μ_1 (SAMe vs. placebo)	0.70	(0.12)	0.52	(0.11)
μ_2 (SAMe vs. standard)	0.00	(0.09)	0.08	(0.09)
β (placebo vs. standard)	0.70	(0.14)	0.44	(0.10)
τ^2	1.01	—	1.02	—
σ^2	1.06	—	1.71	—

For each such trial, let the corresponding element of $\mathbf{y}$ be the proportion responding to the standard minus the proportion responding to placebo. The corresponding row of $\mathbf{X}$ would have elements $(1, -1)$, since $\mu_1 - \mu_2$ represents the difference between the overall response rates to standard and placebo. In all other respects, the metaanalysis would then proceed exactly as in Section 4.1.

However, suppose for this example that the specific data from these other trials were not available, but that it was desired to incorporate subjective information about the relationship between the standard and placebo treatment into the analysis. For example, the scientist might believe that the difference $\boldsymbol{\beta} = \mu_1 - \mu_2$ is probably about 0.3 and almost certainly between 0.1 and 0.5. Or, approximately, that $\boldsymbol{\beta}$ has a normal prior distribution with mean 0.3 and standard deviation 0.1. Then, if we let $\mathbf{X}_0$ be a 10×1 matrix of all ones, and $\mathbf{Z}$ be a 10×1 matrix with 0 for the comparisons of SAMe with placebo, and -1 for the comparisons of SAMe with the standard, the model for $\boldsymbol{\theta}$ can be represented as

$$\boldsymbol{\theta} = \mathbf{X}_0\mu_1 + \mathbf{Z}\boldsymbol{\beta} + \boldsymbol{\delta}. \tag{28}$$

Since $\boldsymbol{\beta} = \mu_1 - \mu_2$, (27) and (28) are equivalent parametric equations for $\boldsymbol{\theta}$. However, the two statistical models for $\boldsymbol{\theta}$ differ in the prior distributions on the parameters. In (27), $\boldsymbol{\mu}$ has a two-dimensional diffuse distribution. In (28), μ_1 has a diffuse distribution but $\boldsymbol{\beta}$ has a $N(0.3, 0.01)$ distribution. In both models $\boldsymbol{\delta}$ has a $N(\mathbf{0}, 0.0225\mathbf{I})$ distribution, independent from $\boldsymbol{\mu}$.

Next we use (20) and (21) to define $\mathbf{d}$ and $\mathbf{V}$ for this example, using the values $b = 0.3$ and $\mathbf{V}_\beta = 0.01$, and also use $\mathbf{X}_0$ instead of $\mathbf{X}$ in the formulas for performing the Bayesian analysis. For example, we get $\mathbf{d} = (0, 0, -0.3, -0.3, -0.3, -0.3, -0.3, -0.3, 0, -0.3)^T$ and a revised $\mathbf{V}$, 49 of whose elements have been increased by 0.01. The rightmost columns of Tables 4 and 5 display the results of using this alternative prior distribution.

Comparing the estimates in Table 4 from the two prior specifications, the general patterns are quite similar. The estimates for comparisons with a placebo are all a bit smaller for the second analysis, while those for comparisons with the standard have almost all increased. This is in accord with the extra prior information that the two types of controls are not expected to differ by as much as they did in the data. There is a conflict between the fact that $\mu_1 - \mu_2$ is estimated to be 0.7 [with a standard deviation of 0.14, found by considering the covariance matrix of $\boldsymbol{\mu}$ in (16)] in the absence of prior information about $\boldsymbol{\mu}$, and to have a prior mean of 0.3 with a prior standard deviation of 0.1. Also, 9 out of 10 of the posterior standard deviations in the later analysis are as large or larger than those from the first analysis. This is in spite of the fact that the second prior specification was more informative—it replaced a diffuse prior by a rather narrow proper prior! This is an example of how the hierarchical prior can react to a situation where the data conflict with prior beliefs.

Table 5 shows that when the data are analyzed under the second set of prior assumptions, the posterior expectation of σ^2 is 1.71, compared to 1.06 from the first analysis. This larger estimate of variance contributes to the increased posterior standard deviation of many of the estimates. The estimate of μ_1 has also decreased substantially, from 0.70 to 0.52, and the estimate of μ_2 has increased from 0.00 to 0.08, in accordance with the information in the prior specification that $\boldsymbol{\beta} = \mu_1 - \mu_2$ is small. Note that the posterior standard deviation of $\boldsymbol{\beta}$ is about the same as the prior standard deviation, 0.10, even though seemingly precise data on $\boldsymbol{\beta}$ were analyzed. If a traditional Bayesian analysis combined a normally distributed estimate having a standard error of 0.14 with a normally distributed prior having a standard deviation of 0.10, the resulting posterior distribution would have a standard deviation of 0.08. Having seen the incompatibility between the assumed accuracies of the estimate and the prior distribution of the parameter, the scientist can either revise his or her opinion as to their accuracies, or merely explain the discrepancy as the occurrence of a rare event, but at least the analysis gives insight as to just how discrepant are the two assumptions.

5 CONCLUSION

In this chapter we have developed and refined a Bayesian hierarchical model for combining results from different studies. Using the formulas set out in Section 3, step-by-step instructions are given for defining the necessary components of the model and carrying out the calculations to arrive at the posterior means and variances of the parameters of interest. Section 2 includes a discussion of the data requirements for use of the methodology, and Section 4 provides a two-part example of the procedure in action.

The procedure is not as completely automatic as, say, fitting a classical least squares regression model has become with the aid of modern software. First, programs to perform the calculations laid out in Section 3 are not yet generally available. The Bayesian computations need to be integrated into a statistical package so that the entire process of data analysis, including data entry, data management, exploratory graphics, and other statistical procedures besides Bayesian inference, are conveniently available. (The reader should contact the author to ascertain the current availability of software.)

Second, forming a Bayesian hierarchical model will never be as automatic as running a classical regression analysis because the need to tailor the model to the situation will always require careful consideration. This in an inevitable cost of having a method that makes use of all available information. It takes effort to make use of the information appropriately. It might help if we included more practice in setting up statistical models as part of university statistics and data analysis courses. The purpose of this chapter has been to show that there can be a systematic approach to performing a Bayesian metaanalysis, especially if we standardize on a particular simple but flexible version of the Bayesian hierarchical framework.

Acknowledgment. Research for this paper was supported by the National Cancer Institute and l'Institut National de la Santé et la Recherche Médicale, France.

REFERENCES

Box, G. E. P., and G. C. Tiao (1973). *Bayesian Inference in Statistical Analysis.* Addison-Wesley, Reading, Mass.

Cohen, J. (1977). *Statistical Power Analysis for the Behavioral Sciences.* Academic Press, New York.

Dempster, A. P., D. B. Rubin, and R. K. Tsutakawa (1981). Estimation in covariance components models. *J. Amer. Statist. Assoc. 76*, 341–353.

DuMouchel, W. (1988). A Bayesian model and a graphical elicitation procedure for multiple comparisons. *Proceedings of the Third Valencia Meeting on Bayesian Statistics* (J. Bernardo et al., eds.). University Press, Valencia, Spain.

DuMouchel, W., and P. Groër (1987). A Bayesian methodology for combining radiation studies. *Proceedings of the Conference on Modeling for Scaling to Man*, Richland, Wash., Battelle Memorial Institute. (To be published in *Health Physics*, 1989.)

DuMouchel, W., and J. Harris (1983). Bayes methods for combining the results of cancer studies in humans and other species (with discussion). *J. Amer. Statist. Assoc. 78*, 293–315.

Efron, B., and C. Morris (1973). Combining possibly related estimation problems (with discussion). *J Roy. Statist. Soc. B 35*, 379–421.

Good, I. J. (1980). Some history of the hierarchical Bayesian methodology. *Bayesian Statistics* (J. M. Bernardo et al., eds.). Valencia University Press, Valencia, Spain.

Harville, D. A. (1977). Maximum likelihood approaches to variance components estimation and to related problems (with discussion). *J. Amer. Statist. Assoc. 72*, 320–340.

Hedges, J. V., and I. Olkin (1985). *Statistical Methods for Metaanalysis.* Academic Press, Orlando, Fla.

Janicak, P. G., J. Lipinski, J. M. Davis, J. E. Comaty, C. Waternaux, B. Cohen, E. Altman, and R. P. Sharma (1988). S-Adenosyl-methionine (SAMe) in depression: a literature review and preliminary data report. *Alabama J. Medical Sciences 25*, 306–312.

Laird, N. M., and J. H. Ware (1982). Random-effects models for longitudinal data. *Biometrics 38*, 963–974.

Light, R. J., and D. B. Pillemer (1984). *Summing Up: The Science of Reviewing Research.* Harvard University Press, Cambridge, Mass.

Lindley, D. V., and A. F. M. Smith (1972). Bayes estimates for the linear model (with discussion). *J. Roy. Statist. Soc. B 34*, 1–41.

Louis, T. A., H. V. Fineberg, and F. Mosteller (1985). Findings for public health from metaanalyses. *Annual Rev. Public Health 6*, 1–20.

Rubin, D. B. (1980). Using empirical Bayes techniques in the law school validity studies (with discussion). *J. Amer. Statist. Assoc. 75*, 801–827.

Sacks, H. S., J. Berrier, D. Reitman, V. A. Ancona-Berk, and T. C. Chalmers (1987). Metaanalyses of randomized controlled trials. *New England J. Med. 316*, 450–455.

Smith, A. F. M. (1973). Bayes estimates in one-way and two-way models. *Biometrika 60*, 319–329.

16

Inferential Problems In Postmarketing Surveillance

DAVID A. LANE University of Minnesota, Minneapolis, Minnesota

NIGEL S. B. RAWSON* Drug Safety Research Unit, Southampton, England

1 INTRODUCTION

Many serious adverse effects of drugs cannot be identified in the clinical trials required to demonstrate efficacy prior to marketing, either because they occur too rarely, or because there is too long a time delay between the initial use of the drug and the appearance of the adverse event. As a result, these adverse effects are first encountered in the uncontrolled world of everyday clinical practice. To detect and quantify these serious adverse effects, on the basis of information captured from everyday practice, is the task of *drug safety postmarketing surveillance* (PMS).

The difficulties that face PMS workers are formidable:

1. *The range of possible PMS problems.* There are many possible drug-event connections, and almost as many have actually been observed at

*Current affiliation: Institute of Cancer Research, Royal Cancer Hospital, Belmont, Surrey, England

least once in a potentially causal chronological sequence: the drug is administered to a patient, who subsequently experiences the adverse event. So PMS must cast a broad net.

2. *The size of PMS study populations.* Serious adverse effects that are not detected in clinical trials are generally quite rare, with incidences of the order of 1 per 1000 exposed patients or less (D'Arcy, 1986; Inman, 1985; Jick, 1977, 1984), yet they may still have important public health consequences. Thus, to accrue adequate data on these effects, PMS systems must monitor very large patient populations.
3. *The profusion of confounders and effect modifiers.* The population of patients who are prescribed a particular drug in everyday practice is often very heterogeneous, contributing to a profusion of possible confounders and effect modifiers. In particular, the patients may suffer from a wide variety of clinical conditions and take a number of other drugs, and these conditions and drugs may themselves cause the adverse effect under study. In addition, the chance that the drug of interest (and the other possible causes as well) will cause the event in question can depend strongly on many different demographic, genetic, behavioral, and medical characteristics, such as age, sex, race, acetylation rate, alcohol consumption, and concomitant medication [see, e.g., D'Arcy (1986)].
4. *The nonstationarity of drug-event connections.* PMS workers cannot rely on spatial or temporal stationarity in the drug-event relationships they study. The propensity for particular drugs to cause particular adverse events can vary across time (as with the outbreak of bismuth salts-associated neuropathies in France, described by Martin-Bouyer et al. (1980), after over 75 years of widespread and problem-free use) and place (as with the singular clioquinol-associated SMON epidemic in Japan (Gent and Shigematsu, 1978).

Discussions of these and other PMS problems, and some of the methods that have been developed to cope with them, can be found in several excellent reviews of PMS activities, including Carson and Strom (1986), Castle et al. (1983), Faich et al. (1987), Feinstein (1974), Finney (1971), Inman (1986), Jick et al. (1979), Jones (1985), Rawson (1989), and Wardell et al. (1979). In this chapter, rather than summarize the *statistical* techniques commonly used in PMS research, which are covered elsewhere in this volume and in some of the previously referenced survey articles, we focus on some *inferential* problems that arise as a result of the difficulties of PMS listed above. Section 2 is concerned with the *objectives* of PMS inference: What aspects of a particular drug-event connection should PMS try to find out about, and in what form should the resulting conclusions be expressed? The appropriate *objects* about which PMS inferences ought to be made are also discussed in this section. Section 3 categorizes the various possible *sources of data* on which PMS inference can be based and examines what each can contribute to the achievement of PMS objectives.

2 INFERENTIAL OBJECTIVES AND OBJECTS FOR PMS

2.1 The Objectives of PMS Inference

PMS research is applied science; its aim is to produce information that can be used to guide clinical and public health decisions about the proper use of marketed drugs. All these decisions depend on the answers to questions of the following form: Should a particular drug be used in a particular way for a particular class of patients? To answer this question, it is necessary to evaluate the net health benefit that the patients can expect to experience with drug use, taking into account both beneficial and adverse effects, compared with what they can expect with alternative treatments. According to the normative theory of decision making under uncertainty, two features of the connection between a specified drug use and a particular adverse effect determine the contribution it makes to evaluating net benefit: how frequently the event occurs among the patients who use the drug in the specified way (to be compared with the same frequencies among those who do not use the drug), and how seriously the event compromises the health of those who do experience it [see Lane (1987) and Lane and Hutchinson (1987)]. The seriousness of the event is a question of values, which the decision makers have to come to grips with somehow; the frequency with which the drug and the event are associated is the subject of PMS research.

Inference from PMS research has a qualitative and a quantitative component. Qualitatively, the first (and most basic) problem is to determine whether a drug D can in fact cause an event E to occur. Second, if D can cause E, it is important to understand who is at risk, and in what circumstances, since the risk posed by D for an event E may differ widely depending on the dosage and duration of usage and on various clinical, genetic, demographic, or behavioral patient characteristics. Once the relevant determinants of risk have been identified, the quantitative problem comes to the fore: to estimate the probability that a patient who uses D will experience the event E as a function of the characteristics that determine this risk. It is of course also important to keep track of how much uncertainty there is about estimates of the risk for E, taking all the available information into account, in order to see how well founded are decisions that depend on analyses that use the estimates. After all, one decision that public health regulatory bodies may take is to obtain additional information intended to reduce their uncertainty about the risk of a drug's adverse effects, before any action restricting the use of the drug is taken.

2.2 The Objects of PMS Inference

One of the most important determinants of risk is *time* relative to first drug use. For any particular schedule of drug use, the risk faced by the user changes throughout the time the patient is on the drug, and then decreases monotonically at some point after drug use ceases. The way in which risk varies with time depends on the mechanism whereby the drug causes the effect to happen. For example, if a drug taken chronically causes an adverse effect by an immunologic mechanism, the probability that the effect will become manifest at time t to a new user is initially nearly zero, but increases with t as susceptible users become sensitized and react, and then decreases with further increasing t, since nonsusceptible users increasingly predominate among the relevant using population. Other mechanisms can be associated with quite different patterns of risk variation with time.

Because of this dependence of risk on the time course of drug use, O'Neill (1987) and Miettinen (1987) have emphasized the importance of incorporating time directly into the definition of the primary quantitative object about which PMS inferences ought to be made. We agree with them and suggest that the proper representation for the primary PMS inferential object is the *event onset density function*, $p_{E|A,D,T}(t)$. Here D specifies the dosage and schedule according to which the drug is to be taken over some time interval $[0, T]$; A specifies a set of patient attributes that determines a risk class of interest; E is an adverse event type; and p is a nonnegative function on $[0, T+S]$, such that the area under p between a and b gives the probability that a user with attributes A and use pattern D will (first) experience an event of type E in the time interval (a, b), and S is the longest time interval in which it is supposed that the drug used in the specified way can continue to cause E after the discontinuation of its use. The probability that a patient with attributes A who uses D will ever experience the event E in the interval $[0, T + S]$ is the integral of p over this interval. The event onset density function $p_{E|A,D,R}$ for a patient who uses the drug as specified by D only during the time interval $[0, R]$, where $R < T$, is equal to $p_{E|A,D,T}$ *up to* R; however, the tail of this density, from R to $R + S$, cannot be obtained from $p_{E|A,D,T}$, except in quite special circumstances.

It is not yet standard practice in formal PMS studies to estimate the event onset density function. In fact, techniques for doing so need to be developed. Some ideas and procedures may be borrowed from those used in survival analysis (see Chapter 11) and density estimation, while specific parametric models for event onset density functions will have to be tailored according to specifications based on pharmacological, immunological, and pathophysiological principles.

The most popular objects for PMS inference in current use, unlike the event onset density function, ignore time as a determinant of risk. These objects include three categories of risk: absolute risk, attributable risk, and relative risk. Absolute risk is the probability that a patient exposed to the drug D will develop the event E; this is just the area under the onset density function between 0 and $T + S$. Attributable risk is the difference between the absolute risk and the background risk (the probability that the same patient will develop the event E if he is not exposed to D), while relative risk is the ratio of the absolute and background risks.

What are the consequences of ignoring time in these concepts of risk? Consider the absolute risk, the most basic of the three. It is generally thought of (and estimated) in terms of a ratio. The numerator in this ratio is the number of cases of E in the reference population. But what should the denominator be? One possibility is the number of patients exposed; another is the total quantity of drug used by the patients in the population, measured in such units as defined daily dose or cumulative time on drug. Either of these indices presents difficulties, whose origin lies in the fact that both give an inadequate summary of the *population distribution* for duration of exposure (assuming a fixed dosage and frequency of administration). Duration of exposure depends on many factors, including the condition for which the drug is prescribed and its severity, patient compliance and tolerance of minor side effects, and changing fashion in physician prescribing behavior. The exposure duration distribution among patients in everyday clinical practice can be spread quite widely, and the distributions for different populations of patients (or even the same population at different points in time) can differ substantially. Since the cumulative risk to a patient depends on the duration of his exposure, the exposed patients in the reference population may face very different risks for E from one another, depending on the duration of their exposures; thus the absolute risk (with either number of patients exposed or total drug consumed in the denominator) represents an odd sort of averaged risk.

Moreover, if different populations have different distributions for duration of exposure, their absolute risks will differ, even if the individuals in the two populations share the same event onset density function. Thus it is difficult to see how to use the observed ratio of cases of E to patients exposed (or total drug consumed) in a study population as a direct estimate of the reference population's absolute risk, without verifying (or simply assuming) that the two populations have the same distributions for duration of exposure, which is typically quite unrealistic. Without this assumption, to adjust the estimate properly would require knowledge of the duration distributions for the two populations, as well as the common event onset density function! Under these circumstances, the absolute risk is difficult to interpret, and thus it is even more difficult to see how it can be used to guide clinical and public health drug management decisions. Similar considerations apply to attributable risk and relative risk.

When it is reasonable to suppose that a population whose members have been treated with D has an exposure duration that has very little variation, the absolute risk (with number of exposed patients in the denominator) is the right object to use in any decision analysis about the use of the drug. If the decision in question is whether to use D or no drug for a particular individual, and that individual's values are measured on the utility scale, the attributable risk is the multiplier of the utility of the adverse event E in the expression for the difference between the expected utility given D and the expected utility given no drug, and thus it too has a natural role to play in making decisions. Similarly, when comparing two different drugs, the difference in their attributable risks multiplies the utility of E in the expression for the relevant difference in expected utilities.

In contrast, in the absence of knowledge of the background risk for E without D, the relative risk has no obvious role in decision making, except in the trivial situation in which there are two possible treatments of which one is at least as beneficial as the other and has lower relative risk than the other for each possible adverse event. Once trade-offs enter the picture, it is essential to consider the actual magnitudes of the relevant probabilities. Of course, estimating relative risk may have value in the *qualitative* component of PMS inference, since a high relative risk suggests that D can in fact cause E (assuming that the members of the study population who did not receive D are otherwise exchangeable with those who did, except for the occurrence of E). However, it is important to realize that a careful analysis of single cases, as described in Chapter 14, can also lead to the same conclusion, much less expensively in terms of money and human suffering than would be the case if a study was mounted whose purpose was merely to estimate relative risk.

In this section we have emphasized the role of time as a determinant of risk. Of course, there may be other important determinants, and whenever possible the reference population should be stratified into risk classes defined by the values of these determinants, in such a way that all the individuals in a given class are regarded as exchangeable with respect to their risk for E. In the definition of the event onset density function, the attribute set A determines such a class. The more heterogeneous with respect to risk are the populations for which any of the effect measures discussed in this section are defined, the more difficult to interpret are the measures and the more restricted is the class of possible decisions to which these measures may be applied.

2.3 Expressing Uncertainty

Just as it is the aim of PMS *research* to generate information that affects opinions about whether, to whom, under what circumstances, and how frequently a drug D causes an adverse event E to occur, it should be the aim of PMS *inference* to measure the plausibility of propositions about these matters in the light of all the available evidence. Many accounts of PMS research in the published literature do not attempt to engage in this inferential endeavor. Instead, they simply describe the conditions under which the research was carried out and provide summaries of the data obtained. Such accounts provide part of the raw material on which PMS inference should be based. However, increasingly, researchers carrying out formal PMS studies are relying on conventional frequentist statistical procedures to generate inferential statements based on the data they collect. They use significance tests to address the problem of whether or not D can cause E, they construct confidence intervals around one of the three risk measures discussed above (usually the relative risk) to express uncertainty about how frequently D causes E, and they are even beginning to infer about "to whom" and "under what circumstances" based on the estimation of parameters in logistic regression models.

For the following three reasons, we believe that the use of these frequentist modes of inference to express uncertainty about the propositions of primary PMS interest is misguided:

1. The propositions whose plausibility it is the aim of PMS inference to measure refer to predictions about what will happen to a reference population consisting of the drug users who will be affected by some contemplated clinical or public health action. On the other hand, the frequentist inferential statements described above refer only to the population observed in a particular PMS study. The study results are not directly generalizable, unless the study and reference populations match with respect to each determinant of risk. Thus the critical question of the external validity of the study results is not addressed in frequentist inference, yet it introduces a major—often a dominating—source of uncertainty about the relevance of the study results to the predictive problem of primary interest. What is the point of reporting a *quantitative* inferential statement in the form of a confidence interval for relative risk, only to qualify its relevance with a lengthy *qualitative*

discussion of possible biases arising from the study design and execution? Unfortunately, this is the typical form of "inference" reported in current formal PMS studies [see e.g., IAAAS (1986)].

2. Even if the results of a single study were directly generalizable to the reference population of interest, there is typically additional information from other sources—including other formal studies, data from spontaneous reports, even theoretical considerations regarding pharmacology or pathophysiological mechanism—that can have an effect on the predictions of interest. The kind of frequentist inferential statements described above cannot be combined with this other information to yield overall inferences about what will happen in the reference population. What role, then, do these statements play in the decision-making process that is the whole *raison d'être* of PMS? Rational decision making in the face of uncertainty requires inferences based on all the available evidence; quantifying each piece of evidence in a form that can only be combined with the rest by the crude qualitative process of global introspection is not much help.
3. Frequentist inferential statements derive from probabilistic models that purport to describe the procedures whereby the study data were generated. If these models do not reflect the real opinions of the inferrers about what actually happened in the study, neither do the resulting inferences. Some of the models describe the way in which the study populations were selected from some larger population (often assumed to be the reference population of interest) or the way in which "treatments" (i.e., drugs) were assigned to subjects. These descriptions rarely provide literal descriptions of the conditions under which PMS studies are carried out, and even as metaphors they have serious and obvious flaws to anyone who takes the trouble to interpret the underlying probabilistic statements into ordinary language. Some models, for example the increasingly popular logistic regression model, purport to describe the way in which adverse events are actually determined by various patient attributes and other factors. However, these models may completely misrepresent what experts think about the mechanisms by which drugs cause adverse events. For example, Kramer et al. (1987) point out the biological implausibility of a multiplicative model for the risk accruing from multiple drug use, as posited by IAAAS (1986). The key point is that unless the models actually *represent* what the experts think, the inferences based on them omit a critical source of uncertainty, uncertainty about the validity of the models themselves.

More extended discussions of the limitations and lack of relevance of study-based formal frequentist inferences to PMS can be found in Jesdinsky (1977), Finney (1971, 1977), and Johnson (1984). These authors offer no other alternative than a kind of numerate skepticism: what Jesdinsky calls "dialectic control" and the "sure eye," and Finney "a critical outlook on numbers." These are no doubt important in formulating reasonable qualitative responses to the results of PMS research and the other information that can affect decisions about the postmarketing management of drugs. But are there any quantitative alternatives?

We believe that Bayesian analysis can provide a framework in which to give a formal expression to the uncertain predictions that are necessary to guide drug use decisions. Bayesian analysis is an attempt to quantify Jesdinsky's "dialectic control." The advantages that derive from this quantification, compared to the qualitative approach advocated by Jesdinsky and Finney, are discussed by Lane (1986).

Two attributes distinguish Bayesian analysis from frequentist inference. The first is the broad view that it takes of what evidence can be assimilated into an analysis. All the modes of knowledge available to experts—theory, data from formal studies, observation and experience—can yield evidence that can be incorporated into a Bayesian analysis. Second, in a Bayesian analysis, all uncertainty, from whatever source, is measured in the same scale, that of subjective probability. This makes it possible to use the laws of probability to combine the uncertainty about propositions that arises from different sources and to merge different streams of evidence to obtain an overall measure of the plausibility of the propositions of primary inferential interest. The use of the laws of probability in this way is supported by a normative theory for reasoning in the face of uncertainty, the theory of coherent inference developed by de Finetti [see de Finetti (1974)]. These two attributes make Bayesian analysis well suited for dealing with the uncertainty that arises in PMS inferential problems, as discussed above (see also Chapters 14 and 15).

3 DATA SOURCES FOR PMS INFERENCE

PMS draws its data from the world of everyday clinical practice. This world has two features that make PMS inference difficult. First, everyday clinical practice is *unmonitored*; consequently, PMS investigators have to adopt an *active* information-gathering strategy if they are to obtain any information at all. In this section we review some of these strategies, focusing on the choice of the PMS study population and the implications of this choice for PMS inference. Second, everyday clinical practice is *nonexperimental*; thus PMS investigators cannot decide which of the individuals that they study receive which treatments—all they can do is to decide whom to watch and what to watch for. This creates inferential problems for each type of study that we discuss.

In any PMS study population, there will be individuals who have received a drug D and subsequently experienced an adverse event E. In a sense, these individuals provide the inferential core of the PMS study. PMS inferential problems have to do with qualitative and quantitative comparisons between this group of individuals and other groups who do not experience D and E in a potentially causal chronological sequence. In particular, to estimate the event onset density function or the absolute risk, it is necessary to compare the "core individuals" with those who take D and do not subsequently experience E, while determining the attributable risk or relative risk requires a further comparison with a group of individuals who do not receive D (but are otherwise fungible with those who do).

How the core individuals get included in the study population, and who else is there with whom they can be compared, are critical factors that set the upper limit to what can be learned about the connection between D and E from the study. There are four possibilities for how these individuals can come into the study population. First, the condition for entry may be that an individual belongs to the core group; then the population consists only of individuals who have taken D and subsequently experienced E. Second, the study population can be recruited by identifying individuals who experience E; the study will then determine which of these had previously been exposed to D. Third, the study population can comprise a group of individuals who take D, and the study will discover which of these subsequently experience E. Finally, the study population may consist of a group of individuals whose medical histories are under surveillance for other purposes, and the study can identify the subpopulation whose members have taken D, the subpopulation whose members have experienced E, as well as the core individual subpopulation whose members have taken D and subsequently experienced E.

Each recruitment procedure has implications regarding how completely the core group can be ascertained, what comparisons between core individuals and others can be made, and how extensive and reliable is the information collected about each individual in the study population. We will discuss some of these implications for each recruitment procedure in turn, and point out how they affect how useful the resulting study data will be toward achieving the PMS goals of determining relevant risk classes and quantifying the extent of risk.

3.1 Recruiting Core Individuals: Suspicion-Based Studies

There are two types of PMS studies in which an individual must have taken D and then experienced E before his case is admitted to the study population. The first type describes a (generally quite small) case series of patients assembled by an individual practitioner; these case descriptions provide information about patients of the practitioner who have been prescribed D and then experienced E. The second type is based on similar data, obtained from so-called spontaneous case reports submitted by practitioners to an industrial or national monitoring agency. In both these study types, cases are subjected to a more or less explicit causal prefiltering before they are admitted to the study population; a practitioner who does not believe that D *can* in fact cause E—and may well *have* done so, in the cases at hand—will not submit a report or construct a series. Thus it is fair to say that *suspicion of a causal drug-event connection* is the primary condition that a case must satisfy before it is admitted to these study populations, and we shall refer to studies of these two types as *suspicion-based studies.*

Because the study population is composed entirely of core individuals in suspicion-based studies, it is not possible to make any PMS inferences, even qualitative ones, solely on the basis of study data. However, it is sometimes possible to synthesize these data together with other available information to draw strong qualitative conclusions about the nature of the $D-E$ connection and even in some circumstances to develop useful bounds on the frequency with which D causes E. Here is an example, based on Fagius et al. (1985), where such bounds were obtained and regarded as strong enough to justify regulatory action. During 1982 and 1983, the Swedish Adverse Drug Reaction Advisory Committee (SADRAC) received 13 reports of the occurrence of Guillain-Barré syndrome in patients treated with zimeldine, a new antidepressive drug. All the reported events had a fairly similar onset time in relation to the commencement of therapy, which seemed biologically consistent with zimeldine causation. To determine whether the drug-event connection was in fact causal, the analysts first obtained information about the total sales of zimeldine in Sweden and inferred the total time on treatment for all patients exposed to the drug. They then estimated the background incidence of Guillain-Barré syndrome from several epidemiological studies of different populations, including one in Sweden. They concluded that the zimeldine users in Sweden experienced Guillain-Barré syndrome at least 20 times more frequently than expected from the estimated background incidence. Finally, they argued that there was no other plausible explanation for this increase, in terms of the attributes of the patient population or exposures to other known etiological agents. This argument gives strong support to the proposition that zimeldine can cause Guillain-Barré syndrome.

One additional ingredient is necessary to produce an estimate of the attributable risk for zimeldine-induced Guillain-Barré syndrome: What fraction of all the cases of Guillain-Barré syndrome that occurred subsequent to zimeldine therapy were reported to the committee? Fagius and his coworkers did not attempt to estimate this reporting fraction, since their estimate of attributable risk based on the assumption that all cases were reported was deemed already sufficiently high to justify the withdrawal of zimeldine from the market. In general, the reporting fraction depends on many factors in a complicated way [see Faich et al. (1987)], but in some situations it can be estimated (and the uncertainty about this estimate can be assessed, too). For example, by examining hospital records to ascertain all cases of hospitalized cytopenias, following up to obtain information about drug use, and comparing these data with the spontaneous reports they had received, SADRAC workers were able to estimate the reporting fraction for drug-induced cytopenias in the early 1970s to be about 0.3 [see Böttiger and Westerholm (1973) and references therein]. There is a need for much more work on the problem of estimating the reporting fraction, since multiplication by the fraction's reciprocal converts the number of cases received by a monitoring agency to an estimate of the number of times patients taking D subsequently experience E. To solve this problem, it is essential to generate a distribution describing uncertainty about the actual value of the reporting fraction; a point estimate is not good enough.

Inferences based on data from suspicion-based studies must take into account uncertainties from many sources, including the following:

1. *Multiple sources of evidence.* To carry out the kind of synthetic inference that is required with suspicion-based studies, many estimates using data from different sources must be used: for example, exposure estimates based on drug sales, background incidence estimates based on epidemiological studies of different populations, and reporting fraction estimates based on special validation studies. Each of these introduces uncertainty into the overall inference, from sampling variability in the source studies, as well as about the relevance of these studies to the problem at hand.
2. *Data quality.* Spontaneous reports are submitted by busy practitioners who are not themselves experts in adverse drug reactions, and there are inevitably problems with missing, misleading, and erroneous data.
3. *Case selection.* For new adverse reactions that have unique features compared to well-established reactions, causal prefiltering can intro-

duce biases, as only cases that conform to familiar drug-event patterns are likely to be reported. More generally, any of the reasons for reporting or not reporting can introduce correlations between the propensity of practitioners to report and the frequency with which their patients experience the adverse event in question.

It is nevertheless important to get the most out of the relatively fast and cheap information that comes from suspicion-based studies. The kind of synthetic inference described above seems the only way to do so. However, this kind of inference can be convincing only to the extent that such factors as those listed above are explicitly taken into account in the analysis and some attempt is made to measure the uncertainty introduced by each of them. Such a program is daunting, but there has been a lot of progress recently in implementing it [see Shaw et al. (1988) for a particularly impressive example].

3.2 Event-Based Studies

Event-based studies start with the problem of identifying a "representative" group of individuals who have experienced a particular event E. Virtually the only practical way to solve this problem is to identify those individuals who receive medical care for E. In particular, if E is sufficiently serious that afflicted individuals generally require hospitalization, the so-called "cases" that make up the study population are recruited from among those admitted to hospital for E, or whose condition (E) is subsequently diagnosed in hospital. This identification, and the collection of information about the individuals identified, may be carried out retrospectively from hospital records, or prospectively as new patients are admitted to hospital. Prospective event-based studies offer an important potential advantage over retrospective event-based studies or suspicion-based studies: the investigators themselves can take responsibility for data acquisition, rather than relying on secondary sources such as physician reports or hospital records, so they can enforce standardization of the meaning of data elements and the conditions under which the data are collected. In particular, it is possible to ensure that the information obtained about individuals who had taken D before they experienced E is truly comparable with that obtained about those who had not.

How complete is the ascertainment of core individuals in an event-based study? First, not every case of E may be identified, either because an afflicted individual who lives in the catchment area of a hospital taking part in the study may not present for treatment at that hospital, or because, even if he does, his condition may not be recognized as a case of E. For example, suppose that E is agranulocytosis, as in IAAAS (1986). Cases of agranulocytosis are identified when the afflicted neutropenic individuals develop infections that require hospitalization. However, individuals who suffer from a transient neutropenia may fail to develop such an infection; the more time-limited the neutropenia, the more probable it is that this will be so, and therefore that this source of underascertainment will operate differently for different causes of the neutropenia. Even if individuals present at hospital, blood counts may not be carried out or may be erroneous [see Offerhaus (1987)]. Finally, an infection may develop of such virulence that the patient may die before neutropenia is diagnosed. In none of these situations would the E-afflicted individual be admitted to the study population.

Cases that are not ascertained will of course affect estimates of the event onset density function or the absolute and attributable risk that are derived from the study. They may even affect estimates of the relative risk, if the probability of ascertaining a case depends on whether or not the afflicted individual had received D prior to experiencing E. This situation can easily occur, since for many conditions ascertainment depends on the extent to which an individual has access to the medical system, and receiving D can be both a sign and a cause of a greater than average degree of medical access. That is, patients who are prescribed drugs see doctors; and patients who take drugs for serious underlying medical conditions may see doctors frequently. In addition, diagnostic tests required to identify E may be carried out more frequently if the patient is known to have received a drug that can cause E.

However troublesome the uncertainty about the extent of case ascertainment in event-based studies, the situation with respect to information about the use of D by the cases that have been identified is much more problematic. Consider the IAAAS, which in this respect is typical of most event-based studies: information about what drugs the agranulocytosis "cases" had taken prior to the onset of their disease was obtained only from patient interviews. The ability of people to remember what drugs they have taken, even in the recent past, has been probed in a few studies, and the results are not very encouraging [see, e.g., Mitchell et al. (1986) and Klemetti and Saxén (1967)]. The problem is compounded when it is important to recall just *when* the drugs were taken in relation to the onset of an event that may have begun well before the hospitalization that led to case identification. For example, some of the analgesics investigated by the IAAAS as possible causes of agranulocytosis are taken in response to the early symptoms of the infections to which the patient's neutropenia predispose them. Thus the exact timing relationship of drug taking and the onset of E is critically important, and it may relate to events occurring months before the patient is interviewed. Analyzing the results of such interviews without accounting for uncertainty introduced by the fallibility of memory is just folly. The attitude of the IAAAS to this question is unfortunate, and sadly not atypical for such studies; after discussing the possibilities of underascertainment of cases and exposures to D, among other difficulties, they conclude that "on balance, we judge that the results are not materially biased" (IAAAS, 1986, p. 1755)—and proceed to estimate relative and attributable risk, along with "confidence bounds" for these estimates, as though they had ascertained every case, drug use, and timing relationship with complete accuracy.

The only individuals in an event-based study population with whom the core individuals may be compared have experienced E, but have not taken D. This comparison cannot be used to estimate any of the quantities that are the objects of PMS inference. Thus, to carry out PMS inference from event-based studies, it is necessary to augment the study population. The usual strategy is to form a control group comprised of individuals who have *not* experienced E. There is a lot of controversy about how to select this group—in particular, about how closely it should be matched to the group of cases. One thing, however, is clear: it is not possible to estimate absolute or attributable risk unless the controls are chosen in such a way that they may be regarded as a random sample, with *known sampling proportion*, from a well-defined population at risk for E (e.g., the general population in the study hospitals' catchment areas, or the population of individuals in these areas with specified demographic or clinical attributes who form a risk class of interest to the investigators). This situation rarely obtains in so-called case-control or case-referent studies. When it does not, it is still possible to estimate the relative risk, following an observation of Cornfield (1951) that if E is rare both among those exposed to D and those not so exposed, the odds ratio (the ratio of the proportions exposed to unexposed among cases and the same ratio of proportions among controls) can serve as an estimate of the relative risk. (Just *what* relative risk this odds ratio estimates depends on the population from which the controls were selected; in particular, if controls are selected to match cases with respect to particular demographic or clinical attributes, as is frequently the case, the relevant relative risk is one for a population of individuals whose relevant attributes are distributed as they are among the cases, which may be difficult to interpret prospectively).

It is generally very difficult to select a control group as an actual random sample from some population of interest, especially considering how important it is that the information about the individuals in the control group be elicited in such a way that it is comparable with that elicited from the cases. A common solution is that adopted by the IAAAS: controls are selected from among the patients who are admitted to the hospitals in which cases are identified for conditions supposed by the study investigators to be unrelated to the use of the drugs of interest. For example, the IAAAS used as controls patients admitted for acute conditions "not known to be caused, prevented by, or otherwise associated with analgesic use (e.g., trauma and acute infections)" and patients "admitted electively for long-standing conditions thought not to influence analgesic use (e.g., hernia)" [IAAAS (1986) p. 1751]. These patients can then be subjected to exactly the same interviews about drug use as are the cases; that is the advantage of this approach. Are such patients really like a "random sample" from the population at large with respect to their patterns of drug use and their distribution for characteristics that predispose to blood dyscrasias? There are fairly evident reasons to doubt that they are, described by Kramer et al. (1987) and Offerhaus (1987). Even if these hospitalized control patients do represent the general population, are the relevant comparisons of cases really with the general population, or with individuals who are otherwise clinically and demographically exchangeable with users of a drug D, except that they do not use the drug? Attributable risk is clearly about the latter comparison (see Chapter 14 for a detailed discussion of this point in the context of the meaning of the proposition that "drug D causes event E"), so it is difficult to see how to interpret the IAAAS' "excess risk" estimate based on a control group that is supposedly representative of the general population in their study catchment areas.

There are certainly some advantages to event-based studies. Information collected in such studies is more reliable (or at least, consistently interpretable) than data obtained from suspicion-based studies. In addition, because most serious conditions that can be drug-caused are quite rare, event-based studies are usually cheaper and less unwieldy than are drug-based studies. It is, however, wrong to analyze the results of these studies with methods of inference that are premised on the completeness of case ascertainment, the accuracy of information obtained from patient recall, and the "representativeness" of the ascertained cases and controls. It is essential to come to grips with all the sources of uncertainty about the meaning and significance of the data, and this will require the integration of many judgments that rely on information and opinion beyond the study data themselves. It is not sufficient merely to announce that "the results are not materially biased" and then compute significance probabilities and confidence intervals based on sampling models bearing little relation to either the aims or the methods of the event-based study itself.

3.3 Drug-Based Studies

Drug-based studies begin by assembling a collection of patients who have been prescribed a particular drug D. These cohorts of D-takers must be very large, since only a small percentage of patients taking D will experience serious adverse events. Thus drug-based studies face difficult logistic and quality control problems. On the other hand, they have one important advantage over event-based or suspicion-based studies: the relevant group to compare with the core individuals to estimate the event onset density function and the absolute risk are, at least in principle, included in the study population—namely, those individuals who take D and do not experience E. In actual practice, since drug-based studies recruit those who are *prescribed* D, it is hard to see how to carry out a drug-based study investigating nonprescription drugs such as dipyrone, the primary target of the IAAAS. Even for prescription drugs, it is important to determine the extent to which those prescribed D may fail to take it, as well as the extent to which they may share their drug with individuals who have no prescriptions, and to take these estimates of the difference between those prescribed D and those who take D into account in carrying out PMS inference from drug-based studies.

How do drug-based studies recruit their cohorts of those prescribed D? The most direct access is through dispensing pharmacies. Thus, in a prototype study carried out by the Upjohn Company, pharmacists at 11 participating clinics recruited patients who presented prescriptions for antibacterials (Borden and Lee, 1982). It is also possible to identify patients through the prescribing physician, as in a postmarketing study of ketotifen in the United Kingdom, described by Maclay et al. (1984). A less direct but more centralized model is provided by the Drug Safety Research Unit (DSRU), an independent organization in Southampton, United Kingdom, which runs an ongoing series of drug-based studies organized into a system called Prescription-Event Monitoring (PEM). PEM relies on the national clearing house for all pharmaceutical prescriptions in England, the Prescription Pricing Authority (PPA), to supply the DSRU with photocopies of all the prescription forms issued by general practitioners for a specific set of drugs. Thus a PEM cohort should consist of every individual prescribed a drug D in England, until a selected number of patients have been assembled, currently 20,000 for a drug newly released for use in general practice [Inman (1987)]. Whichever of these identification methods are used, because the individuals in a drug-based study population are identified at the time they are first prescribed the target drug, it is possible to ascertain the time at which drug treatment begins with considerably more accuracy than in a typical event-based study that relies on patient recall.

Once a drug-taking cohort is assembled, a drug-based study faces its most daunting task: how to obtain standardized, reliable information on all the adverse events experienced by each of the many (typically 10 to 20,000) individuals in the cohort. The data may be obtained directly from patients, perhaps with follow-up from medical personnel, as in Borden and Lee (1982). Or the prescribing practitioner may serve as the primary data source, as is the case in PEM, which identifies the prescriber from the photocopy supplied by the PPA. In the PEM procedure, each such practitioner is sent a questionnaire—the so-called green form—usually on the first anniversary of the initial prescription for the drug. The green form asks for information about any adverse medical and social events that the patient has experienced since the drug was prescribed; the physician is specifically urged to refrain from causally prefiltering the events that he or she reports. While the information supplied by the practitioner in PEM is of course obtained retrospectively, it is based on written documentation: the practitioner's case notes and reports relating to the hospitalization of patients.

How good are the data received by PEM? There is a lot of missing information. About a third of the questionnaires in each study are note returned to the DSRU, despite the unremitting efforts of the Unit's staff to encourage compliance and the promise of complete confidentiality in DSRU treatment of the data. From those practitioners who do cooperate, not all relevant information is received. The patient may have experienced an event without seeking treatment for it, or may be lost to follow-up because he left the physician's practice, or the practitioner himself may have retired or relocated. In addition, the busy physician may decide that some events are not sufficiently interesting to bother reporting or simply omit them inadvertently. It is important to realize that all these missing data cannot be modeled as though they were "missing at random"; for example, elderly patients are more likely to be lost to follow-up than younger patients, since they may enter old persons' homes or terminal care hospitals.

To illustrate the extent of the missing data problem, in a recent study of enalapril (Inman et al., 1988), of 15,169 green forms received by the DSRU, 1456 were void, mainly because the patient had left the prescriber's practice. Another 1170 responses in the enalapril study gave no dates for the duration of treatment, and the date of the event was omitted for 11% of the recorded events. For 809 of the 1109 reported deaths in the study, it could not be determined from information on the green form whether the patient was still taking enalapril at the time of his death, and no cause was recorded on the form for 598 of the deaths.

A further difficulty arises with data actually received. They are not uniformly reliable; a follow-up of all 1109 patients who were reported to have died during the course of the enalapril study revealed that 11 had in fact *not* died. Moreover, the data elements in PEM studies are difficult to interpret consistently, because each participating practitioner makes individual choices about the terminology he employs and the extent of detailed case information he returns to the DSRU. As a result, the data collected in PEM can only be standardized by workers at the DSRU, who have no direct access to the patients in question. As of yet, no validation study had been carried out to measure the quality and reliability of the data obtained from green forms, nor is it possible to evaluate the direction or extent of nonresponse bias introduced by the noncooperating practitioners. Without some plausible estimates of the magnitude of the uncertainty introduced by these data quality problems, it is difficult to generate reasonable inferential conclusions from PEM data.

Suppose that the problems of data completeness and reliability described above could be solved. What could then be inferred from the information collected in PEM? First, it would be possible to discover how the incidence of adverse events varies as a function of whatever baseline data (demographic characteristics, underlying clinical condition, other medications prescribed) that practitioners were asked to submit about patients prescribed D, up to the constraints imposed by the frequency of the events and the size of the D-prescribed cohort. Second, if information was collected about the time at which events begin and the periods during which patients are on and off drug treatment (as PEM currently attempts to do), it would be possible to estimate the event onset density function and the absolute risk, as functions of characteristics defining (sufficiently large) risk classes of D-takers. As stated above, none of these inferences can be carried out from suspicion-based or event-based studies, without augmenting the study population and making (and justifying!) some delicate judgments of partial exchangeability between individuals in the original and augmented populations.

To estimate relative and attributable risks, it is necessary to compare the experiences of those who take D with those who do not. Since individuals get included in drug-based study populations only when they are prescribed a drug, it is not clear that it is possible to generate such comparisons without augmenting the study population. However, the DSRU has developed two strategies that may be applied to this problem in special circumstances. The first of these may be used for inferences relevant to decision problems that require comparison of adverse event risks for patients who take a particular drug with otherwise exchangeable patients who take a different drug. Such comparisons are relevant particularly when "no treatment" is simply not a feasible option for the class of patients under consideration [Kramer et al. (1987)]. In these situations it may be possible to recruit drug-based cohorts for each of the drugs under consideration and then to estimate the ratio or difference of the risks for adverse events for the patients in these different, drug-defined cohorts. It is of course necessary to check the extent to which the cohorts are similar with respect to other attributes that can affect the patients' propensities to experience the events in question from causes other than the drugs, and perhaps to make adjustments for differences in the distributions of these attributes when necessary. An example of the construction of such comparable drug-based cohorts by the DSRU, involving five nonsteroidal anti-inflammatory drugs, has been presented by Rawson (1987), although, due to limited facilities, the analysis was not carried as far as that suggested here.

The second DSRU strategy is an observational version of a crossover trial (Chapter 8). The practitioners in PEM are asked to report on adverse events experienced by their patients during at least one calendar year after the drug is first prescribed; where appropriate, this year can be divided up into periods in which the patient is on and off drug treatment. The incidence of adverse events in these two (variable-length) periods can then be compared across all the patients in the cohort. Clearly, there are many questions that must be addressed about a particular drug-event connection before it is possible to decide whether this procedure can yield meaningful comparisons that could be used to estimate interpretable relative or attributable risks. For example, why do patients stop taking the drug? Are they healthier than when they were treated, or have they become worse and require different, perhaps "stronger" treatment? Is the reason for ceasing treatment related to their propensity to experience adverse events due to the drug or to other causes? How long after the patients stop treatment are they still at risk for events caused by the drug? Although DSRU workers are presently carrying out analyses based on their crossover strategy, they have not developed any theory that could be used to determine what inferences can be drawn from this strategy, and in what circumstances. Nevertheless, the idea is intriguing, and there may well be a class of situations in which it can be usefully applied.

3.4 Record-Linkage Studies

Imagine an ideal world in which to practice PMS. In this world, all the individuals in a particular geographic area would be identified, and all the interesting events of everyday clinical practice relating to each of these individuals would be coded into a standardized and fully informative language and entered into a master database as they occurred. The events recorded would include summaries of every visit of a patient to a practitioner: details about patient complaints, tests administered with results, physician diagnoses and management decisions, including drugs prescribed (and pharmacy records of those prescriptions actually dispensed would be in the system as well). Similarly, all hospital admissions would be recorded, with details of in-hospital diagnoses, treatments, and discharge summaries. The system would also include a vital statistics registry containing such information about each individual in the population as birth date, sex and, at death, date and presumed cause. The data base would be organized in such a way that the records corresponding to groups of individuals defined by any recorded attribute or experience could be abstracted and statistically analyzed. Moreover, it would be possible to identify the individuals in these groups and locate paper versions of their medical records, as well as the patients themselves.

Such a system, extended over a sufficiently populous area, would make all the PMS information-gathering methods described in the previous three subsections obsolete, at least for prescription drugs. Spontaneous reports would serve no purpose, since the system could be used on a routine basis to monitor the connection between every event requiring medical attention and every prescribed drug. There would be no need to set up special and expensive prospective event-based studies, as in IAAAS (1986), since, if needed, the relevant populations could be identified retrospectively; nor would it be necessary to rely on patient recall to discover which patients had been prescribed which drugs. Clearly, the system would supplant PEM, since it would not be restricted in the number of drugs it could study at one time and it would not require the long lag-time of PEM to study effects of interest, nor would it suffer from PEM's problems of missing information and unstandardized terminology. With such a system, every potentially relevant comparison between cohorts could be carried out whenever scientific or policy interest required.

Of course, no such system exists, and there are great obstacles standing in the way of creating one: programming problems including the formidable difficulty of constructing the standardized language to describe all relevant clinical events, quality control problems of ensuring (or at least precisely estimating the extent of) the validity of the information in the system, ethical problems of guaranteeing confidentiality to the individuals in the population, political problems of establishing the degree of centralization in health care implied by the system, and the economic problems posed by the tremendous startup and operating costs of such a system. Nevertheless, there are some record linkage systems already in place that offer some of the advantages of the ideal system. For example, the Group Health Cooperative of Puget Sound (GHC), a health maintenance organization with about 300,000 members, has computerized, linkable records of its pharmacy prescriptions, of all hospital discharge diagnoses of its members, and of the deaths of its members. In addition, GHC patients can be interviewed by telephone. GHC has cooperated with the Boston Collaborative Drug Surveillance Program on a number of PMS studies [for discussion and examples: Jick (1985), Porter et al. (1982), and Jick et al. (1987)]. However, even a population size as large as that of GHC is not sufficient to resolve some of the important problems that face PMS researchers, such as the possible association between nonsteroidal anti-inflammatory drugs and peptic ulceration (Jick et al., 1987).

Another potentially useful and larger system, which also links pharmacy data with hospital discharge information and includes a vital statistics registry and a cancer registry, records information on the approximately 1 million residents covered by the Saskatchewan Health Services (Strand, 1985). A prototype study based on this system is reported by Guess et al. (1987). Somewhat similar systems exist for other centralized health systems, particularly in the Scandinavian countries [see, e.g., Aromaa et al. (1976)].

Several PMS investigators in the United States use data obtained from the Medicaid system. While this system contains observations on a much larger group of people than those mentioned above, it is primarily a billing system and there is good reason to mistrust much of its diagnostic data. In addition, the population that it monitors is very unstable, as individuals' eligibility status changes. Nevertheless, some very interesting studies have been carried out based on Medicaid data [see, e.g., Morse (1985), Ray et al. (1987), and Avorn et al. (1986)].

We believe that record linkage systems will be the most important source of PMS study populations in the future. If careful attention is paid to defining data elements and ensuring data quality, record linkage systems based on *sufficiently large* patient populations can provide the information needed to discover relevant risk classes and to estimate event onset density functions and attributable risks for virtually any drug-event pairs. They raise the exciting possibility that in the future, everyday clinical practice may well no longer be unmonitored. However, it will continue to be nonexperimental, and the PMS inferential problems associated with this fact will remain.

REFERENCES

Aromaa, A., M. Hakama, T. Hakulinen, E. Saxén, L. Teppo, and J. Idänpään-Heikkilä (1976). Breast cancer and use of rauwolfia and other antihypertensive agents in hypertensive patients: a nationwide case-control study in Finland. *Internat. J. Cancer 18*, 727–738.

Avorn, J., D. Everitt, and S. Weiss (1986). Increased antidepressant use in patients prescribed beta-blockers. *J. Amer. Med. Assoc. 255*, 357–360.

Borden, E., and J. Lee (1982). A methodologic study of post-marketing drug evaluation using a pharmacy-based approach. *J. Chronic. Dis. 35*, 803–816.

Böttiger, L., and B. Westerholm (1973). Drug-induced blood dyscrasias in Sweden. *British Med. J. 3*, 339–343.

Carson, J., and B. Strom (1986). Techniques of postmarketing surveillance: an overview. *Med. Toxicol. 1*, 237–246.

Castle, W., J. Nicholls, and C. Downie (1983). Problems of post-marketing surveillance. *British J. Clin. Pharmacol. 16*, 581–585.

Cornfield, J. (1951). A method of estimating comparative rates from clinical data. Applications to cancer of the lung, breast and cervix. *J. Nat. Cancer Inst. 11*, 1269–1275.

D'Arcy, P. (1986). Epidemiological aspects of iatrogenic disease. In *Iatrogenic Diseases*, 3rd ed. (P. D'Arcy and J. Griffin, eds.). Oxford University Press, Oxford, pp. 29–58.

de Finetti, B. (1974). *Theory of Probability*, English translation. Wiley, New York.

Fagius, J., P. Osterman, A. Sidén, and B. Wiholm (1985). Guillain-Barré syndrome following zimeldine treatment. *J. Neurol. Neurosurg. Psychiatry 48*, 65–69.

Faich, G., H. Guess, and J. Kuritsky (1987). Postmarketing surveillance for drug safety. In *Clinical Trials and Tribulations* (A. Cato, ed.). Marcel Dekker, New York.

Feinstein, A. (1974). Clinical biostatistics. XXVIII. The biostatistical problems of pharmaceutical surveillance. *Clin. Pharmacol. Ther. 16*, 110–123.

Finney, D. (1971). Statistical logic in the monitoring of reactions to therapeutic drugs. *Methods Inform. Med. 10*, 237–245.

Finney, D. (1977). Discussion of Jesdinsky. In *Drug Monitoring*, F. Gross, and W. Inman, eds. Academic Press, London, pp. 97–98.

Gent, M., and I. Shigematsu, eds. (1978). *Epidemiological Issues in Reported Drug-Induced Illnesses—SMON and Other Examples.* McMaster University Library Press, Hamilton, Ontario, Canada.

Guess, H., R. West, L. Strand, D. Helston, E. Lydick, U. Bergman, and K. Wolski (1987). Fatal upper gastrointestinal hemorrhage or perforation among users and nonusers of nonsteroidal anti-inflammatory drugs in Saskatchewan, Canada 1983. *J. Clin. Epidemiol. 41*, 35–45.

IAAAS (International Agranulocytosis and Aplastic Anemia Study) (1986). Risks of agranulocytosis and aplastic anemia. A first report of their relation to drug use with special reference to analgesics *J. Amer. Med. Assoc. 256*, 1749–1757.

Inman, W. (1985). Risks in medical intervention. In *Risk: Man-Made Hazards to Man* (M. Cooper, ed.). Oxford University Press, Oxford, pp. 35–53.

Inman, W., ed. (1986). *Monitoring for Drug Safety*, 2nd. ed. MTP Press, Lancaster, England.

Inman, W. (1987). Prescription-Event Monitoring. Its strategic role in post-marketing surveillance for drug safety. *PEM News 4*, 16–29.

Inman, W., N. Rawson, L. Wilton, G. Pearce, and C. Speirs (1988). Post-marketing surveillance of enalapril: I. Results of Prescription-Event Monitoring. *British Med. J. 297*, 826–829.

Jesdinsky, H. (1977). Use and abuse of statistical data. In *Drug Monitoring* (F. Gross and W. Inman, eds.). Academic Press, London, pp. 91–97.

Jick, H. (1977). The discovery of drug-induced illness. *New England J. Med. 296*, 481–485.

Jick, H. (1984). Adverse drug reactions: the magnitude of the problem. *J. Allergy Clin. Immunol. 74*, 555–557.

Jick, H. (1985). The Boston Collaborative Drug Surveillance Program and the Puget Sound Health Maintenance Organization. *Drug Inform. J. 19*, 237–242.

Jick, H., A. Walker, and C. Spriet-Pourra (1979). Postmarketing follow-up. *J. Amer. Med. Assoc. 242*, 2310–2314.

Jick, S., D. Perera, A. Walker, and H. Jick (1987). Non-steroidal anti-inflammatory drugs and hospital admission for perforated peptic ulcer. *Lancet 2*, 380–382.

Johnson, A. (1984). Postmarketing surveillance: statistics and augury. *J. Chronic Dis. 37*, 949–952.

Jones, J., ed. (1985). International adverse reaction surveillance, Proceedings of the Drug Information Association Workshop Oct. 18–20, 1984, Bethesda, Md. *Drug Inform. J. 19*, 205–393.

Klemetti, A., and L. Saxén (1967). Prospective versus retrospective approach in the search for environmental causes of malformations. *Amer. J. Public Health 57*, 2071–2075.

Kramer, M., D. Lane, and T. Hutchinson (1987). Analgesic use, blood dyscrasias, and case-control pharmacoepidemiology. A critique of the IAAAS. *J. Chronic Dis. 40*, 1073–1081.

Lane, D. (1986). The logic of uncertainty: measuring degree of belief. *Drug Inform. J. 20*, 445–453.

Lane, D. (1987). Utility, decision and quality of life. *J. Chronic Dis. 40*, 585–591.

Lane, D. and T. Hutchinson (1987). The notion of "acceptable risk": the role of utility in drug management. *J. Chronic Dis. 40*, 621–625.

Maclay, W., D. Crowder, S. Spiro, and P. Turner (1984). Postmarketing surveillance: practical experience with ketotifen. *British Med. J. 288*, 911–914.

Martin-Bouyer, G., B. Foulon, H. Guerbois, and C. Barin (1980). Aspects épidémiologiques des encéphalopathies après administration de bismuth par voie orale. *Therapie 35*, 307–313.

Miettinen, O. (1987). Principles of risk assessment for adverse drug reactions, unpublished manuscript. Prepared under the auspices of Hoechst AG, Frankfurt, West Germany.

Mitchell, A., L. Cottler, and S. Shapiro (1986). Effect of questionnaire design on recall of drug exposure in pregnancy. *Amer. J. Epidemiol. 123*, 670–676.

Morse, M. (1985). The COMPASS data base. *Drug Inform. J. 19*, 249–252.

Offerhaus, L. (1987). Letter to the editor. *Nederl. Tijdschr. Geneeskd. 131*, 1681–1683.

O'Neill, R. (1987). Statistical analyses of adverse event data from clinical trials: special emphasis on serious events. *Drug Inform. J. 21*, 9–20.

Porter, J., J. Hunter, D. Danielson, H. Jick, and A. Stergachis (1982). Oral contraceptives and nonfatal vascular disease—recent experience. *Obstet. Gynecol. 59*, 299–302.

Rawson, N. (1987). Prescription-event monitoring: a new method for studying drug safety, unpublished Ph.D. thesis. Faculty of Medicine, University of Southampton, Southampton, England.

Rawson, N. (1989). Post-marketing surveillance. In *Comprehensive Medicinal Chemistry*, Vol. 1: *General Introduction* (P. Kennewell, ed.). Pergamon Press, Oxford.

Ray, W. and M. Griffin (1989). Use of Medicaid data for pharmacoepidemiology. *Amer. J. Epidemiol. 129*, 837–849.

Shaw, F., D. Graham, H. Guess, J. Milstien, J. Johnson, G. Schatz, S. Hadler, J. Kuritsky, E. Hiner, D. Bregman, and J. Maynard (1988). Postmarketing surveillance for neurologic adverse events reported after hepatitis B vaccination: experience of the first three years. *Amer. J. Epidemiol. 127*, 337–352. .

Strand, L. (1985). Drug epidemiology resources and studies: the Saskatchewan data base. *Drug Inform. J. 19*, 253–256.

Wardell, W., M. Tsianco, S. Anavekar, and H. Davis (1979). Postmarketing surveillance of new drugs: I and II. *J. Clin. Pharmacol. 19*, 85–94, 169–184.

Index